Wolff's
HEADACHE
and other head pain

Edited

by

DONALD J. DALESSIO, M.D.

Chairman, Department of Medicine
Head, Division of Neurology/Psychiatry/Psychology
Scripps Clinic & Research Foundation
La Jolla, California

FOURTH EDITION

New York • Oxford
OXFORD UNIVERSITY PRESS
1980

Copyright © 1948, 1963, 1972, 1980 by Oxford University Press, Inc.

Library of Congress Cataloging in Publication Data

Wolff's Headache and other head pain.

Bibliography: p.
Includes index.
1. Headache. 2. Pain. I. Dalessio, Donald J.,
1931–   II. Title. III. Title: Headache and
other head pain.
RB128.W67   1980   616'.047   79-14021
ISBN 0-19-502624-1

Printed in the United States of America

To Isabel Bishop Wolff
and
Jane Dalessio

PREFACE TO THE FOURTH EDITION

The life of this book now spans three decades and more, the breadth of a professional career for most men. That it is still extant is a source of reassurance to the current reviser, who has now been responsible for two of the four editions.

This fourth edition departs from the previous volumes by introducing a series of writers to review topics within their special expertise. A serious attempt has been made to integrate new material with that still applicable from the older editions. Where this is not possible, then entirely new chapters have been created, such as those on the surgical treatment of head and neck pain, and the inheritance and epidemology of headache. Another new chapter on radiologic investigations of headache makes use of the rapid developments in technology in diagnostic radiology which have been so helpful in improving the diagnostic precision of clinicians.

In any revision there are problems, particularly in integrating new and old material. We have attempted to maintain continuity by restricting contributors to staff and consultants of a single institution. Inevitably, given writing styles and variations in the approach to the patient, differences have arisen and may be evident to the reader. I hope that these will not be jarring. Diagnosis and treatment of headache is an ongoing process, and yesterday's heresy may be tomorrow's dogma. There is always room for discussion and consultation between reasonable physicians, especially where therapy is indicated. Perhaps this will be one of the strengths of the new edition, rather than a weakness.

The first two editions of this book were, in a sense, a personal memoir of Dr. Wolff and data in those volumes were set down in detail from his New York Hospital studies. Some of these studies have not ever been repeated. (Some would probably not be acceptable to Human Research Committees now.) I have retained these data where applicable and identified them as the work of the Wolff group, either directly or simply as the "New York Hospital studies."

I am indebted to many persons for help with this revision. Several deserve special mention. The administrative officers of the Scripps Clinic, including Charles Edwards, Edmund L. Keeney, and John L. Smith, have been a source of constant support. Others have been consistently encouraging, especially the members of the Division of Neurology/Psychiatry/Psychology including Shirley Otis, M. Aung, Jack Sipe, Richard Smith, Richard Anderson, Edward Mohns, Varda Backus, Richard Sternbach and Dee Jacobsen. I have learned much from my colleagues including J. Alfred Berend, Richard Conroy, Richard Kahler, Donald Stevenson, David Mathison, Thomas Waltz, and Kenneth Ott. I have been the beneficiary of vigorous stimulation from the members of the Neuroscience Department of the University of California at San Diego Medical School, especially Burt Wiederholt and Robert Livingston, A. Baird Hastings, and Reginald Bickford. Seymour Diamond, of Chicago, a constant friend and colleague, is another to whom I express gratitude.

The faithful application and work of Mrs. Camille Mead made preparation of this manuscript possible.

I have been encouraged to complete this work by Mrs. Isabel Bishop Wolff, and by Miss Helen Goodell, and I acknowledge the editorial help of Jeffrey House and Brenda Jones of the Oxford University Press.

The following journals, publications, and publishers have kindly permitted use of material: AMA Archives of Internal Medicine, AMA Archives of Neurology and Psychiatry, Annals of Internal Medicine, Archives of Neurology, Archives of Surgery, Bulletin of the New York Academy of Medicine, International Archives of Allergy and Applied Immunology, Journal of the American Medical Association, Journal of Chronic Diseases, Journal of Dental Medicine, Journal of Psychosomatic Research, Headache, Mayo Clinic Proceedings, Medical Clinics of North America, Proceedings of the Association for Research in Nervous and Mental Disease, Psychosomatic Medicine, Science, Transactions of the American Neurological Association, Transactions of the Association of American Physicians, Academic Press, Charles C. Thomas, Inc., S. Karger, and the Williams & Wilkins Co.

La Jolla   D. J. D.
April 1979

PREFACE TO THE FIRST EDITION

Since the human animal prides himself on "using his head," it is ironic and perhaps not without meaning that his head should be the source of so much discomfort. Though pain always means "something wrong," with headache it most often means "wrong direction" or "wrong pace"—a biologic reprimand rather than a threat. Thus, the vast majority of discomforts and pains of the head stem from readily reversible bodily changes, and are accompaniments of resentments and dissatisfactions. On the other hand, the headaches of brain tumor, brain abscess, fever, arteritis, meningitis, subdural and subarachnoid hemorrhage, and the pains of major neuralgias and neuritides, which call for prompt and often heroic measures, constitute only a minor proportion of the total number of pains of the head. Headache may be equally intense whether its implications are malignant or benign, and though there are few instances in human experience where so much pain may mean so little in terms of tissue injury, failure to separate the ominous from the trivial may cost life or create paralyzing fear.

Some fifteen years ago, during attempts to learn about the cerebral circulation, it was noted that the major cerebral blood vessels are covered by a network of nerve fibers having to do with pain. From these elementary observations has grown a series of investigations on headache. One part of the head after the other has been explored, and thus, piece by piece, the headache picture has been put together. Happily, in the intervening years the curiosity of bold and able workers has been aroused by the problem, and the chapters that follow are mainly the results of their efforts.

Headache as a subject for investigation has fared badly through being divided among "specialists." In an effort to unify the topic, the author and his colleagues have had the temerity to transgress divisions. By thus approaching the problem from many angles and with a variety of tools, we have tried to increase the knowledge of the natural history of headaches and other head pains, and to track down some of their mechanisms, to the end that suffering may be prevented or relieved. Doubtless there is much to correct and to clarify, but here is the account as far as it has gone.

New York Hospital   H. G. W.

CONTENTS

CONTRIBUTORS

John F. Alksne, M.D.
Professor of Neurosurgery
University of California, School of Medicine
San Diego, California
Consultant in Neurosurgery
Scripps Clinic & Research Foundation
La Jolla, California

Richard W. Anderson, M.D.
Member, Division of Neurology/Psychiatry/Psychology
Scripps Clinic & Research Foundation
La Jolla, California

Donald J. Dalessio, M.D.
Chairman, Department of Medicine
Head, Division of Neurology/Psychiatry/Psychology
Scripps Clinic & Research Foundation
La Jolla, California

Frank V. Howell, D.D.S.
Chairman, Department of Oral Medicine & Stomatology
Scripps Clinic & Research Foundation
La Jolla, California

Ronald J. Ignelzi, M.D.
Assistant Professor of Neurosurgery
University of California, School of Medicine
San Diego, California

Consultant in Neurosurgery
Scripps Clinic & Research Foundation
La Jolla, California

Edward B. Mohns, M.D.
Member, Division of Neurology/Psychiatry/Psychology
Scripps Clinic & Research Foundation
La Jolla, California

Charles A. Robinson, M.D.
Member, Division of Rheumatology
Scripps Clinic & Research Foundation
La Jolla, California

Stanley G. Seat, M.D.
Chairman, Department of Radiology
Head, Division of Diagnostic Radiology
Scripps Clinic & Research Foundation
La Jolla, California

Richard A. Smith, M.D.
Member, Division of Neurology/Psychiatry/Psychology
Scripps Clinic & Research Foundation
La Jolla, California

Richard A. Sternbach, Ph.D.
Director, Pain Treatment Center
Member, Division of Neurology/Psychiatry/Psychology
Scripps Clinic & Research Foundation
La Jolla, California

Donald D. Stevenson, M.D.
Member, Division of Allergy/Immunology
Scripps Clinic & Research Foundation
La Jolla, California

David M. Worthen, M.D.
Professor of Ophthalmology
University of California, School of Medicine
San Diego, California
Consultant in Ophthalmology
Scripps Clinic & Research Foundation
La Jolla, California

HEADACHE AND OTHER HEAD PAIN

1

A CLINICAL CLASSIFICATION OF HEADACHE

DONALD J. DALESSIO

Headache has been called the most common medical complaint of civilized man, yet severe and especially chronic headache is only infrequently caused by organic disease. Hence it may be inferred that for the most part chronic headache represents an inability of the individual to deal in some measure with the uncertainties of life, a symptom of an underlying disorder of thought or behavior rather than structural disease of the nervous system. Nonetheless, headache may also be the presenting complaint of catastrophic illness such as brain tumor, cerebral hemorrhage, or meningitis, and to ignore the symptom in this context is to risk the life of the patient. Headache may be equally intense whether its source is benign or malignant.

What makes headaches hurt? What are the underlying mechanisms of headache? How can headaches best be classified?

These questions are basic to an understanding of headache. If the clinician appreciates how and why headache generally occurs, he will proceed more directly to a specific diagnosis, and a decision on therapy will follow as a natural consequence.

First, one must take the time to get a reasonable history. If the physician thinks "analgesic" as soon as the patient describes headache, nothing will be accomplished. All pain is subjective; no pain can be measured effectively. All symptoms are subjective, and must be described by the patient. Many patients are not good observers of their own complaints, even when those complaints are chronic. Some patients, and physicians as well, have difficulty verbalizing

precisely what they are feeling. So the chances are the physician will need time to probe and find out where the patient's head pain is, what it feels like, when it occurs, how it is provoked, whether it runs in the family, and so on, before any tests are done, and most of all, before anything is prescribed.

Remember, then, that the diagnosis of headache often depends upon the patient's description of his symptoms. There are *no* precise clinical tests for many specific pain syndromes, including classic and common migraine, cluster headache, and the major neuralgias.

Since all physicians may be called upon to treat patients with headache, it is important to have a simple classification which may give clues to appropriate therapy. We have divided headache into three main groups, rather than a series of disparate headache syndromes which may tax the memory. These groups are: vascular, muscle contraction, and traction and inflammatory (Table 1-1).

VASCULAR HEADACHE

Vascular headache includes classic and common migraine, hemiplegic migraine, ophthalmoplegic migraine, cluster (histamine) headache, and toxic vascular headache. Common to all these is a tendency to vascular dilatation, which represents the headache phase of the migraine attack. Vasoconstriction may also be evident and may be responsible for painless sensory phenomena prior to the onset of head pain. Hemiplegic and ophthalmoplegic mi-

1

TABLE 1-1   Classification of Headache

VASCULAR HEADACHE	MUSCLE CONTRACTION HEADACHE	TRACTION AND INFLAMMATORY HEADACHE

Migraine
1. Classic
2. Common
3. Hemiplegic } complicated
4. Ophthalmoplegic } migraine
Cluster (histamine)
	Cervical osteoarthritis
	
	Chronic myositis
		Mass lesions (tumors,
		    edema, hematomas,
		    cerebral hemorrhage)
		
		Diseases of the eye, ear,
		    nose, throat, teeth

Toxic vascular Hypertensive		Infection Arteritis, phlebitis (Cranial neuralgias) Occlusive vascular disease

graine are considered more severe forms of classical migraine. Toxic vascular headache is evoked by a systemic vasodilatation and may be produced by fever, alcohol, CO_2 retention, agents such as nitrites, and the like.

Classic and Common Migraine

This is the most troublesome form of headache, and it may be viewed as a symptom complex, for migraine represents a whole spectrum of body alterations of which headache is only a single part. Classic migraine is considered to be the prototype of vascular headache. Thus, in addition to headache pain that may last from a few hours to a few days, the patient may also suffer photophobia, nausea, vomiting, constipation or diarrhea, weight gain and fluid retention followed by diuresis, scotoma or field defects, paresthesias or defects in motility, vertigo, and elevation of blood pressure. Many of these symptoms provide the basis for migraine "equivalents." These are paroxysmal, recurrent symptom complexes, occurring in patients with a previous history or familial history of migraine, often replacing headache by the equivalent syndrome; they may be relieved with appropriate therapy, often similar to that which is used to abort the headache attack itself. Migraine equivalents may take many forms involving the abdomen, chest, pelvis, eye, cerebral cortex (hemiplegic), and perhaps other organs as well. It has been estimated that migraine equivalents occur in approximately 20% of subjects with migraine.

In classic migraine, painless sensory experiences precede the headache phase. In common migraine they do not. Most often these stimuli are expressed as scotomata or field defects. Rarely do paresthesias and defects in motility, usually unilateral, occur. These phenomena are usually attributed to intracranial vasoconstriction. It has been demonstrated that the cranial arteries of patients with migraine are especially reactive; any one of a number of stimuli may set off a migraine attack, with the vasoconstrictor phase representing the initial vector of vascular activity. In some patients, especially young women, the prodromal symptoms may be of unusual intensity and complexity. In this set of symptoms, considered by some to be related to migraine involving the basilar-vertebral arterial system, visual loss and scotomata may involve both sides of the field of vision, with associated vertigo, dysarthria, loss of consciousness, and bilateral, peripheral symptoms and signs. In at least one episode of this type, death following migraine has been described.

The initial phase of vasoconstriction is followed by vasodilatation, which provokes the headache phase of the migraine attack. The vessels involved become painful; the pain is usually described as aching and throbbing, frequently coincides with the pulse beat, and is sometimes relieved by extra-arterial pressure. After a period of vasodilatation a sterile inflammatory reaction begins about the vessel wall, so that edema and inflammation of the affected arterial wall and the surrounding tissues may develop. By now the migraine process is in full swing. The patient is often nauseated, may vomit, and usually seeks to avoid sensory stimuli of all types, especially light. Hence, he retires to a dark room, goes to bed, and attempts to sleep or, at the least, to shut out the world. The pain lasts from 8 to 24 hours and sometimes longer, but eventually the patient recovers, often after a period of sleep.

Cluster Headache

There are several synonyms for cluster headache including histamine headache, Horton's headache, and migrainous neuralgia. This type of vascular headache has features which are specific enough to justify separate description, and the diagnosis can often be made on the basis of history alone. The pain occurs in attacks, is constant, of high intensity, burning, and "boring" in character. It involves the region of the eye, the temples, the neck, and often the face, and may extend into the shoulder on the involved side. It may spread to the upper teeth and occasionally to the lower teeth. Attacks often begin after middle age. Generally the attacks last less than one hour, commence, and often terminate suddenly, and often awaken the patient at night. The pain is so severe that the patient frequently jumps out of bed before he is fully awake.

The pain is associated with certain other characteristic manifestations that appear on the affected side. These are profuse watering and "congestion" of the conjunctiva, rhinorrhea and nasal obstruction, increased perspiration, and frequently evidence of vasodilatation in the skin. Swelling of the temporal vessels may be noted. During and after the attacks, marked tenderness is frequently found when pressure is applied over the branches of the external and common carotid arteries. The pain is not confined to the distribution of any cranial nerve but conforms to the ramifications of the external carotid artery.

Cluster headache occurs predominantly in males, with a 5:1 sex ratio. Often these are middle-aged men, commonly heavy smokers, without a family history of recurrent vascular headache. The term "cluster" is used because of the unique tempo of the recurring attacks, which vary from patient to patient but often exhibit a striking periodicity. Despite this periodicity, attempts to implicate allergen(s) in this form of headache have not been successful.

Patients with cluster headache are extremely sensitive to vasodilating agents, especially drugs such as nitroglycerin or histamine, alcohol, and the aged cheeses which contain tyramine. Sensitivity to oral nitroglycerin can be used as a provocative test if the diagnosis is suspected.

Hemiplegic Migraine

The vascular reactions of classical migraine also occur in hemiplegic migraine. Here they may be exaggerated to the point that long-lasting ischemia of brain tissue occurs. This form of migraine may be familial, suggesting again that an inherited instability of vascular control is present. Whether the sequelae of this form of migraine are related to the prolongation of the vasodilator or of the vasoconstrictor phases of migraine is unknown; possibly both factors are implicated.

Ophthalmoplegic Migraine

In ophthalmoplegic migraine ocular palsy is associated with headache. Those structures served by the third cranial nerve are most often involved. This is attributed to the pressure on the nerve exerted by the dilated and edematous wall of the internal carotid artery and its branches. Segmental narrowing of all or part of the intracranial portion of the internal carotid artery has been demonstrated by arteriography in patients during a migraine attack. It has also been suggested that brain edema produced by migraine may provoke herniation of the hippocampal gyrus sufficient to compress the third nerve, but this concept is speculative.

In patients who suffer repeated attacks, ocular palsies are usually transitory. In rare instances, however, these palsies may become persistent. It is important to differentiate between the mechanisms of ophthalmoplegic mi-

TABLE 1-2   Causes of Toxic Vascular Headaches

PATHOLOGICAL CONDITIONS		TOXIC SUBSTANCES		WITHDRAWAL FROM DRUGS
Febrile	Others	Nonpharmacological	Pharmacological	
Pneumonia	Alcohol	Carbon monoxide	Nitrates	Ergot
Tonsillitis	Hypoglycemia	Lead	Indomethacin	Caffeine
Septicemia	Hypoxia	Benzene	Oral progestational	Amphetamines
Typhoid fever	Altitude	Carbon tetrachloride	Oral vasodilators	Many phenothiazines
Tularemia	Hypercarbia	Insecticides		
Influenza	Effort	Nitrates		
Measles				
Mumps				
Poliomyelitis				
Infectious mononucleosis				
Malaria				
Trichinosis				

graine and those which produce similar symptoms but are related to intracranial aneurysms, particularly of the posterior communicating artery. The sudden appearance of third-nerve signs in a patient not subject to migraine may be an indication for arteriography.

Toxic Vascular Headache (Table 1-2)

This category includes all of the diseases and conditions which produce headache of a vascular nature as part of their overall symptomatology. The most common nonmigrainous vascular headache is that which is produced by fever. Generalized vasodilatation may occur as a consequence of any significant fever, usually becoming more intense as the fever rises. Particularly intense vascular headaches may occur with pneumonia, tonsillitis, septicemia, typhoid fever, tularemia, influenza, measles, mumps, poliomyelitis, infectious mononucleosis, malaria, and trichinosis. The vasodilatation in these diseases is often intracranial as well as extracranial. Nonmigrainous headache may also occur in a whole series of miscellaneous disorders including such diverse entities as hangover headache and headache associated with hypoglycemia regardless of cause. In hypoxic states headache may be a persistent complaint, especially in those in which an increased CO_2 tension in the

blood exists concurrently. Exposure to carbon monoxide may provoke a very severe form of vascular headache. Headaches may be produced by the administration of nitrates, either as medicament or unintentionally, as an industrial hazard. Many poisons may evoke headache, including lead, benzene, carbon tetrachloride, and insecticides. Treatment with monamine oxidase inhibitors may cause a serious headache, especially when small amounts of catecholamines are ingested at the same time. The headache produced may be catastrophic, and cerebrovascular accidents as well as deaths have been reported as a result of this combination.

Withdrawal from many pharmacologic agents may provoke headache. This is especially likely after prolonged therapy with ergot derivatives but may also follow the discontinuation of caffeine, benzedrine, and many of the phenothiazines. Treatment of arthritis with indomethacin may evoke headache, presumably by producing a chemical vasodilation.

Headache Associated with Arterial Hypertension, and Toxemia of Pregnancy

Several kinds of headache are associated with hypertension and deserve discussion. A sudden rise in blood pressure during violent exercise, anger, or sexual excitement, may be associated with bilateral pounding headache, usually short-lived or transient, which is rarely of diagnostic or therapeutic importance. Effort migraine occcuring in athletes after a long race, or in mountain climbers experiencing anoxia, is a related phenomenon. Such episodes do not usually require specific therapy.

Sudden and extreme elevations of the blood pressure may occur with toxemia of pregnancy, in the malignant state of essential hypertension, and with end-stage renal disease. The syndrome termed hypertensive encephalopathy consists of severe headache, nausea, vomiting, and convulsions, proceeding to confusion and coma. Papilledema is always present as a primary sign of increased intracranial pressure. The headache is more or less continuous, is generalized, pounding, and difficult to relieve with simple analgesics. It is assumed that brain edema in some form produces the headache associated with hypertensive encephalopathy. The intravenous injection of osmotically active agents such as mannitol will reduce its intensity. Oral glycerol is also effective. These agents produce relative dehydration of the brain, subsequent to which traction and displacement of pain-sensitive structures is reduced.

The neurological signs of hypertensive encephalopathy occurring in toxemia are probably related to cerebral vasospasm, thereafter producing cerebral ischemia and cerebral edema. The primary therapeutic aim in hypertensive encephalopathy is to reduce the blood pressure, which is the only effective way to relieve the symptoms.

Vascular headache may also be associated with a paroxysmal rise of blood pressure as seen in a patient with a pheochromocytoma, but other physical findings should lead rapidly to that diagnosis.

What remains are those headaches associated with essential hypertension. With this common disease, the pain is vascular in nature and is related to the contractile state of the extracranial and intracranial arteries. Should these arteries dilate, for whatever reason, hypertensive vascular headache will occur. Usually the pain is described as dull and aching with a pounding component, often present in the morning, and improving as the patient stirs, gets up, and moves about. The pain is frequently increased by effort, stooping, and by jolts to the head. Hypertensive headache is rarely present unless the diastolic blood pressure exceeds 110 mm Hg.

Patients with minimal hypertension who complain of headache need careful evaluation. Often the tendency is to blame the headache on the hypertension when this may not be the case. As mentioned above, unless the diastolic blood pressure exceeds 110 mm Hg, another etiology should be sought in this situation.

MUSCLE CONTRACTION HEADACHE

Perhaps the most common form of headache is that related to chronic muscular contraction occurring about the head and neck. This produces dull, band-like, persistent pain, which may last for days or months. In treating this type of pain, a search should be made for tender and painful areas of the head and neck, as well as significant arthritis of the spine.

In chronic muscle contraction, skeletal muscle spasm is related to local pathologic processes and their central influences and involves three independent reflex arcs and four consecutive steps:

1. A multisynaptic reflex of withdrawal usually initiates muscle spasm. A local pathologic process produces stimulation of nerve fibers. The impulse is transmitted directly to the spinal cord and thence to the ventral roots. From there, the stimulus passes via the efferent nerves to the neuromuscular junction. The muscle contracts acutely, and movement from the painful stimulus occurs.

2. Polysynaptic spinal pathways and the lemniscal system are also stimulated. By these paths the initial stimulus is conducted up the spinal cord to thalamic and central levels, where the stimulus is appreciated as painful.

3. The brain then sends impulses through the reticulospinal system to activate the gamma efferent neurons which contract the muscle spindle.

4. The contracting muscle spindle evokes a monosynaptic stimulus which travels directly to the ventral horn and augments the discharge

in the efferent peripheral nerve and, more importantly, augments muscle contraction.

The contraction of the muscle spindle itself (third reflex arc) is in fact a monosynaptic pathway and thus is related to the simple tendon-stretch reflexes evoked in a neurologic examination. In ordinary circumstances the contracting muscle inhibits firing of the muscle spindle and terminates the third-arc stretch reflex, allowing the muscle to relax. The degree of muscle tone is thus largely determined by the state of activity of the gamma motor system. If the gamma efferent system continues to fire, because of cortical influences or local or systemic disease, the muscle spindle remains tight and the muscle contracts continually until the contraction itself becomes painful. Thus arises the cycle of pain, spasm, anxiety, and pain known as muscle contraction headache.

TRACTION AND INFLAMMATORY HEADACHE

This category comprises headache evoked by organic disease of the skull or its components, including the brain, meninges, arteries, veins, eyes, ears, teeth, nose, and paranasal sinuses. The term *traction headache* is used to describe the often nonspecific headache seen with mass lesions of the brain, such as tumors, hematomas, abscesses, or brain edema from whatever cause. Traction headache of a particularly intense type occurs in subarachnoid and intraventricular hemorrhage, and in cortical venous thromboses. Traction headache is associated with inflammatory disease of the meninges, and intracranial or extracranial arteritis or phlebitis. Inflammatory headache evoked by disease of the special sense organs and the teeth, and the major cranial neuralgias including tic douloureux, are included here.

Mass Lesions

A traction headache can be elicited by hematomas of any sort, abscesses, nonspecific brain "edema," and lumbar puncture. It is especially a symptom of brain tumors. Local traction on adjacent pain-sensitive structures by the tumor may occur, as well as distant traction related to the tumor mass indirectly when internal hydrocephalus and ventricular obstruction occur. For this reason localization of a brain tumor by determining the site of headache can be unreliable. It has also been possible to demonstrate localized skull tenderness at the site of meningiomas, or in the mastoid area with a cerebellopontine angle tumor, presumably due to local involvement and extension into the skull or its structures by the tumor.

Arteritis and Infections

Headache may be produced by inflammatory processes within or outside the skull, particularly meningitis, intracranial arteritis, phlebitis, and those associated with subarachnoid hemorrhage. The pain is evoked by an inflammatory response which includes the pain-sensitive structures of the head. The head pain in most instances coincides with the course of the disease, usually abating as the disease is brought under control, and is not recurrent or paroxysmal.

Extracranial inflammation may also produce headache. The mechanism responsible is inflammation of the extracranial arteries. The condition may be seen in a localized form as it occurs in cranial (temporal) arteritis, or in a more generalized disease as part of a widespread collagen-vascular syndrome. The intracranial arteritis occurs in systemic lupus erythematosus or periarteritis nodosa and can produce excruciating headache pain of a generalized nature.

In polyarteritis nodosa, there are multiple areas of arterial necrosis and inflammation affecting many organs. The arterial lesion appears to be identical to that found in serum sickness arteritis. Gamma globulin may be identified in areas of fibrinoid necrosis. The role of gamma globulin in producing this lesion is under intensive investigation.

A rather common form of rheumatism that affects the elderly with pains in the head, neck, back, and proximal areas of the limbs may be associated with systemic signs of disease, an elevated sedimentation rate, and a prompt therapeutic response to corticosteroids. This

TABLE 1-3   A Classification of Facial Neuralgias

Classic neuralgia
  Trigeminal neuralgia
  Glossopharyngeal neuralgia

Other neuralgias
  Geniculate (intermedius) neuralgia of Hunt
  Postherpetic facial neuralgia
  Sphenopalatine neuralgias
    vidian neuralgia of Vail
    ciliary neuralgia (Charlin) } probably cluster
    petrosal neuralgia   } headache variants
    erythroprosopalgia
  Paratrigeminal syndrome of Raeder

Facial pain related to craniofacial pathology
  Temporomandibular joint pathology (Costen's
    syndrome)
  Intracranial pathology
  Orofacial pain—burning tongue

Lower-half headache
Atypical facial pain
Carotidynia

---

condition is best known as polymyalgia rheumatica. A significant number of patients with polymyalgia rheumatica will eventually develop temporal arteritis in the course of their illness, suggesting that the two diseases are in fact one, and that the myalgias of polymyalgia rheumatica may represent an early stage of cranial arteritis.

In temporal arteritis there is a similar pathologic picture, except that the inflammatory reaction tends to be relatively limited to the temporal arteries, though it may involve other arteries as well. It is often acute and self-limited, and may be associated with the development of multinucleate giant cells in media of the blood vessel (giant-cell arteritis).

Recent studies employing immunofluorescence techniques have demonstrated that patients with temporal arteritis have anticapillary antibodies in their sera, as well as deposits containing IgG and complement components which are localized to the arterial wall in temporal artery biopsies procured for diagnosis. The capillary antibodies in sera of these patients are present in significant titer. Such antibodies are also found in certain rheumatic diseases, some of which, such as rheumatoid arthritis and systemic lupus erythematosus, are characterized by an arteritis. Capillary antibodies are discovered infrequently in normal controls or in blood donors.

It is suggested that temporal arteritis represents an example of immunologic vasculitis wherein antibodies deposited within the walls of blood vessels produce localized vascular injury and inflammation, with the consequent signs and symptoms which are identified by clinical means. Capillary antibodies may be a primary factor contributing to the vascular injury or may aggravate the process by reacting with vessels already damaged by another mechanism.

Cranial Neuritis and Neuralgias, Temporomandibular Joint (TMJ) Disease

This category includes those forms of facial pain that are mediated by the cranial nerves, excluding the trigeminal and glossopharyngeal neuralgias (Table 1-3). It commonly includes the atypical facial neuralgias, lower-half headache, sphenopalatine neuralgias, orofacial pains, and carotidynia. Some of these syndromes are poorly developed and may not deserve separate status. Some of them probably represent vascular pain or a form of migraine perceived in an unusual location (Table 1-3). This is particularly true of lower-half headaches, which may respond to prophylaxis with such lysergic acid derivatives as methysergide.

CATEGORIZING CHRONIC FACIAL PAINS

Perhaps the best way to categorize chronic facial pain is to separate out those specific syndromes which have a neuroanatomical basis and deal with the rest as atypical facial neuralgias. Certain discrete facial pain syndromes can be recognized by the clinician. These include especially the major neuralgias; postherpetic neuritis; cluster headache in its anatomic and verbal variations; diseases of the eyes, ears, nose, teeth, and throat; cranial arteritis; and pseudotumor of the orbit (see Tables 1-1 and 1-3).

TEMPOROMANDIBULAR JOINT (TMJ) DISEASE

Are there symptoms related to temporomandibular joint (TMJ) disease? The question is moot. We believe that facial pain can occur with temporomandibular joint (TMJ) disease which is usually felt in the face adjacent to the joint, with radiation to the jaw, the neck, and behind the ear, not neuritic in character. In our view, the syndrome consists of localized facial pain, limitation of motion of the jaw, muscle tenderness, and joint crepitus. Usually the joint itself has a normal radiologic appearance.

There is no evidence that hearing loss, damage to cranial nerves, disturbances of equilibrium, development of Ménière's syndrome, or difficulty with the eustachian tubes are in any way related to this syndrome. The current view of etiology is that occlusal disharmony and psychophysiological factors play primary roles, with most of the dysfunction resident in the masticatory muscles rather than in the TMJ itself. Those pathologic changes which affect the joint, such as rheumatoid arthritis, may cause similar complaints, but they are, by definition, different problems which need not be discussed here. The syndromes delineated as trigeminal neuralgia (tic douloureux) and glossopharyngeal neuralgia are better characterized.

Trigeminal Neuralgia (Tic Douloureux)

In tic douloureux, pain is experienced chiefly in areas of the face supplied by the second and, to a lesser extent, the third and first divisions of the fifth cranial nerve. It may be felt in any part of the face, but never below the ramus of the jaw or in back of the ear and rarely in the entire distribution of the fifth nerve at any one time. The pain is of an aching and burning quality and may occur spontaneously, but it is more often initiated by cold air or light touch on the skin of the cheek, or by biting, chewing, laughing, swallowing, talking, yawning, sneezing, or similar movements. The pain is usually described as a high-intensity "jab" of 20–30-sec duration, followed by a period of abatement lasting from a few seconds to a minute, and followed again by another jab of high-intensity pain. The spasms do not last longer than a minute. The entire attack or series of such brief pains usually lasts one or more hours.

A familiar characteristic of trigeminal neuralgia is the patient's ability to point out trigger zones. These zones are 2–4 mm in diameter and are hyperexcitable areas of skin or mucous membrane which, when given a minimal stimulus, are capable of producing paroxysmal pain in one or more divisions of the trigeminal nerve. These zones are clustered around the mouth and nares. The type of stimulus needed to evoke pain in the trigger zone is interesting. A painful stimulation of the trigger zone may not be effective. Thermal stimuli also seem to be ineffective. Pressure from a tactile stimulus or a vibratory stimulus on a trigger zone almost always evokes an attack in patients with tic douloureux. This accounts for the behavioral modification seen in susceptible patients: they develop elaborate protective mechanisms to guard their trigger zones by chewing or speaking out of one side of the mouth.

Glossopharyngeal Neuralgia

Glossopharyngeal tic is a related phenomenon. Severe pain similar to that described for tic douloureux is experienced in the tonsillar area and ear. It is often initiated by eating, yawning, or swallowing. Syncope may occur during the painful episode, presumably due to cardiac asystole.

2

MODERN CONCEPTS OF PAIN

RICHARD A. STERNBACH

An understanding of the evolving concepts of pain and analgesic mechanisms is obviously fundamental to a specialized interest in face and head pain. In the following discussion, neurophysiological and psychological processes in pain and analgesia will be described, irrespective of body locus. The head participates with the rest of the body in spinal and supraspinal mechanisms, sharing in the spinal events by virtue of the innervation from the first and second cervical roots. In addition, as is well known, there is innervation by the three branches of the trigeminal (fifth cranial) nerve. Despite the transmission of pain along these fibers, in other respects the information below regarding receptors, fibers, descending inhibitory mechanisms, etc. is applicable to pains of the head and face as well as other parts of the body.

In this area of rapidly changing information about pain and analgesic mechanisms, it is obviously difficult to be exhaustive or even thorough in a single chapter. Furthermore, when psychological factors as well are considered, the task becomes nearly impossible. In what follows, only brief highlights are given of relevant topics and information. Readers who are interested in a more comprehensive reference to both neurophysiological and personality factors in pain mechanisms may consult Sternbach (1978). Specific syndromes, conditions, and clinical entities of head pain are presented elsewhere in this volume.

NEUROPHYSIOLOGICAL MECHANISMS
Pain Receptors and Fibers

Recent developments in dissection and recording techniques have made it possible to show that there are three general classes of nociceptors (pain receptors): high-threshold mechanoreceptors, heat nociceptors, and "polymodal" nociceptors responsive to both noxious mechanical and noxious thermal stimuli (Bessou and Perl, 1969). Polymodal and heat nociceptors can be sensitized after repeated or prolonged stimulation, or during regeneration following section of nerve, so that their thresholds for activation can be lowered to levels of stimulus intensity which are ordinarily innocuous. This may account for the pain states following burns or nerve injury.

Perl and his colleagues (Bessou and Perl, 1969; Burgess and Perl, 1967; Perl, 1968; Perl, 1971) found that a large proportion of both A-delta and C fibers in cutaneous nerve of both cat and monkey were specifically responsive to tissue damage. That is, these fibers responded only to intensities of peripheral stimulation which were at or near levels sufficient to produce injury.

Several investigators have used microelectrode recording techniques in normal human subjects, and have recorded from single cutaneous C fibers (Torebjork and Hallin, 1973, 1974a; Van Hees and Gybels, 1972). These reports, along with the work of Price

(1972, 1976), suggest that the activation of A-delta fibers is associated with the experience of "first" pain: fast, sharp, and well-localized. Activation of C fibers is associated with the experience of "second" pain: slow, aching, burning, long-lasting, and poorly localized.

From these studies it appears that pain is a specific sensory event (Perl, 1971), and not merely excessive stimulation of other sensory modalities as was formerly supposed (Keele, 1957). It would seem that there are specialized nociceptors whose information is transmitted to the spinal cord over specific A-delta and C fibers.

Spinal Cord

There appear to be two types of pain-related sensory neurons in the dorsal horn of the spinal cord. Christensen and Perl (1970) described a Class 1 nociceptive cell, located in the marginal zone or most superficial layer of the dorsal horn (lamina 1). Class 1 cells are specifically responsive to injurious or near-injurious levels of stimulation.

Class 2 nociceptive cells are located primarily in lamina 5, and respond to low-intensity stimulation, but as the intensity of stimulation is increased to noxious levels these cells follow with more vigorous and sustained discharge (Hillman and Wall, 1969; Price and Browe, 1973; Willis et al., 1974).

Class 2 cells are impinged upon by inputs from both visceral and somatic sources; they may thus be involved in visceral referred pain (Pomeranz et al., 1968). They show "windup" or temporal summation with repetitive C-fiber activation (Price and Wagman, 1970), and they also show prolonged afterdischarges to noxious heat stimuli (Handwerker et al., 1975).

The axons of many Class 1 and Class 2 cells project directly to the brain, others ascend multisynaptically or contribute to reflex paths (Kerr, 1975). A large proportion of both types of cells ascend in the contralateral anterolateral quadrant and terminate in the thalamus. Mayer et al. (1975) studied the effects of direct stimulation of the anterolateral columns in

conscious patients undergoing cordotomy for relief of pain. These results were compared with similar data on Class 1 and Class 2 cells projecting to the anterolateral columns in monkeys (Price and Mayer, 1975). Refractory periods and electrical thresholds for Class 2 cells in the monkey were more similar to the periods and thresholds which caused sensations of pain in man. These authors suggest that while Class 1 cells may be involved in pain perception, activation of Class 2 cells alone may be a sufficient condition for some kinds of human pain.

GATE CONTROL THEORY

The gate control theory of pain proposed by Melzack and Wall (1965) suggests a dynamic interaction among large and small afferent fibers, mediated through the small cells of the substantia gelatinosa (laminas 2 and 3 in the dorsal horn of the spinal cord). Substantia gelatinosa cells are proposed to exert presynaptic inhibition on both large and small fiber terminals as they synapse on dorsal horn transmission cells whose axons project to the brain. Large fibers excite the substantia gelatinosa, thus increasing presynaptic inhibition (closing the gate) to noxious impulses incoming via small fibers. Small fibers inhibit the substantia gelatinosa, thus decreasing presynaptic inhibition (opening the gate). Pain is perceived when a threshold level of firing is attained by the central transmission cells. The gating mechanism could be influenced also by higher centers via descending fibers projecting to spinal cord cells.

The gate theory has been modified and expanded to encompass recent developments in neurophysiology, including evidence that postsynaptic is more important than presynaptic inhibition (Melzack, 1973). The theory has been criticized from an anatomical point of view (Kerr, 1975), as well as conceptually (Perl, 1971), but many clinical observations, as well as experimental studies, are compatible with it. The gating mechanism, susceptible to influence from centrifugal as well as centripetal sources, appears a useful concept.

Supraspinal Mechanisms

The anterolateral columns project to a number of discrete regions of the brain. The one most thoroughly studied is the nucleus gigantocellularis (NGC) of the bulbar reticular formation. Casey and his colleagues have found that many cells of this nucleus respond maximally to activation of A-delta and C fibers or to intense natural stimuli of the skin (Casey, 1971a,b,c; Morrow and Casey, 1976). There do not appear to be any significant number of nociceptive cells in the NGC. Rather, the great majority appear to have properties like those of Class 2 and not Class 1 dorsal horn cells, in that they respond maximally but not uniquely to noxious stimuli. Also, like Class 2 cells, the NGC cells have large, peripheral receptive fields, and thus are not likely to have a significant sensory discriminative role in nociception. The NGC cells may be part of an affective component of pain.

Most studies of more rostral brain regions have used anesthetized animals and may be misleading with respect to nociception. For example, Poggio and Mountcastle (1960) found that 60% of the units studied in the posterior nuclear region of the thalamus responded specifically to noxious stimuli. But Casey (1966), using an unanesthetized animal, found that none of these cells were specifically nociceptive during waking. He also found that many cells throughout the diencephalon and rostral midbrain responded differentially to noxious and nonnoxious stimuli, and most of these had wide peripheral receptive fields.

Attempts have been made to postulate brain mechanisms based upon studies of the effects of lesions designed to relieve pain in chronic pain states. These studies are fraught with difficulties. Changes in emotionality typically follow limbic system lesions, and these alterations in the affective component of pain make an assessment of its severity difficult. Furthermore, such lesions are seldom placed in those with a long life expectancy, thus long-term follow-up is rare. Even highly successful anterolateral cordotomies frequently fail after 12-18 months in chronic pain states. Casey and

Melzack (1967) note that the progressive divergence of the pain signals at higher levels makes it unlikely that focal lesions will significantly or permanently interrupt the sensory-discriminative aspects of nociception.

ANALGESIC MECHANISMS
Peripheral Stimulation
ACUPUNCTURE

This technique has long been known in this country as well as in Asia, for Osler (1912) cites it (and electrical stimulation) as a treatment for neuralgias. Travell and Rinzler (1952) long ago reported the special effect of dry needling of certain trigger points for myofascial syndromes, and Melzack et al. (1977) have shown the similarity of traditional acupuncture points and trigger points for referred pain sites.

Well-controlled studies of the efficacy of acupuncture are few, and their outcomes are frequently contradictory. Some studies report a strong analgesic effect (Gaw et al., 1975; Mann et al., 1973), others only a weak effect (Day et al., 1975; Li et al., 1975). The mechanism of action is unclear, but the typical 20-min delay of analgesia suggests a humoral process. This is supported by the finding that naloxone reverses acupuncture analgesia, but not hypnotic analgesia, suggesting a chemical rather than psychological mechanism (Goldstein and Hilgard, 1975; Mayer et al., 1976).

TRANSCUTANEOUS ELECTRICAL NEUROSTIMULATION (TNS)

Melzack and Wall's (1965) gate control theory of pain predicted that activation of large fibers by somatosensory stimulation would "close the gate" to noxious input along small fibers. Wall and Sweet (1967) confirmed that direct electrical stimulation of peripheral fibers relieved pain due to peripheral neuropathy for many minutes or hours after the brief stimulation.

The mechanism of this analgesic effect may indeed involve a central closing of a gate; this is supported by the finding that TNS can relieve the pain of postherpetic neuralgia, which involves pathologic lesions of dorsal root ganglia and dorsal columns (Nathan and Wall, 1974). However, studies by Taub and Campbell (1974), Torebjork and Hallin (1974b), and Ignelzi and Nyquist (1976) also suggest a direct "fatiguing" effect on small peripheral fibers, in evoked potential studies. Somatosensory changes in patients using TNS successfully for pain relief also suggest the effect to be primarily peripheral (Ignelzi *et al.*, 1976). The notion that suggestion, or a placebo effect, is not important is shown in follow-up studies, which show continued increased activity levels after one year of regular daily use (Sternbach *et al.*, 1976a). There is no clear habituation effect with TNS as with narcotic analgesia, and there may even be increasing sensitivity to electrical analgesia (Melzack, 1975).

Central Stimulation

Liebeskind *et al.* (1974) have shown that electrical stimulation of mesencephalic periaqueductal gray matter, in the region of the dorsal raphe nucleus, produces a very significant analgesia. This stimulation-produced analgesia (SPA) has been obtained using many different pain tests in many species, including man (Adams, 1976; Giesler and Liebeskind, 1976; Goodman and Holcombe, 1976; Hosobuchi *et al.*, 1977; Mayer and Liebeskind, 1974; Melzack and Melinkoff, 1974; Richardson and Akil, 1976 a,b; Soper, 1976). After only a few seconds of stimulation, the analgesia may last as long as several hours. The analgesia may be subtotal, so that the animal completely ignores a strong pinch to one limb but responds normally to a pinch to another limb. The analgesia can be equivalent to large doses of morphine (Mayer and Liebeskind, 1974), but the animals are normally reactive to other stimuli and can engage in normal behaviors (Mayer *et al.*, 1971).

SPA appears to result from stimulation of medial structures from the nucleus raphe magnus in the rostral medulla, through midbrain central gray, to the caudal diencephalon. It can completely inhibit the pain-evoked discharges of Class 2 dorsal horn cells, without affecting their responsiveness to nonpainful stimuli (Oliveras *et al.*, 1974). Akil has shown that this is a serotonergic system (Akil and Mayer, 1972; Akil and Liebeskind, 1975). Either chemical or dietary depletion of brain serotonin levels increases sensitivity to pain, which can be restored to normal levels by administration of the precursors tryptophan or 5-hydroxytryptophan. SPA can be blocked by selective destruction of the spinal cord dorsolateral funiculus in which the serotonin-containing fibers descend from the nucleus raphe magnus (Basbaum *et al.*, 1976).

NEUROHUMORAL SUBSTRATES

A number of pain-related behaviors are also serotonergically mediated; sleep is one of these (Jouvet, 1969). Sleep disturbance is one of the symptoms most frequently complained of by patients with chronic pain (Sternbach, 1974a). It is now reported that patients with painful fibromyositis syndrome have abnormal stage 4 sleep patterns (Moldofsky *et al.*, 1975). Normal subjects whose stage 4 sleep pattern is experimentally interrupted develop painful fibrositis symptoms (Moldofsky and Scarisbrick, 1975).

Patients with chronic pain typically develop depressive reactions (Sternbach, 1974a,b). There is some evidence which suggests that there may be two kinds of depression, associated with underactivity of brain norepinephrine or brain serotonin (Maas, 1975; Asberg *et al.*, 1976); pain patients seem to have the serotonin-type of depression. Akil and Liebeskind (1975) had shown that brain norepinephrine tended to antagonize the analgesic promoting effects of brain serotonin. We showed that administration of chlorimipramine, a tricyclic antidepressant which acts primarily to block reuptake of brain serotonin, reduced pain in chronic pain patients more than amitryptyline, which did no better than placebo; chlorimpramine exerted its effect by increasing pain tolerance (Sternbach *et al.*, 1976b).

OPIATE SYSTEM

The sites where microinjections of morphine are effective in producing analgesia are virtually identical to the effective sites of SPA

(Mayer and Murfin, 1976), and cross-tolerance develops between morphine- and stimulation-induced analgesia (Mayer and Hayes, 1975). Alteration of brain monoamine levels alter SPA and morphine analgesia similarly (Akil and Liebeskind, 1975). The morphine antagonist, naloxone, reverses SPA (Adams, 1976; Akil et al., 1976; Hosobuchi et al., 1977; Oliveras et al., 1975). These reports suggest that SPA responds to pharmacologic manipulations as does morphine.

There are also anatomical and electrophysiological studies to suggest that the opiate system is involved in a pain-inhibiting mechanism. Microinjection of morphine in the central gray results in a greater analgesia than injection in the ventricles or elsewhere (Jacquet and Lajtha, 1974; Pert and Yaksh, 1974), and stereospecific binding sites for opiates have been found in central gray (Kuhar et al., 1973). Both morphine and SPA selectively suppress nociceptive responding units in the dorsal horn (Kitahata et al., 1974) and in the brainstem (Oleson and Liebeskind, 1976).

Most recently, an endogenous opiate, an apparent ligand of morphine, has been identified and synthesized (and termed "enkephalin") and found to have analgesic properties (Hughes, 1975; Hughes et al., 1975). It appears to be one of the class of endorphins known as the opioid peptides, which have clear morphine-like activity and which are apparent neurotransmitters present in the limbic system but especially in the pituitary, central gray, and substantia gelatinosa (Goldstein, 1976). Injection of these peptides into the fourth ventricle or periaqueductal gray causes physical dependence, as shown by withdrawal symptoms precipitated by naloxone (Wei and Loh, 1976). Although the naturally occurring endorphins have analgesic properties lasting only a few minutes before enzymatic breakdown, molecular changes incorporated into synthetic enkephalin result in long-lasting effects (Pert et al., 1976; Walker et al., 1977). The electrophysiological effects of enkephalin include the ability to depress single neurons in the opiate system in anesthetized animals (Frederickson and Norris, 1976) and to increase spontaneous multiple-unit activity in the periaqueductal gray matter in awake animals (Urca et al., 1977). Both of these findings suggest that enkephalin is a neurotransmitter actively involved in endogenous mechanisms of analgesia.

Mayer and Price (1976) have reviewed the literature on central mechanisms of analgesia, and have proposed a model involving both a serotonergic and an enkephalin-like neurotransmitter system. Both ascending and descending serotonin pathways are involved with periaqueductal-periventricular structures of the brainstem, especially the nucleus raphe magnus, being critical loci or funnels in this system. In series or in parallel with this system is an enkephalin system. Electrical or chemical stimulation of either produces analgesia, while chemical or surgical blockade of either prevents analgesia. This powerful descending pain inhibitory mechanism is still being unraveled.

Psychological Mechanisms

One of the compelling arguments for a gating model of pain is the lack of a 1:1 relationship between stimulus intensity and the subjective experience of stimulus magnitude. Pain does not involve a straight-through transmission system, but is subject to ascending and descending modulating processes (Melzack, 1973). Some of these processes show consistent patterns, or "lawfulness," and we will consider those which have been best documented.

Perceptual Parameters
PAIN THRESHOLDS

This is the lowest intensity of stimulation at which pain is perceived; or, the least intensity of stimulation which can be called painful. It is the "absolute threshold" for pain in the same sense that the term is used for vision and hearing. In operational psychophysical terms, it is the point of stimulus intensity at which pain is reported 50% of the time in a series of ascending and descending (!) stimulus presentations.

Unlike the other modalities, in which a judgment of "present" or "not present" is made, the decision of "painful" versus "not painful" usually involves comparing the quality of two stimuli, rather than detecting the presence of one stimulus. That is, the point at which a warm stimulus becomes a pricking pain, or a cold one becomes an ache, or a pressure becomes painful, is rather different from noting whether a flash or a tone appears or not. The nature of the comparative judgment depends on what form of painful stimulation is used. With any noninvasive technique, it is arguable whether "pure" pain can occur: sensations of heat, cold, or pressure are also usually involved, taking on the added quality of pain.

Using the radiant heat technique, Hardy *et al.* (1952) found that physiological factors such as site, skin temperature, blackness, wetness, injury, repetition, and duration were important determinants of threshold, whereas race, sex, age, fatigue, and emotional state seemed not to be marked influences. Similar findings have been obtained with electric shock techniques. Although thresholds can be modified somewhat by acquired attitudes toward pain (Sternbach and Tursky, 1965), they are relatively stable and apparently a function of physiological parameters (Tursky, 1974).

Attempts have been made to measure deep somatic pain as well as superficial cutaneous pain. Wolff and Jarvik (1965), using hypertonic saline injections in the gluteus medius muscle, found that age increases the pain threshold, particularly for men; and women have a slightly (not significantly) lower threshold than men. The authors also compared radiant heat, ice water, and hypotonic as well as hypertonic saline, and obtained some significance in correlations of thresholds which ranged from .42 to −.53. They concluded that different stimuli applied to different body loci can elicit correlated pain thresholds under certain conditions.

PAIN TOLERANCE

This is the maximum pain level, the point at which the subject no longer voluntarily accepts pain; it is thus the upper threshold for pain. In several respects the pain tolerance level may be a more useful concept for clinical applications than is the pain threshold, although it is more

difficult to measure. One of the technical difficulties is that humanitarian and ethical considerations make it necessary to employ only an ascending series of stimuli, and precludes use of a descending series. This introduces a measurement error which is avoided by using both series in determining the lower pain threshold.

Hardy *et al.* (1952) admitted to difficulties with assessing pain tolerance to radiant heat because of resultant tissue damage, and an inability to obtain repeated measures within a reasonable period of time. In studies with electric shock, pain tolerance was found to be easily influenced by coaxing subjects, and was more susceptible to attitudes associated with ethnic membership than was pain threshold (Sternbach and Tursky, 1965). In a very large sample of over 40,000 subjects subjected to pressure on the Achilles tendon delivered by a calibrated motor-driven device, it was found that: pain tolerance decreases with age, more so for men than women; pain tolerance at every age is greater for men than women; and whites tolerate more pain than blacks who tolerate more pain than orientals (Woodrow *et al.*, 1972).

Several authors using different techniques have noted significant correlations between pain thresholds and pain tolerances. Wolff and Jarvik (1963), using radiant heat, obtained a correlation of .91 between the two levels. Merskey and Spear (1964), using the pressure algometer, obtained correlations in three groups of subjects of .70, .82, and .84. Tursky and O'Connell (1972), using electric shock, obtained within-day correlations of .97 to .99, and day-to-day correlations ranging from .73 to .85.

Clearly there is a significant association between pain threshold and pain tolerance. One reason why the correlations are not better, however, is that the latter is more readily influenced by subjects' sets (attitudes). Among the factors which have been shown to influence pain tolerance are suggestion, distraction, manipulation of anxiety, and motivation (Sternbach, 1968). Recently, social modeling has also been shown to alter tolerance; that is, if a model appears to endure more or less pain, this influences the subject's tolerance in the same direction (Craig, 1975). In general, when studies have examined the effects of experimental variables on both pain threshold and pain tolerance, the effects on tolerance are more marked.

PAIN SENSITIVITY RANGE

This is the difference between the pain threshold and pain tolerance. Other terms have been used, such as "pain interval" and "pain duration," but they imply a time scale. Wolff's (1971) suggestion of the term *"pain sensitivity range"* (PSR) is becoming more widespread. Wolff and Jarvik (1963) noted that the PSR correlated more highly with pain tolerance than with pain threshold, and Merskey and Spear (1964) did also.

Wolff (1971) performed a factor analysis on data he obtained from 60 chronic arthritis patients, using several different experimental pain techniques: cold pressor, radiant heat, cutaneous shock, deep muscle shock, and hypertonic saline. For each stimulation method the pain threshold, pain tolerance, and the PSR were calculated.

The factors obtained in analysis comprised a "cutaneous sensitivity" factor, containing all the cutaneous parameters except the PSR responses, and two "gluteal (deep) sensitivity" factors. However, a separate PSR factor emerged, representing the PSR measures independent of type of pain or depth of pain or body locus. Wolff (1971) termed this the *pain endurance factor*. This factor had a small but significant positive correlation with successful postoperative painful rehabilitation in the patients. Thus the PSR is an experimental factor with clinical relevance.

In an application of this concept, ischemic pain has been used to match the intensity of clinical pain experienced by patients, and is expressed as a percentage of the patient's ischemic pain tolerance. In a factor analysis of pain and personality measures, the matched level and maximum tolerance level emerged as a separate factor, confirming the concept of pain endurance as a specific pain factor related to clinical pain experience (Timmermans and Sternbach, 1974). A canonical correlation analysis of patients' ischemic pain scores, their numerical estimates of clinical pain severity, and personality measures, showed that patients' pain estimates were associated with the impact of pain on daily activities, but that ischemic pain scores were associated with level of depression (Timmermans and Sternbach, 1976).

JUST NOTICEABLE DIFFERENCE

This measure, the JND, represents the traditional psychophysical difference limen, which is the smallest interval that can be discriminated between levels of pain intensity. Hardy *et al.* (1952), using the radiant heat method, found 21 JNDs from pain threshold to pain tolerance. From this they created a Dol scale, in which a Dol represented two JNDs, so that there were 10½ clearly discriminable dols from threshold to tolerance. They used the Weber ratio $\Delta I/I$ in which I = stimulus intensity, and found that it did not remain constant as expected, but increased from .03 at threshold to .29 at tolerance, and concluded that the Weber law was not obeyed for pricking pain.

Interest in psychophysics shifted from JNDs to the power function. Stevens *et al.* (1958), using electric shock and a magnitude estimation technique, obtained a slope whose exponent was 3.5. Sternbach and Tursky (1964) obtained exponents of 1.8–1.9 in four different magnitude estimation studies, much closer to slopes for other sensory modalities, and a range of slopes of 1.25–2.68, depending on the psychophysical technique used.

Craig *et al.* (1975) found that social modeling can influence the psychophysical relationship. This is impressive because previously cited studies have shown that the pain threshold can be only slightly influenced by psychological factors, and pain tolerance easily influenced by these factors, but there had been no suggestion that social context could influence the psychophysical exponent. In fact, Sternbach and Tursky (1964, 1965) failed to find significant differences among ethnic groups in their magnitude estimation exponents. But Craig *et al.* (1975) found that their pain tolerant model had the effect of significantly reducing the size of the exponent in certain groups, as compared with control groups with pain intolerant models.

SIGNAL DETECTION

One of the difficulties with traditional psychophysical analyses is that error variances cannot be parceled out into those which are due to errors of sensory discrimination and those which are due to other biasing factors. This difficulty has been overcome by the relative operating characteristic (ROC) technique which emerged from statistical decision theory and electronic signal detection theory (Swets, 1973). The approach has important implications for experimental pain research, because it provides a measure of "sensory discriminability," and a measure of affective and motivational factors reflecting "response bias" (Clark, 1974). Analgesic effects of placebo and suggestion result only from a change in response bias (Clark, 1969, 1974; Feather et al., 1972), whereas nitrous oxide alters both bias and discriminability (Chapman et al., 1973). Recent studies of the effectiveness of acupuncture analgesia have also shown changes in bias and discriminability (Chapman et al., 1977), although there is some dispute about whether pain can be assessed by this technique (Rollman, 1977).

Personality Parameters
ANXIETY

There are now many experimental and clinical studies to show that anxiety enhances sensitivity to pain, or increases pain responsiveness (Sternbach, 1968). This is one of the major aspects of the "reaction component" of pain described by Beecher (1959). He showed that the significance of the injury suffered (anxiety) determined the degree of pain more than the extent of tissue injury.

When studies are made of those whose anxiety is very great—psychiatric patients—it is found that complaints of pain occur most frequently in those diagnosed as having anxiety neurosis or anxiety hysteria. And medical pa-

tients with complaints of pain are more likely to be diagnosed as anxious than medical patients without pain symptoms (Merskey and Spear, 1967). Furthermore, the severity of postoperative pain and complications in surgical patients are in large measure a function of neurotic anxiety (Parbrook et al., 1973 a,b).

Although anxiety is highly associated with the occurrence and severity of pain, it should be noted that in both the experimental and clinical situations it is acute pain that is correlated with anxiety; chronic pain is associated with depression, as described below (Sternbach, 1978).

EXPRESSIVENESS

Clinicians have long held that the patient who complains about pain more than the average has a "low pain threshold." This is an error. The readiness to communicate the experience of pain is a function of expressiveness, and this in turn is associated with degree of extraversion and also with group membership.

In experimental studies, Lynn and Eysenck (1961) found that the pain tolerance of college students to radiant heat was negatively correlated with neuroticism, and positively correlated with extraversion. Eysenck (1961) found that among 100 married and 100 unmarried women having their first babies, extraversion correlated significantly with experienced pain; the more extraverted the woman, the more she recalled her labor as having been painful. Neuroticism was not related to the pain ratings.

In several studies of groups of patients with advanced cancer, Bond and his colleagues (Bond and Pilowsky, 1966; Bond and Pearson, 1969; Pilowsky and Bond, 1969; Bond, 1971, 1973) have shown rather convincingly that the experimental findings on extraversion apply as well to the clinical situation. To sum these studies, it appears that the degree of *pain experienced* is positively correlated with the degree of neuroticism, but the *complaint* of pain (and the receipt of analgesics) is associated with the degree of extraversion. Of those with the greatest amount of pain (by rating), the amount of pain expression seemed to be a function of extraversion, so that neurotic intraverts might suffer silently, with little relationship between pain severity and pain complaint, but those with high extraversion scores had little difficulty communicating.

Social learning influences expressiveness as well, including that related to pain communication. Zborowski (1969) interviewed "Old American," Irish, Italian, and Jewish veterans who were surgical patients in pain, and their families, to determine their attitudes toward pain and pain expression. He found that Old Americans have a phlegmatic, matter-of-fact, doctor-helping orientation associated with their not complaining. The Irish, who also do not complain much, have a fearful, lonesome attitude with a great concern not to appear weak. The Italians and Jews are not inhibited in their pain expression. The Italians express a desire for immediate pain relief. The Jews express a concern for the meanings of pain as a symptom and the future implications of the pain.

Sternbach and Tursky (1965) interviewed and tested Yankee, Irish, Italian, and Jewish housewives, and corroborated the differences in attitudes toward pain and its expression. The Yankees felt one simply "took it in stride." The Irish were similarly undemonstrative, but anxious, and felt it important to "keep a stiff upper lip" and "don't be a baby." The Italians felt pain was an accident of fate and not to be endured, and pain expression helped to rally support and obtain relief. The Jews were similarly demonstrative, in part because of a belief in the cathartic value of "getting it out of your system," and because of a concern to direct attention to the underlying disease the pain represented. These various attitudes were associated with differences in laboratory findings. Italian women had significantly lower pain tolerance to electric shocks, and the Yankees demonstrated a more rapid and complete adaptation of diphasic palmar skin potentials to repeated strong shocks. In addition, there were significant group differences in a number of autonomically innervated variables (Tursky and Sternbach, 1967).

These findings indicate that culturally acquired attitudes toward pain and its expression can modulate the physiological responses to pain. There are many anecdotal reports which suggest even greater differences among various cultures in defining what constitutes pain (Melzack, 1973). However, almost all such observations lack any semblance of methodological rigor (Wolff and Langley, 1968).

DEPRESSION

In clinical situations, anxiety is associated with the *anticipation* of pain (body harm), or of loss (separation). Depression is associated with the *consequence* of these, in the form of intropunitive anger, or of mourning. In view of this relationship it might be expected that anxiety will be found in acute pain states, as noted above, and depression in chronic pain states. Sternbach *et al.* (1973) found that patients with low back pain of less than six months' duration obtained MMPI profiles within normal limits, whereas those with low back pain of longer duration had markedly elevated scores for depression, hypochondriasis, and hysteria.

Merskey and Spear (1967) found that in 200 consecutive admissions to a psychiatric clinic, pain was a symptom in 53%. Depression was the most common diagnosis, and pain occurred in 56% of the 85 depressives. Pilling *et al.* (1967) reported on 562 patients seen in psychiatric consultation at the Mayo Clinic; 32% had a pain as a presenting symptom. In both men and women, about 64% of those with pain were thought to have depressive symptoms. This supports the inference from Kenyon's (1964) study of hypochondriasis that pain can "stand for" an affective disorder, as in "masked" depressions.

Bradley (1963) studied the response to antidepressant treatment of 35 patients with pain and depression. In 16 whose pain preceded the depression, depression alone responded to treatment, but there was an increased tolerance to the pain. In the 19 whose pain and depression occurred together, both were relieved by treatment of the depression. Others have also reported on the effects of antidepressants in relieving chronic pain, sometimes in combination with other psychotropic agents (Merskey and Hester, 1972; Taub and Collins, 1974).

HYPOCHONDRIASIS

A frequent accompaniment of the depression is hypochondriasis, which often "masks" the depression so that the patient and observer are unaware of the depressed affect, but focus instead on physical symptoms. Hypochondriasis is the "fascinated absorption by the experience of a physical or mental impairment" (Ladee, 1966).

Pilowsky (1967) found three factors basic to the concept of hypochondriasis: bodily preoccupation; disease phobia; and conviction of the presence of disease with nonresponse to reassurance. Any one or combination of these factors may be present in a pain patient.

Kenyon (1964) examined the records of all patients seen at Bethlem Royal and Maudsley Hospitals in the ten-year period from 1951–1960, and chose those receiving an only or primary diagnosis of hypochondriasis ($N = 301$) to compare with those diagnosed as hypochondriacal secondary to some other diagnosis ($N = 211$). The symptom most often presented was pain, occurring in 75% of the primary group and in 62% of the secondary group. Affective symptoms of anxiety and depression were next most frequent, occurring in about 40% of the primary group and in 60% of the secondary group. Of those receiving a secondary diagnosis of hypochondriasis, 82% received a primary diagnosis of an affective disorder.

Pilowsky (1968) found that anxiety and depression were correlated with a good outcome in hypochondriacal patients; treatment of the associated affective disorder diminished the hypochondriasis. Poor treatment outcome was associated with the presence of organic pathology, among other variables. He also found that older males and younger females did less well in treatment.

SUMMARY

Pain is a specific sensory event normally initiated by tissue damage or impending tissue damage. There are specialized nociceptors whose information is transmitted to the spinal cord over specific A-delta and C fibers. Class 1 nociceptive cells, located in lamina 1 of the dorsal horn, respond specifically to injurious stimuli; Class 2 cells in lamina 5 respond to the full range from low intensity to noxious levels of stimulation. The gate control theory predicts that such responses can be inhibited both by large-fiber input and centrifugal mechanisms. Peripheral analgesic stimulation, whether from acupuncture, transcutaneous neurostimulation, or other mechanisms, seems to involve both a direct effect on peripheral fibers, and a central inhibitory mechanism which is partly dependent on a serotonin system in the periaqueductal gray and periventricular areas, and partly dependent on an enkephalin system in overlapping areas which also involves other structures of the limbic system. Direct stimulation of these areas produces analgesia which is reversible by naloxone. Other forms of central analgesia, such as motivation, attention, and hypnosis, are not reversible by naloxone.

Pain threshold and pain tolerance can be determined fairly accurately by several experimental techniques, and show high reliability. Age, sex, race, ethnic group and other factors can influence both, but pain tolerance is especially susceptible to these. Men have a higher tolerance than women, and with aging there is a slight increase in pain threshold and a marked decrease in pain tolerance, especially for men, and thus a narrowing of the pain sensitivity range with age. This pain sensitivity range has been shown to be a significant pain endurance factor of relevance to clinical pain, and a version of it has been used to measure the severity of clinical pain. The slope of the psychophysical relationship (stimulus intensity versus perceived sensation) depends on the technique used to assess it, but seems to have a slightly larger exponent in pain than in most of the other perceptual modalities; it is also susceptible to such influences as the social context of the experimental situation. Signal detection techniques are useful in separating pain sensitivity from biasing factors such as placebo effects.

In both laboratory and clinical situations, the intensity of the subjective pain experience is almost directly proportional to the individual's degree of neuroticism. This neuroticism consists chiefly of anxiety in the acute pain situation, and of depression in the chronic situation. Experimentally, the pain experience may be made less intense by extraversion, and by the presence of a model who is pain tolerant. Clinically, the pain experience may be potentiated by hypochondriasis. In both the laboratory and clinical situations the readiness to describe the pain experience appears to depend upon both the degree of extraversion, and on ethnic or cultural membership. Certain groups encourage the expression of pain, albeit for different reasons, and others inhibit such expression, also for different reasons. The clinical pain complaint appears to be an endpoint of both the pain experience and pain expression. As such it seems to be a function of neuroticism, extraversion, and social learning. In cases of "psychogenic" pain, these seem to be adequate causes. In cases of "somatogenic" pain, these seem to be the factors which make the pain intractable, and the patient demanding and manipulative (Sternbach, 1978).

REFERENCES

Adams, J. E. (1976). Naloxone reversal of analgesia produced by brain stimulation in the human. *Pain* 2, 161-166.

Akil, H., and J. C. Liebeskind (1975). Monoaminergic mechanisms of stimulation-produced analgesia. *Brain Res. 94*, 279-296.

Akil, H., and D. J. Mayer (1972). Antagonism of stimulation-produced analgesia by p-CPA, a serotonin synthesis inhibitor. *Brain Res. 44*, 692-697.

Akil, H., D. J. Mayer, and J. C. Liebeskind (1976). Antagonism of stimulation-produced analgesia by naloxone, a narcotic antagonist. *Science 191*, 961-962.

Asberg, M., P. Thoren, L. Traskman, L. Bertilsson, and V. Ringberger (1976). "Serotonin depression"—a biochemical subgroup within the affective disorders? *Science 191*, 478-480.

Basbaum, A. I., N. Marley, and J. O'Keefe (1976). Spinal cord pathways involved in the production of analgesia by brain stimulation. In *Advances in Pain Research and Therapy, Vol. 1, Proceedings of the First World Congress on Pain* (J. J. Bonica and D. Albe-Fessard, eds.), pp. 511-515. Raven Press, New York.

Beecher, H. K. (1959). *Measurement of Subjective Responses: Quantitative Effects of Drugs.* Oxford University Press, New York.

Bessou, P., and E. R. Perl (1969). Response of cutaneous sensory units with unmyelinated fibers to noxious stimuli. *J. Neurophysiol. 32*, 1025-1043.

Bond, M. R. (1971). The relation of pain to the Eysenck Personality Inventory, Cornell Medical Index and Whiteley Index of Hypochondriasis. *Brit. J. Psychiatry 119*, 671-678.

Bond, M. R. (1973). Personality studies in patients with pain secondary to organic disease. *J. Psychosom. Res. 17*, 257-263.

Bond, M. R., and I. B. Pearson (1969). Psychological aspects of pain in women with advanced cancer of the cervix. *J. Psychosom. Res. 13*, 13-19.

Bond, M. R., and I. Pilowsky (1966). Subjective assessment of pain and its relationship to the administration of analgesics in patients with advanced cancer. *J. Psychosom. Res. 10*, 203-208.

Bradley, J. J. (1963). Severe localized pain associated with the depressive syndrome. *Brit. J. Psychiatry 109*, 741-745.

Burgess, P. R., and E. R. Perl (1967). Myelinated afferent fibres responding specifically to noxious stimulation of the skin. *J. Physiol. (Lond.) 190*, 541-562.

Casey, K. L. (1966). Unit analysis of nociceptive mechanisms in the thalamus of the awake squirrel monkey. *J. Neurophysiol. 29*, 727-750.

Casey, K. L. (1971a). Responses of bulboreticular units to somatic stimuli eliciting escape behavior in the cat. *Intern. J. Neurosci. 2*, 15-28.

Casey, K. L. (1971b). Escape elicited by bulboreticular stimulation in the cat. *Intern. J. Neurosci. 2*, 29-34.

Casey, K. L. (1971c). Somatosensory responses of bulboreticular units in awake cat: relation to escape-producing stimuli. *Science 173*, 77-80.

Casey, K. L., and R. Melzack (1967). Neural mechanisms of pain: a conceptual model. In *New Concepts in Pain and Its Clinical Management* (E. L. Way, ed.), pp. 13-31. Davis, Philadelphia.

Chapman, C. R., T. M. Murphy, and S. H. Butler (1973). Analgesic strength of 33 percent nitrous oxide: a signal detection theory evaluation. *Science 179*, 1246-1248.

Chapman, C. R., A. C. Chen, and J. J. Bonica (1977). Effects of intrasegmental electrical acupuncture on dental pain: evaluation by threshold estimation and sensory decision theory. *Pain 3*, 213-227.

Christensen, B. N., and E. R. Perl (1970). Spinal neurons specifically excited by noxious or thermal stimuli: marginal zone of the dorsal horn. *J. Neurophysiol. 33*, 293-307.

Clark, W. C. (1969). Sensory decision theory analysis of the placebo effect on the criterion for pain and thermal sensitvity (d'). *J. Abnormal Psychology 74*, 363-371.

Clark, W. C. (1974). Pain sensitivity and the report of pain: an introduction to sensory decision theory. *Anesthesiology 40*, 272-287.

Craig, K. D., H. Best, and L. M. Ward (1975). Social modelling influences on psychophysical judgments of electrical stimulation. *J. Abnormal Psychology 84*, 366–373.

Day, R. L., L. M. Kitahata, F. F. Kao, E. K. Motoyama, and J. D. Hardy (1975). Evaluation of acupuncture anesthesia: a psychophysical study. *Anesthesiology 43*, 507–517.

Eysenck, S. B. G. (1961). Personality and pain assessment of childbirth of married and unmarried mothers. *J. Mental Science 107*, 417–430.

Feather, B. W., C. R. Chapman, and S. B. Fisher (1972). The effect of a placebo on the perception of painful radiant heat stimuli. *Psychosom. Med. 34*, 290–294.

Frederickson, R. C. A., and F. H. Norris (1976). Enkephalin-induced depression of single neurons in brain areas with opiate receptors—antagonism by naloxone. *Science 194*, 440–442.

Gaw, A. C., L. W. Chang, and L.-C. Shaw (1975). Efficacy of acupuncture on osteoarthritic pain. *New Eng. J. Med. 293*, 375–378.

Giesler, G. J. Jr., and J. C. Liebeskind (1976). Inhibition of visceral pain by electrical stimulation of the periaqueductal gray matter. *Pain 2*, 43–48.

Goldstein, A. (1976). Opiois peptides (endorphins) in pituitary and brain. *Science 193*, 1081–1086.

Goldstein, A., and E. R. Hilgard (1975). Lack of influence of the morphine antagonist naloxone on hypnotic analgesia. *Proc. Nat. Acad. Sci. 72*, 2041–2043.

Goodman, S. J., and V. Holcombe (1976). Selective and prolonged analgesia in monkey resulting from brain stimulation. In *Advances in Pain Research and Therapy, Vol. 1, Proceedings of the First World Congress on Pain* (J. J. Bonica and D. Albe-Fessard, eds.), pp. 495–502. Raven Press, New York.

Handwerker, H. O., A. Iggo, and M. Zimmermann (1975). Segmental and supraspinal actions on dorsal horn neurons responding to noxious and non-noxious skin stimuli. *Pain 1*, 147–165.

Hardy, J. D., H. G. Wolff, and H. Goodell (1952). *Pain Sensations and Reactions*. Williams and Wilkins, Baltimore.

Hillman, P., and P. D. Wall (1969). Inhibitory and excitatory factors influencing the receptive fields of lamina 5 spinal cord cells. *Exp. Brain Res. 9*, 284–306.

Hosobuchi, Y., J. E. Adams, and R. Linchitz (1977). Pain relief by electrical stimulation of the central gray matter in humans and its reversal by naloxone. *Science 197*, 183–186.

Hughes, J. (1975). Isolation of an endogenous compound from the brain with pharmacological properties similar to morphine. *Brain Res. ii*, 295–308.

Hughes, J., T. W. Smith, H. W. Kosterlitz, L. A. Fothergill, B. A. Morgan, and H. R. Morris (1975). Identification of two related pentapeptides from the brain with potent opiate agonist activity. *Nature 258*, 577–579.

Ignelzi, R. J., and J. K. Nyquist (1976). Direct effect of electrical stimulation on peripheral nerve evoked activity: implications in pain relief. *J. Neurosurg. 45*, 159–165.

Ignelzi, R. J., R. A. Sternbach, and M. Callaghan (1976). Somato-sensory changes during transcutaneous electrical analgesia. In *Advances in Pain Research and Therapy, Vol. 1, Proceedings of the First World Congress on Pain* (J. J. Bonica and D. Albe-Fessard, eds.), pp. 421–425. Raven Press, New York.

Jacquet, Y. F., and A. Lajtha (1974). Paradoxical effects after microinjection of morphine in the periaqueductal gray matter in the rat *Science 185*, 1055–1057.

Jouvet, M. (1969). Biogenic amines and the states of sleep. *Science 163*, 32–41.

Keele, K. D. (1957). *Anatomies of Pain*. Blackwell, Oxford.

Kenyon, F. E. (1964). Hypochondriasis: a clinical study. *Brit. J. Psychiat. 110*, 478–488.

Kerr, F. W. L. (1975). Neuroanatomical substrates of nociception in the spinal cord. *Pain 1*, 325–356.

Kitahata, L. M., Y. Kosaka, A. Taub, K. Bonidos, and M. Hoffert (1974). Lamina-specific suppression of dorsal-horn unit activity by morphine sulfate. *Anesthesiol. 41*, 39–48.

Kuhar, M. J., C. B. Pert, and S. H. Snyder (1973). Regional distribution of opiate receptor binding in monkey and human brain. *Nature 245*, 447–450.

Ladee, G. A. (1966). *Hypochondriacal Syndromes*. Elsevier, Amsterdam.

Li, C. L., D. Ahlberg, H. Lansdell, M. A. Gravitz, T. C. Chen, C. Y. Ting, A. F. Bak, and D. Blessing (1975). Acupuncture and hypnosis: effects on induced pain. *Exp. Neurol. 49*, 272–280.

Liebeskind, J. C., D. J. Mayer, and H. Akil (1974). Central mechanisms of pain inhibition: studies of analgesia from focal brain stimulation. In *Advances in Neurology, Vol. 4*. (J. J. Bonica, ed.), pp. 261–268. Raven Press, New York.

Lynn, R., and H. J. Eysenck (1961). Tolerance for pain, extraversion and neuroticism. *Perceptual and Motor Skills 12*, 161–162.

Maas, J. W. (1975). Biogenic amines and depression: biochemical and pharmacological separation of two types of depression. *Arch. Gen. Psychiat. 32*, 1357–1361.

Mann, F., D. Bowsher, J. Mumford, S. Lipton, and J. Miles (1973). Treatment of intractable pain by acupuncture. *Lancet 2*, 57–60.

Mayer, D. J., and R. Hayes (1975). Stimulation-produced analgesia: development of tolerance and cross-tolerance to morphine. *Science 188*, 941–943.

Mayer, D. J., and J. C. Liebeskind (1974). Pain reduction by focal electrical stimulation of the brain: an anatomical and behavioral analysis. *Brain Res. 68*, 73–93.

Mayer, D. J., and R. Murfin (1976). Stimulation-produced analgesia (SPA) and morphine analgesia (MA): cross-tolerance from application at the same brain site. *Fed. Proc. 35*, 385.

Mayer, D. J., and D. D. Price (1976). Central nervous system mechanisms of analgesia. *Pain* 2, 379-404.

Mayer, D. J., T. L. Wolffe, H. Akil, B. Cardr, and J. C. Liebeskind (1971). Analgesia from electrical stimulation in the brainstem of the rat. *Science* 174, 1351-1354.

Mayer, D. J., D. D. Price, and D. P. Becker (1975). Neurophysiological characterization of the anterolateral spinal cord neurons contributing to pain perception in man. *Pain* 1, 51-58.

Mayer, D. J., D. D. Price, J. Barber, and A. Rafii (1976). Acupuncture analgesia: evidence for activation of a pain inhibitory system as a mechanism of action. In *Advances in Pain Research and Therapy, Vol. 1, Proceedings of the First World Congress on Pain* (J. J. Bonica and D. Albe-Fessard, eds.), pp. 751-754. Raven Press, New York.

Melzack, R. (1973). *The Puzzle of Pain*. Basic Books, New York.

Melzack, R. (1975). Prolonged relief of pain by brief, intense transcutaneous somatic stimulation. *Pain* 1, 357-373.

Melzack, R., and D. F. Melinkoff (1974). Analgesia produced by brain stimulation: evidence of a prolonged onset period. *Exp. Neurol.* 43, 369-374.

Melzack, R., and P. D. Wall (1965). Pain mechanisms: a new theory. *Science* 150, 971-979.

Melzack, R., D. M. Stillwell, and E. J. Fox (1977). Trigger points and acupuncture points for pain: correlations and implications. *Pain* 3, 3-23.

Merskey, H., and R. N. Hester (1972). The treatment of chronic pain with psychotropic drugs. *Postgraduate Med. J.* 48, 594-598.

Merskey, H., and F. G. Spear (1967). *Pain: Psychology* of the pressure algometer. *Brit. J. Soc. Clin. Psych.* 3, 130-136.

Merskey, H., and F. G. Spear (1967). *Pain: Psychological and Psychiatric Aspects*. Bailliere, Tindall, and Cassell, London.

Moldofsky, H., and P. Scarisbrick (1975). Induction of neurasthenic musculoskeletal pain syndrome by selective sleep stage deprivation. *Psychosom. Med.* 38, 35-44.

Moldofsky, H., P. Scarisbrick, R. England, and H. Smythe (1975). Musculoskeletal symptoms and non-REM sleep disturbance in patients with "fibrositis syndrome" and healthy subjects. *Psychosom. Med.* 37, 341-351.

Morrow, T. J., and K. L. Casey (1976). Analgesia produced by mesencephalic stimulation: effect on bulboreticular neurons. In *Advances in Pain Research and Therapy, Vol. 1, Proceedings of the First World Congress on Pain* (J. J. Bonica and D. Albe-Fessard, eds.), pp. 503-510. Raven Press, New York.

Nathan, P. W., and P. D. Wall (1974). Treatment of post-herpetic neuralgia by prolonged electric stimulation. *Brit. Med. J.* 3, 645-647.

Oleson, T. D., and J. C. Liebeskind (1976). Modification of midbrain and thalamic evoked responses by analgesic brain stimulation in the rat. In *Advances in Pain Research and Therapy, Vol. 1, Proceed-*

ings of the First World Congress on Pain (J. J. Bonica and D. Albe-Fessard, eds.), pp. 487-494. Raven Press, New York.

Oliveras, J. L., J. M. Besson, G. Guilbaud, and J. C. Liebeskind (1974). Behavioral and electrophysiological evidence of pain inhibition from midbrain stimulation in the cat. *Exp. Brain Res.* 20, 32-44.

Oliveras, J. L., F. Redjemi, G. Guilbaud, and J. M. Besson (1975). Analgesia induced by electrical stimulation of the inferior centralis nucleus of the raphe in the cat. *Pain* 1, 139-145.

Osler, W. (1912). *The Principles and Practice of Medicine* (8th ed.), pp. 1092-1093. Appleton, New York.

Parbrook, G. D., D. G. Dalrymple, and D. F. Steel (1973a). Personality assessment and postoperative pain and complications. *J. Psychosom. Res.* 17, 277-285.

Parbrook, G. D., D. F. Steel, and D. G. Dalrymple (1973b). Factors predisposing to postoperative pain and pulmonary complications. *Brit. J. Anaesthesia* 45, 21-33.

Perl, E. R. (1968). Myelinated afferent fibres innervating the primate skin and their response to noxious stimuli. *J. Physiol. (Lond.)* 197, 593-615.

Perl, E. R. (1971). Is pain a specific sensation? *J. Psychiat. Res.* 8, 273-287.

Pert, C. B., A. Pert, J.-K. Chang, and B. T. W. Fong (1976). (D-Ala²)-met-enkephalinamide: a potent, long-lasting synthetic pentapeptide analgesic. *Science* 194, 330-332.

Pert, A., and T. Yaksh (1974). Sites of morphine induced analgesia in the primate brain: relation to pain pathways. *Brain Res.* 80, 135-140.

Pilling, L. F., T. L. Brannick, and W. M. Swenson (1967). Psychologic characteristics of psychiatric patients having pain as a presenting symptom. *Can. Med. Assoc. J.* 97, 387-394.

Pilowsky, I. (1967). Dimensions of hypochondriasis. *Brit. J. Psychiat.* 113, 89-93.

Pilowsky, I. (1968). The response to treatment in hypochondriacal disorders. *Australian and New Zealand J. Psychiat.* 2, 88-94.

Pilowsky, I., and M. R. Bond (1969). Pain and its management in malignant disease: elucidation of staff-patient transactions. *Psychosom. Med.* 31, 400-404.

Poggio, G. F., and V. B. Mountcastle (1960). A study of the functional contributions of the lemniscal and spinothalamic systems to somatic sensibility. *Bull. Johns Hopkins Hosp.* 106, 266-316.

Pomeranz, B., P. D. Wall, and W. V. Weber (1968). Cord cells responding to fine myelinated afferents from viscera, muscle and skin. *J. Physiol. (Lond.)* 199, 511-532.

Price, D. D. (1972). Characteristics of second pain and flexion reflexes indicative of prolonged central summation. *Exp. Neurol.* 37, 371-387.

Price, D. D. (1976). Modulation of first and second pain by peripheral stimulation and by psychological set. In *Advances in Pain Research and Therapy,*

Vol. 1, Proceedings of the First World Congress on Pain (J. J. Bonica and D. Albe-Fessard, eds.), pp. 427-431. Raven Press, New York.

Price, D. D., and A. C. Browe (1973). Responses of spinal cord neurons to graded noxious and nonnoxious stimuli. *Brain Res. 64*, 425-429.

Price, D. D., and D. J. Mayer (1975). Neurophysiological characterization of the anterolateral quadrant neurons subserving pain in *Macaca mulatta. Pain 1*, 59-72.

Price, D. D., and I. H. Wagman (1970). Physiological roles of A and C fiber inputs to the spinal dorsal horn of *Macaca mulatta. Exp. Neurol. 29*, 383-399.

Richardson, D. E., and H. Akil (1977a). Pain reduction by electrical brain stimulation in man. I. Acute administration in periaqueductal and periventricular sites. *J. Neurosurg. 47*, 178-183.

Richardson, D. E., and H. Akil (1977b). Pain reduction by electrical brain stimulation in man. II. Chronic self-administration in the periventricular gray matter. *J. Neurosurg. 47*, 184-194.

Rollman, G. B. (1977). Signal detection theory measurement of pain: A review and critique. *Pain 3*, 187-211.

Soper, W. Y. (1976). Effects of analgesic midbrain stimulation on reflex withdrawal and thermal escape in the rat. *J. Comp. Physiol. Psychol. 90*, 91-101.

Sternbach, R. A. (1968). *Pain: A Psychophysiological Analysis.* Academic Press, New York.

Sternbach, R. A. (1974a). Pain and depression. In *Somatic Manifestations of Depressive Disorders* (A. Kiev, ed.), pp. 107-119. Excerpta Medica, Princeton, N.J.

Sternbach, R. A. (1974b). *Pain Patients: Traits and Treatment.* Academic Press, New York.

Sternbach, R. A. (ed.) (1978). *The Psychology of Pain.* Raven Press, New York.

Sternbach, R. A., and B. Tursky (1964). On the psychophysical power function in electric shock. *Psychonomic Science 1*, 217-218.

Sternbach, R. A., and B. Tursky (1965). Ethnic differences in psychophysical and skin potential responses to electric shock. *Psychophysiology 1*, 241-246.

Sternbach, R. A., S. R. Wolf, R. W. Murphy, and W. H. Akeson (1973). Traits of pain patients: the low-back "loser". *Psychosomatics 14*, 226-229.

Sternbach, R. A., R. J. Ignelzi, L. M. Deems, and G. Timmermans (1976a). Transcutaneous electrical analgesia: a follow-up analysis. *Pain 2*, 35-41.

Sternbach, R. A., D. S. Janowsky, L. Y. Huey, and D. S. Segal (1976b). Effects of altering brain serotonin activity on human chronic pain. In *Advances in Pain Research and Therapy, Vol. 1, Proceedings of the First World Congress on Pain* (J. J. Bonica and D. Albe-Fessard, eds.), pp. 601-606. Raven Press, New York.

Stevens, S. S., A. S. Carton, and G. M. Shickman (1958). A scale of apparent intensity of electric shock. *J. Exp. Psych. 56*, 328-334.

Swets, J. A. (1973). The relative operating characteristic in psychology. *Science 182*, 990-1000.

Taub, A., and J. N. Campbell (1974). Percutaneous local electrical analgesia: peripheral mechanisms. In *Advances in Neurology Vol. 4* (J. J. Bonica, ed.), pp. 727-732. Raven Press, New York.

Taub, A., and W. F. Collins, Jr. (1974). Observations on the treatment of denervation dysesthesia with psychotropic agents: postherpetic neuralgia, anesthesia dolorosa, peripheral neuropathy. In *Advances in Neurology, Vol. 4* (J. J. Bonica, ed.), pp. 727-732. Raven Press, New York.

Timmermans, G., and R. A. Sternbach (1974). Factors of human chronic pain: an analysis of pain and personality measures. *Science 184*, 806-807.

Timmermans, G., and R. A. Sternbach (1976). Human chronic pain and personality: a canonical correlation analysis. In *Advances in Pain Research and Therapy, Vol. 1, Proceedings of the First World Congress on Pain* (J. J. Bonica and D. Albe-Fessard, eds.), pp. 307-310. Raven Press, New York.

Torebjork, H. E., and R. G. Hallin (1973). Perceptual changes accompanying controlled preferential blocking of A and C fibre responses in intact human skin nerves. *Exp. Brain Res. 16*, 321-332.

Torebjork, H. E., and R. G. Hallin (1974a). Identification of afferent C units in intact human skin nerves. *Brain Res. 67*, 387-403.

Torebjork, H. E., and R. G. Hallin (1974b). Excitation failure in thin nerve fiber structures and accompanying hypalgesia during repetitive electric skin stimulation. In *Advances in Neurology, Vol. 4* (J. J. Bonica, ed.), pp. 733-736. Raven Press, New York.

Travell, J., and S. H. Rinzler (1952). The myofascial genesis of pain. *Postgraduate Med. 11*, 425-434.

Tursky, B. (1974). Physical, physiological, and psychological factors that affect pain reaction to electric shock. *Psychophysiology 11*, 95-112.

Tursky, B., and D. O'Connell (1972). Reliability and interjudgment predictability of subjective judgments of electrocutaneous stimulation. *Psychophysiology 9*, 290-295.

Tursky, B., and R. A. Sternbach (1967). Further physiological correlates of ethnic differences in responses to shock. *Psychophysiology 4*, 67-74.

Urca, G., H. Frenk, J. C. Liebeskind, and A. N. Taylor (1977). Morphine and enkephalin: analgesic and epileptic properties. *Science 197*, 83-86.

Van Hees, J., and J. M. Gybels (1972). Pain related to single afferent C fibers from human skin. *Brain Res. 48*, 397-400.

Walker, J. M., G. G. Berntson, C. A. Sandman, D. H. Coy, A. V. Schally, and A. J. Kostin (1977). An analog of enkephalin having prolonged opiate-like effects in vivo. *Science 196*, 85-87.

Wall, P. D., and W. H. Sweet (1967). Temporary abolition of pain in man. *Science 155*, 108-109.

Wei, E., and H. Loh (1976). Physical dependence on opiate-like peptides. *Science 193*, 1262-1263.

Willis, W. D., D. L. Trevino, J. D. Coulter, and R. A. Maunz (1974). Responses of primate spinothalamic tract neurons to natural stimulation of the hindlimb. *J. Neurophysiol. 37*, 358–372.

Wolff, B. B. (1971). Factor analysis of human pain responses: pain endurance as a specific pain factor. *J. Abnormal Psych. 78*, 292–298.

Wolff, B. B., and M. E. Jarvik (1963). Variations in cutaneous and deep somatic pain sensitivity. *Can. J. Psychol. 17*, 37–44.

Wolff, B. B., and M. E. Jarvik (1965). Quantitative measures of deep somatic pain: further studies with hypertonic saline. *Clin. Sci. 28*, 43–56.

Wolff, B. B., and S. Langley (1968). Cultural factors and the response to pain: a review. *Am. Anthropologist 70*, 494–501.

Woodrow, K. M., G. D. Friedman, A. B. Siegelaub, and M. F. Collen (1972). Pain tolerance: differences according to age, sex and race. *Psychosom. Med. 34*, 548–556.

Zborowski, M. (1969). *People in Pain.* Jossey-Bass, San Francisco.

3

PAIN-SENSITIVE STRUCTURES WITHIN THE CRANIUM

REVISED BY DONALD J. DALESSIO

To understand what causes or influences headache, it is essential to know which of the structures of the head are sensitive to pain. Postmortem studies, however thorough, have not yielded adequate data, for the demonstration of nerve fibers or nerve endings in a given structure does not in itself justify the inference that the structure is sensitive to pain or produces pain when stimulated. This is because afferent fibers cannot, with certainty, be distinguished from efferent fibers in a morphological study, nor can pain-conducting afferent fibers in end organs be differentiated from other afferent nerves. Some clinical studies on man and the lower animals have shown that portions of the cranial blood vessels are pain sensitive (Chorobski and Penfield, 1932; Clark, S., 1934; Graham and Wolff, 1937; Gulland, 1898; Huber, 1899; McNaughton, 1938; Pickering, 1939; Wolff, 1959). In addition, brain surgery in humans offers a direct approach to the problem and it has been possible to obtain, through the use of general and local anesthesia, a considerable body of data on the sensitivity of intracranial structures to pain (Cushing, 1908, 1909; Fay, 1931, 1936, 1937; McNaughton, 1938; Penfield, 1932, 1935; Putnam, 1937).

The basic reference for this chapter is the monumental paper of Ray and Wolff (1940) who systematically stimulated multiple intracranial sites in 30 patients, in most of whom multiple observations were made. These were surgical patients in whom necessary surgical exposure of the brain afforded an opportunity to make careful observations on the sensitivity of the structures within and outside the cranium to pain. The use of a variety of stimuli resulted in a data base of knowledge to which all students of head and neck pain still refer. For the most part, this work has not been repeated, although additional observations have been made.

As a basis for this study, 30 patients were selected from a large group. The following conditions were required:

1. The patients were intelligent and cooperative, so that not only could pain be reported but its site and nature could be described.

2. The patients were relatively free of apprehension and of preoccupation with pain, so that a minimal amount of local and general analgesia was required.

3. The operative procedures were such that the patients were not too prostrate or inarticulate to describe their sensations.

4. The structures in every case were free of disease. This was necessary to ensure normal responses to stimulation.

5. The observations were recorded in the operating room in detail and by appropriate charts at the time they were being made.

PERIOSTEUM OF THE SKULL (EPICRANIUM)

One hundred observations were made on 30 subjects.

The periosteum had a variable sensitivity to pain. On the whole it was not particularly sensitive, and in small areas over the vertex it was entirely insensitive. In general, the degree of sensitivity increased in the regions just over

24

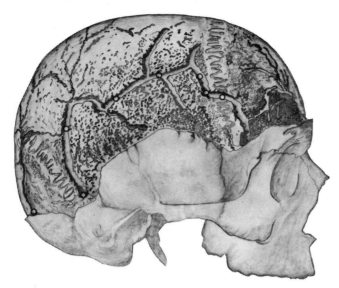

FIG. 3-1. Diploic and emissary veins of the cranium; ○ indicates the point of stimulation without pain.

the brow, low in the temporal regions, and low in the occipital regions. Always when a periosteal elevator was used to strip up the periosteum around the base of the skull there was a complaint of moderate pain somewhere in the neighborhood of the point of stimulation.

CRANIAL BONE, INCLUDING DIPLOID AND EMISSARY VEINS

The cranial bone was everywhere insensitive. This was demonstrated many times in the process of drilling, sawing, rongeuring, and coagulating at all points of the skull. This general statement is valid for the inner and outer tables and the cancellous central portion. It may further be stated that when there was occasion to test for pain in regions of endostoses and exostoses, which were sometimes highly vascularized, there was still no evidence of sensation (3 subjects, 12 observations). The venous channels (diploic veins) of the bone were also insensitive on faradic stimulation (3 subjects, 12 observations). There was occasion to stimulate directly the walls of some of the larger diploic veins both with faradic current

and by the coagulating endothermy; no pain was elicited. Specifically, the principal diploic veins just outside the skull Fig. (3-1) were directly stimulated with faradic current and found to be insensitive (3 subjects, 12 observations).

Clinical Application. Osteomyelitis or other destructive disease of the cranial bone does not in itself produce pain. But rapid elevation, stretch, and acute inflammation of the periosteum do result in pain of moderate or high intensity, depending on the site. Thus, periostitis at the base, over the mastoid bone, over the frontal sinuses, or, in general, below the hairline is usually more painful than that above the hairline. Slow expansion and low-grade or chronic inflammation (as in some instances of syphilis), may not be associated with pain. Also metastatic invasion of the skull by involving the periosteum may be the cause of much or little pain, depending in general on the site and the speed of growth. When metastases (notably from breast or thyroid cancer) cause pain, X-ray therapy, by stopping or slowing the expansion, reduces or eliminates pain.

Rarely and for short periods headache results from the stretch of the periosteum during phases of rapid growth in patients with acromegaly, Paget's disease, and osteomas.

Hyperostosis frontalis interna, a complex of signs

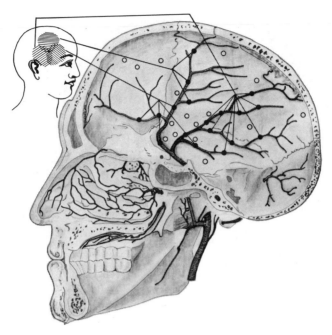

FIG. 3-2. Middle meningeal artery, ○ indicates the point of stimulation of the dura without pain; ● indicates the point of stimulation causing pain. The diagram shows three overlapping areas of pain in the parietotemporal region resulting from stimulation of different portions of the artery and its branches.

and symptoms also called Morgagni's syndrome, often has headache as a prominent manifestation. Circumscribed areas of increased density in the frontal bone and thickness of the orbital plate may be found on X-ray. Headache, obesity, and evidence of anxiety, fear, depression, and other behavior and mental disorders are common. The condition occurs chiefly in women of middle age. It rarely is found in men. With increasing age the orbital plate in this disorder gradually becomes thinner and approaches the normal. The author has never been convinced that the headache of which these patients complain is due to the bony changes. Other explanations and mechanisms appear more likely.

DURAL ARTERIES

The principal dural artery is the middle meningeal, a branch of the external carotid artery which supplies all the supratentorial dura except for the dura of the floor of the anterior fossa and that over the anterior pole of the brain. The latter dura is supplied by the anterior meningeal artery, a branch of the cavernous portion of the internal carotid artery, and by the anterior and posterior ethmoidal arteries. The latter are branches of the ophthalmic artery, itself a branch of the internal carotid artery. The subtentorial dura is supplied by the posterior meningeal arteries, branches of the occipital, vertebral, or ascending pharyngeal arteries.

It was demonstrated that the main trunks of all the dural arteries were sensitive to painful stimuli.

The stimuli employed included faradizing, burning, distending, stroking, stretching, and crushing the middle meningeal artery and its branches (see Fig. 3-2). Distention was affected as follows. On one occasion the tip of a clamp was introduced into the lumen of the middle meningeal artery and spread, and on another a series of silk sutures equally placed about the circumference of the artery were simultaneously pulled on (Fig. 3-3). The pain produced was localized fairly accurately in the area of disten-

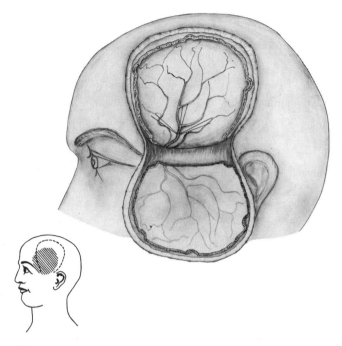

Fɪɢ. 3-3. Traction sutures symmetrically placed in the wall of the middle meningeal artery. The mechanical distention of the artery resulting from simultaneous traction on all three sutures caused pain in the hatched area on the diagram.

tion and also was commonly described as being in the back of the eye. It was aching, similar to that resulting from distention of the temporal artery. It also was accompanied by nausea.

A few of the smaller branches arising from the main divisions of the middle meningeal artery, even within a few centimeters of the midline at the vertex, were found to be sensitive to pain. The area in which the pain was felt was usually fairly discrete and was somewhere in the region of stimulation. In general, the pain experienced from stimulation of the middle meningeal artery was within the homolateral temporoparietal region and was deep and aching. It could be shown that there was a slight discrepancy in the exact localization when different parts of the artery were stimulated. Thus, pain arising from the main trunk of the artery and the more proximal part of the anterior branch was felt in the mid-temporal region; pain arising from the more distal divisions of the anterior branch was more parietal in its location, and pain arising from the posterior branches of the artery was localized behind both of the other two sites.

The usual experience associated with reflection of a temporoparietal osteoplastic flap was the occurrence of sharp pain in that general region as a result of stretching the middle meningeal artery or tearing it from its groove in the bone (24 subjects, 24 observations). The severity of the pain was variable but usually comparable to that from painful superficial structures and more severe than that arising from stimulation of most pain-sensitive intracranial structures. This impression was substantiated by application of other stimuli to the artery. Although distention of a main trunk of the artery by some mechanical means repeatedly caused pain, vigorous constriction of the arterial wall after local application of epinephrine was unaccompanied by pain. These findings conformed to those made on

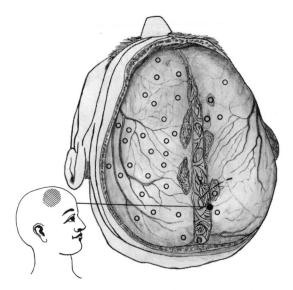

FIG. 3-4. Superior sagittal sinus and the adjacent venous lacunae and arachnoid granulations; ○ indicates the point of stimulation without pain; ● indicates the point of stimulation causing pain. The diagram shows the area of pain following stimulation of the margin of the superior sagittal sinus.

similarly testing the superficial temporal artery.

Transection, ligation, or procaine hydrochloride infiltration of the middle meningeal artery anywhere along its course, even as far proximal as the foramen spinosum, was always followed by anesthesia of the artery distal to that point. This finding plus the further observation that the dura which lies between the branches of the midmeningeal artery was insensitive to pain indicates that the pain-conducting fibers join the artery near its origin and travel adjacent to it.

The localization of pain from stimulation of the anterior meningeal arteries was limited to the forehead and the region of the eye on the same side (12 subjects, 48 observations). That from the posterior meningeal arteries was limited to the back of the head on the same side (4 subjects, 16 observations). The sensitivity to pain of the anterior and posterior meningeal arteries was limited to the most proximal portions of these quickly arborizing vessels, and the small distal branches in the dura over the frontal poles of the cerebrum and over the cerebellar lobes were insensitive to pain.

DURA, SUPRATENTORIAL

The supratentorial dura (Fig. 3-4) covering the convexities of the cerebrum and exclusive of the base was found to be entirely insensitive to all forms of stimulation except along the margins of the dural sinuses and along the course of the middle meningeal artery (11 subjects, 148 observations).

The entire dural floor of the anterior fossa (12 subjects, 48 observations), on the contrary, while inconstantly sensitive to pressure, was almost uniformly sensitive to faradic stimulation, and the pain arising from this region was localized to the homolateral eye, that is, over, within, behind, or beside the eye. Sometimes, stimulation of the floor of the anterior fossa at widely separated points caused pain at slightly different sites within the general region about the eye. The dura of the olfactory groove was found to be unusually sensitive to pain, while the dura that forms the roof of the orbit was perhaps slightly less so. The dura along the superior aspect of the sphenoidal ridge, in the region of the dorsum sellae, and at the base of the anterior clinoids was but moderately sensi-

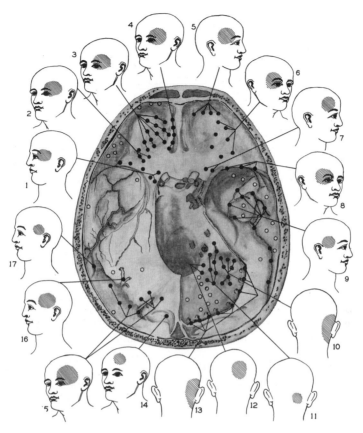

FIG. 3-5. The dural floor of the skull, the tentorium cerebelli, and the adjacent venous sinuses and venous tributaries; ○ indicates the point of stimulation without pain; ● indicates the point of stimulation causing pain. The diagrams show the area of pain following stimulation of (1 to 8) the dura of the floor of the anterior fossa; (9 and 17) the middle meningeal artery; (10 to 12) the dura of the floor of the posterior fossa; (13) the inferior wall of the transverse sinus; (14) the superior wall of the torcular Herophili; (15) the superior wall of the transverse sinus and upper surface of the tentorium cerebelli; and (16) the inferior cerebral veins.

tive. At the lateral and anterior margins of the floor of the fossa, that is, lateral and anterior to the roof of the orbit, the dura became progressively less sensitive to pain and was finally insensitive at points 2 cm or more above the floor (Fig. 3-5).

As an example of the occasional variation from the normal in the presence of a local disease process, the following experience deserves mention. The dura several centimeters above the floor of the anterior fossa was found to be sensitive in the presence of a large meningioma of this region which had a wide attachment to the dura of the floor of this fossa and above. Furthermore, arteries over the convexity and within the substance of the tumor which had doubtless grown in from the anterior meningeal arteries were sensitive to pain. The pain arising from stimulation of these arteries and from the dura about the upper margins of the tumor's attachment was experienced in the region about the eye, just as was noted after stimulation of the normal dura and dural arteries on the floor of the anterior fossa.

It should be emphasized that, not only were the visible portions of the dural arteries of the floor of the anterior fossa sensitive to pain, but the dura that lies between these vessels was itself sensitive to pain. The tests were made when the tissue was dry, so that spread of the stimulation was minimal. A similar arrangement was found to exist in the posterior fossa. But the same was not true for any part of the floor of the middle fossa. Here the dura was insensitive. While all the principal branches of the middle meningeal artery were sensitive to pain, the dura at all points more than 2 mm away from such vessels was insensitive to all the aforementioned forms of stimulation. The floor of the middle fossa (Fig. 3-5) was examined as far medially as the foramen lacerum and the cavernous sinus (4 subjects, 20 observations).

Stimulation of the dural capsule of the components of the fifth cranial nerve resulted in pain usually distributed over the face, and it was impossible to determine whether the nerve itself rather than its capsule was receiving the stimulus. Suffice it to say that whatever served to stimulate the capsule doubtless stimulated the nerve also.

White and Sweet (1955) advised that an accessory pathway for pain from supratentorial structures which may be referred to the ear or to the ipsilateral frontotemporal region is contained in the nervous intermedius of the facial nerve. Kerr (1967) has investigated referral of pain produced by dural irritation or inflammation. He finds that dural pain may be independent of specific dural innervation. Kerr notes that the intraspinal portion of the descending trigeminal tract and nucleus contained in the upper two segments of the cervical cord make up the main relay center for head pain. Sensory fibers from the upper three cervical dorsal roots also pass through this region and may synapse with trigeminal neurons in the spinal nucleus. This intermingling of trigeminal and cervical pathways permits referral of pain from the upper neck to the head and vice versa. After the initial synapse, sensory impulses cross the midline and ascend through the brainstem as the quintothalamic tract to the posteroventromedial nucleus of the thalamus. Some of these trigeminal fibers may also cross the midline and terminate in the opposite dordal horn. These anatomic variations account for the contralateral and bilateral referral of dural pain.

DURA OF THE SELLA TURCICA AND DIAPHRAGMA SELLAE

There was opportunity to make observations on the dura and diaphragma of the sella only when tumors existed in the region, and in these instances the dura was more or less attenuated from distortion and compression by the tumor. Faradic stimulation of the thinned-out diaphragma in a case of pituitary adenoma failed to cause pain. Pressure on this structure and also tearing it by spreading its fibers with a clamp produced pain experienced just behind the eye, yet crushing the torn edge did not cause pain. It appeared that the pain induced by pressure and tearing was the result of distortion of the pain-sensitive carotid artery nearby (3 subjects, 20 observations).

The only opportunity for studying the dura lining the sella occurred upon introduction of a suction tube into the depths of the sella or traction with forceps on the deep fragments of a pituitary adenoma. Both of these methods of stimulation in one subject produced pain near the top of the head. Furthermore, when the stimulus was applied to the left side of the sella the pain was felt to the left of the midline at the vertex; the opposite was true for the other side. In this case it was known that the roof of the sphenoid sinus had collapsed, and it is possible that the membranous lining of the sinus was being stimulated and was the cause of the pain at the vertex.

DURA OF THE POSTERIOR FOSSA

The dura over the convexity of the cerebellar hemispheres was everywhere insensitive to pain except along the margins of the occipital and transverse sinuses (6 subjects, 150 observations). The floor of the posterior fossa, on the other hand, was uniformly sensitive in a fashion comparable to that of the anterior fossa. Roughly, the floor of the posterior fossa was taken to be that more or less triangular region that lies between the rim of the foramen magnum and the lateral attachment of the ten-

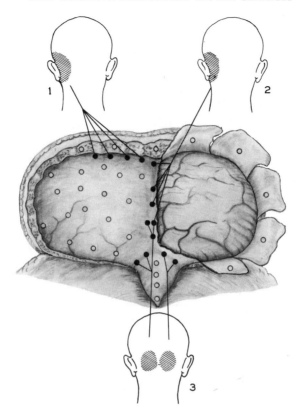

FIG. 3-6. The venous sinuses and the dura over the cerebellum and the upper part of the cord; ○ indicates the point of stimulation without pain; ● indicates the point of stimulation causing pain. The diagrams show the area of pain following stimulation of (1) the transverse sinus; (2) the torcular Herophili and upper part of the occipital sinus; and (3) the lower part of the occipital sinus.

torium cerebelli. Observations with closely spaced stimulation of the dura of this region revealed that, while the entire area was sensitive to pain, from some points the pain was felt just behind the homolateral ear, and from other points it was felt in the back of the head (Fig. 3-6).

That portion of the dura that lay over or was near the margins of the lateral (sigmoid) sinus when stimulated caused pain behind the ear (2 subjects, 8 observations). Section of the ninth and tenth cranial nerves in one of the patients made it impossible to elicit pain on subsequent stimulation of these dural and sinal structures. Stimulation of the remaining and more mesial portion of the dura, extending to the rim of the

foramen magnum, caused pain low in the back of the head (2 subjects, 14 observations). This region of the dura was sometimes seen to be traversed by small branches of the posterior meningeal arteries, and the localization of the pain following stimulation was the same for both the dura and the arteries (2 subjects, 8 observations). Section of the posterior roots of the first three cervical nerves in one of the patients made it impossible to elicit pain on subsequent stimulation of the abovementioned dural and arterial structures.* There was no

*F. L. McNaughton (1938) who made morphologic studies of the posterior fossa and upper cervical region, was never able actually to visualize the en-

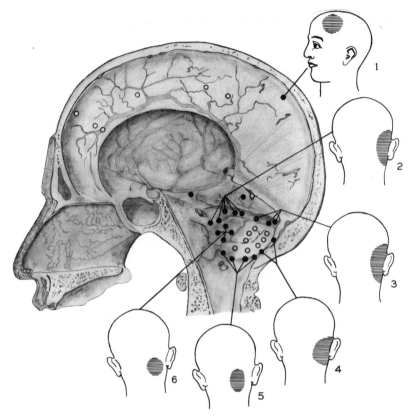

FIG. 3-7. The falx cerebri, the dura, and venous sinuses of the posterior fossa; ○ indicates the point of stimulation without pain; ● indicates the point of stimulation causing pain. The diagrams show the area of pain following stimulation of (1) the superior sagittal sinus; (2) the sigmoid sinus; (3) the transverse sinus; (4) the upper part of the occipital sinus; (5) the lower part of the ccipital sinus; and (6) the dura of the floor of the posterior fossa.

occasion to visualize or stimulate the dura that lies beneath the brainstem and covers the clivus blumenbachii (Figs. 3-5, 3-7, 3-8).

FALX

It was found that burns, cuts, faradic stimulation, and pressure along the anteroposterior

extent of the falx failed to produce pain unless the margins of the superior sagittal sinus were displaced or encroached on (5 subjects, 35 observations). An exception to this general finding on the sensitivity of the falx was the observation that faradic stimulation of the first few centimeters above its attachment to the crista galli caused pain in and about the homolateral eye (2 subjects, 6 observations). There was opportunity to explore the inferior margin of the falx only along the anterior half of its border with the inferior sagittal sinus; this much of it was found to be insensitive. Lateral pressure against the falx with a blunt ventricular needle was exerted to a degree sufficient almost to puncture this tough structure, without causing

trance of branches from cervical roots into the posterior fossa; he did, however, frequently see such cervical root branches traverse the uppermost cervical region of the dura and its arteries, and tissue contiguous to the foramen magnum and adjacent structures (personal communication; see also Penfield and McNaughton (1940).

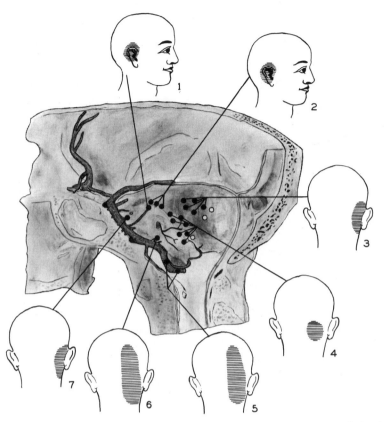

FIG. 3-8. The arteries and dura of the posterior fossa; ○ indicates the point of stimulation without pain; ● indicates the point of stimulation causing pain. The diagrams show the area of pain following stimulation of (1) the internal auditory artery; (2) the dura at the porus acusticus; (3) the wall of the sigmoid sinus and the adjacent dura; (4) the dura near the rim of the foramen magnum; (5) the vertebral artery; (6) the posterior inferior cerebellar artery; and (7) a pontile artery.

pain. Sometimes the point of pressure was within 2 cm of the superior sagittal sinus, yet pain did not result (Figs. 3-7 and 3-9).

TENTORIUM CEREBELLI

On the superior surface of the tentorium it was found that pressure against its central portion caused pain in the homolateral side of the forehead and the region of the homolateral eye. Faradic stimulation of this surface in spotty areas of apparently fortuitous distribution (Fig. 3-5) caused pain in the same region (4 subjects, 20 observations).

On the inferior surface of the tentorium the findings at first appeared variable but eventually permitted inferences to be drawn. Slight or even moderate pressure upward usually failed to cause pain unless the margins of the venous sinuses were approached, in which case pain was usually experienced behind the homolateral ear. When pressure on the center of the tentorium was increased, pain occurred behind the ear in the region of the forehead and eye on that side or in both regions. Strong pressure applied at a point near the free edge at the side of the pons in one case caused pain low in the back of the head on the same side, apparently because of secondary displacement of some other pain-sensitive structure. Faradic

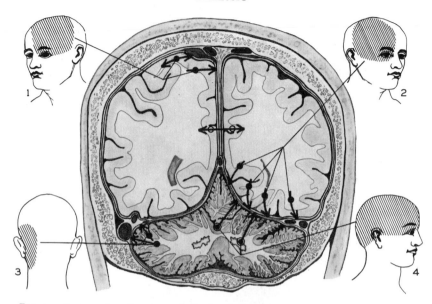

Fɪɢ. 3-9. A coronal section through the head, showing the falx cerebri, the tentorium cerebelli, and the associated venous sinuses; ∅ indicates the point of stimulation of the falx cerebri without pain; ✦ indicates the point of stimulation causing pain; ⊙ indicates the point at which stimulation of greater intensity than usual is required to produce pain. The diagrams show the area of pain following stimulation of (1) the superior sagittal sinus and tributary veins; (2) the superior surface of the tentorium cerebelli and wall of the transverse sinus; (3) the inferior wall of the transverse sinus; and (4) the inferior surface of the tentorium cerebelli, resulting in secondary effects on (2) and (3).

stimulation of sufficient intensity to induce pain in the structures with well-established sensitivity to pain (Figs. 3-9 and 3-10) failed to cause pain when applied to points on the undersurface of the tentorium more than 5 mm from the venous sinuses. It was found further, however, that if the intensity of the stimulus was increased sufficiently, pain was experienced in the forehead and in the region of the eye on that side, suggesting that the stimulus was transmitted through the tentorium to its superior surface (5 subjects, 35 observations).

DURAL SINUSES AND THEIR TRIBUTARY VEINS
Superior Sagittal Sinus

The walls of the major extent of this sinus were found to be sensitive to pain, although in general the pain produced was only moderately intense as compared with that resulting from stimulation of the middle meningeal artery or of the large arteries at the base of the brain.

Pressure, traction, and faradic stimulation were used. In addition, it was discovered that stripping the dural wall away from its attachments to the cranial vault produced slight pain. In its more anterior portion, that is, along its first 7 or 8 cm, the sinus was either insensitive or much less sensitive than in its middle and posterior thirds. Pain in the frontal part of the head and in the region of the eye usually followed stimulation of the sensitive regions. Sometimes the pain arising from the more anterior half of the sinus was localized in the parietal region, near the vertex. It was also noted, although it was impossible to define the area accurately, that the middle third of the sinus lost some of its sensitivity after an incision through the dura that traversed the main trunk of the midmeningeal artery and the nerves traveling along with the artery. The side of the head on which pain was felt (Figs. 3-4 and 3-11) was always the same as the side on which the wall of the sinus was stimulated (8 subjects, 32 observations).

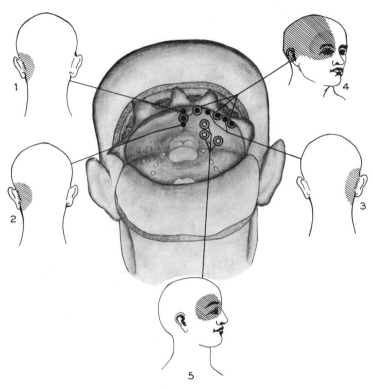

FIG. 3-10. Undersurface of the tentorium cerebelli; ● indicates the point at which stimuli of usual intensity cause pain; the diagrams show the area of pain following stimulation of (1) the torcular Herophili; (2) the straight sinus; and (3) the transverse sinus. ◎ indicates the point at which stimuli of usual intensity cause no pain whereas stimuli of increased intensity cause frontal pain; (4) shows the area of pain following stimulation of the transverse and straight sinuses; (5) shows the area of pain following stimulation of the undersurface of the tentorium cerebelli. ◉ indicates the point at which stimuli of usual intensity cause pain behind the homolateral ear whereas stimuli of increased intensity cause pain over the entire homolateral side of the head.

Tributary Veins to the Superior Sagittal Sinus (Superior Cerebral Veins)

These veins, which pass from the cerebral cortex to the sinus, were found to be insensitive to coagulation, crushing, and faradic stimulation except for the few millimeters of vessel next to the sinus. However, traction on the vessels at all points along the extent of the sinus produced pain in the same sites as that caused by direct stimulation of the adjacent wall of the sinus (8 subjects, 32 observations). There was variability in the occurrence and degree of the pain resulting from traction on these veins; but sometimes, and particularly along the posterior third of the sagittal sinus, very slight traction caused moderately intense pain. With the sudden collapse of a dilated lateral ventricle, all the veins passing from the cortex to the sagittal sinus were observed to be put on stretch, and at the same time there was pain in the homolateral frontoparietal and ocular regions (Figs. 3-4, 3-9, and 3-11). Penfield and McNaughton (1940) were able to show that the dural nerves derived from the trigeminal nerve formed the major contribution to innervation of dural structures. They also demonstrated that the nerve supply of the anterior

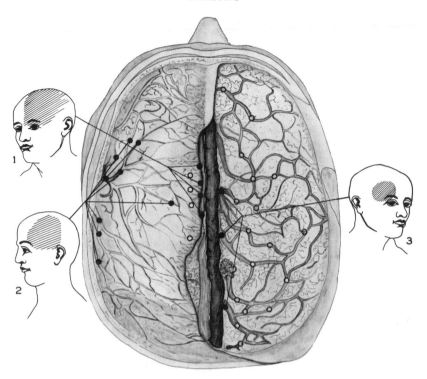

FIG. 3-11. The calvarium removed. The dura and the meningeal arteries are shown on the left; the cerebral and tributary veins are shown on the right. ○ indicates the point of stimulation without pain; ● indicates the point of stimulation causing pain. The diagrams show the area of pain following stimulation of (1) the margin of the superior sagittal sinus; (2) the middle meningeal artery; and (3) the tributary veins to the superior sagittal sinus.

fossa is meager. A few small branches run toward the cribriform plate and upward in the anterior leaf of the falx. Several more branches of variable size and number can be traced along the sphenoid wing. All these branches originate in the ophthalmic division of the trigeminal nerve. More numerous bundles take a course across the floor of the middle fossa to continue as a perivascular plexus about the middle meningeal artery. These nerves remain closely related to the artery and its branches. The most widespread of the trigeminal supply to intracranial structures is provided by the rich plexus of tentorial nerves that course back along the tentorium and sweep forward and upward in the dura of the falx.

McNaughton (1938) studied carefully the tentorial nerves and their relevance to intra-cranial pain in man. He pointed out that the tentorial nerves contain many myelinated fibers of medium size. He suggested that they have functions in addition to subserving pain sensibility as yet unknown. The tentorial nerves, in contrast with the middle meningeal nerves, supply venous rather than arterial structures. Subjects experience pain when cerebral veins entering the longitudinal and transverse sinus are stimulated. These venous structures are subserved by branches of the tentorial nerves coming from the first division of the trigeminal nerve. Included are the nerves in the tentorium, torcular, falx cerebri, occipital dura, and the venous sinuses enclosed by these dural septa. Some nerve bundles derived from the tentorial nerves have been traced directly onto the cerebral veins draining into the transverse and longitudinal sinus. Many other nerve branches are distributed to the venous sinuses themselves and can be traced as far forward as the anterior third of the superior longitudinal sinus. Nerve bundles along the inferior sagittal sinus have been identified as coming from tentorial nerve branches. On the other hand, branches from the dural nerves of the posterior fossa extend upward to supply the transverse sinus and the occipital dura. Local anesthetic solutions injected into the dura of the falx and torcular regions abolish the pain that results from stimulation of the lateral and superior longitudinal sinuses. Pain induced by traction of the venous structures of the middle fossa and by traction of the middle cerebral arterial vessels can be eliminated by injection of procaine into the trigeminal ganglia, the first division of the trigeminal nerve being mainly implicated. Noxious stimulation of the tentorial nerves inside the head results in pain experienced in the eye or forehead, regions supplied by the main cutaneous branches of the ophthalmic division of the trigeminal nerve.

As an accompaniment of severe dysentery or colitis, venous thrombosis in various parts of the body may occur. Cerebral venous thromboses, notably of the longitudinal sinus and its tributary veins, under such circumstances occur more commonly in infants than in children or adults. However, such thromboses do occur in both during exacerbations of ulcerative colitis. The initial complaint may be a palsy of both legs, followed by weakness in the arms and aphasia. Headache is usually in the front of the head during the first few hours, but may become generalized and severe. Confusion and delirium are conspicuous features.

Pacchionian Granulations and Venous Lacunae

Pacchionian granulations were stimulated with faradic current without producing pain (3 subjects, 12 observations). It seemed likely that all such arachnoid extensions were insensitive. The walls of the venous lacunae at various points along the lateral margins of the sagittal sinus (Fig. 3-4) also were insensitive to burning,

pressure, and faradic stimulation (3 subjects, 12 observations).

Inferior Sagittal Sinus

The inferior sagittal sinus was stimulated only along its anterior 5 to 6 cm., and in this region the channel is of smaller caliber and has few or no tributaries from the cerebrum (see Fig. 3-7). When this anterior portion of the sinus was crushed or stimulated with faradic current it was found to be insensitive (4 subjects, 12 observations).

Transverse Sinus, Torcular Herophili, and Straight Sinus (Supratentorial Surfaces)

Stimulation of the walls of the transverse sinuses and torcular Herophili on their supratentorial surfaces by faradic current uniformly caused pain in the region of the homolateral side of the forehead and the homolateral eye (4 subjects, 16 observations). The stimulation that resulted from pressure and gentle friction in the same region was insufficient to cause pain. Only a short segment of the straight sinus near the torcular was available for study (3 subjects, 6 observations). Pain resulting from stimulation was felt in the homolateral side of the forehead and the homolateral eye. It was not possible to stimulate that part near the free edge of the tentorium, nor were the veins of Galen investigated (Figs. 3-5 and 3-9).

Inferior Cerebral Veins

The veins on the inferior surface of the temporal lobe were not sensitive to pain. But the main veins that pass from the undersurface of the temporal lobe to the lateral end of the transverse sinus and to the superior petrosal sinus were invariably found to be sensitive to crushing, burning, stretching, and faradic stimulation. These veins, several in number and sometimes referred to as the veins of Labbé, were as long as 1.5 to 3 cm in their

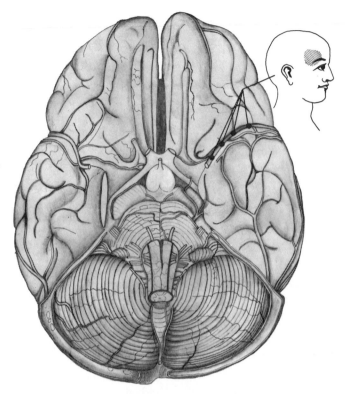

FIG. 3-12. Veins at the base of the brain; ● indicates the point of stimulation causing pain. The diagram shows the area of pain following stimulation of the deep segment of the sylvian vein.

extracerebral course (Figs. 3-5 and 3-12). When they were stimulated, the pain was experienced in the homolateral temporal region (3 subjects, 10 observations).

Occipital Sinus

That portion of the sinus that lies in the midline and extends from the torcular to the rim of the foramen magnum was uniformly sensitive to faradic stimulation, and the pain was experienced in one or both of two regions of the head (Figs. 3-6 and 3-7). Stimulation of the sinus near the torcular caused pain behind the ear, while stimulation near the foramen magnum caused pain low in the back of the head. After section of the posterior roots of the first three cervical nerves it was impossible to elicit pain on stimulation of the sinus near the

foramen magnum. Just as was the case with the other midline sinuses, the superior sagittal and the straight, the side of the head on which pain was felt was homolateral to the side on which the wall of the sinus was stimulated. The divisions of this sinus which partly encircle the foramen magnum were also sensitive, and the pain was felt low in the back of the head (4 subjects, 20 observations).

Transverse Sinus, Torcular Herophili, and Straight Sinus (Infratentorial Surfaces)

Stimulation of the walls of these sinuses on their infratentorial surfaces by faradic current uniformly caused pain in an area behind the homolateral ear (6 subjects, 24 observations). (Faradic stimulation of the petrosal vein caused pain behind the homolateral ear.) In addition,

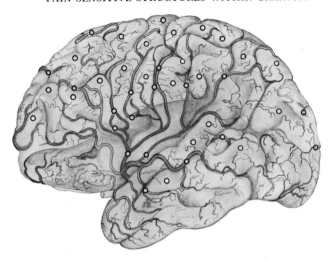

FIG. 3-13. Arteries over the cerebral cortex; ○ indicates the point of stimulation without pain.

it was found that if a current of greater intensity was employed, pain was also felt in the homolateral side of the forehead and near the homolateral eye. The tributary veins from the cerebellum to these sinuses were found to lack sensitivity to pain when stimulated with faradic current, crushed, or put on slight traction (Figs. 3-6, 3-7, and 3-10).

The wall of the lateral portion of the transverse sinus (sigmoid sinus) was stimulated from the inside of the posterior fossa (Figs. 3-5, 3-7, and 3-8). The margins of the sinus here are indistinct, but faradic stimulation of the dura overlying the sinus, from the margin of the tentorium to the jugular foramen, uniformly caused pain behind the homolateral ear (see the section on the dura of the posterior fossa).

The wall of the cavernous sinus in one subject was stimulated at the point where the midcerebral vein joined it. Faradic stimulation here caused pain in the homolateral ocular and maxillary region. Since the ophthalmic and maxillary nerves lie in the lateral wall of the sinus, it is probable that they were being stimulated directly.

There was no opportunity to stimulate directly the more inaccessible venous channels, which include the petrosal sinuses and the basilar plexus.

PIA-ARACHNOID

The pia-arachnoid covering the convexity of the cerebral and cerebellar hemispheres was found to be insensitive to crushing, burning, stretching, and faradic stimulation, with the possible exception of the pia-arachnoid very near to the great arteries at the base of the brain (30 subjects, 120 observations). It was found that tearing the pia-arachnoid surrounding the carotid arteries and the anterior part of the circle of Willis caused subjects to complain of pain, but this might well have been the result of secondary pull on these sensitive arteries (Figs. 3-13 and 3-14A). It is likely, however, that the pia-arachnoid is itself pain sensitive in the regions adjacent to the basal arteries, and that these pain-sensitive pial structures above the tentorium when stimulated cause pain to be experienced in the front of the head. Thus, Von Storch et al. (1940) found that the introduction of air into the cisterna magna produced a severe generalized bilateral headache, into the cisterna interpeduncularis a dull bifrontal headache, into the cisterna ambiens (body and horns) a dull bifrontal headache, and into the prechiasmatic and postchiasmatic cistern and the left horn of the cisterna ambiens a dull bifrontal headache.

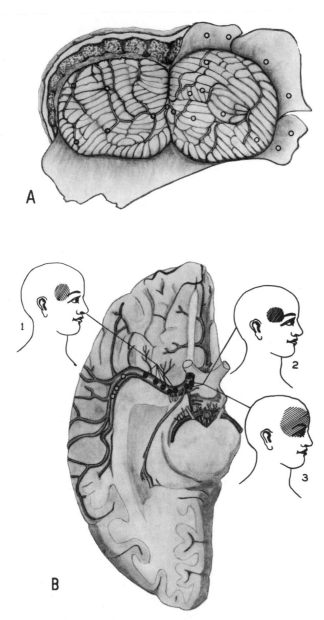

FIG. 3-14. A, arteries and veins over the cerebellar cortex. ○ indicates the point of stimulation without pain. B, intracranial portion of the internal carotid artery and the proximal part of the middle cerebral artery. ○ indicates the point of stimulation without pain. ● indicates the point of stimulation causing pain. The diagrams show the area of pain following stimulation of: (1) the middle cerebral artery and (2) and (3) the intracranial portion of the internal carotid artery.

The arachnoid forming the roof of the cisterna magna was found to lack sensitivity to pain (4 subjects, 12 observations).

ARTERIES AND VEINS OF THE BRAIN

The pial arteries and veins over the superior and lateral convexities of the cerebrum (24 subjects, 300 observations) and the cerebellum (16 subjects, 150 observations) were found to lack sensitivity to pain with all forms of stimulation (Figs. 3-13 and 3-14A).

However, as will be described, when pain resulted from stimulation of certain cerebral and pial arteries at the base, it was deep, intense, dull, and aching. It was diffuse, yet grossly localizable, and it became throbbing when the stimulus was repeated. The pain, when prolonged, was associated with a feeling of nausea. When different pain-sensitive arteries were stimulated, the quality and intensity of pain that ensued were approximately of the same order, but the sites varied.

The intracranial segment of the internal carotid artery was consistently sensitive to stretching, stroking, and faradic stimulation (three subjects, ten observations). The pain was felt behind the eye and low in the temporal region on the same side (Fig. 3-14B).

The middle cerebral artery was found to be similarly sensitive along its proximal 1 to 2 cm (3 subjects, 10 observations). The pain was gion, where the artery lies hidden in the lateral cerebral fissure and where it courses over the parietal lobe, it was not sensitive (20 subjects, 60 observations). Pain arising from the proximal segment had the same distribution in and behind the eye as did that from the internal carotid artery.

The anterior cerebral artery was found to be sensitive to crushing, stretching, burning, and faradic stimulation from its point of origin to a point 1 cm beyond the genu of the corpus callosum, a segment several centimeters in length (3 subjects, 12 observations). Beyond this point the artery was insensitive. The pain arising from the proximal segment was experienced in a rather poorly localized area behind and above the homolateral eye (Fig. 3-15A).

One of the principal pontile arteries at a point about 1.5 cm from its origin (Figs. 3-8 and 3-15B) was found to be sensitive to pain on crushing, traction, coagulation, and faradization, and the resulting pain was experienced behind the homolateral ear (1 subject, 4 observations).

The internal auditory artery, which accompanies the seventh and eighth cranial nerves (Figs. 3-8 and 3-15B), was sensitive to stretching and faradic stimulation, and the pain was experienced in and just behind the homolateral ear (2 subjects, 8 observations).

The posterior-inferior cerebellar artery was sensitive to faradic stimulation and stretching in the proximal 1 to 2 cm of its course (2 subjects, 8 observations); beyond this it was insensitive (6 subjects, 20 observations).

The pain arising from the proximal segment was felt in a rather diffuse area in the homolateral occipital and suboccipital regions (Figs. 3-8 and 3-15B).

The vertebral artery, when stimulated by crushing, traction, and faradic current, was sensitive to pain. The pain was slightly more intense but had the same distribution as that following stimulation of the posterior-inferior cerebellar artery (Figs. 3-8 and 3-15B), that is, in the homolateral side of the occiput and subocciput (1 subject, 5 observations).

Traction on numerous arteries at the base of the brain occurred when there was displacement of the brainstem by retraction during the removal of angle tumors. The pain associated with this maneuver was widespread, but for the most part was experienced on the side of the head where vessels were being stretched. The pain associated with traction on the circle of Willis and its branches after distention of the third ventricle will be discussed later (see section on the third ventricle).

The middle cerebral vein, or sylvian vein, which runs in the lateral cerebral fissure to the cavernous sinus, was found on faradic stimulation to be uniformly sensitive to pain in the 3 to 4 cm nearest the sinus but inconstantly sensitive higher. In one subject the vein was sensitive to pain well up on the lateral aspect of the brain. Retraction of the temporal lobe for the purpose of exposing the segment of the vein near the cavernous sinus did not put the vein

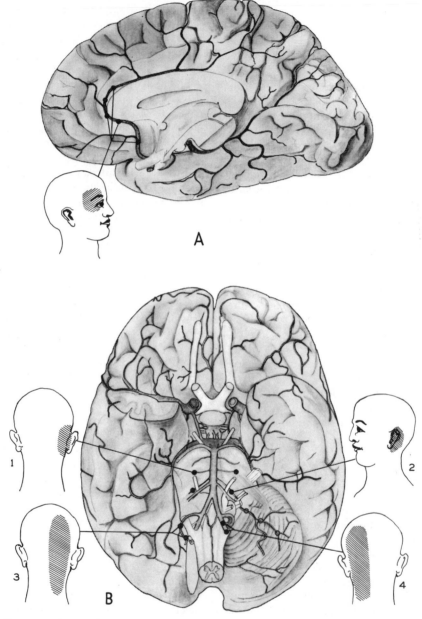

FIG. 3-15. A, anterior cerebral artery. The diagram shows the area of pain following stimulation of the proximal segment of the artery. B, arteries at the base of the brain. The diagrams show the area of pain following stimulation of: (1) a pontile artery; (2) the internal auditory artery; (3) the proximal portion of the posterior-inferior cerebellar artery; and (4) the vertebral artery. ○ indicates the point of stimulation without pain. ● indicates the point of stimulation causing pain.

on obvious traction, since it was rather closely adherent to the frontal lobe; the effect of traction on the vein was therefore not ascertained. The pain following stimulation of all sensitive points (Fig. 3-12) was felt in the anterior temporal region and in the outer angle of the brow on the same side (4 subjects, 20 observations).

Dahl (1975) studied the morphological differences in extracerebral and intracerebral arteries by light microscopy, transmission electron, and scanning electron microscopy. He found that all of the extracerebral vessels examined had a similar structure consisting of the three usual coaxial coats; the tunica intima, tunica media, and tunica adventitia. The vascular endothelium forms a continuous layer with no fenestration. The internal elastic lamina appears to be made up of a homogeneous matrix in which elastic tissue is deposited. In the basilar artery the media is constructed of 10 to 12 layers of smooth muscle cells. As the vessels diminish in size, the muscular coat is reduced until finally, in the small pial arteries, only a single layer of muscle cells is observed. At regular intervals, membranous contacts between the endothelial cells and the smooth muscle cells are seen. A typical feature of the extracerebral arteries is the outer border of the vessel wall which has a sharply defined boundary, made up of thin cellular processes. Where the vessels enter the cerebral cortex, a membranous junction between this outer lining of the vessel wall and the cytoplasmic processes of the pia occurs. The outer layer of the intracerebral arteries is thin and differs to some extent from the adventitial cost of the extracerebral vessels. Most importantly, while the extracerebral arteries are provided with an abundant nerve supply including periadventitial, segmental, and adventitial nerves, the intracerebral vessels are devoid of enervation. This makes it reasonable to suggest that while the extracerebral vessels may be subjected to both a nervous or segmental and chemical control, the tone of the intracerebral vessels is regulated by chemical mechanisms only.

The entire parenchyma of the cerebrum and cerebellum, including the vessels found in it, was insensitive to pain under all forms of stimu-

lation (30 subjects). The olfactory, optic, and auditory nerves were not sensitive to pain.

The cranial ninth and tenth nerves were each found, when stimulated, to cause pain behind the homolateral ear and in the throat. Stimulation of the eleventh cranial nerve caused pain low in the back of the head and in the upper cervical region on the same side. Stimulation of an inconstantly present posterior root of the first cervical nerve caused pain near the vertex of the head, while stimulation of the second and third posterior roots caused pain at the vertex and back of the head and neck.

VENTRICLES, AQUEDUCT OF SYLVIUS, AND CHOROID PLEXUSES
Lateral Ventricles

Although sudden collapse and overdistention of the lateral ventricles produced pain, direct stimulation of various parts of the ventricular walls (with their vessels as well as the choroid plexuses) did not result in pain. Specifically, it was found that coagulation, compression, and faradic stimulation of the ependymal lining of the entire lateral ventricle produced no pain. The large terminal vein that passes along the floor of the body of the lateral ventricle was insensitive to crushing, coagulation, and faradic stimulation. The same was true for the choroid plexus at the glomus and in the region of the foramen of Monro. Spreading the lumen of the foramen of Monro and cutting its margins with the endothermy were painless. Firm pressure against the part of the ventricular wall nearest the thalamus was not followed by pain (4 subjects, 24 observations).

That a bilateral and diffuse type of headache resulted from rapid emptying or overdistention of the ventricular system was repeatedly demonstrated during ventriculographic studies. In the case of a tumor filling the third ventricle, the changes in pressure of the lateral ventricles alone produced the same type of pain.

A balloon placed through a small opening into the anterior horn and body of a lateral ventricle when inflated sufficiently to cause overdistention of the ventricle produced a diffuse frontal pain on the homolateral side of the head. This was done with the brain exposed, so that there was no possibility of stretching or compressing the dural arteries. Sudden deflation of the balloon produced a transitory and intense but poorly localized pain, again over the frontal area of the same side (Figs. 3-16 and 3-17).

Third Ventricle

Manipulation of a paraphysial cyst lying in the third ventricle and traction and coagulation of its stalk in the region of the roof of the ventricle were all painless. The choroid plexus of this ventricle was also not sensitive to coagulation.

In a case of hydrocephalus due to obstruction of the aqueduct of Sylvius, an opening made into the third ventricle through the lamina terminalis was unaccompanied by pain. Cutting, crushing, and coagulation of the ependyma of the ventricular wall here were painless. A balloon introduced into the third ventricle through this opening was inflated under moderate pressure and caused a diffuse pain over all parts of the head, variously said to be most intense in the back of the head, in the forehead and eyes, and in the ears. Release of the pressure was accompanied by prompt cessation of the pain. In this respect it was unlike the pain that came with both distention and deflation of the balloon in the lateral ventricle. Pressure from the inside on the floor of the third ventricle, behind the chiasma, produced pain of similar distribution and nature to that following distention of the ventricle, yet cutting and stretching of the floor alone in this region produced no pain. The conclusion was that the pain accompanying distention of the ventricle was due to traction by displacement of the large arteries in the region of the circle of Willis (Fig. 3-18).

Aqueduct of Sylvius

The ependymal walls of the aqueduct were found to be insensitive when a snugly fitting catheter was used to stimulate them by pres-

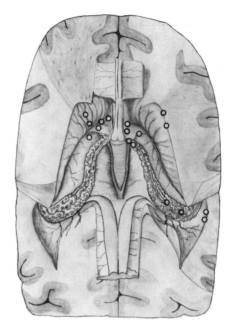

FIG. 3-16. The lateral ventricles, the terminal veins, the choroid plexuses, and the foramens of Monro. ○ indicates the point of stimulation without pain.

sure, stretching, and traction. All parts of the walls of the aqueduct from the fourth to the third ventricle (Fig. 3-19) were thus explored (1 subject, 4 observations).

Fourth Ventricle

The ependymal walls of this ventricle lack sensitivity to pain just as do those of the other ventricles. It was found that cutting, coagulating, and faradizing the roof of the ventricle caused no pain. Manipulation, traction, and stroking of the floor of the ventricle likewise were painless (4 subjects, 16 observations). The choroid plexuses of this ventricle (Fig. 3-19) were insensitive to coagulation, crushing, traction, and faradic stimulation (4 subjects, 16 observations).

Comment: This study does not purport to determine whether structures found to be sensitive to pain on stimulation actually possess sensory endings or are only traversed by pain-conducting fibers. This differentiation is dif-

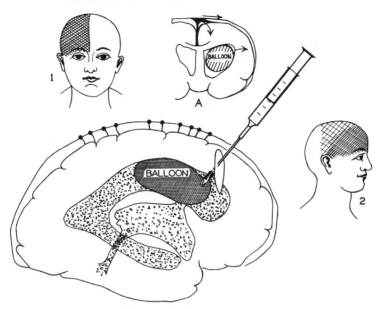

FIG. 3-17. Schematic representation of a balloon in the lateral ventricle and the tributary veins passing from the cerebral cortex to the superior sagittal sinus. ● indicates the point at which the tributary veins were put on traction, causing pain with both inflation and deflation of the balloon. The insert (a) demonstrates the outward traction on the tributary veins, with inflation of the balloon, and the downward traction, with deflation. The diagrams (1) and (2) show the area of pain resulting from both distention and collapse of the body and frontal horn of one lateral ventricle.

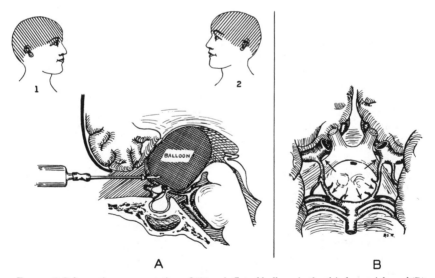

FIG. 3-18. Schematic representation of (A) an inflated balloon in the third ventricle and (B) the resulting traction on pain-sensitive arteries of the circle of Willis. The arrows indicate the lines of force, with distention of the ventricular floor. Diagrams (1) and (2) show the diffuse area of pain following inflation of the balloon.

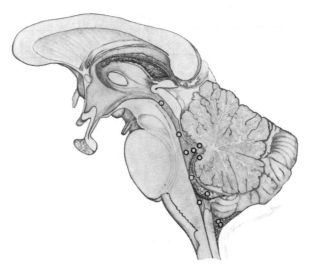

FIG. 3-19. The aqueduct of Sylvius, the fourth ventricle, the choroid plexus, and the cisterna magna. O indicates the point of stimulation without pain.

ficult at best even with histologic methods, and conclusions must be deferred. Thus McNaughton (1938) who failed to find nerve endings in the walls of venous sinuses in man, indicated that the question of their presence "may well be a problem of adequate staining methods." Also, it is conceivable that the methods of stimulation employed may not have been adequate in every instance to stimulate sensory endings for pain. In this respect a specific instance, particularly important to consider, is that of the pial arteries over the convexity of the hemispheres, which were found to be insensitive. It may be that the stimulus used was inadequate at one point or was not widespread enough to stimulate sparsely distributed end-organs.

"Pain Pathways" of the Head

The sensory innervation of the extracranial structures will not be considered here. A discussion of the innervation of pain-sensitive intracranial structures readily falls into a consideration of (1) the structures supplied by the fifth cranial nerve and (2) those supplied by other nerves. The fifth and the tenth cranial nerves are widely conceded to be the principal afferent nerves of the intracranial structures,

but, in addition, the ninth, eleventh, and twelfth cranial and the upper cervical nerves play a role, as, perhaps, do other cranial nerves as well.

1. The sensory fibers of the fifth nerve supply the superior surface of the tentorium cerebelli and all the pain-sensitive structures that lie above it. The subtentorial structures probably receive few, if any, fibers from the fifth nerve.

Many fibers of the fifth nerve accompany the middle meningeal artery and its branches. The "nervus spinosus" described by von Luschka (1850) as a branch of the third division and the "nervus meningeus medius" described by Arnold (1851) as a branch principally of the second division of the trigeminal nerve are fairly constant. But McNaughton (1938) has indicated that there are also fine unnamed branches of all divisions of the fifth nerve accompanying the artery. It is hardly possible or even necessary to attempt to allocate all these fine connections to one of the three divisions; suffice it to say that they are all components of the fifth nerve.

The nerve fibers follow the main divisions of the middle meningeal artery and form a network in the adventitia. Branches of the nerves have been seen to extend out into the dura, away from the artery. The failure to find the dura itself sensitive to pain suggests that either the nerve fibers and endings are sparsely distributed or that such nerves as the dura possesses include no pain-conducting fibers. The nerves diminish in number as the vessels divide, but occasionally arteries of small caliber near the sagittal sinus have been found sensitive to pain. It is likely that some of the fibers extend even to the sagittal sinus and form a part of its sensory supply, particularly in its middle third.

There is less certainty about the nerves to the anterior meningeal arteries and the dura of the anterior fossa, but it is probable that the anterior meningeal branch of the internal carotid artery is accompanied by fibers that connect directly with the first division of the fifth nerve, near the gasserian ganglion. It is also probable that the meningeal branches of the ethmoidal arteries are accompanied by nerves that pass through the cribriform plate as branches of the intraorbital portion of the ophthalmic nerve (McNaughton, 1938). Whereas the sensory tests indicate that the pain-conducting fibers accompanying the middle meningeal artery do not supply any part of the dura traversed by that artery, the facts that the dura of the floor of the anterior fossa is uniformly sensitive to pain and that the quality and site of reference of pain are identical, suggest that it and its arteries have a common nerve supply.

The nervus tentorii, a branch of the first division of the trigeminal nerve, was first described by Arnold in 1851, and its existence has been repeatedly verified since. This nerve is made up of afferent fibers from at least the posterior extent of the superior sagittal sinus, passing by way of the falx to join afferent fibers from the superior surface of the tentorium cerebelli, the superior walls of the transverse and the straight sinuses, and the torcular Herophili. The collected fibers pass anteriorly from the margin of the tentorium, in or close to the sheath of the trochlear nerve (McNaughton, 1938), to join the first division of the fifth nerve about 1 cm from its ganglion. The nervus tentorii, therefore, carries painful impulses from the general region of the posterior and medial aspects of the supratentorial fossa.

The same nerve (nervus tentorii) in all probability supplies the pain-sensitive venous tributaries from the parietal and occipital lobes to the venous sinuses, but by virtue of the different location of the pain following stimulation of the group of inferior cerebral veins that drain the temporal lobe, it is suggested that these latter tributary veins have another innervation, perhaps from fibers that accompany the posterior branch of the middle meningeal artery.

The arteries of the brain, including the parenchymal branches and also the choroid plexuses, have been shown to be equipped with nerve fibers and endings (Chorobski and Penfield, 1932; Clark, S. L., 1934; Gulland, 1898; Penfield, 1932; Stohr, 1922, 1932). Even though Huber's (1899) original conception of the myelinated fibers as sensory and the unmyelinated as vasomotor must now be modified, it is conceivable that many of these are pain-conducting fibers. Under the conditions of these investigations, however, stimulation of the large arteries at the base of the brain and only the most proximal portions of their cerebral branches caused pain. The nerve plexuses about these larger arteries are said to have connections with various cranial nerves (Arnold, 1851) (the third, the fifth, the sixth, the seventh, the eighth, the ninth, the tenth, the eleventh, and the twelfth). It seems unlikely that all of these cranial nerves serve as pathways from the pain-sensitive vessels, but at present definite information about these afferent pathways for pain is limited.

Studies on experimentally induced "histamine headache" indicate that the fifth cranial nerve is undoubtedly the chief afferent nerve for headache arising from dilatation of the pial and cerebral arteries of the supra-tentorial fossae. It is also clear that stimulation of the intracranial portion of the internal carotid artery, the proximal 1 or 2 cm of the midcerebral and postcerebral arteries, and the anterior cerebral artery as far up as the genu of the corpus callosum results in pain in the region of the homolateral eye. Since the pain resulting from stimulation of these larger arteries of the forebrain is experienced in the region of the eye, there is further reason to assume that at least the major part of the innervation of these vessels is by the fifth cranial nerve.

2. The arrangement of nerves beneath the tentorium is more complicated, but a few inferences regarding pathways for pain seem justifiable. The ninth, tenth, and eleventh cranial nerves were shown to be sensitive to pain on direct stimulation intracranially, and the pain was felt in the general region of the back of the head and subocciput; the twelfth cranial nerve is said to be similar in this regard. The studies with experimentally induced "histamine headache" indicate that the ninth and tenth cranial and upper cervical nerves are the chief afferents for headache resulting from dilatation of pial and cerebral arteries of the infratentorial fossa. Further differentiation of the specific innervation of the structures is afforded by the observation that the area of pain following stimulation of the undersurfaces of the transverse sinus, the torcular Herophili, the straight sinus, the upper end of the occipital sinus, and the dura in the region of the sigmoid sinus is largely in and behind the homolateral ear and in the same area after direct stimulation of the ninth and tenth nerves. Since in this region pain could not be elicited on stimulation of the aforementioned structures after section of the ninth and tenth cranial nerves, the deduction that these two cranial nerves include afferent fibers for pain from these structures is further supported.

Similarly, it is inferred that the upper cervical nerves possess fibers for pain from the lower part of the occipital sinus, the vertebral and posterior inferior cerebellar arteries, the posterior meningeal artery, and the dura of the floor of the posterior fossa near the rim of the foramen magnum, since stimulation of the structures after section of the upper cervical nerves did not elicit pain.*

Finally, it is to be emphasized that the innervation by sensory fibers of all the structures investigated is strictly unilateral. The line of

*Careful observations during surgical operations on the contents of the posterior fossa in man led F. W. L. Kerr (1962) to infer that the first cervical root frequently exists as an independent afferent pathway and as regards pain sensation, subserves the foramen magnum and perhaps other regions.

demarcation is sharp, so that even structures in the midline have half their innervation from one side and half from the other.

EFFECTS OF INFLAMMATION ON THE PAIN-SENSITIVE STRUCTURES WITHIN THE CRANIUM

It has been indicated above that traction and displacement of certain intracranial structures cause head pain. Many of the nerve endings involved in noxious stimulation are on or near the surface of structures that would be surrounded by microorganisms and the products of inflammation in the event of meningeal infection. Furthermore, the effects on pain threshold of inflammatory processes within the cranium are relevant to the understanding of headache from meningitis.

The headache is probably due to inflammation in and about the wall of the pain-sensitive internal carotid artery, exacerbated at intervals with the recurrence of headache and other clinical manifestations. A secondary factor may be that irritation of the internal carotid artery near or at the bifurcation of the common carotid artery reflexly incites painful vasodilatation in the temporal and orbital regions. Also direct effect of tissue ischemia may be pertinent.

Indeed striking effects on the blood vessels of the region have been demonstrated. Since the conjunctiva receives its blood supply from branches (dorsal, nasal, and lacrimal) of the ophthalmic artery, study of the bulbar conjunctival blood vessels makes possible the examination of the terminal parts of a vascular tree whose origin is the same as that which supplies a large part of the cerebral hemisphere. Retinal artery pressures are significantly lower on the side of a thrombosed or surgically ligated internal carotid artery. However, after ligation of the common carotid, probably because of a more adequate establishment of collateral circulation, the lowering of the retinal arterial pressure persists for a shorter time than with occlusion of an internal carotid artery.

During routine observations of the bulbar conjunctival blood vessels of patients with a variety of vascular diseases, differences in appearance of the vessels of the two eyes were noted by Pavlou and Wolff (1959) in those having unilateral thrombosis of the internal carotid artery. Evidence of insufficiency of circulation in the central retinal artery, indicating thrombosis of the internal carotid artery, was clinically manifested in these patients by disturbances in vision, such as blurring and transient blindness, and by the low blood pressure (often less than half the normal) in the retinal artery on the side of the occlusion. This suggested that impairment of the bulbar conjunctival circulation might be detected by examination of these blood vessels, since both retinal and uveal circulation are of common origin (from the ophthalmic artery), and the blood pressure normally is about the same in these two arterial systems of the eye.

A. T. Pavlou and H. G. Wolff (1959) studied the changes in appearance and behavior of the bulbar conjunctival vessels accompanying unilateral occlusion of the common or internal carotid artery in a series of 11 patients by examination of the eyes with a slit lamp.

Headache and Cerebral Thrombosis

Fisher (1968) has reviewed the association of headache and cerebrovascular disease. He makes the following points. The basic atherosclerotic process which characterizes stroke, regardless of its site, is always or almost always painless. Cerebral arteriosclerosis thus is not a cause of headache. Occlusion may involve arteries from the largest to the smallest, and occlusion of the larger vessels usually evokes well-recognized clinical syndromes. However, the infarct itself does not give rise to pain unless hemorrhage occurs or there is associated severe edema leading to displacement of cerebral structures.

When the internal carotid artery was occluded, 35 of 109 patients (31%) had some pain or discomfort, with the headache most prominent in the frontal area and lateralized in ten cases, frontal but nonlateralized in five, frontal and occipital in five, cervical occipital in three, and not further described in nine patients.

The typical pain of middle cerebral artery

thrombosis is located behind, in, or above the corresponding eye. Fisher notes that middle cerebral embolism is more likely to produce headache on the side of the head above the temple. The great majority of his cases did not have headache.

Headache in Patients with Cerebral Embolism

Headache was the most prominent premonitory symptom among 120 patients at the New York Hospital with evidence of cerebral embolism. Although the incidence is far lower than that of patients with thromboses of the internal carotid artery, this remarkable phenomenon occurred in ten patients. The headache preceded the hemiplegia by 2 to 48 hr; in most of the patients it was 10 to 12 hr. In five of the ten, the headache was localized to the side of the head that later became the seat of an embolus; in five the headache was generalized. It is suggested that the headache is induced by direct or indirect stimulation by the embolus of the pain-sensitive internal carotid artery or arteries of the circle of Willis before finally becoming lodged in the small vessels of the parenchyma (Wells, 1961).

Headache in Patients with Meningitis

It is probable that the acute inflammation of the meninges, involving the structures within the cranium equipped with afferent nerve endings for noxious stimuli, lowers the pain threshold (Bilisoly et al., 1954; Schumacher, 1943). The pia, dura, and the blood vessels about the base, as well as the aforementioned cervical and cranial nerves, are provided with these nerve endings. The lowering of the pain threshold by a product of inflammation thus gives rise to headache by sensitizing to mechanical disturbances pain nerve endings which would otherwise be inadequate.

It was reported by Pickering (1939) and repeatedly confirmed by Wolff and associates that the headache associated with meningitis is increased by raising the intracranial pressures to 500 to 700 mm of saline, and is also increased by reducing the pressure to zero. Meningitis may be accompanied by a mild or moderate elevation of intracranial pressure, which is probably not an important factor in the production of the headache. These experiments on the effect of modifying the pressure upon the intensity of the headache indicate that the afferent impulses already arising from inflamed intracranial structures are increased in number by the traction and displacement effects resulting from adding fluid to or withdrawing it from the lumbar sac.

The involvement of the upper cervical roots, as well as structures in the posterior fossa, causes the muscles of the occipital region and the neck to maintain contraction, resulting in the stiff and often rigid neck, and flexion of the thigh and legs when the neck is passively flexed (Brudzinski's sign). The involvement of the sensory roots of the remaining portion of the cord and secondary contraction of the skeletal muscle cause the Kernig sign, scaphoid abdomen, and tripod position. The noxious stimuli from within the head dominate, so that even though noxious stimuli from sustained contraction of muscle of the head and neck also give rise to pain, this is secondary to the pain from intracranial sources.

The headache is usually generalized, though more intense in the occipital region. It is of high intensity, continuous, and throbbing, and associated with photophobia. The intensity of the pain is increased by bodily effort, such as walking, ascending stairs, or rising from a chair, by shaking the head, flexing the neck, by jugular compression, and by the sitting-up position. It is reduced in intensity by lying flat in bed. The neck rigidity associated with meningitis is greater than that from any other cause. Codeine in 60-mg amounts given repeatedly will usually give the patient sufficient support until specific therapeutic agents can exert their effects on the inflammation, or until the patient lapses into coma as the result of his infection.

In short, the features of the headache of meningitis, namely its throbbing, its relation to variations in intracranial pressure, the increase in intensity by shaking the head, bodily effort, and jugular compression, all indicate that minor traction, displacement, and distention, incapable of causing pain under normal conditions, will do so when the threshold for pain is lowered by the products of inflammation.

These statements concerning the headache in meningitis are valid regardless of the etiologic agent, and especially when the inflammation is acute.

JOLT HEADACHE

Experimental force, induced by a jolt, has been applied by Wolff, Kunkle, Lund, and Maher (1947) to the head in the study of headache mechanism.

A jolt headache can be self-induced in many individuals by sudden brief rapid rotary movement of the head. It is common experience, moreover, that certain clinical headaches are aggravated by even mild head movement. In these studies the standard technic was a quick rotary snap of the head to one side and back to mid-position. The forces exerted upon the head and indirectly upon the cranial contents were measured by a miniature accelerometer gripped between the teeth (see Fig. 3-20). The forces exerted in a jolt were recorded in units of g (gravity) by the deflection of the accelerometer stylus in contact with a smoked glass. The jolt threshold, defined as that force which just produces a transient mild anterior headache or accentuates a headache already present, was estimated by analysis of a series of jolts of graduated intensities.

In a series of 35 adult subjects, including normal individuals and others with structural brain disease or various types of headache, the following were found.

1. The mean threshold value of jolt headache in normal subjects was approximately 6 g; the inter-individual range was wide, and the threshold varied moderately and unpredictably in the same individual from day to day with a range as broad as ± 2.7 g.

2. The threshold of jolt headache was found to be significnatly lowered during states in which pain-sensitive vascular structures anchoring the brain to the cranium were distended or inflamed. Moreover, since the jolt headache threshold was greatly lowered when intracranial arteries were dilated (notably after the injection of histamine), but was not lowered during procedures inducing distention of intracranial veins (by straining or jugular com-

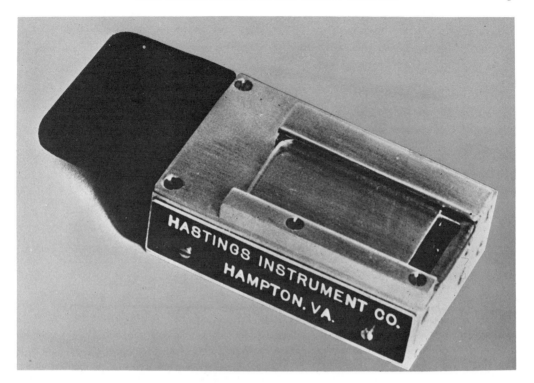

FIG. 3-20. Instrument for recording force of head jolt in g units.

pression) it is inferred that jolt headache arises chiefly or entirely from traction upon the major pain-sensitive arteries which anchor the brain at the base.

3. When headache arising from structures on the outside of the head (e.g., muscle contraction headache) was present, jolt headache threshold was not significantly altered.

4. In individuals with histories of migraine, the jolt headache threshold in headache-free periods was within the normal range; in such subjects during an attack of migraine the threshold was usually not altered, but in a few the threshold was moderately depressed. When from other evidence it appeared likely that the intracranial arteries were painfully involved, the jolt threshold was lowered.

5. The jolt headache threshold was moderately lowered in subjects with headaches known or presumed to arise primarily from dilation of pain-sensitive intracranial vessels, particularly arteries, e.g., the headache in-

duced by histamine given intravenously, and the headache of caffeine-withdrawal, anoxia, hunger, induced hypoglycemia, fever, some systemic infections, "hangover," post-puncture reaction, and the early post-concussion state.

6. The threshold was greatly lowered in subjects with headaches known or presumed to arise primarily from inflammation of pain-sensitive intracranial vessels, e.g., headache accompanying meningitis or following ventriculography or pneumoencephalography.

7. In patients with space-occupying intracranial masses, e.g., subdural hematoma (Fig. 3-21) or brain tumor, the threshold was usually moderately depressed and the location of the headache induced by jolting sometimes indicated the side on which the lesion lay.

It is concluded that the measurement of the threshold of jolt headache may indicate whether a headache arises from intracranial structures, offer indirect evidence for the presence of dilatation of intracranial arteries,

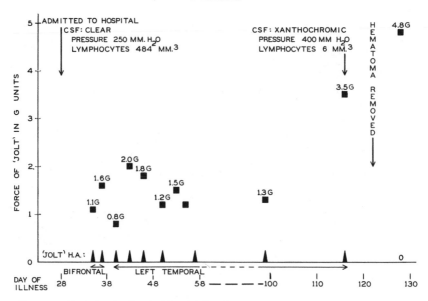

FIG. 3-21. Variation in threshold to jolt headache in a patient with left temporoparietal subdural hematoma.

or suggest the presence and location of a space-occupying intracranial mass.

COUGH HEADACHE

Headache that is either initiated by or is worsened by coughing has been carefully studied by Symonds (1956). He described six patients with intracranial tumors or structural displacements who exhibited this phenomenon. Severe pain in the head initiated on coughing, sneezing, laughing, stooping, or straining at stool was for 15 months the only symptom of a patient with a posterior fossa meningioma arising from the undersurface of the tentorium. A second patient experienced for two years transient severe pain in the head notably upon coughing, sneezing, or straining at stool. It was revealed that he had a cyst of the midbrain within the incisura tentorii. Three patients had for two to three years severe headache on coughing, lifting, laughing, or straining at stool as the predominant or only symptom of Paget's disease of the skull with basilar impression. After continuing for several months in one patient this liability ended; but four years later recurred and continued for six years; basilar impression of an extreme degree was demonstrated. A sixth patient developed transient severe headache upon coughing, sneezing, laughing, stooping, or straining at stool. This had its onset several weeks after the removal of an acoustic neuroma and persisted for at least a year. All six patients had or had had disease within the posterior

fossa. Symonds pointed out that lumbar puncture headache which is aggravated by jugular compression may be provoked, when temporarily absent, by coughing. He also called attention to the immediate aggravation by coughing of pre-existing headache in many patients with any variety of intracranial-space-occupying lesion, and suggested that the headache is due to displacement of traction upon pain-sensitive intracranial structures. He then analyzed the data of 21 patients who had cough headache without evidence of gross structural alterations within the cranium. Thirteen of the 21 patients were male. The earliest age of onset was 37, the latest 77, with an average age of 55. Several patients had low-grade infections, and 5 of the 21 had had migraine headaches from time to time. In nine patients after shorter or longer periods of the cough headache, the symptom disappeared. In four the headache occurred only with provocation, and in five headache was sometimes present without such provocation. Two patients volunteered that quick rotation of the head would similarly cause headache.

From experience with cough headache at the New York Hospital it was noted that the phenomenon may occur with systemic illness that alters vascular tone within the head, such as infectious or post-infectious states, or the reduced vascular tone that occurs from time to time in patients with vascular headaches. The patients without demonstrated intracranial disease who have exhibited this phenomenon are those, usually in the middle-age or older-age group, who during one or another period in their past lives have had complaints of vascular headaches of the migraine type. The cough headache has then made its appearance after a period of exhaustion, prolonged sleep loss, or during a mild depression, coupled with a respiratory illness and cough that induced the symptoms. The cough headache has spontaneously disappeared with recovery of general health, energy, and better spirits.

Thus, cough headache results from traction upon and displacement of pain-sensitive intracranial structures due to the rise in venous pressure, and has features in common with the jolt headache studied by Wolff *et al.* (1947).

FORMULATION OF THE PATHOPHYSIOLOGY OF HEADACHE FROM INTRACRANIAL SOURCES

From these data, inferences concerning headache from intracranial sources may be formulated. Inflammation, traction, displacement, and distention of pain-sensitive structures are the disturbances primarily responsible for headache. It is noteworthy that as a source of pain the cranial vascular structures far outweigh in number and distribution all others and will often be implicated. Yet it is obvious that no single structure or disturbance is entirely responsible for the headache. Hence, the following brief summary is presented.

1. Traction on veins that pass to the sagittal and transverse sinuses from the cerebral cortex results in a dull, aching pain over a wide area on the front, top, and side of the head. Not only are most of these veins sensitive to pain at the site of juncture with the sinus, but secondary traction on the walls of the sinuses to which they are attached causes pain. Since many of these veins bridge a gap of 1 to 3 cm between the cortex of the brain and the sinus, swelling of the brain puts them under tension. Hence, tumors of the brain may produce headache either by displacement and direct traction on these veins or through secondary hydrocephalus. Unusually low intracranial pressure, e.g., after lumbar puncture, may similarly result in traction on the tributary veins, principally those to the sagittal sinus, and thus induce headache. Air in the subarachnoid spaces after pneumoencephalographic procedures may likewise produce headache by causing traction on these anchoring veins.

2. Traction on the middle meningeal arteries causes headache as far forward as the eye and as far back as the ear, depending on whether the stress is primarily on the more anterior or the more posterior branches. Dural, extradural, or subdural tumors causing traction on these arteries in any part of their extent, from their origin at the foramen spinosum in the middle fossa to their terminal branches near the sagittal sinus, may thus cause headache.

3. Traction on the large arteries at the base of the brain and their main cerebral branches or on the pia-arachnoid in immediate contact with them causes headache. When the traction is on the intracranial portion of the internal carotid arteries and the major components of the circle of Willis, the headache occurs in the region of the eyes or in the front, top, or sides of the head. Traction on the basilar and vertebral arteries and their branches produces headache in the back of the head and neck. Displacement of this entire arterial system from right to left causes a generalized headache, chiefly on the right, from the eye to the neck. Distention of the third ventricle causes traction on numerous arteries at the base of the brain and results in pain all over the head (see Fig. 3-18). Tumors in the region of the sella turcica or above it may cause pain by traction on the pain-sensitive arteries at the anterior end of the circle of Willis. The anterior cerebral artery, when under traction even as high as the genu of the corpus callosum, causes pain over or within the eye. Hence, tumors in the frontal lobe or in the corpus callosum causing traction on one or both of these arteries may produce pain in the region of the eye as described.

Since traction on pontile and internal auditory arteries causes pain within and behind the ear, tumors of the eighth nerve and others within the cerebellopontile angle or in the region of the internal auditory meatus may cause pain in the region about the ear.

4. Distention and dilatation of the intracranial arteries result in headache. The arteries responsible for such pain are: pial arteries (chiefly at the base, as has been described) and dural arteries (chiefly the middle meningeal). Included in this category are headaches due to intravenous histamine, amyl nitrite inhalation,

fever, sepsis, etc. These headaches will be discussed in detail in later chapters.

5. Inflammation involving the pain-sensitive structures at the base and the convexity of the brain causes severe headache. When inflammation is limited to the posterior fossa the headache is chiefly over the back of the head. When the inflammation is in the supratentorial fossa the headache is primarily frontal or vertical. The headaches associated with meningitis, subarachnoid hemorrhage, or meningeal invasion by tumor are examples of headaches due to local tissue reaction or inflammation.

6. Direct pressure by tumors on nerves possessing many pain-conducting fibers may cause pain. Thus, compression of the intracranial portion of the sensory division of the fifth cranial nerve results in pain in the front, top, and side of the face and head. Similarly, compression of the intracranial portions of the ninth and tenth cranial nerves produces pain in and behind the corresponding ear, while compression of the upper cervical roots results in pain in the back of the head and neck.

Tumors probably do not commonly cause headache through circumscribed pressure on the dura even in the pain-sensitive areas. Thus, mere downward pressure on the dura of the floor of the anterior fossa, for example, does not cause headache. Although neoplastic invasion of the dura with the usual inflammatory reaction may be a cause of headache, as has been mentioned, traction and displacement of arterial and venous structures are the mechanical disturbances more likely to be responsible for headache in the presence of a tumor.

Summary

1. The sensitivity to pain of most of the intracranial structures has been ascertained from a series of 45 patients during surgical procedures on the head. Some of the pain pathways and the pathophysiology of headache are defined.

2. Of the intracranial structures, the great venous sinuses and their venous tributaries from the surface of the brain, parts of the dura at the base, the dural arteries, and the cerebral arteries at the base of the brain are sensitive to pain.

3. The cranium (including the diploic and emissary veins), the parenchyma of the brain, most of the dura, most of the pia-arachnoid, the ependymal lining of the ventricles, and the choroid plexuses are not sensitive to pain.

4. With the exception of those sensations that result from stimulation of the parenchyma and nerves, the only sensation that is experienced on stimulation of the intracranial structure is pain.

5. Stimulation of the pain-sensitive intracranial structures on or above the superior surface of the tentorium cerebelli results in pain in various regions in front of a line drawn vertically from the ears across the top of the head. The pathways for this pain are contained in the fifth cranial nerve.

6. Stimulation of the pain-sensitive intracranial structures on or below the inferior surface of the tentorium cerebelli results in pain in various regions behind the line just described. The pathways for this pain are contained chiefly in the ninth and tenth cranial nerves and the upper three cervical nerves.

7. From the data available, six basic sources of headache from within the cranial cavity have been formulated. Headache may result from (1) traction on the veins that pass to the venous sinuses from the surface of the brain and displacement of the great venous sinuses; (2) traction on the middle meningeal arteries; (3) traction on the large arteries at the base of the brain and their main branches; (4) distention and dilatation of intracranial arteries; (5) inflammation in or about any of the pain-sensitive structures of the head; and (6) direct pressure by tumors or adjacent tissue on the cranial and cervical nerves containing many pain-afferent fibers from the head.

References

Arnold, F. (1851). *Handbuch der Anatomie des Menschen.* A. Emmerling and Herder, Freiberg, Germany.

Bilisoly, F. N., H. Goodell, and H. G. Wolff (1954). Vasodilation, lowered pain threshold, and increased tissue vulnerability; effects dependent upon peripheral nerve function. *Arch. Intern. Med.* *94*, 759.

Chorobski, J., and W. Penfield (1932). Cerebral vasodilator nerves and their pathway from the medulla oblongata, with observations on the pial and intracerebral vascular plexus. *Arch. Neurol. Psychiat.* *28*, 1257.

Clark, D., J. Hughes, and H. S. Gasser (1935). Afferent function in the group of nerve fibres of slowest conduction velocity. *Am. J. Physiol.* *114*, 69.

Clark, S. L. (1934). Innervation of the choroid plexus and the blood vessels within the central nervous system. *J. Comp. Neurol.* *60*, 21.

Cushing, H. (1908). Surgery of the head. In *Surgery: Its Principles and Practice* (W. W. Keen, ed.), Vol. 3, Chap. 36. W. B. Saunders, Philadelphia.

Cushing, H. (1909). A note upon the faradic stimulation of the post-central gyrus in conscious patients. *Brain* *32*, 44.

Dahl, E. (1975). Intracranial arteries, morphologic differences in extracerebral and intracerebral muscles. *The Bergen Migraine Symposium (Supp. I)*, 24.

Fay, T. (1931). Certain fundamental cerebral signs and symptoms and their response to dehydration. *Arch. Neurol. Psychiat.* *26*, 452.

Fay, T. (1936). Mechanisms of headache. *Trans. Am. Neurol. Assoc.* *62*, 74.

Fay, T. (1937). Mechanism of headache. *Arch. Neurol. Psychiat.* *37*, 471.

Fisher, C. M. (1951). Occlusion of the internal carotid artery. *Arch. Neurol. Psychiat.* *65*, 346.

Fisher, C. M. (1968). Headache and cerebrovascular disease. In *Handbook of Clinical Neruology* (P. J. Vinken and G. W. Bruyn, eds.), pp. 124–156. North Holland, Amsterdam.

Gardner, W. S., Stowell, A., and Dutlinger, R. (1947). Resection of the greater superficial petrosal nerve in the treatment of unilateral headache. *J. Neurosurg.* *4*, 105.

Graham, J. R., and H. G. Wolff (1937) (1938). Mechanism of migraine headache and action of ergotamine tartrate. *Assoc. Res. Nerv. Dis. Proc.* *18*, 638. *Arch. Neurol. Psychiat.* *39*, 737.

Gulland, L. (1898). The occurrence of nerves on intracranial blood vessels. *Brit. Med. J.* *2*, 781.

Huber, G. C. (1899). Observations on the innervation of the intracranial vessels. *J. Comp. Neurol.* *9*, 1.

Kerr, F. W. L. (1967). Evidence for a peripheral etiology of trigeminal neuralgia. *J. Neurosurg.* *26* *(Suppl.)*, 168.

Kerr, F. W. L. (1962). Facial, vagal and glossopharyngeal nerves in the cat: afferent connections. *Neurol.* *6*, 264.

McNaughton, F. L. (1938). The innervation of the intracranial blood vessels and dural sinuses. *Assoc. Res. Nerv. Dis. Proc.* *18*, 178.

Pavlou, A. T., and H. G. Wolff (1959). The bulbar conjunctival vessels in occlusion of the internal carotid artery. *Arch. Intern. Med.* *104*, 53.

Penfield, W. (1932a). Intracerebral vascular nerves. *Arch. Neurol. Psychiat.* *27*, 30.

Penfield, W. (1932b). Operative treatment of migraine and observations on the mechanism of vascular pain. *Trans. Am. Acad. Ophthalmol.* *37*, 50.

Penfield, W. (1935). A contribution to the mechanism of intracranial pain. *Assoc. Res. Nerv. Dis. Proc.* *15*, 399.

Penfield, W., and F. McNaughton (1940). Dural headache and innervation of the dura mater. *Arch. Neurol. Psychiat.* *44*, 43.

Pickering, G. W. (1939). Experimental observations on headache. *Brit. Med. J.* *1*, 4087.

Pickering, G. W. (1948). Lumbar puncture headache. *Brain* *71*, 274.

Pickering, G. W., and W. Hess (1933). Observations on the mechanism of headache produced by histamine. *Clin. Sci.* *1*, 77.

Putnam, T. J. (1931). Cerebral circulation: some new points in its anatomy, physiology and pathology. *J. Neuropath. Psychopath.* *17*, 193.

Ray, B. S., and H. G. Wolff (1940). Experimental studies on headache. Pain-sensitive structures of the head and their significance in headache. *Arch. Surg.* *41*, 813.

Schumacher, G. A. (1943). The influence of inflammation on the pain threshold in man. *Assoc. Res. Nerv. Dis. Proc.* *23*, 166.

Stohr, P. J. (1922). Ueber die Innervation der Pia Mater und des Plexus Choriodens des Menschen. *Z. Ges. Anat.* *63*, 562.

Stohr, P. J. (1932). Nerves of the blood vessels, heart, meninges, digestive tract and urinary bladder. In *Cytology and Cellular Pathology of the Nervous System* (W. Penfield, ed.) Vol. 1, Sect. 8, p. 383. Hoeber, New York.

Sweet, W. H. (1959). Pain. In *Handbook of Physiology*, Sect. 1, Neurophysiology, Washington, D.C. Am. Physiol. Soc. *19*, 450.

Sweet, W. H., and J. C. White (1952). Pain fibers in the petrosal nerves. *Trans. Am. Neurol. Assoc.* *77*, 87.

Symonds, C. P. (1956). Cough headache. *Brain* *79*, 557.

Von Luschka, H. (1850). *Die Nerven in der Harten Hirnhaut.* H. Laupp, Tubingen, Germany.

Von Storch, T. J. C., L. Secunda, and C. M. Krinsky (1940). Production and localization of headache with subarachnoid and ventricular air. *Arch. Neurol. Psychiat.* *43*, 326.

Wells, C. E. (1961). Pemonitory symptoms of cerebral embolism. *Arch. Neurol.* *5*, 490.

White, J. C., and W. H. Sweet (1955). *Pain: Its Mechanisms and Neurosurgical Control.* Charles C. Thomas, Springfield, Ill.

Wolff, H. G. (1959). The nature and causation of headache. *J. Dent. Med.* *14*, 3.

Wolff, H. G., E. C. Kunkle, D. W. Lund, and P. J. Maher (1947). Studies on headache: induced mechanical stresses in the analysis of headache mechanisms. *Trans. Am. Neurol. Assoc.* *72*, 93.

4

MIGRAINE

REVISED BY DONALD J. DALESSIO

Although the headache is but part of a widespread disturbance, it is this symptom that is characteristic of migraine and most relevant to this discussion. It will therefore be considered in detail.

According to Riley (1932), Aretaeus of Cappodocia, at the end of the first century A.D., isolated from the general group of headaches a type distinguished by its paroxysmal nature, its severity, its one-sidedness, and its association with nausea, the crises of pain being separated by intervals during which the patient is free from all discomfort. About a half century later, Galen introduced the term *hemicrania*. During the following centuries the word was gradually modified, to *hemigranea, emigranea, migranea, megrim,* and finally the word *migraine*.

DESCRIPTION OF MIGRAINE

The outstanding feature of the migraine syndrome is periodic headache, usually unilateral in onset, but which may become generalized. The headaches are associated with irritability and nausea, and often with photophobia, vomiting, constipation, and diarrhea. Not infrequently the attacks are ushered in by scotomata, hemianopia, unilateral paresthesia, and speech disorders. The pain is commonly limited to the head, but it may include the face and even the neck. Often other members of the patient's family have similar headaches. Cranial artery dilatation occurs during the attack, but permanent structural damage is rare.

Other bodily accompaniments are abdominal distention, cold cyanosed extremities, vertigo, tremors, pallor, dryness of the mouth, excessive sweating, and chilliness. Many patients have noticed either just before or during the migraine headache attack that rings on the fingers are difficult to remove. Others describe and call attention to the "thickness of the skin," which appears and feels edematous. Pale urine of low specific gravity also bespeaks a widespread disturbance in water metabolism as an accompaniment of the headache.

The evening before the onset of an attack is often characterized by a feeling of especial well-being with excessive talkativeness and high spirits, unwillingness to retire, and increased appetite for food. The duration of attacks is from a few hours to several days and the headache can be of any degree of severity. After an attack, again patients often experience a period of buoyancy and well-being. In the interval between headaches, gastrointestinal disturbances, notably constipation, may occur. Diarrhea is less frequent. Migraine may begin at any age, though commonly it begins during adolescence. No age, social, intellectual, or economic group is immune. There are many variants of the migraine attack and some phase of the syndrome other than headache may become the presenting complaint. Periodic or cyclic vomiting may occur in infancy, although the child may not complain of headache until the age of six.

Some prefer to limit the use of the word *migraine* to headaches that are always strictly unilateral throughout the attack. There is no objection to such a precise use of the term except that it results in profitless subdivisions of overlapping headache syndromes. Many persons with strictly unilateral periodic headaches also have, from time to time, attacks that become bilateral, or are bilateral from the start. It seems justifiable to include such kindred headaches in one general class called migraine or migraine variants, the members having in common vascular mechanisms and clinical phenomena to be described below.

A patient with a migraine headache attack looks ill, and often very ill. His features imply dejection and suffering. He may be supporting his head with his hand pressed against the painful region, or against the corresponding side of his neck. His face is occasionally red, but usually it is pale, sallow, with the skin sweaty or greasy. Regardless of superficial color, the temporal, frontal, or supraorbital vessels on the painful side appear distended and conspicuous. The tone of the skin is usually poor, with evident wrinkles and folds, but there may be puffiness or edema of the face, as well as elsewhere. His extremities are usually cold, he complains of feeling chilly, he smells of stale sweat, and his breath is foul. The patient may be moaning, groaning, or tearful. He looks and acts as though prostrated and speaks slowly, without vigor. If ambulatory, he seems drooped, or lacking in the usual muscle tone. When the attack is so mild as to permit the patient to work, he gives the impression of being very tired and irritable. He may yawn repeatedly.

Migraine shares with other vascular headaches the features of depth, diffusion, and aching, and the rhythmic features of throbbing and pulsating. The quality of the headache is throbbing and aching early in its course, but it may, with the passage of hours, become a steady ache. Although there is some predictability concerning the site of duration of headache in a given individual, the intensity and associated phenomena vary greatly. Intensity may vary from a barely perceptible, or what is called by some the "background headache" to a headache of fierce intensity. It is increased in intensity by walking, by bodily effort, or by any sudden change in position. It is also increased in intensity by bright light, loud sounds, and mental effort. It is diminished by pressure on superficial scalp arteries and the common carotid artery on the affected side. A high-intensity headache is often made worse by the lying-down position and is slightly reduced by sitting upright.

The attack may be of any duration, from a few minutes to several weeks. There may be short-duration, high-intensity attacks; long-duration, low-intensity attacks; or any combination of the two. Usually the attack lasts from sunup to sundown, i.e., the commonest time of onset is the early morning hours, and the commonest time of dissipation is in the early evening. On the other hand, attacks may begin at any time of the day or night. Commonly the headache is not of such severity as to prevent sleep, which, though fitful or broken, is a state of optimal comfort for the patient. On the other hand, headache of high intensity does awaken the patient and make sleep impossible, and forces him to "jump out of bed." Photophobia and phonophobia almost always accompany high-intensity headaches.

The sites of the migraine headache are notably temporal, supra-orbital, frontal, retrobulbar, parietal, postauricular, and occipital. However, as will be indicated later, they may occur as well in the malar region, in the upper and the lower teeth, at the base of the nose, and in the median wall of the orbit. They are usually unilateral in onset and most commonly vary from side to side in successive attacks. Some patients have generalized headaches from their onset, and most unilateral headaches become generalized during the attack. Rarely, patients will report that all headaches are experienced on the same side.

Anorexia is an accompaniment of most migraine headaches. Anorexia may be slight when the headache is of mild intensity, but severe headache is always associated with anorexia and usually with nausea. Vomiting, though common with severe headache, is usually absent, even with severe headache, if the duration is short. Emesis sometimes immediately precedes the termination of the attack. On the other hand, it may occur throughout the attack. The vomitus often is tasteless or bitter, becoming more acid toward the end of the attack. Dry retching is common in patients who have prolonged vomiting with their attacks. Vomiting may constitute the most serious aspect of the headache attack, causing prostration during the attack and delay in recovery after its termination. Patients with such severe emesis are least likely to feel the usual buoyancy immediately following the termination of the attack.

Also, after some hours of headache the face, the head, and especially the lids may become edematous and blotchy, the edema usually outlasting the headache for hours. Nasal, skin, eye, vasomotor, and other smooth muscle and gland phenomena, such as the degree of blanching or blushing, sweating, vasomotor rhinitis, nasal obstruction, and lacrimation, are extremely variable. The attacks in which pain is most marked in the face are accompanied by the most disturbance in smooth muscle function. The pattern of the headache may change from time to time.

Of extreme variability and conspicuousness are the preheadache phenomena. Some patients with migraine headache never have clearly defined prodromes. Many have feelings of mounting tension, hunger, and wakefulness, often followed by profound sleep just preceding the attack. Still others are aware of declining energy and drive, and a few of extreme buoyancy, talkativeness, and well-being just before the attack. On the other hand a small group predictably have visual and other sensory disturbances immediately before the onset of the headache. Some patients have visual disturbances not always followed by headache, and another group have headache frequently, with visual disturbances perhaps only three or four times during a lifetime.

These visual disturbances precede the headache and have a duration of a few minutes to an hour. Rarely they may persist for hours. When they are short-lived they usually terminate before the onset of the headache and between the visual disturbance and the headache phase there is a symptom-free phase when the patient feels relatively well. Then, however, the headache begins and becomes gradually worse. On the other hand, if the visual disturbances have been of 30 to 60 minutes' duration they may only gradually dwindle off, overlapping the beginning of the headache and persisting for a few minutes or even hours during the headache phase.

The preheadache visual disturbances may be blind spots arranged in visual field quadrants or in isolated areas of blindness. There may be homonymous, quadrantic, or hemianopic field defects. Such defects are usually contralateral to the side of the headache.

Also, there may be areas of bright flashes of light, geometric designs, wavy visions, golden balls, stars, tessellations, serrations, and so-called fortification phenomena, and most of these visual hallucinations are mobile and interfere with vision. These disturbances are not to be confused with visual difficulties such as photophobia, large pupil with blurred vision, focusing difficulties, increased lacrimation, and edema of the lids, or the ophthalmoplegic phenomena that accompany the headache itself and usually occur later in its course after the headache is well established or receding.

Other prodromes occurring along with but independent of these disturbances, and sometimes occurring as isolated events, are paresthesias of the face and hand and even of the foot on the contralateral side. Rarely aphasia or anomia occurs. Another relatively common preheadache phenomenon is vertigo. This may begin suddenly as a violent spinning with nausea, vomiting, sweating, prostration, and even syncope, followed by intense headache and further nausea and vomiting.

The mood disorders that accompany the headache are often outstanding. The patient complains of feeling prostrated, dejected, and often seriously depressed. At such times he is unsocial, rejecting companionship or the presence of others, irritable and irascible, and often unwilling to assume his usual responsibilities, especially rejecting any demand to make a decision. His judgment is poor, and he is impulsive, hostile, and sometimes destructive, often directing his hostility at those who are dependent upon him. Memory, attention, concentration, and retention are usually poor during the headache, and cooperation is denied.

After a migraine attack the patient may feel

relaxed, in good spirits, filled with energy and drive, enthusiastic about his work, and sometimes even overactive and in ebullient spirits. Or he feels depleted for a day or two, especially if there has been a great deal of vomiting or diarrhea.

Some common metabolic disturbances that precede and overlap the headache have been mentioned, the chief of these being the disturbance in water metabolism, which causes the patient to become edematous, usually just before and during the early part of the headache. Dehydration occurs during the headache with urinary frequency and the passage of a large amount of pale urine. Though the appetite for food is minimal, the patient may be interested in salty or sour foods. Commonly there is constipation, though diarrhea may also occur. There may be leukocytosis and fever, though this is rare.

Variability of symptoms and periodicity is a characteristic feature of the syndrome. Some patients have attacks predictably once or twice a week, others once a month, still others have only three or four attacks in a lifetime. Further, some patients have headache attacks once or twice a week for a period of four to six months, and then they are free of attacks for from three to five years. Still other patients have frequent, even daily, attacks for a week every three or four months during twenty years or more, with freedom from attacks on the interims. Some have headache attacks preceded by scotomata, paresthesias, and speech disorders three or four times in 30 years or more, and in the interims, at intervals of once a month, have attacks of mild hemicrania or generalized headaches without antecedent visual or other sensory disturbances. Some women have migraine headache attacks with or preceding menstruation, and at no other time. Often migraine headache attacks end with the onset of pregnancy, but sometimes they persist or become more frequent and intense. Many women patients lose their headache attacks with the menopause; in others their headaches persist, and a few women begin having migraine headache attacks at this time, which then recur for many years. Some patients have one short period (about six months) when migraine headaches recur frequently and are severe, and after which all headache attacks are permanently absent. Although migraine headache attacks commonly begin in adolescence, they can begin at any age, and they often start in late middle life.

Another outstanding feature of the migraine attack is its occurrence in relation to the period of "let down." Headache attacks often occur on week ends, the first days of a holiday, Sundays, and on the occasion of a planned social engagement or travel.

Not only are duration, frequency, and occurrence extremely variable, but intensity varies, sometimes in the same person, from an intolerable pain causing the patient to border on prostration or coma, to a discomfort so slight as to be compatible with gaiety and laughter. Further, the type of clinical disorder may vary in the same person, so that a different part of the head becomes involved, and the duration of the attack changes from hours to 20 or 30 min.

Because of this variability of migraine headache attacks, a long list of names has been attached to the variants such as: menstrual headach; relaxation headache; Sunday headache; weekend headache; vacation headache; ordinary or common headache; menopausal headache; spring headache; summer headache; fall headache; winter headache; humidity headache; barometric pressure headache; hot-weather headache; tropical headache; wash-day headache; cleaning-day headache; inventory headache; constipation headache; indigestion headache; sick headache; bilious headache; and so forth.

ALTERATIONS IN REGIONAL BLOOD FLOW IN MIGRAINE

A limited number of measurements of cerebral blood flow (CBF) during attacks of migraine have been made by the intracarotid injection of radioactive xenon-133 performed at the time of angiography. O'Brien made the first such measurement in 1967, using an inhalation technique. In his initial series of observations, the measurements were primitive. The patient breathed a mixture of xenon-133 which, after 5 min on a closed circuit system, presumably saturated the tissues. Then the xenon inhalation was stopped and the desaturation curve produced by arterial washout was followed over a period of 40 min, using two scintillation counters placed on either side of the head. O'Brien suggested that the half-life of the fast component of the washout curve was an index of the cerebral cortex perfusion rate.

During these early experiments, because there were only two scintillation counters, it was impossible to isolate the intracranial from the extracranial circulation, a major deficiency, since in migraine it is well known that there may be marked alterations in intracranial and extracranial blood flow. Nonetheless, the observations were important and have stimulated a whole series of radioactive measurements of cerebral blood flow in migraine.

In his original observations, O'Brien noted a mean decrease in blood flow of 20% during the headache period with no asymmetry between the cerebral hemispheres, even though the patients might be having unilateral headaches. From studies of a larger series of patients, he reported in 1971 that cerebral blood flow measured during headache showed a small increase of 8%, whereas during the painless preheadache aura it was reduced by 23%. Perhaps more interesting, patients studied during the aura showed a generalized reduction in blood flow which was not limited to a small area of the cerebral hemisphere related to the symptoms. Also, the alterations in blood flow did not correspond exactly in time with the patients' estimation of the length of the aura.

In the intracarotid xenon technique a polyethylene catheter is inserted into the internal carotid artery and a bolus of 2–3 mci of xenon-133 and saline is injected. In this situation the rate of xenon washout from the carotid circulation does reflect cerebral blood flow. Further, a very large number of external counters are positioned over over the hemicranium, from 16 to more than 200, so that regional cerebral blood flow values can be calculated from the slope of the washout curves and expressed as ml of blood/100 gm of brain/min. Obviously, this technique is invasive and is suited only to patients with migraine who are

having carotid arteriograms. Usually, also, intracarotid xenon is injected unilaterally, this having the disadvantage of measuring blood flow through one hemisphere only. The advantages of this method are that it is rapid and accurate, and extracranial vascular function and blood flow can be excluded, thus providing the first clear information on hemispheric blood flow during migraine.

Using intracarotid xenon, in 1969 Skinhoj and Paulson noted that regional cerebral blood flow was reduced in one patient during an aura, while the angiogram was normal, suggesting that the alteration in blood flow was in vessels which were too small to be visualized angiographically. In another patient the regional cerebral blood flow increased during a migraine episode. Then in 1973 Skinhoj reported regional cerebral blood flow measurements in six patients during headache and in four during auras. During the painless preheadache experiences regional blood flow was markedly reduced, though not uniformly throughout the hemisphere, in all four patients. At times the regional blood flow fell to critical levels. Five of the six patients measured during the headache phase showed increased regional blood flow, the sixth being a patient who was hyperventilating so that cerebral blood flow could have been altered by absence of a steady state for carbon dioxide. Skinhoj noted that patients with increased blood flow during headache had decreased bicarbonate and increased lactate in the cerebral spinal fluid, suggesting intracranial acidosis, and he hypothesized that the vasoconstriction and the ischemia of the aura produced hypoxia and lactic acidosis which led thereafter to compensatory vasodilatation, both intracranial and extracranial.

Edmeads (1977) has measured regional cerebral blood flow in four patients with migraine and one with cluster headache, using the intracarotid xenon-133 technique with 16 extracranial probes. In four of the five patients cerebral blood flow declined during the migraine aura. In one patient it was normal. Edmeads felt that in this patient the aura was probably due to dysfunction of the occipital cortex supplied by the vertebral basilar system, which was not within the capacity of his system to measure. His patients had increased cerebral blood flow during headache, which he attributed to a compensatory response to the hypoxia of the aura. The distribution of the increased regional cerebral blood flow did not correlate with the location of headache. The increased blood flow was often bilateral even in strictly unilateral headaches. Ergotamine, when given intramuscularly, did not alter regional cerebral blood flow, which is a point of practical therapeutics, in that the traditional prohibition of this drug for patients with severe vasoconstrictor auras does not appear to be necessary, at least when the aura involves the territory supplied by the carotid arteries.

It seems evident, therefore, that the symptomatic manifestations of migraine reported by the patient do not correlate well with the alterations in blood flow observed in experimental studies. Further, disordered cerebral vasoreactivity may persist for prolonged asymptomatic periods as has been observed in Doppler studies.

F. Sakai and J. J. Meyer (1978) measured regional cerebral blood flow (rCBF) by the ^{133}Xe inhalation method in 71 patients with different types of headache and 32 age-matched normal controls.

During the headache phase, mean cerebral blood flow in a group of patients with classic and common migraine was significantly higher than that of a comparable group measured in the headache-free interval. Serial measurements made as the migraine headaches became more severe showed accompanying increases in the mean blood flow. In 24 patients with severe migraine studied 2–48 hr after the headache subsided, the blood flow values remained significantly increased compared with patients who were headache-free for six days or longer. Subsequent measurements made after the headache showed progressive reduction of cerebral blood flow values to normal within six days after the headache subsided. Reduction of the head pain by administering codeine decreased hemispheric rCBF values but did not change the high flow in the basilar artery territory. Conversely, administration of ergotamine did not change hemispheric flow

values but reduced rCBF in brainstem and cerebellar regions. Significant regional reductions of blood flow correlating with the neurological deficit were measured during the prodrome of classic migraine, and during the headache and postheadache intervals of complicated migraine.

During cluster headaches, mean rCBF values were also significantly increased and the extracerebral flow indices showed marked increases; these were at the site of the headache.

Sakai and Meyer concluded that cerebral hyperperfusion during migraine headaches is mainly due to postischemic reactive hyperemia.

Doppler Studies, Regional Blood Flow, and Migraine

We have had considerable experience in the use of the Directional Doppler study of the orbital circulation, and this procedure will be described in detail. We call it the *Doppler Ophthalmic Test* (DOT).

If patients experience occlusion, partial stenosis, or spasm of the internal carotid artery, there is almost always an increase in blood flow through collateral channels including the superficial temporal, facial, and angular branches of the external carotid artery which anastomose with terminal branches of the internal carotid. Blood will then flow in retrograde fashion through these arteries, through the ophthalmic artery, and into the internal carotid artery circulation. The direction of this flow can be assessed by compressing those branches of the external carotid artery which are accessible, particularly the superficial temporal artery. Thus, for example, if orbital flow decreases when the superficial temporal artery is compressed, it can be assumed that the internal carotid artery is either compromised, occluded, or in a state of persistent vasoconstriction, and that the external carotid artery is the major source of the collateral supply.

Several specific DOT patterns have been identified (Fig. 4-1). The normal record is characterized by augmentation of the supraorbital pulse upon temporal artery compression. The abnormal record is characterized by oblit-

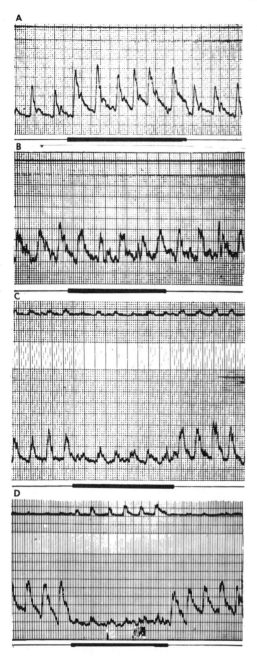

eration of the pulse during the temporal artery compression. Obliteration of the pulse is also seen in a third type of record but, in addition, a pulse appears in the channel recording flow away from the probe at the time of temporal artery compression. The fourth type of recording is termed inconclusive. Here there is no change in the supraorbital signal upon temporal artery compression.

Nine of 96 patients with vascular headaches were found to have an abnormal DOT, implying persistent alteration of blood flow in the internal carotid artery or its tributaries (Dalessio et al., 1978). In three of these cases, the DOT was abnormal on both sides. This finding was noted when patients were headache-free and it persisted in most patients with serial observations. Angiograms were normal. Bilaterally abnormal DOT's in a patient with hemiplegic migraine gradually reverted to normal when anovulatory drugs were discontinued. In order to evaluate the effect of vasoactive drugs on the DOT, five normal subjects and ten patients with vascular headaches (five with normal and five with abnormal DOT's) were studied after administration of amylnitrate, CO_2 by inhalation, and ergotamine tartrate. The abnormal DOT of one headache patient transiently returned to normal configuration with administration of amylnitrate. We interpret the abnormal DOT in a minority of migraine patients as evidence of persistent vasospasm in the carotid circulation.

Coupling the DOT with oral administration of nitroglycerin, Kaneko et al. (1978) have studied the intracerebral and extracerebral hemodynamics of migraine headaches. The headache produced by nitroglycerin is not, of course, strictly comparable with the naturally occurring migrainous episode. In particular, it lacks any preheadache or vasoconstrictor phenomena. After nitroglycerin administration the external carotid flow increased rapidly

FIG. 4-1. Doppler cerebral blood flow studies, supraorbital arterial pulse recordings. A, the record is normal. Note the augmentation of the supraorbital pulse upon temporary artery compression. B, the record is inconclusive. C, the record shows obliteration of the pulse during temporal artery compression, suggesting that the internal carotid artery on the same side is compromised. D, a similar finding, but here, in addition, a pulse appears in the channel recording flow away from the probe at the time of temporal artery compression, suggesting only partial obstruction of the internal carotid artery.

in migraine patients but did not increase in normal subjects, and the internal carotid flow decreased slightly in all subjects. The vertebral flow decreased significantly in seven patients who had neurologic symptoms in addition to headache.

Biochemical, Hematologic, and Hormonal Variable in Migraine

Though migraine is unquestionably a vasomotor phenomenon, it should be remembered that vasomotor disorders are not necessarily painful unless accompanied by ischemia or inflammation. This is no better illustrated than by the painless preheadache pheromena of migraine itself, wherein profound intracranial blood flow changes may occur without any pain whatsoever. Nor does a patient complain of head pain after overheating, prolonged exercise (although at high altitude this may occur), or after sitting in a tub of hot water. Yet extracranial vasodilation is obvious at these times. Thus, it has been suggested that the symptomatic manifestations of migraine (or as the patient appreciates it, the pounding headache associated with extracranial vascular dilation) are related to vasodilation associated with a sterile local inflammatory reaction. In other terms, it has been suggested that migraine is a clinical syndrome of self-limited neurogenic inflammation. Furthermore, when one begins to study inflammation, blood clotting, and complement system, and immune mechanisms cannot be avoided, for all these systems are intertwined and seemingly are included in migraine.

Inflammation begins with a series of cellular events. Usually an injury occurs, provoked by multiple factors including ischemia, the deposition of immune complexes, activation of Hageman factor, deposition of bacterial toxins, and possibly stress and/or higher nervous activity. Vasoactive amines such as histamine and serotonin are released from platelets, basophils, and tissue mast cells. Other tissues, when injured, may release prostaglandins. All increase vascular permeability. Serum components come in contact with extravascular proteins, modifying them. The complement cascade is stimulated. Fixation of complement, for example to immune complexes, attracts polymorphonuclear leukocytes which localize in the area. Upon rupture of their lysosomal membranes, a series of enzymes is elaborated. Kinins are produced when the coagulation system is activated. Prostaglandins are released by antigen/antibody reactions and by bradykinin; prostaglandins aggregate platelets, causing their disruption and increasing the concentration of vasoactive substances.

Present evidence implicates at least five groups of vasoactive substances associated with inflammation: (1) catecholamines, (2) other bioactive amines including histamine and serotonin, (3) the peptide kinins, (4) the prostaglandins, which are fatty acids, and (5) slow reactive substance (SRS-A), an acidic lipid.

All have potent biologic properties, such as: (1) contraction or relaxation of smooth muscle, (2) constriction or dilation of arteries and veins, (3) induction of water and sodium diuresis, (4) production of fever, (5) production of wheal and flare reactions, and (6) induction of pain, including headache.

The evidence for the role of vasoactive substances in migraine is fragmentary and can best be summarized as follows:

1. Serotonin levels in the plasma, which are related to platelet aggregation, fall at the onset of a migraine attack (Lance et al., 1967). Platelets of patients with migraine exhibit specific abnormalities, which will be discussed below. Serotonin constricts scalp arteries in man (Sicuteri, 1966). An increase in the major metabolite of serotonin, 5-hydroxyindole acetic acid (5HIAA), has been inconsistently demonstrated during migraine attacks (Curzon et al., 1966).

2. Local accumulation of a vasodilator polypetide, similar to bradykinin, can be demonstrated in the subsurface tissues of patients with migraine (Chapman et al., 1960).

3. Tyramine and phenylethylamine, found in certain foods, can evoke migraine in susceptible subjects (Smith et al., 1970; McCulloch and Harper, 1978). Tyramine liberates norepinephrine from tissues. A defect in the conjugation of tyramine has been reported in migraine patients which has genetic implica-

tions, since migraine is at least a familial if not a genetic disorder (Smith *et al.*, 1970).

4. Temporal arteries removed from humans during the painful stage of migraine have increased capacity to manufacture norepinephrine. Conversely, infusions of norepinephrine can be used to treat migraine (Ostfeld and Wolff, 1955).

5. Prostaglandins have not been measured in humans with migraine, but injections of prostaglandins may produce headache in susceptible subjects (Carlsen *et al.*, 1968).

6. In cluster headache, related to migraine, an increase in whole blood histamine levels has been demonstrated at the onset of an attack (Anthony and Lance, 1971). Injection of histamine and other vasodilators may provoke an attack in susceptible subjects with migraine and cluster headaches.

The prophylaxis of migraine has come to depend upon the use of drugs that inhibit vasodilating substances. These agents also tend to stabilize membranes and interfere with the chemical mediators of inflammation. Thus, for example:

1. Antihistamine and antiserotonin compounds interfere with the actions of vasoactive amines, or inhibit their elaboration from their respective depots.

2. Nonsteroidal antiinflammatory drugs, including aspirin and phenylpropionic acid derivatives, stabilize proteins and inhibit the formation of active prostaglandins from their precursors. Aspirin and other compounds will reduce platelet aggregation and indirectly affect the release of vasoactive substances. This will be discussed more fully below.

3. Corticosteroids reduce inflammation at several levels, enhance the vasoconstrictor actions of naturally occurring catecholamines, and stabilize lysosomal membranes.

4. Some of the antiinflammatory drugs such as butazolidin will interfere with kinin functions.

5. Some drugs have multiple effects. Ergot, for example, is both a vasoconstrictor and an alpha adrenergic blocker, and reduces vascular overactivity.

No single drug will inhibit all components of inflammation or vasomotor activity. Effective therapy may require the use of several. It seems evident that the specific antiserotonin activity of a compound has little to do with its efficacy in migraine. It simply is not enough to block the peripheral actions of serotonin alone and expect adequate migraine prophylaxis to be accomplished. Cyproheptadine, which blocks both serotonin and histamine is an example of a drug with multiple actions. Methysergide, advertized initially as a serotonin antagonist, has complex pharmacologic effects (Dalessio et al., 1961). It also blocks histamine indirectly by interfering with histamine liberators, at least *in vivo*. Furthermore, as suspected early on, it has significant vasoconstrictor properties. Recent studies in the dog have shown that it produces profound vasoconstriction of the external carotid artery (Saxena, 1972).

These results raise questions regarding the etiologic role of serotonin in the pathogenesis of migraine. The changes in the level of plasma serotonin observed before the onset of migraine probably represent only one aspect of the migraine process.

What seems likely is that histamine, serotonin, the plasma kinins and perhaps other vasoactive substances participate in a sterile inflammatory reaction involving painful and distended blood vessels. Such substances are, then, an integral but peripheral part of the migraine process, and certainly one part of the process which can be measured and toward which therapy can be directed. But they are important primarily in that part of the migraine episode wherein *an increase in vascular permeability occurs.*

Saxena (1972) has studied the effects of antimigraine drugs on the vascular responses of the external carotid bed of dogs. He found that both ergotamine and methysergide caused a dose-dependent decrease in the pulsations and blood flow of the external carotid artery without much increase in blood pressure, unless very large amounts of ergotamine were used. Methysergide did not effect the blood pressure but decreased the external carotid blood flow, thereby increasing resistance in the arterial tree. When cyproheptadine was given there were no appreciable changes elicited in the external carotid artery. Saxena concluded that ergotamine was more active than methysergide in increasing resistance in the external carotid bed of the dog, whereas cyproheptadine was without effect.

Saxena also studied the effects of 5-hydroxytryptamine (5HT) and noradrenalin on the same animal preparation. Injections of 5HT and noradrenalin caused vasoconstriction of the carotids, while histamine and bradykinin produced vasodilatation. Saxena concludes that the usefulness of the antimigraine drugs is not related to their antiserotonin action. The selective vasoconstriction elicited by ergotamine and to some extent by methysergide in the external carotid bed is a more likely explanation for their therapeutic effectiveness. Saxena suggests further that the central vasomotor depressant actions of methysergide and ergotamine, though they may be important in the prophylaxis of headache, may also be secondary to the flow changes discussed before.

Spira et al. (1978) have investigated the effects of antimigraine drugs on the cranial circulation of the monkey. They showed that the external carotid vasculature of the monkey is dilated by prostaglandins, bradykinin, histamine, and acetylcholine and is constricted by adrenalin, noradrenalin, serotonin, and other prostaglandins. In the internal carotid circulation, serotonin and prostaglandin F2 produced constriction, whereas bradykinin, histamine, and acetylcholine resulted in dilatation. These authors suggested that, with the exception of bradykinin, these humoral agents in normal circulating levels are unlikely to modify cranial vascular tone directly, although in pathologic states circulating levels may be sufficiently elevated to produce vascular effects.

Their results using antimigraine drugs at dose levels approximating those used clinically, suggest that the antagonism of cranial vascular effects of serotonin may be important in the antimigraine activity of methysergide and pizotifen (BC-105).

Spira et al. (1978) confirmed that intravenous ergotamine has a marked vasoconstrictor action in the external carotid territory, without a concomitant systemic vasopressor effect.

Welch et al. (1977) have investigated transient cerebral ischemia and brain serotonin with relevance to migraine. Their experimental model used Mongolian gerbils. The right common carotid artery of these animals was dissected and occluded by the application of two aneurysm clips. Some animals were sacrificed under liquid nitrogen. In others, the arterial clips were removed after 30 min of ischemia and reflow in the carotid artery was confirmed visually.

Serotonin levels were reduced in the occluded hemispheres and the contralateral nonoccluded hemispheres throughout ischemia. The levels remained reduced in both hemispheres during one hour of reperfusion. The authors suggest that depletion of serotonin may be responsible for some of the pain supersensitivity seen in the migraine syndrome. Sicuteri (1974) has also suggested that depletion of serotonin in the central nervous system is of fundamental importance in the migraine syndrome.

Sandler et al. (1974) have described a phenylethylamine oxidizing defect in migraine. McCulloch and Harper (1978) have shown that phenylethylamine will significantly reduce cerebral blood flow in migrainous patients. The threshold for this effect can be further reduced by inhibiting monoamine oxidase, type B. The cerebral circulation is unresponsive to systemically administered monoamines probably because of the existence of blood/brain mechanisms that limit the access of the monoamines to the brain. In contrast to serotonin, noradrenalin, and tyramine, phenylethylamine readily crosses the blood/brain barrier. It seems likely therefore that phenylethylamine, a constituent of many foods, can initiate migraine-type headaches in susceptible individuals.

Gamma-aminobutyric Acid (GABA) and Migraine

Welch and his colleagues (1976), have made biochemical comparisons between migraine and stroke. They measured gamma-aminobutyric acid (GABA) and 3',5'-cyclic adenosine monophosphate (cyclic AMP) in the cerebrospinal fluid (CSF) of patients with stroke and vascular headache of the migraine type. GABA was elevated in CSF of patients with recent onset of thromboembolic occlusive cerebrovascular disease (CVD) and within 48 hr of an attack of vertebral basilar ischemia (VBI). Similarly, GABA was elevated in CSF of all patients studied during a migraine attack but not in asymptomatic migraine patients or patients with muscle contraction (tension) headache. CSF cyclic AMP was also elevated in patients with recent onset of thromboembolic occlusive CVD and in patients studied during or within 48 hr of a migraine attack. Since the biochemical abnormalities reported herein were common to occlusive CVD and migraine headache, it seems probable that they are due to the ischemia associated with both conditions and possibly related to a resultant disorder of cerebral energy metabolism produced by anoxia.

Platelets and Platelet Antagonists

Recent studies suggest that there are abnormalities of aggregation of platelets in migraine patients which may be unrelated to the type of migraine (Couch, 1976). There is a significant increase in platelet aggregation during the preheadache phase of migraine, and this parallels the increase in plasma serotonin level during the headache prodromata (Deshmukh and Meyer, 1977). During the headache phase platelet aggregation and plasma serotonin fall. It seems likely that the alterations in platelet aggregation are responsible for the observed changes in the plasma serotonin levels, since, at least in humans, platelets contain virtually all of the total plasma serotonin. Couch and Hassanein (1977), could not correlate platelet hyperaggregability with the severity of migraine, but they do suggest that the platelet changes may help explain the increased incidence of stroke and coronary artery disease in migrainous patients reported elsewhere.

Pathophysiology of Platelet Aggregation and Its Prevention

Platelets aggregate in three waves (Mustard et al., 1972). Initially they stick to foreign substances, usually nonendothelial in character. A second wave of aggregation occurs immediately thereafter, associated with release of several platelet substances, including ADP (adenosine diphosphate), serotonin, platelet factor IV, and perhaps others, thus increasing the number of clumped platelets (Weiss, 1975). A third phase of platelet aggregation is related to the deposition of fibrin as a part of the clotting mechanism.

Platelet antagonists such as aspirin inhibit the agglutination response in several different ways (Majerus, 1976). They interfere with the initial phase of platelet aggregation to foreign substances, and they also inhibit activation of platelet factors III and IV and ADP in the second wave of platelet aggregation. Finally, aspirin interferes with the reaction whereby platelet arachidonic acid is transformed into several forms of prostaglandins, a reaction which may be critical to platelet aggregation. Interestingly, only the acetyl form of salicylic acid is affective in this activity. For example, sodium salicylate has no effect on platelet clumping (Weiss, 1978).

In addition to aspirin, a variety of other drugs are effective as platelet antagonists, including dipyridamole, sulfinpyrazone, and the phenylpropionic acids such as fenoprofen (Fig. 4-2). Many of these compounds interefere with prostaglandin actions. Others prevent ADP release in the second wave of aggregation. Most of those mentioned above are currently being evaluated in the prophylaxis of transient ischemic attacks, stroke, and coronary artery disease.

Our preliminary studies on the effects of platelet antagonists in the prophylaxis of migraine suggest that sulfinpyrazone and fenoprofen may be particularly effective in reducing the intensity and frequency of headache attacks. The well-established use of aspirin in various headache syndromes may in part be related to its effect upon platelets although it is, in addition, an analgesic drug. Substances which interfere with platelet aggregation thus provide yet another avenue for the prophylaxis of recurrent vascular headache.

Immunologic Events Including Allergic Reactions

The complex relationship of allergy to headache is a source of continuing confusion in

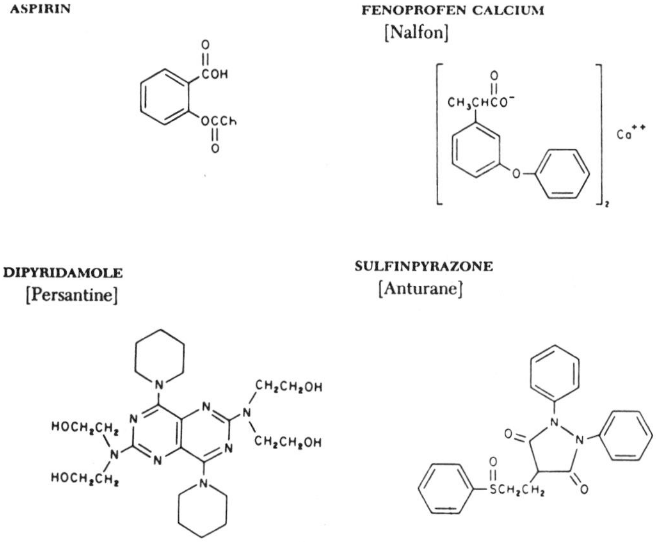

ASPIRIN

FENOPROFEN CALCIUM
[Nalfon]

DIPYRIDAMOLE
[Persantine]

SULFINPYRAZONE
[Anturane]

FIG. 4-2. Several useful platelet antagonists.

medicine. A wide range of hypotheses exists, ascribing allergy to a major, minor, or even non-existent role in the pathogenesis of headache. The problem has arisen in part from a lack of precision in definition. What sort of headaches are being described in patients who are also allergic? What is the relationship, if any, between these two very common disorders, allergies and headaches? (See Chapter 12.)

Allergic reactions may be divided into four types of hypersensitivity, as defined by Gell and Coombs (1968). Type I reactions are antigen/antibody immediate hypersensitive reactions, including allergic rhinitis, asthma, anaphylactic reactions to insect bites, and reactions to certain foods and drugs. In man, antigen combines with IgE, a unique immunoglobulin, to initiate mediator release from storage cells and thus, Type I reactions. In Type II hypersensitivity reactions, antigens are bound to the cell wall or cells, and cytotoxic or cytolytic reactions occur as a consequence of activation of complement. A prime example is hemolytic anemia. In Type III reactions, antigen and antibody form immune complexes and fix complement. Acute inflammation then occurs which may become chronic and frequently involves vascular endothelium or media. Serum

sickness is an example of this form of allergic reaction, as is vasculitis and nephritis. In Type IV delayed hypersensitivity reactions, antigen-sensitized lymphocytes react with antigens, producing chronic inflammation. Contact dermatitis is a classic example.

Although others choose to include nonimmunologic untoward "reactions," this is imprecise and diagnostically confusing, frequently leading to overutilization of immunologic diagnostic and therapeutic programs of symptoms not truly allergic in origin.

Migraine and Allergy

There is a long medical history of attempts to relate migraine to Type I or IgE-mediated immediate hypersensitivity reactions. For the most part these reports are anecdotal and appear in the older medical literature. Some obviously report dietary migraine, in which vasoactive substances are ingested in food which in turn directly stimulates cranial vascular spasm and headache in susceptible patients. This subject will be discussed later.

The best and most recent studies of the lack of relationship between the allergic state and migraine are those of Lance and Anthony (1966), Medina and Diamond (1976), and

Ziegler (1972). Lance and Anthony studied 500 patients with migraine and 100 with tension headaches at their hospital in Australia. Seventeen percent of the migraine patients were found to have allergic diseases including asthma, hay fever, hives, and eczema. Thirteen percent of patients with tension headaches had similar allergies. The allergy rates for the two groups are not statistically different nor do they vary from the incidence of allergic diseases in the general population. Ziegler studied 289 patients in a headache clinic and found no significant association between hay fever or asthma and migraine. Medina and Diamond surveyed 89 cases of migraine and 27 with muscle contraction headaches in whom serum IgE levels were obtained. Elevated serum IgE levels were found in 5.7% of migraine and 3.7% of muscle contraction headache patients, an incidence not significantly different from each other or the nonatopic general population. The authors concluded that migraine does not depend upon an IgE-mediated hypersensitivity reaction (Type I).

In addition, positive wheal and flare cutaneous reactions occur in about 20% of the asymptomatic, nonatopic general population, emphasizing that the presence of specific IgE antibodies (as detected by allergy skin testing) does not prove that IgE-mediated reactions are occurring at that time.

Finally, antihistamines which are quite effective in blocking the actions of histamine in allergic rhinitis and urticaria are not effective in the prevention of migraine headaches.

To summarize, it has not been possible to demonstrate that migraine results from a true antigen/antibody reaction, regardless of whether the antigen is an inhalant pollen, an injected material, or a food. There is no correlation between positive skin tests of various allergens and the appearance of migraine. Hyposensitization to presumed allergens is not indicated in the clinical treatment of migraine. Hives, allergic rhinitis, atopic eczema, bronchial asthma, and other manifestations of true Type I allergic reactions cannot be equated with the migraine episode. No well-controlled clinical study has yet shown that migraine headache is an allergic reaction or has proved that decreased migraine attacks occur during

prescribed diets which are due to elimination of offending food allergens.

Dietary Migraine

However, dietary migraine may occur, related to the ingestion of food containing vasoactive substances, including alcohol (Dalessio, 1972). Patients with cluster headache are notoriously sensitive to even small amounts of alcohol and they learn to avoid alcohol during the period of cluster headache recurrence. Alcohol is a nonspecific vasodilator, which probably accounts for its precipitation of the vascular headache process. The vasodilatation is assumed to result from depression or alteration of the central vasomotor centers, since the direct action of alcohol on blood vessels is insignificant. Moderate amounts of alcohol do not affect cerebral blood flow, but severe intoxication causes a significant increase in cerebral blood flow with diminished cerebrovascular resistance.

Foods which contain tyramine, a vasoactive amine, may precipitate headache, particularly in patients who are treated with monoamine oxidase (MAO) inhibitors (Hanington and Harper, 1968). Tyramine-rich foods include strong or aged cheese, pickled herring, chicken livers, canned figs, and the pods of broad beans. Recent studies have cast doubt on the importance of this finding, some confirming and some denying that ingestion of oral tyramine *without* MAO inhibitors may provoke headache in patients subject to migraine (Medina and Diamond, 1978).

We have adopted a pragmatic approach to this problem and suggest that those foods and beverages which have been shown to have vasoactive properties be eliminated from the diet of migraineurs (Table 4-1). Thus, our recommendations include avoidance of alcohol, particularly some wines which contain large amounts of histamine, aged or strong cheese, pickled herring, chicken livers, pods of broad beans, canned figs, and chocolate. We do not suggest avoidance of milk products. Large amounts of monosodium glutamate (MSG) may produce a generalized vasomotor reaction which may include headache (the Chinese restaurant syndrome) (Reif-Lehrer, 1976). Use of

TABLE 4-1 Dietary Suggestions for Headache Patients

1. No alcohol, particularly red wines and champagne.
2. No aged or strong cheese, particularly cheddar cheese.
3. Avoid chicken livers, pickled herring, canned figs, pods of broad beans.
4. Use monosodium glutamate sparingly.
5. Avoid cured meats such as hot dogs, bacon, ham, and salami, if these can be demonstrated to evoke vascular headache.
6. Eat three well-balanced meals per day. Avoid skipping meals, prolonged fasting, or excessive ingestion of carbohydrates at any single sitting.
7. Avoid chocolate.
8. Avoid fatty or fried foods.

(All of these foods contain vasoactive materials of varying types and all have, in specific circumstances, evoked headache in patients predisposed to headache.)

excessive amounts of monosodium glutamate is unwise.

Hypoglycemia

A word should be said about the quality and amount of food consumed by the patient with migraine. Hypoglycemia exerts a profound effect on the tone of the cranial blood vessels (Dexter *et al.*, 1978). If the sugar content of the blood is reduced by insulin or by other means, conspicuous cerebral vasodilatation occurs. Headache is a prominent symptom of insulin shock, for example. Furthermore, in migraine patients, the relative hypoglycemia produced by fasting may evoke typical vascular headaches. Even reactive hypoglycemia occurring after ingestion of an excessive carbohydrate load may precipitate vascular headache in a susceptible person. For these reasons we suggest that the patient with migraine eat three well-balanced meals a day and avoid an overabundance of carbohydrates at any single meal.

Other Dietary Studies

Medina and Diamond (1978) have conducted a prospective long-term dietary study. In order to determine the role of the diet in migraine, patients were randomly placed on three sequential diets: A, B, and C. Each diet was given for six weeks. During the dietary period A, the patients were allowed two items daily of a list of foods containing tyramine and other vasoactive substances. During diet B, they consumed tyramine-free foods and excluded tyramine-containing ones. During diet C, they ate and drank ad lib. At the end of the 18 weeks, the frequency, duration, and intensity of the headaches and the amount of symptomatic medication used during the three diets were compared. The results showed no significant difference with any particular diet.

Medina and Diamond also determined whether the headaches were time-locked to any specific food or fasting by evaluating, in all patients as a unit, the specific food scores. The scores were obtained by rating the headaches that occurred within 12 hr from the time of particular food ingestion and relating them to the total number of days that the specific food was consumed. Similarly, the fasting score was obtained by considering the headaches timelocked to fasting if they occurred during fasting after 6 hr during the day or 12 hr overnight without food consumption. The three maximum scores were reached by alcoholic drinks, chocolate, and fasting. The foodstuff with the highest tyramine content, aged cheese, had a low score similar to immature cheeses or hamburgers. Medina and Diamond conclude that diet is a relatively unimportant provoking factor in migraine except perhaps for alcoholic drinks, chocolate, and fasting.

Dexter, Roberts, and Byer (1978) also investigated the relationship between dietary habits and migraine. Over a three-year period the authors studied 222 new patients with migraine. Of these, 74 patients related many of their attacks to either fasting in midmorning or midafternoon, and were therefore evaluated with a 5-hr glucose tolerance test. Of 74 patients, six had a diabetic glucose tolerance test and 56 had reactive hypoglycemia, i.e., serum glucose less than 69 mg %, or a drop of 50 mg % within one hour.

All patients with either hypoglycemia or diabetic glucose tolerance curves were instructed in a 1,000–2,500 calorie diet with a protein: fat: carbohydrate ratio of 20:45:35 distributed in six feedings 2-1-2-1-2-1. The calories were calculated for weight maintenance or reduction, whichever was applicable. After dietary therapy the six patients with a diabetic glucose tolerance test showed improvement in headaches of greater than 75% and three were headache-free. Of 56 patients with reactive hypoglycemia, 43 returned after dietary instruction. Twenty-seven (63%) of the 43 showed greater than 75% improvement, 17 (40%), 15 to 75% improvement, and 4 (9%), 25 to 50% improvement.

The authors noted that this investigation has the difficulties inherent in a retrospective uncontrolled study, but they feel, nonetheless, that it is a basis for further prospective studies into the possibility that glucose intolerance is a trigger to migraine.

Immune Complex Disease and Headache

Lord and Duckworth (1977) have suggested that a Type III allergic reaction, that is, an immune-complex-mediated response, might account for some migraine phenomena which cannot be explained by a Type I response.

Serum complement components and immunoglobulins were measured in migraineurs. Patients were assigned to several groups: Group 1 (prodromal migraineurs), and Group 2 (nonprodromal). The latter group was subdivided into Group 2A (common) and Group 2B (with focal neurologic symptoms commencing after headache onset). In the immunoglobulin study: (1) Group 1 had an elevated IgA level, (2) Group 2A had elevated IgG and IgA, 2B elevated IgG, IgA, and IgM when compared with appropriate controls. The IgM in Group 2B was significantly higher than in Groups 1 and 2A, supporting the division of patients with focal neurologic symptoms into two groups.

The complement study compared patients during headache and when headache-free. The "in headache" patients were further subdivided into early and late groups. The complement results are from patients in Group 2 only. During headache, samples were obtained from 18 migraineurs. In nine patients,

headache-free specimens were collected enabling paired analysis of results.

Reductions in levels of complement components C_4 and C_5 in the paired study, and lower levels of C_4, during early headache in the unpaired study are evidence of complement activation associated with migraine. Demonstration of complement breakdown products in three patients at least three hours before headache onset, and absence of difference in component levels between headache-free and late headache migraineurs, indicates complement activation of short duration.

Lord and Duckworth mention that the elevated immunoglobulin levels and complement activation suggest a late-onset immune reaction of short duration. They propose that this mechanism provides an explanation for many of the features of nonprodromal migraines including platelet release of serotonin, basophil and mast cell degranulation, increased whole blood histamine during an attack, fluid retention, and an increased thrombotic tendency.

There may be similar processes operative in cranial (temporal) arteritis. Edgington and Dalessio have performed immunofluorescence microscopy on serial sections of temporal arteries in which typical cranial arteritis was found (see Chapter 10). The sections were cut in a transverse plane and demonstrated extensive but incomplete thrombotic occlusions of the arteries. Several areas of the intima were heavily laden with fibrinogen, gamma globulin, and other serum proteins. The disruption of the internal elastic lamella was easily recognized. The media was heavily infiltrated with plasma proteins, including fibrinogen and immunoglobulin G, as well as some of the complement components. At certain loci there were usually dense or lumpy deposits of immunoglobulin G with an increase in the first component of complement, C1q. This localization of immunoglobulin G and complement at the sites of arteritic injury was suggestive of an immunologically mediated arteritis.

Monoamine Oxidase and Fatty Acid Changes

A transitory but significant decrease in platelet monoamine oxidase activity was observed by Sandler (1975) during headache attacks in migrainous subjects, which reverted to normal during attack-free periods. This phenomenon did not stem from the action of drugs commonly used for the treatment of migraine.

The cause of the temporary decrease in platelet MAO activity during an attack is unknown. Whether this decrease contributes to the attack, or results from it, is unclear. As mentioned before, since there is a decrease in platelet serotonin content during migraine, it is conceivable that a relatively nonspecific circulating platelet-damaging agent appears briefly in the circulation during an attack.

Anthony (1976) suggests that free fatty acids (FFA) may release platelet serotonin *in vitro*. He has measured the four most commonly occurring acids in plasma: linoleic, oleic, palmitic, and stearic, using gas liquid chromatography in ten patients, before, during, and after a migraine attack. Total plasma FFA were also estimated in the same group of patients under similar circumstances.

Comparison of the preheadache and headache mean values, shows a marked rise of linoleic (135.8%), oleic (95.0%), and palmitic (80.9%) acids; this rise being less prominent with stearic acid (36.0%). Similar comparison of total plasma FFA shows a mean rise of 52%, the rise in both cases being statistically significant.

Since the highest elevation of plasma FFA during migraine occurs in the levels of unsaturated acids (linoleic and oleic), which are also the most potent releasers of platelet serotonin *in vitro*, he suggests that FFA play a role in serotonin release in migraine.

Hormones and Pregnancy

Kudrow (1975) finds that since migraine is a vasomotor disorder, and since estrogens alter vasomotor stability, an effect of estrogens on migraine is to be anticipated, particularly during the cyclical changes of the menstrual cycle. Headaches associated with menses (menstrual migraine) are characterized by decreasing estradiol levels, and menstrual migraine can be delayed by administering estradiol (Somer-

ville, 1972). In contrast, manipulation of blood progesterone levels does not effect menstrual migraine. Not unexpectedly then, in pregnancy, characterized by persistently high estrogen levels, remission of migraine almost always occurs.

There is an increased incidence in vascular headaches in young women using oral contraceptives, as well as an increased incidence of stroke. Some authorities feel that progressive migraine in a patient taking oral contraceptives is a harbinger of stroke. Those who continue to use oral contraceptives in this situation should be advised of the relative risk involved.

Are estrogens then useful in the clinical management of migraine? Only rarely, in the author's opinion, and then in women of menopausal age who experience excessive vasomotor phenomena. In general, it is best to avoid hormonal tinkering with the normal menstrual cycle of young women with migraine.

Cerebrovascular Alterations in Migraine
RESPONSE OF PREHEADACHE SCOTOMATA TO AMYL NITRITE AND CARBON DIOXIDE

To ascertain whether dysfunction of the cerebral vasculature is responsible for scotomata, a vasodilator agent, amyl nitrite, known to affect cerebral vessels, was employed by Wolff and colleagues. It is justifiable to infer that cerebral vasodilatation induced without a fall in blood pressure increases cerebral blood flow, whereas a sharp drop in blood pressure, regardless of the state of the cerebral arteries, decreases the cerebral blood flow. Symptoms due to cerebral vasoconstriction should be overcome by cerebral vasodilatation in the presence of a sustained normal level of blood pressure, but they should be augmented by a fall in blood pressure with accompanying decrease in cerebral blood flow. The experiments to be described were based on these two potential actions of the vasodilator drug amyl nitrite.

Method. The subject's preheadache scotomata lasted approximately 40 to 45 min. For the most part, visual fields were charted with a standard perimeter, though the subject was sufficiently familiar with

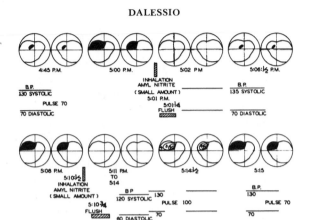

FIG. 4-3. Effect of inhaling a small amount of amyl nitrite on preheadache scotomata in a subject with migraine. The amount was insufficient to cause a drop in blood pressure or "lightheadedness."

perimetric methods to be able to chart his visual fields on an improvised screen. In the absence of scotomata, the subject familiarized himself with the effect of amyl nitrite and prepared for two experiments. (1) He learned to inhale just enough amyl nitrite to induce a head flush without appreciable change in blood pressure. Under such circumstances no "lightheadedness" or syncope occurred, though slight headache and pulse acceleration did. (2) By rapidly inhaling larger amounts of amyl nitrite he caused a precipitous fall in blood pressure, with lightheadedness. Nevertheless, it remained possible for him under these circumstances to define accurately his visual fields. The following results are representative of the two types of experiment.

Experiment 1. The subject noted a quadrantic defect at 4:45 P.M. (Fig. 4-3). By 5 P.M. this quadrantic defect became a complete right upper quadrant defect. In the manner just described, a small amount of amyl nitrite was inhaled at 5:01 P.M. Fifteen seconds later the subject experienced a flush, and by 5:02 P.M. visual defects had entirely disappeared. The blood pressure, which had been 130 systolic and 70 diastolic, remained approximately the same for the next 4 min. By 5:06½ P.M., or 4½ min after the disappearance of the defect, it began to return, and within a minute and a half the visual defect had returned to its former size. At 5:10½ P.M. the experiment was repeated. Again small amounts of amyl nitrite were inhaled, and 15 sec after inhalation came the flush, which was soon followed by complete disappearance of the visual defect. Blood pressure dropped very slightly, and the pulse rate accelerated from 70 to 100. At 5:14½ P.M. the visual defect began to return in the manner indicated in the figure,

beginning at the center and progressing peripherally. By 5:15 P.M., or within half a minute, the visual defect had again returned. Examination of the fundus before and during the visual defect revealed no change in the appearance of the retina or retinal vessels. During the action of amyl nitrite all the retinal vessels were dilated.

Experiment 2. The subject first noted a right lower quadrantic field defect at 7:25 P.M. After initial blood pressure readings he inhaled repeatedly and deeply of amyl nitrite. Within 10 sec the subject experienced the flush, and soon thereafter the visual fields became normal. Three seconds later multiple visual field defects became manifest, and within 15 to 20 sec of the beginning of inhalation the subject complained of feeling faint and said that only central vision remained. At this point the blood pressure was so low that an accurate reading could not be made. Within about a minute the blood pressure had again risen to 130 systolic and 70 diastolic, the visual fields had again lost all defects and the subject was no longer lightheaded. Within 3 min a quadrantic defect began to manifest itself—now, however, in the right upper quadrant. Within a minute this had become larger, and within 2 min it obliterated the right upper quadrant (Fig. 4-4).

Comment. It is apparent from these experiments that cranial vasodilatation associated with a sustained normal level of blood pressure caused symptoms to disappear, whereas a procedure that decreased cranial blood flow caused the symptom to become worse. From this it may be deducted that cranial vaso-

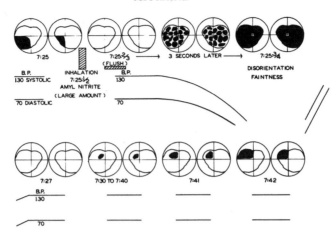

FIG. 4-4. Effect on preheadache scotomata of inhaling a larger amount of amyl nitrite. Here a sufficient amount was inspired to cause an abrupt fall in blood pressure, with amblyopia and faintness.

constriction was responsible for the visual defect in this patient with migraine. It is also likely that the cause of the visual defect was not in the retina or orbit but within the cranial cavity.

There are several reasons for making the latter inference. First, during an attack there was sparing of central vision. Second, homonymous quadrantic defects could readily result from a single defect in the visual cerebral cortex, whereas it would be necessary to postulate a bizarre arrangement of multiple defects in the retina. Third, the progression of the scotomata from center to periphery also suggests cortical involvement, since such a defect could result from occlusion of the branches of the posterior cerebral arteries, causing ischemia of the most peripheral portions of the artery's blood supply, namely, that area near the occipital pole and spreading ultimately to involve the areas more anterior. If the defect resulted from retinal ischemia, the opposite would hold. Hence it is inferred that visual preheadache phenomena result from dysfunction of cerebral vessels, in contrast to the headache phenomena which result mainly from dilatation of extracerebral vessels, and which will be considered below. Very careful studies of the progression of scotomata were made by Lashley (1941) and further suggest that cortical disturbances are the basis of the defects.

Effects of Carbon Dioxide—Oxygen Mixtures Given during the Preheadache Phase of the Migraine Attack

In an attempt to study the vasoconstrictor phase further, a number of patients were given carbon dioxide by inhalation in New York Hospital. Carbon dioxide was used in these studies, primarily because it is known to exert a potent vasodilator influence on cerebral arteries. In their reactions to carbon dioxide, the cerebral vessels are sensitive, as well as prompt, and the magnitude of their response is great. All sizes of vessels in all parts of the brain respond to the drug. Second, carbon dioxide itself does not produce headache, as does histamine administered intravenously. Third, carbon dioxide is a physiologic agent and appears to play an integral part in the normal vasoregulatory mechanism of the head. A fourth consideration in its selection is the important fact that it is simple to administer and is easy for the patient to accept.

Method. Carbon dioxide in 10% concentration was administered by face mask to recumbent patients for three periods of 5 min each. Five to 15 min was allowed between trials to permit observation of the effects of the procedure and to allow the patient to rest after the exertion of the profound hyperventilation produced. The same technique was used in each experiment. If no effect was obtained after three trials, the procedure was discontinued. Mixtures of 10% carbon dioxide in air and of 10% carbon dioxide with 90% oxygen were used in these experiments. The mixture used was not known to the patient. The pulse and blood pressure remained within the range of normal throughout all the trials.

The carbon dioxide mixtures were administered during one of three phases of the migraine attack: during the vasoconstrictor stage before the headache, during the interval when vasoconstrictor phenomena overlapped the painful, vasodilator phase, and when the headache alone was present.

Observations. A total of 25 trials were carried out on 15 patients. In five instances only vasoconstrictor phenomena were present. In these, carbon dioxide-air mixtures produced transient clearing of the visual disturbances, with return of symptoms to their former intensity within five minutes after inhalation of the gas was discontinued. When the carbon dioxide-air combination was followed by the carbon dioxide-oxygen mixture similar amounts or when the carbon-dioxide-oxygen mixture was used alone, vision cleared completely and remained so. The expected headache did not follow.

One subject experienced extreme sleepiness and nausea as preheadache manifestations. Ordinarily these disappeared as the headache developed. During inhalation of the carbon dioxide-oxygen mixture the patient became alert; nausea disappeared in less than the usual interval, and the expected headache did not follow. When headache was present, the results were so unpredictable that no conclusions could be drawn. Except in one subject, the headache was not increased by the procedure.

Comment. From these experiments two inferences may be drawn: First, a powerful physiologic intracranial vasodilator, carbon dioxide, is effective in decreasing or abolishing the intracranial vasoconstrictor phenomena of the migraine attack. Second, oxygen when used in conjunction with carbon dioxide makes these effects more pronounced and may prevent the progression of the attack.

The effect of carbon dioxide-oxygen mixtures observed here is similar to, but more pronounced than, the effect of oxygen when used alone, as reported by others (Alvarez, 1934). Furthermore, the effects on the preheadache phenomena are more predictable. The results as regards the termination of already existing headache were no more predictable than those reported by Alvarez. The

latter pointed out that the therapeutic effect in his series appeared to be better when oxygen was administered early in the attack. In his series, complete relief was noted in 42% of patients with "apparently typical migraine" and 44% were helped. He found that 100% oxygen had to be inhaled for periods ranging from 15 to 120 min to produce these effects.

The superiority of the combination of carbon dioxide and oxygen may rest on a dual effect. Inhalation of carbon dioxide in 10% concentration alone was found to double the cerebral blood flow in one series. Kety and Schmidt (1946) reported that 5.7% carbon dioxide produced a 75% increase in blood flow as measured by the nitrous oxide technique. It is therefore postulated that the greatly increased amount of blood which is maximally saturated with oxygen corrects an underlying oxygen deficiency in a strategic area of the brain, where the neural impulses which set up the compensatory vascular dilatation of the migraine attack may originate. This postulation fits into the broader concept that the stage of painful vasodilatation is an attempt on the part of the organism to restore cranial circulatory homeostasis.

Although these experiments have not shown that the use of carbon dioxide-oxygen mixtures is entirely predictable in its effects, they indicate that the migraine attack can sometimes be interrupted before the headache develops. Further, they suggest that vasoconstriction is a feature of the type of attack studied and may persist into the period of painful vasodilatation.

The Study of Bulbar Conjunctival Vessels during the Preheadache Phase

The small vessels of the bulbar conjunctivae were studied during the preheadache phase of the migraine syndrome by means of an opthalmic slit lamp at a magnification of 47.5× and appropriate photographs made. The observation that the conjunctival vessels were very often involved in migraine as well as the ready accessibility of this vascular bed suggested that a visual and pharmacologic examination of these vessels would serve further to elucidate the pathophysiology of the pre-headache and headache phenomena (Ostfeld and Wolff, 1957).

The approximate caliber of arterioles and venules, the number of patent capillaries, the intrinsic rhythmic activity and the periodic interruption of flow of arterioles, the approximate rate of flow, and the presence or absence of sludging of blood were observed. The sensitivity of the arterioles and minute vessels to the topical application of norepinephrine, a potent vasoconstrictor agent with minimal metabolic effects, and to acetylcholine was assayed. These agents were in earlier experiments dissolved in sterile 5% dextrose in water, and in later experiments in an isotonic phosphate buffer at a pH of 7.4 and were used immediately after preparation. The concentration required in the case of norepinephrine to blanch capillaries and in the case of acetylcholine to produce significant increase in the diameter of arterioles was called the sensitivity.

As will be described later, no defect in the bulbar conjunctival vessels could be detected during the headache-free periods between attacks.

Seven patients were studied just before and at intervals of several hours preceding the headache attack. In five of these seven subjects, the appearance and behavior of these minute vessels were normal. Specifically, the rate of flow was moderately rapid, there was no sludging, and minimal periodic interruption of flow. The sensitivity to norepinephrine was in the range of 1:50,000 to 1:100,000 and to acetylcholine 1:400 to 800 (two subjects were tested with acetylcholine, all with norepinephrine). In two subjects, however, there was arteriolar constriction, sludging, an increased rate of rhythmic interruption of flow, and the norepinephrine sensitivity increased to 1:200,000 and 1:400,000. Acetylcholine was not used in either of these subjects. These observations support the inference that in many subjects an euvascular state in the cranial vessels is usual during the interval between and even shortly before migraine attacks.

In the subject examined while she was experiencing unilateral scotomata, there were on the side of the scotomata 4+ arteriolar spasm, 3+ rhythmic interruption of arteriolar flow with 1:6000,000 morepinephrine which was required to blanch capillaries. The scotoma-free eye showed 3+ arteriolar

spasm and 3+ rhythmic interruption of arteriolar flow with 1:300,000 topical norepinephrine blanching capillaries. This degree of bulbar conjunctival ischemia and sensitivity to topical norepinephrine was unusual and not exhibited by this subject during scotoma-free periods.

Although cranial vasoconstriction does not invariably precede the subsequent migraine type of vascular headache, an attempt was made to ascertain whether there might be a causal relationship between the preheadache vasoconstriction and the subsequent cranial vasodilatation of migraine. Norepinephrine was infused intravenously at rates which caused conjunctival minute-vessel ischemia and a high degree of extracranial artery narrowing. Although such infusions were continued for periods up to three hours in four persons subject to headache, no headache occurred after cessation of infusion. Hence it is unlikely that the painful vasodilatation of headache is an inevitable sequel of or reaction to previous ischemia. Apparently another element must be present.

State of Bulbar Conjunctival Vessels during the Migraine Headache

The appearance and behavior of the small vessels of the bulbar conjunctivae were studied in 33 patients during the headache attack. At onset of headache there was almost invariably dilatation of arterioles and venules and an increase in the number of visible capillaries on the headache side as compared with the headache-free side (Fig. 4-5). When dilatation was great, a slowing of flow with sludging occurred. On five occasions small hemorrhages were noted along the course of dilated venules. During periods of conjunctival vascular dilatation there was haziness of the conjunctival tissues and an indistinctness of vascular structure which was compatible with and probably due to conjunctival edema. At these times the complaints of a burning sensation in the eye were most prominent. The sensitivity of vessels of the bulbar conjunctivae on the side of the headache as compared with that on the headache-free side to the topical application of norepinephrine solutions was ascertained. Sensitivity was assayed by defining that concentration of norepinephrine in diluent which produced a blanching of capillary beds. In nine subjects who seldom

Right Eye    Left Eye

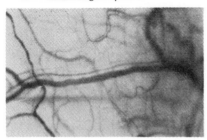   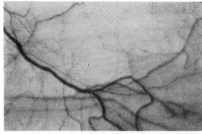

FIG. 4-5. Contrast in appearance of vascular structures in right and left bulbar conjuctivae during right-sided headache. Conjunctival vessels in the eye on the headache side are increased in diameter and exhibit great tortuosity. On inspection through the slit-lamp the walls of these vessels are "blurred," there are relatively few red cells within their lumina, and blood flow is slow.

had headaches, the usual range of sensitivity was 1:50,000 to 1:100,000. In the interval between headache in patients subject to migraine headache the sensitivity ranged from 1:37,500 to 1:100,000. The changes that occurred during the preheadache period have already been discussed (Ostfeld and Wolff, 1955).

During the headache, the sensitivity fell in both bulbar conjunctivae. It fell especially on the side of the headache with values ranging from 1:5,000 to 1:25,000, and a fall of lesser degree occurred in the contralateral eye with values varying between 1:10,000 to 1:50,000. Although the threshold values in headache-free intervals and during headache varied from patient to patient, the fall in sensitivity predictably occurred at the beginning of those headaches in which vasodilatation was present (Fig. 4-6).

A 2½% cortisone ophthalmic suspension was topically applied to the bulbar conjunctivae in an attempt to ascertain whether augmentation of the effect of norepinephrine could be produced in these minute vessels. Cortisone, while in itself not changing vessel caliber, increased vascular sensitivity to norepinephrine approximately twofold in both headache and headache-free subjects.

The bulbar conjunctivae of two patients with "atypical facial neuralgia" were examined during attacks of pain. There was dilatation of the vascular structures on the side of the pain. In one of these patients, a concentration of 1:5,000 norepinephrine topically applied on the side of the pain was required to blanch capillaries, thus demonstrating a great reduction of sensitivity of the vessels of the bulbar conjunctivae.

Whereas seven headache-free and six headache

subjects showed an acetylcholine sensitivity of 1:200 to 1:800 during the interval between headache attack and in the headache-free eye during attack, the eye on the side of headache exhibited a sensitivity of 1:800 to 1:600 during such attacks.

Bulbar conjunctival minute vessels during headache are less readily constricted and more easily dilated than during headache-free periods. This supports the theory that the vasodilatation is an active process maintained by the local effects of a pain-threshold-lowering and vasodilatating substance or substances whose actions are antagonized directly by norepinephrine and indirectly by cortisone. The nature of these agents is still undefined; but it is unlikely that histamine is relevant, since 50 mg diphenhydramine hydrochloride (benadryl) given intravenously, and tripellenamine administered topically, just before the onset of two attacks, modified the subsequent headache and function of the bulbar conjunctival vessels in no way.

Dilatation of conjunctival vessels similar in appearance to that observed in patients having vascular headache of the migraine type was produced experimentally in three subjects by two methods.

The local application of soap emulsion in one eye was followed by marked vasodilatation, tears, and pain. The dilated arterioles were only one-third to one-half as sensitive to topical norepinephrine as they were in the unirritated control eye. Local cortisone pretreatment of the irritated eye was associated with a partial restoration of sensitivity to norepinephrine in two subjects.

Vasodilatation of the conjunctival vessels of one eye was produced by inhalation of ammonium carbonate through one nostril while

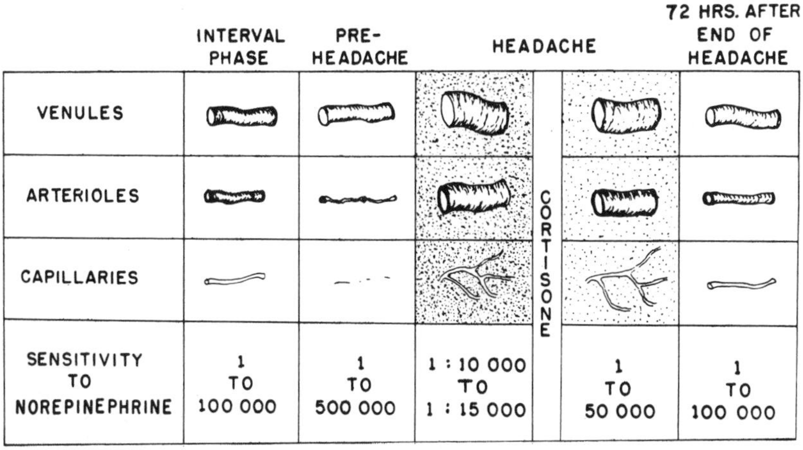

	INTERVAL PHASE	PRE-HEADACHE	HEADACHE		72 HRS. AFTER END OF HEADACHE
VENULES					
ARTERIOLES				C O R T I S O N E	
CAPILLARIES					
SENSITIVITY TO NOREPINEPHRINE	1 TO 100 000	1 TO 500 000	1 : 10 000 TO 1 : 15 000	1 TO 50 000	1 TO 100 000

FIG. 4-6. Schematic representation of function and sensitivity to topical norepinephrine of bulbar conjunctival blood vessels on side of migraine headache.

both eyes were kept closed to prevent direct stimulation. In this experiment, vasodilatation occurred reflexly as a result of noxious stimulation of afferent fibers in the nasal mucosa. The threshold sensitivity of such dilated arterioles to topical norepinephrine was reduced by one-third to one-half as compared with those of the control eye. Sensitivity to norepinephrine following the application of cortisone was partially restored.

Comment. These results paralleled those seen in chemical irritation and in vascular headache of the migraine type. It seemed possible that local dilatation of minute vessels in migraine headache might be due to reflex effects of noxious stimulation from the large and painfully involved arteries. However, on five occasions, observations in patients with severe muscle-contraction headache have revealed unilateral or bilateral constriction of conjunctival vessels. It was more likely, therefore, that the local dilatation of minute vessels occurred as a part of the migraine attack rather than as a reflex consequence of pain in the head (Ostfeld et al., 1957).

A small proportion of the migraine type of vascular headache is associated with more malignant ocular manifestations. Dunning's (1942) review discusses two cases in which hemorrhage occurred into the retina and/or optic nerve. On 23 occasions, we have observed hemorrhagic accumulations in the frontal or temporal areas of the scalp late in the course of severe attacks. One of the patients who experienced scalp hygromata also bled on two occasions from dilated conjunctival vessels during headache. We have also studied a young man who on four occasions, each time in association with a migraine headache attack, experienced hemorrhage into the vitreous humor of the eye with resultant decrease in visual function.

THE PATHOPHYSIOLOGY OF HEADACHE IN THE MIGRAINE SYNDROME
Analysis of Headache by the Action of Ergotamine Tartrate

Ergotamine tartrate is known to terminate migraine headache attacks. With this effective tool the attack can be sufficiently shortened to permit convenient analysis of certain changes that take place in the transition from the peak to the termination of the headache. Because ergotamine tartrate predominantly affects smooth muscle, inquiry concerning its action during migraine headache was centered on the cranial blood vessels. The following experiments by Graham and Wolff (1938) were performed when the phenomena which characterize the onset of an attack, namely, scotomata, blurring of vision, paresthesias, and aphasia, had already passed and had been supplanted by headache. Hence these results have no bearing on preheadache phenomena. They concern only the origin of migraine pain.

Material. Experimental analyses were made during 52 attacks of migraine occurring in 22 subjects. Fifty series of observations and records were made on 46 volunteer control subjects.

Method. Pulsations of the temporal and occipital branches of the external carotid artery were recorded by means of tambours placed on these arteries where they could be palpated under the skin.

In the same way, pulsations of the intracranial and intravertebral arteries, as reflected in the spinal fluid, were recorded by means of a Frank capsule connected directly with a needle in the lumbar subarachnoid space. A timer was so arranged that it recorded intervals of seconds on bromide paper, thus permitting determinations of pulse rate. Blood pressure readings were made at frequent intervals, and in ten experiments the skin temperatures of the ear, cheek, temple, and hand were measured by a Hardy radiometer.

Changes in the intensity of the headache were estimated by the patient and recorded in terms of "plusses," with the understanding that 10+ represented the "most severe" headache. The patient allotted a suitable number of 'plusses' to the intensity of his pain at the beginning of the period of observation and subsequently reported in terms of "plusses" such changes in intensity as took place. The subject rested comfortably on a couch, and at least three records of the amplitude of pulsations of the arteries were made at intervals of several minutes, to obtain suitable measurements as controls. With each control measurement the subject was asked to estimate the intensity of his headache in terms of 'plusses,' and simultaneously blood pressure readings were taken.

Experimental Results

1. *Relation of Headache to the Effect of Ergotamine Tartrate on Certain Branches of the External Carotid Artery.* After the observations made as controls, ergotamine tartrate (from 0.37 to 0.5 mg) was injected intravenously and, as already described, records of the pulsations of the temporal or the occipital artery on the affected side were made at frequent intervals until the headache was abolished. In 20 such experiments the injection of ergotamine was followed by decrease in amplitude of the pulsations. The maximal reduction was 84% of the

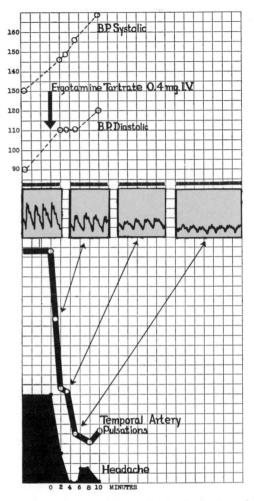

Fig. 4-7. Relation of the amplitude of pulsations of the temporal artery to the intensity of headache after administration of ergotamine tartrate. The sharp decrease in the amplitude of pulsations following injection of ergotamine closely paralleled the rapid decrease in intensity of the headache. Representative sections of the photographic record are inserted. The average amplitude of pulsations for any given minute before and after administration of ergotamine was ascertained by measuring the individual pulsations from the photographic record. The points on the heavy black line represent these averages, expressed as percentages. The initial or "control" amplitude was taken as 100%.

original amplitude, the minimal 18%, and the average approximately 50%. This drop usually began immediately, but in some instances its onset was delayed for from ten to 15 min. The

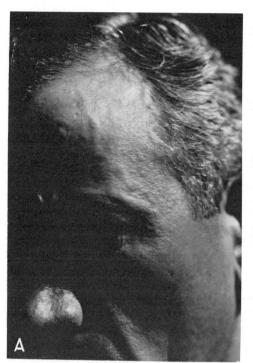 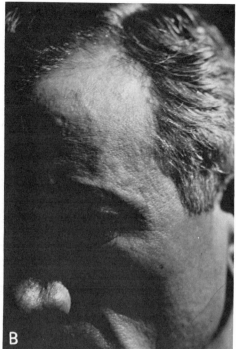

Fig. 4-8. Appearance of the temporal artery before and after termination of migraine headache by ergotamine tartrate. Photograph A was taken while the patient was suffering from a left-sided migraine headache. The temporal arteries stood out clearly. Photograph B was taken under identical conditions 20 min later. In the interim the patient had received ergotamine tartrate (1.4 mg) intravenously, and his headache had been abolished. The temporal vessels were then much less prominent. (Fig. 4-7 is the record of the changes in the amplitude of pulsations of the temporal artery in the subject.)

maximum drop was obtained in from about 30 to 40 min in most instances.

This marked decrease in the amplitude of the temporal or occipital pulsations bore a close relation to the decline in the intensity of the headache. In 16 of the 20 experiments the amplitude of pulsations declined with the diminishing intensity of the headache. If the amplitude of pulsations decreased slowly, headache likewise diminished slowly. If the amplitude dropped precipitously, the headache was ended promptly.

Similar observations made on a group of 34 control subjects showed an almost identical reduction in amplitude of pulsations of the temporal artery, average 52% (see Fig. 4-7).

Nevertheless, to determine directly whether ergotamine tartrate constricted the superficial temporal and occipital vessels, they were photographed during and after attacks under identical conditions. Figure 4-8 shows such photographs. In A, taken when the headache was maximal, the temporal artery stands out prominently. B was taken 20 min after ergotamine tartrate (0.4 mg) had been given intravenously. It is apparent that the artery was less prominent. (A record of the changes in the amplitude of pulsations in this subject is shown in Fig. 4-7.) Likewise, direct observation in man on the middle meningeal artery (a branch of the external carotid artery) during a craniotomy revealed a decrease of approximately 20% in the diameter of the artery following the intravenous injection of 0.5 mg of ergotamine tartrate.

2. *Relation of Headache to the Effects of Er-*

gotamine Tartrate on Branches of the Internal Carotid Arteries. The amplitude of pulsations of the intracranial and intravertebral arteries, reflected in the cerebrospinal fluid, was observed in five patients during five attacks of migraine headache and their subsequent abolition. In two of these subjects, after injection of ergotamine there was an initial decrease in the amplitude of pulsations, followed by an increase of a variable extent. In the other three subjects the initial decrease was not observed, and only an increase was evident. In no instance could a correlation be established between the amplitude of the cerebrospinal fluid pulsations and the state of the headache. Although the intensity of the headache steadily declined, the pulsations might be larger or smaller than during the control period.

In a series of 28 subjects used as controls, the effect of ergotamine on pulsations of the cerebrospinal fluid was also observed to be inconstant.

3. *Effects of Ergotamine Tartrate on Cerebrospinal Fluid Pressure.* Measurements were made of the cerebrospinal fluid pressure in four subjects during four attacks of migraine headache and their abolition. In three instances the pressure was between 130 and 160 mm of saline solution during maximal headache. In none of the four subjects did the termination of the headache by means of ergotamine have any significant effect on the pressure. The average rise in pressure after the injection was about 20%, but in no case was there correlation between the change in pressure and the state of the headache. The pressure was the same at the end of the experiment, when the headache had ended, as it was at the beginning, when the headache was severe. Similar observations were made in 13 control subjects.

4. *Effects of Ergotamine Tartrate on Blood Pressure, Pulse Rate, Pulsations of the Radial Artery, and Skin Temperature.* After the administration of ergotamine tartrate, the average rise in blood pressure in 60 subjects was about 20%. There was no appreciable difference between the responses of the migraine group and those of the control group.

The average decline in the pulse rate in 52 patients was 18%. Here, too, there was no significant difference between the responses of the two groups.

In ten of the control subjects records were made of the amplitude of pulsations of the radial artery by the method already described for the temporal artery. In this small group of subjects the amplitude of pulsations of the radial artery showed an average reduction of 38%.

In three patients with migraine and seven subjects without headache, the skin temperature of the ear and cheek showed a change of no more than 1°C (1.8×F). In one control subject the skin temperature of the hand rose 10°C (18×F).

Comment. The slowing of the pulse, the slight rise in the pressure of the blood and the cerebrospinal fluid, and the state of the headache observed here are in accord with the findings of other investigators (Pool *et al.*, 1936). The maintenance of the skin temperature at a fairly constant level, despite constriction of the arteries, may be attributed to a concomitant rise in the systemic arterial blood pressure sufficient to compensate for the local cutaneous vasoconstriction (Lennox *et al.*, 1935, 1937).

5. *Effects of Ergotamine on Perception and Reflex Activity.* In no instance was the perception of touch, temperature, or superficial or deep pain affected by ergotamine tartrate.

Dilation of the pupil as the result of pinching the skin of the neck was as readily obtained in ten subjects at the height of the ergotamine action as it was before this agent had been given.

6. *Effect of increasing the intracranial pressure:* In six subjects spinal puncture was performed during an attack of migraine headache.

Method. The cerebrospinal fluid pressure was varied by progressively increasing the height of the fluid column from 0 (at the level of the spinal canal) to from 700 to 1000 mm in stages, several minutes between each successive increase being allowed for adjustments in pressure to occur. To reduce pressure, the level of the solution of sodium chloride was dropped to that of the spinal canal, and at the termination of the experiment fluid was allowed to flow freely from the subarachnoid space.

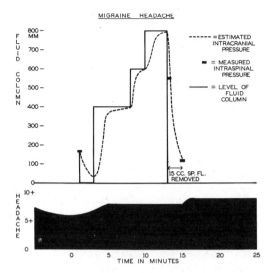

MIGRAINE HEADACHE

----- = ESTIMATED INTRACRANIAL PRESSURE

■ = MEASURED INTRASPINAL PRESSURE

— = LEVEL OF FLUID COLUMN

15 CC. SP. FL. REMOVED

FIG. 4-9. Failure of induced increase in the intracranial pressure to diminish the intensity of an attack of migraine headache.

Results. In six of the subjects no change in the intensity of the migraine headache occurred after increasing subarachnoid pressures to the kevek if 700 to 1000 mm of solution of sodium chloride for 15 to 30 min (Fig. 4-9). In one of these six subjects, a woman aged 33, with recurrent attacks of severe hemicrania for 20 years, hypertension of a mild degree (165 systolic and 100 diastolic to 180 systolic and 120 diastolic) had developed within the preceding six months.

The fact that increased intracranial pressure abolishes cluster headache and has no effect on migraine headache is evidence that the former emanates mainly from intracranial, the latter mainly from extracranial, vessels, at least in many subjects.

If one speaks of vasomotor changes in migraine it is, of course, important to realize that in considering vasoconstriction or vasodilatation, the false impression is created that peripheral vascular resistance is a simple or single physiologic entity, whereas it is well known that the peripheral vascular bed is a sequence of different vascular sections having specialized functions and reacting differently to various physiologic and pharmacologic stimuli. This is perhaps best illustrated with

respect to ergot compounds, many of which have an amphoteric action. That is, they elicit vasoconstriction at low vascular tonicity and vasodilatation at high vascular tonicity. The point of transition between these two reactions is called the "inversion point" and this inversion point is different for various ergot compounds which are tested. Some ergot compounds consistently induce vasodilatation and some always cause vasoconstriction, but most of the common ones in use, such as ergotamine tartrate and methysergide, do show this amphoteric action. There is no correlation between the inversion point and the magnitude of the vasoconstrictor or vasodilator effects of the ergot alkaloids. There is no relationship between their alpha-adrenergic blocking activity and their inversion point.

Many of the ergot drugs will significantly increase the amount of noradrenalin available to maintain vascular tone. On the other hand, methysergide has no effect on noradrenalin uptake. Ergot compounds inhibit serotonin uptake and will prevent the fall in plasma serotonin which is thought to occur at the onset of a migraine attack. Tricyclic compounds such as BC-105 and Periactin also clearly inhibit the uptake of noradrenalin and serotonin, thus maintaining high blood levels of the vasoconstrictor mines and altering the reduction of vascular tone which may lead to the migraine attack.

Fluctuations in Cranial Arterial Tone in Patients Subject to Vascular Headache of the Migraine Type

Graham and Wolff (1938) noted, when histamine was administered to a subject just after a severe headache had been eliminated by ergotamine tartrate, that the headache transiently recurred, especially on the side that had previously been involved in the migraine attack, associated with an increase of amplitude of temporal artery pulsation. McNaughton (1937) confirmed this observation and supplemented it by noting on several occasions that histamine given during a unilateral migraine headache exaggerated the headache on the same side, rather than causing the bilateral headache usual in the headache-free subject.

Pfeiffer and Kunkle (1951) made the interesting observation that there were fluctuations in cranial arterial tone as measured by histamine responsiveness, and that these fluctuations were relevant to the occurrences of vascular headaches of the migraine type.

Kunkle postulated that the intensity of the transient headache which can be induced by histamine would be greater when intracranial arterial tone was low, and vice versa. Accordingly, the responsiveness of human subjects to intravenously injected histamine was observed from day to day, and variations in the intensity of the induced headache were compared with other biologic data, particularly attitudes and feeling states of the subject.

A secondary aim concerned the issue of how readily man can be desensitized to histamine. Although the repeated administration of this agent has been recommended for the purpose of desensitizing patients with vascular headache, little evidence has ever been offered that such a program reliably produces increased tolerance to histamine.

The subjects were eight white adults, ages 21 to 38. Seven were male physicians or medical students, and one was a female hospital technician. Two subjects were prone to migraine headache, one to atypical migraine, and two to muscle-tension headache. Histamine phosphate was given intravenously to each subject in an amount found by preliminary trial to be adequate to induce a brief or mild headache (0.03 mg in six, and 0.04 mg in two subjects). All experiments were carried out at a room temperature of approximately 22°C and at 5:00 to 5:30 P.M. each day. Observations were made of pulse rate and blood pressure of the subject at rest in the seated position before the daily injection, and were repeated at the peak of the induced headache and after its subsidence.

Prior to each injection, notes were made of the subject's activities, of his mood, of his awareness of tension and fatigue, and of any other data concerning the day's events and his attitudes. The statements of the subject were supplemented by observations of his emotional state as indicated by body posture, gestures, facial expression, tone of voice, and random comments. The intensity of the headache induced by the histamine injection was estimated by the subject on a ten-point dol scale for purposes of daily comparisons. This procedure was followed for 14 to 18 consecutive days; in four subjects the injections were briefly resumed later after intermission of 12 to 165 days. As one additional measure of desensitization to histamine, the wheal and flare reactions to a standard amount of histamine by intradermal injection were measured in each subject at the beginning and the end of this experimental series.

The induced headache was bifrontotemporal or generalized in six subjects. In one of the two subjects with a history of typical migraine, always right hemicranial, the experimental headache was usually confined to the right side. On the other hand, in the individual with atypical migraine, also right hemicranial, the experimental headache was uniformly left-sided and often strictly temporal; similar left temporal headache occurred spontaneously twice during the two-week experimental period and returned occasionally thereafter. Day-to-day variations in the intensity of the histamine-induced headache were moderate in all subjects, ranging from no headache to one of four dols. Small daily fluctuations were noted in pulse rate and blood pressure readings in all subjects and were of no demonstrable significance.

Because of the extent of the variations in daily headache responses, in the final review of results attention was focused primarily on the experimental days which were marked by maximum and minimum headaches, for it seemed likely that these occasions would offer the most informative data. Such an analysis revealed apparently significant correlations between the intensity of the induced headache and the type of feeling states in six of the subjects. These correlations were of two kinds.

(1) In nine instances in five of the subjects, injections evoking the mildest headache (0 to trace) were on days on which the individual was rested and relaxed; or if he had been busy at work, felt unusually satisfied with his accomplishments. (2) In four instances in three of the subjects, the injections evoking the most intense headache coincided with feelings of tension and resentment or of discouragement with work performance. In one individual, for example, the only two peak headaches were on days on which his recurrent resentment towards a colleague had flared up; the only two occasions of failure of histamine to evoke headache in this same man were on a weekday spent in highly productive effort preparing for an important conference and on a Sunday devoted to light reading and recreation.

Less noteworthy correlations were seen in a few instances. In two of the subjects, peak experimental headaches followed afternoons of exercise in hot weather, and, in one, the ingestion of alcohol. In one subject, two of his three peak headaches occurred on successive days of a mild laryngitis without fever.

The skin test reaction to histamine was slightly less at the end of the injection series in one subject only.

These data, therefore, support the thesis that the responsiveness of cranial arteries to a vasodilator challenge can in some individuals be affected by multiple factors, including life circumstances and the reaction to them.

Edmund (1952) showed that those with vascular headache were more likely to experience headache after small amounts of histamine than other persons; and furthermore that the headache was more likely to occur on the side that was usually implicated.

Tunis and Wolff (1953) noted that persons who have frequent, severe vascular headaches may have the temporal artery prominent on one or both sides of the head, even when headache free. Major variability occurs in the size and prominence of the temporal artery from day to day, and indeed from hour to hour. Moreover, persons with migraine headache exhibit such cranial vasomotor changes, especially during periods of frequent headache attacks and particularly during the 18 to 72 hr prior to the headache. These observations suggest that there is greater variability in the contractile state of the cranial arteries in subjects with migraine than in those who seldom or never have headache. Accordingly, long-term studies were undertaken with improved amplifying and recording instruments to define more precisely these alterations.

Method. Glycerine tambours (glycerin-filled rubber spheres in an airtight metal case) were placed bilaterally on the skin over selected cranial arteries to "pick up" the pulsations. Pulse-wave tracings were obtained by connecting the tambour through a piezoelectric pulse-wave attachment to a multiple-channel direct writing recorder. Seventy-five persons subject to migraine headache were studied during various phases of headache and during headache-free periods. Cranial-artery pulse waves were recorded two to five times a week at variable intervals for five to 30 weeks. Under these circumstances more than 5000 records were assembled, representing all phases of the patients' headache state and cranial-artery function, i.e., long before, immediately before, during, and after headache attacks.

From this series, records obtained from the frontal branch of the right temporal artery of ten migraine subjects at the midpoint of a headache-free interval of not less than two weeks' duration were selected for special analysis.

For purposes of comparison, six to eight records were obtained from the frontal branch of the temporal artery at random intervals from ten subjects who never or seldom had headaches and who did not have headache during the three-month period of study. A total of 72 records were thus obtained. In this nonheadache group the earlier records differed in no way from the tracings taken during subsequent periods of observation.

All the subjects whose records were selected had stable brachial-artery blood pressures (100/70 to 120/80) and pulse rates (70 to 76 per min). One hundred consecutive pulse waves from the right temporal artery of each subject were measured, and the data from the headache-free migraine group were compared with the data from the nonheadache group.

The components of the cranial-artery pulse wave, as shown in Fig. 4-10, were measured as follows: (1) the height, in millimeters, of the apex of the systolic component from the baseline; (2) the height, in millimeters, of the apex of the dicrotic wave from the baseline; (3) the height, in millimeters, of the apex of the dicrotic wave from its own baseline; (4) the number of the small reflected waves on the diastolic limb of the pulse wave; and (5) the total amplitude of the small reflected waves on the diastolic limb of the pulse wave.

The changes in the amplitude of the arterial pulse wave (systolic apex to base) were taken as evidence of changes in the caliber of the artery. Inferences were drawn concerning the contractile state of the vascular bed under observation, on the basis of these changes, in conjunction with the other measured components of the wave.

Observations. The data for 1000 pulse-wave contours of the ten subjects in each group are shown in Table 4-2. Each measured component of the pulse-wave contour of the headache-free migraine group was significantly greater than the comparable measurement from the nonheadache group. For example, for the migraine subjects the mean amplitude (systole) was 26.4 mm as contrasted with a mean of 12 mm in the nonheadache group.

As compared with the nonheadache group, there was greater variability of the contractile state of the vascular bed under observation in the headache group. This is demonstrated both by the greater range of pulse-wave amplitudes (systole) (16 to 48 mm versus 8 to 17 mm) and by the greater range for

ARTERIAL PULSE-WAVE CONTOUR

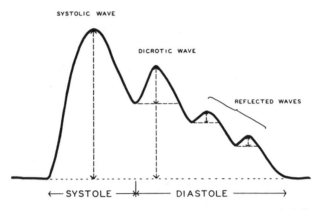

FIG. 4-10. Schematized cranial-artery pulse-wave contour. The vertical distances, indicated by the broken lines and arrows, were measured in millimeters. The total number of reflected waves and their total amplitude also were ascertained for the 100 consecutive pulse waves from the record of each subject.

TABLE 4-2   Analysis of Pulse-Wave Contours for Subjects Who Have Vascular Headaches and for Subjects Who Never Have Headaches

	HEADACHE SUBJECTS		Nonheadache Subjects
	During Headache	Form of Headache	
Systoles			
Wave amplitude			
Range (mm)	17–57	16–48	8–17
Average (mm)	42.7	26.4	12
Standard deviation	±3.1	±2.20	±0.95
Dicrotic, apex to base			
Range (mm)	10–35	6–17	1–12
Average (mm)	18.7	10	6
Standard deviation (mm)	±3.0	±2.07	±0.74
Diastoles			
Dicrotic wave amplitude			
Range (mm)	3.0–20	0.2–7	0–3
Amplitude (mm)	8.1	3.3	1.2
Standard deviation (mm)	±1.0	±1.0	±0.5
Number of reflected waves			
Range	0–4	0–6	0–2
Average	1.4	1.4	0.6
Standard deviation	±0.82	±0.82	±0.53
Size of reflected waves			
Range (mm)	0–16	0.2–2	0.1–1
Average (mm)	1.4	1.4	0.4
Standard deviation (mm)	±1.3	±1.31	±0.4

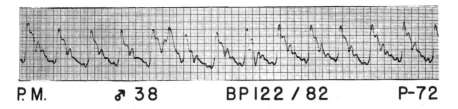

P. M.   ♂ 38   BP 122 / 82   P-72

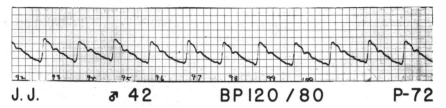

J. J.   ♂ 42   BP 120 / 80   P-72

FIG. 4-11. Representative right-temporal-artery pulse-wave tracings from a headache-free migraine subject (upper), and a subject who never had migraine (lower).
Note the variability of the pulse waves in the tracing from the migraine subject.

the number of the reflected waves (diastole) (o to 6 versus o to 2). The range and average size of the reflected waves were also greater in the headache-free migraine subjects.

When compared with the uniform records of the nonheadache group, the records of subjects in the migraine group exhibited greater variability in the contractile state of the studied artery from subject to subject within the group, and indeed from pulse wave to pulse wave on a given tracing from any individual subject (see Fig. 4-11).

Observations. The long-term records in the migraine group exhibited a further peculiarity. Three to four days before the onset of headache, the pulse-wave records of the migraine subjects showed a decided increase in the variability of the contractile state of the investigated vascular beds. This variability was sustained until the subject was again in a headache-free phase.

A record of the sequence of contour changes in the temporal-artery pulse waves in a representative subject is reproduced in Fig. 4-12. For 36 to 72 hr before the onset of headache, large pulse waves with a variable contour were recorded. The amplitude generally was well above that exhibited in records from prolonged headache-free phases. Transient facial flushing, often unilateral, and/or alternating pallor was also noted. The amplitude diminished, and was minimal when the subject reported scotomata in the hour preceding the onset of head pain and indicated increased vascular resistance and vasoconstriction.

Also, the average, the range, and the standard deviation of the systolic pulse-wave and dicrotic-wave amplitudes were greater during headache than were these data when the same subjects were headache free. Moreover, shortly after the onset of headache, dilatation was evidenced by the appearance of a concave downward diastolic limb, and a marked reduction in size and often disappearance, of reflected waves (Tunis and Wolff, 1952).

The observations indicate that during headache the caliber of the involved vessel is increased, as is its variability. The elevation of the apex of the dicrotic wave from the baseline is also increased, and with the other described changes indicates greater stretch on the wall of the involved vessel during headache than in the headache-free state (Tunis *et al.*, 1951). Variability became more striking 72 hr prior to the onset of headache and was maximal at the height of the headache attack.

GENERAL COMMENT

Even during headache-free phases, persons subject to migraine exhibited significantly greater variability in the contractile state of particular portions of the cranial vascular tree than did persons who are not subject to headache. Such variability during headache-

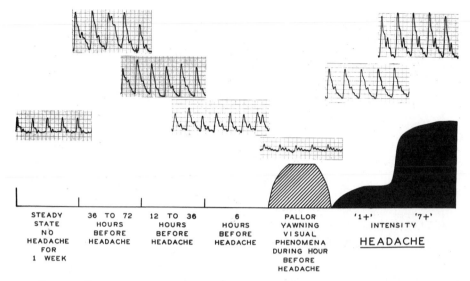

FIG. 4-12. Representative record of the sequence of temporal-artery pulse-wave changes prior to and during a headache attack. Note the variability of the pulse waves in the tracing obtained 72 hr prior to the onset of headache. This variability is sustained until the subject is again headache free.

free phases of persons subject to migraine was especially evident during life periods marred by severe and frequent headache attacks. The striking modifications in cranial-artery function characteristic of the headache attack merely punctuated the more or less continuous series of physiological changes that comprised part of the particular life adjustment of these persons. The observed modifications in cranial-artery function were accompanied by mood alteration, feelings of tension, sustained effort, and restlessness. The concurrence of these changes suggests that these modifications in vascular function and structure are the sequel of sustained adaptive reactions to life stress.

CRANIAL ARTERIES INVOLVED IN MIGRAINE AND DISTRIBUTION OF PAIN

Having demonstrated that the extracranial branches of the external carotid artery are of major significance in inducing the headache of migraine, the role of intracranial arteries, both the internal and external carotid artery branches, will be further discussed.

Some older observations concerning the middle meningeal artery are relevant to this discussion. It has been noted that attacks of migraine headache often fail to recur after subtemporal decompression. Since such a procedure customarily includes ligation of branches or the trunk of the middle meningeal artery, the suggestion presents itself that this artery plays a part in the production of pain. There is also more direct evidence that the middle meningeal artery is implicated, since ligation of this vessel abolished attacks of migraine headache in some subjects. The beneficial effect lasted no longer than six months. In others, however, this procedure diminished the intensity, but did not prevent the recurrence of attacks.

The role of the pial and cerebral arteries in the migraine headache needs further definition. It should be recalled that faradic stimulation of the proximal few centimeters of the anterior, middle, and posterior cerebral arteries and the first few centimeters of the intracranial portion of the internal carotid artery causes pain within, behind, or over the homolateral eye. Furthermore, stimulation of the vertebral and basilar arteries and the proximal portions of their branches causes pain in the occipital and the suboccipital region. These areas are commonly involved in migraine attacks. The evidence from persons who have migraine headache that headache induced by histamine resembles the most intense migraine headache also suggests that the larger arteries at the base of the brain and their immediate branches may be implicated in some patients during severe migraine headache.

On the other hand, there is considerable evidence against this view. If the headache were due primarily to dilatation of the dural and cerebral arteries, raising the cerebrospinal fluid pressure would dampen the pulsations of these vessels and the headache would diminish, as in the case of the headache induced by histamine. Since in some instances even severe migraine headaches have not been modified by these procedures, it is unlikely that pial and cerebral arteries are major contributors to the pain (Schumacher and Wolff, 1941). Yet, some individuals who have the usual features of periodic unilateral headaches for years may, from time to time, develop a somewhat different attack of headache that is bilateral or generalized, intense and long-lasting. In contrast to their usual type of headache, which is not modified by head jolts and is eliminated by ergotamine tartrate, this other type is increased in intensity by even minimal head jolts and is not appreciably modified by ergotamine tartrate. It is, however, decreased in intensity by carotid compression. It would appear that this latter type of headache may involve not only dilated arteries of the dura and outside of the cranium, but also cerebral arteries as well.

The internal and the external carotid artery and the vertebral arteries have branches both in the subcutaneous tissue and in the meninges. The branches of the external carotid artery predominate numerically, both superficially and on the dura. On the other hand, the anterior meningeal artery arises from branches of the internal carotid artery, as do the superficial frontal and the supra-orbital artery. Since the area supplied by the latter structures is commonly involved in migraine headaches, branches of the internal carotid

artery may contribute to the pain. It is obvious, therefore, that it would be arbitrary to contrast these arteries too sharply.

Although most attacks of migraine headache are limited to the temporal, the frontal, or the occipital region, some patients have pain elsewhere. In the face, below the eye, and behind and below the zygoma, severe throbbing pain, which seems to emanate from the back teeth of the upper jaw, occasionally occurs. Another variant is facial pain, which spreads behind the angle of the jaw, down the neck, and into the shoulder. The latter aching sensations are sometimes associated with awareness of unusual throbbing in the neck.

The pains described can and probably do result from dilatation and distention of the extracranial portion of the middle meningeal artery, between its origin and the point of entrance into the skull, the internal maxillary artery, and the trunks of the external and the common carotid artery. It has been shown that the latter structures are sensitive to pain, and the sites in which pain is felt are the face, neck, and shoulder.

Atherosclerosis of the relevant arteries of the head has been suggested as the reason why vascular headaches of the migraine type are relatively uncommon in some older persons who have had them for the better part of their adult lives. It is postulated that the vessel walls, becoming rigid, cannot painfully dilate. This explanation can be immediately dismissed or supported by giving the individual in question a small amount of amyl nitrite to inhale while at the same time measuring the amplitude of the pulsations of his temporal arteries, and if possible, of the intraspinal and cranial arteries via the spinal fluid. In no instance in the experience of the investigators has it been possible to show that the cranial arteries have been incapable of major dilatation.

Factors other than those implicating the elasticity of the peripheral vascular walls must be operating. It would be easier to assume that the reduction in strivings and tensions of older adults might be far more pertinent to the dwindling occurrence of headaches. As a matter of fact, in some older persons where major adaptive problems still persist or are growing more difficult, the headache may become more frequent and severe.

Effect of Prolonged Dilatation upon Cranial Artery Walls

After several hours of headache involving, for example, the temporal artery, the latter may appear prominent and distended, and become more palpable through the skin. Instead of being easily collapsible it becomes rigid, pipelike and less readily compressible by the palpating finger, an observation which has erroneously led to the inference that the artery is in a state of spasm, and that this spasm is causing the headache. Also, the artery may be tender when compressed. Patients so affected report that after the first hour or two of a migraine headache attack the quality of the headache changes, in that the initial pulsating or throbbing is less conspicuous or absent and the pain becomes a steady ache; also, that administration of ergotamine tartrate may fail to give prompt relief.

To account for such changes, it was postulated that following the sustained arterial dilatation of a local artery of the head, there occurs a transient change in the structure of the artery wall, namely, thickening or edema of muscular and adventitial structures. Indeed the sections taken from the temporal artery of patients during attacks of migraine headache involving this structure, microscopically studied, suggested that there was thickening of the arterial wall. The problem was approached through animal studies by ascertaining whether transient changes within the arterial walls, such as are relevant to this discussion, can follow prolonged vasodilatation (Torda and Wolff, 1945).

The ears of cats were subjected to prolonged vasodilatation by infusion for two hours with 10 cc of mammalian Ringer's solution containing a vasodilator agent (0.05 mg acetylcholine). The infused ears were then removed, fixed in Bouin's fluid, and prepared in serial sections. Each ear was compared with the noninfused ear of the same cat, prepared in the same way and used as control. The areas of the walls of all arteries containing visible smooth muscle were measured in cross section.

The measurements showed that cranial arteries exposed to the prolonged effect of a vasodilator agent exhibit an increase in the thickness of the arterial walls. Thus, sustained dilatation of cranial vessels leads to transient structural changes. It is possible that the vasa vasorum in the dilated walls become more permeable and that the tissue spaces within the walls contain more fluid. The relation of these changes to clinical phenomena may be significant.

Furthermore, ergotamine tartrate was found to be less prompt and less effective in constricting arteries with such thickened and edematous walls, as compared with its effect on normal walls.

Similar changes in arterial walls of patients during long migraine headaches may be the explanation for the rigid, pipelike texture of the arteries and the tenderness of these structures, the steady aching pain, and the loss in effectiveness of ergotamine tartrate in reducing headache.

Dunning (1942) has collected evidence concerning structural changes which he and others observed to be associated with the migraine headache attack. In addition to prominent arteries, the defects outside the cranium include edema, echymosis, thrombosis, and hemorrhage; those within include thrombosis and hemorrhage. The facial edema and the results of hemorrhage may outlast the headache by many hours or even days.

Changes in the appearance of capillaries have been observed during migraine headache attacks. These changes are attributed to a swelling of the endothelial cells of the capillary wall and to an increased transudation.

EVIDENCE OF REVERSIBLE TISSUE DAMAGE AND CHANGES IN SENSITIVITY IN THE PAINFUL REGIONS OF MIGRAINE HEADACHE

Conspicuous evidence of damage to vascular walls during headache were 19 spontaneous hygromata in areas of headache in 11 patients during 19 attacks of migraine (Tunis et al., 1953). The hygromata varied in diameter from 1 to 6 cm, and in depth from ½ to 2 cm. They were usually localized in the tissues adjacent to

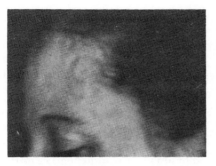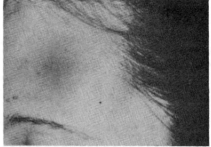

FIG. 4-13. Two views of a hygroma about the left temporal artery that developed 48 hr after onset of headache in subject.

the frontal branch of the involved temporal artery, and made their appearance 10–60 hr after the onset of a severe headache attack. The hygromata were tender on palpation, ecchymotic in appearance, and persisted for a few days to over a week (see Figs. 4-13 and 4-14).

These hygromata have been referred to as hematomata, an unfortunate word since it implies that the mass is a blood clot or cyst containing blood. As a matter of fact, surgical resection of such swellings has revealed only local accumulation of pink-stained fluid without evidence of fresh blood or rupture of a large vessel. Hence, a more suitable term would be hygromata, representing as it does an exaggeration of the edema formation evident to a less degree in many other patients. The massive edema suggests what might occur intracranially in some patients, i.e., in those with transient hemipareses and hemihypesthesias.

Also, evidence of tissue damage, although far less dramatic than such relatively rare hygromata, is the tenderness of tissues on the outside of the cranium, long recognized as a

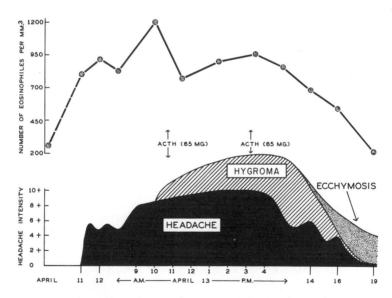

FIG. 4-14. Demonstration of the time of onset and development of a hygroma during a severe long-lasting migraine headache attack. It is doubtful whether the ACTH in this instance altered the course of events.

common feature of vascular headaches involving extracranial arteries. It has been suggested that such hypersensitivity may be a factor in the mechanism of headache, since vasodilation per se does not always induce headache.

Use of Norepinephrine in the Study of Tenderness and Edema of the Head in Migraine Patients

With an increasing awareness of the importance of the visible and palpable tissue changes at the site of headache of the vascular type and the tenderness so commonly mentioned by patients, it became imperative to explore further the nature of these processes. Having learned from the use of ergotamine tartrate a few elementals about the subsurface arteries in relation to the pain of vascular headache, it became desirable to use another powerful and almost pure vasoconstrictor, norepinephrine, to ascertain whether its effect on the headache is the same, and what influence, if any, it has on the edema and tenderness. Should the effect turn out to be much the same as that of ergotamine tartrate, it would add support to the view that the local action on the blood vessels is mainly responsible for the elimination of the headache.

Method. Norepinephrine in a dilution of 4 cc of a 0.2% solution in a liter of 5% dextrose in water was administered intravenously at an average rate of 1 drop per sec, or sufficient to raise the systolic blood pressure 10 to 40 mm Hg. With the patient supine, blood pressure and pulse were determined at intervals of 1–2 min initially and thereafter every 10–15 min. Pulse-wave tracings of the involved cranial arteries were made, and deep pain thresholds of the scalp were assayed (Wolff *et al.*, 1953). When possible, the diameter of relevant dilated cranial vessels was measured directly at intervals during norepinephrine infusion, and observations were made of the accompanying phenomena, such as edema, conjunctival injection, and rhinorrhea. The patient's reports of the effects of the norepinephrine on the intensity of the headache were recorded.

Results. Norepinephrine, in the manner described above, was administered on 116 occasions to 35 patients with vascular headache of the migraine type. On 93 of these occasions the headache began to diminish in 10–60 min, and was either eliminated or much reduced in intensity in an average time of 82 min, the range being from 20 to 160 min. In general, the more intense the headache, the longer was the time required for its elimination. Mild headaches have been terminated in 20 min, severe headaches persisting for as long as 160 min after beginning norepinephrine infusion. In four instances of status hemicranicus this agent was without significant effect.

Ophthalmic involvement, in the form of conjunctival injection, lacrimation, blurred vision, or photophobia, was present in 36 of the 116 headache attacks. Consistently they were terminated more rapidly than other headache phenomena, in 10–15 min of infusion. Nasal mucosal injection and/or rhinorrhea was present in eight headache attacks and also was relieved in every instance. Usually 30–45 min of infusion were required to terminate the nasal symptoms. The degree of scalp edema could be readily estimated by the depth of depression made by applying a standard pressure with the Hardy deep-pain dolorimeter. It was observed that the edema was decreased when a headache had been terminated through the action of norepinephrine. On three occasions the temporal artery was prominent enough for its diameter to be measured directly. As the headache intensity lessened, the diameter decreased. Pulse-wave tracings showed a decrease in amplitude and increase in the number of reflected waves as the headache intensity was dwindling (Fig. 4-15). These contour changes had been observed previously by Wolff and Tunis (1952) to be compatible with vasoconstriction.

In a patient with ophthalmoplegic migraine manifested by diplopia and right sixth cranial nerve weakness, the ocular movements returned to normal, and diplopia and strabismus disappeared after 70 min of norepinephrine infusion. In previous attacks in this patient the usual duration of sixth nerve involvement had been four days. Another patient who had ptosis of the right eyelid for 48 hr during a headache attack was able to raise the lid normally after 90 min of norepinephrine infusion. Irritability, giddiness, and difficulty in thinking were repeatedly eliminated during norepinephrine administration. Feelings of tension and exhilaration were common sequelae, and no depression, prostration, or lethargy was noted.

On seven occasions in four patients with essential hypertension of moderate severity, vascular

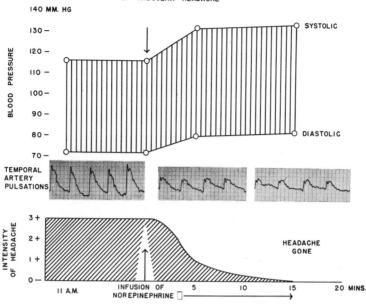

FIG. 4-15.

headaches were similarly eliminated. Optimal effects were noted when norepinephrine was given at rates that induced an average rise in blood pressure of 28 mm Hg systolic and 9 mm Hg diastolic (Fig. 4-15).

Comment. The amount of norepinephrine administered was under control at all times. Its administration required the constant attention of competent personnel. Without ill effect, the agent was infused for as long as 5 hr. It was given as often as three times weekly to three patients. No nausea or vomiting resulted. The agent was used effectively after the administration of repeated ineffective amounts of ergotamine tartrate. Some untoward effects of norepinephrine have been observed. When it was infused too rapidly, there was a sudden, dramatic rise in blood pressure (40 to 60 mm Hg systolic) with intensification of the headache already present, presumably due to further distention of pain-sensitive intracranial arteries. Uncommonly, it produced unpleasant sensations in the neck with mild dysphagia. Muscle-contraction headache, previously shown to be associated with scalp artery constriction, was increased (Tunis and Wolff, 1952). When headache is terminated through the action of norepinephrine or ergotamine tartrate, the lowered deep pain thresholds return to normal more promptly than when the headache ends spontaneously.

When the headache is present in a small head area and deep pain thresholds are lowered over a larger area, pain thresholds in the area involved with headache and in the area free of headache return to pre-attack levels at the same rate during norepinephrine infusion. Moreover, when, after spontaneous ending of a headache, deep pain thresholds remain lowered, the administration of norepinephrine or ergotamine tartrate raises them promptly. In following the dwindling intensity of headache after the vasoconstrictor drugs are given it has been noted that the deep pain thresholds persist at lower levels longer about the painfully dilated large arteries than in scalp tissue more peripheral to these vessels. In three instances when headache was allowed to end spontaneously and marked scalp edema was present, it was observed that deep pain thresholds remained below pre-attack levels as long as edema persisted.

GENERAL COMMENT

The investigations of von Euler (1951) and others have shown that norepinephrine is the substance mediating the effects of stimulation of adrenergic nerves. It has been further shown that norepinephrine acts almost entirely as a vasoconstrictor and does not share with epinephrine the ability to produce marked metabolic changes. While ergotamine tartrate is also a vasoconstrictor, it has other effects, notably on the central nervous system. Thus, it is possible that the vasoconstrictor property of the ergot alkaloids is not the only effective one in the treatment of migraine. However, the fact that an almost pure vasoconstrictor agent, such as norepinephrine, promptly reverses all the painful aspects of migraine headache is further evidence that the genesis of this pain is vasodilatation, granting that local tissue changes do lower the pain threshold so as to make vascular distention more painful.

The following postulated pathophysiology of vascular headache and of the effect of vasoconstrictor agents is in keeping with the foregoing observations. At the onset of headache there is concomitant dilatation of the large arteries, arterioles, and metarterioles. The dilatation of the arterioles and metarterioles increases the capillary hydrostatic pressure. The elevated capillary hydrostatic pressure favors the accumulation of pain-threshold-lowering material in the subcutaneous tissue of the scalp. There is thus present in the tissue, in greater amounts than normal, a substance, postulated as "headache stuff." Dilatation and distention of large arteries coupled with accumulation of this pain-threshold-lowering substance result in headache. A simpler explanation of the abolition of tenderness with the ending of the headache after administration of ergotamine tartrate and norepinephrine is that the vasoconstriction resulting from the action of these agents reduces the permeability of the blood vessel walls at the site of tenderness. It may then be postulated that either (a) pain-threshold-lowering substances themselves are prevented from leaking into the tissues or (b) some substance from the serum essential to the activation of another substance liberated by nerve action is prevented from leaking into the tissue. Of the two, the latter is the more attractive explanation, but as a consequence of either

(a) or (b), pain threshold is raised as permeability diminishes and as the larger arteries constrict. Thus both effects are achieved at the same time, and the headache attack is terminated.

Variations in Fluid and Electrolyte Excretion Associated with Migraine Headache

It has long been recognized that many patients with the migraine type of vascular headache undergo changes in fluid balance and fluid distribution during the headache attack. Local changes in fluid distribution are evidenced by (a) puffiness of the face, (b) periorbital edema, and (c) localized patches of edema about the temporal and frontal regions. More widespread fluctuations in fluid balance are evidenced by (a) swelling of the extremities; (b) weight gain prior to headache; (c) occurrence in some women of headaches in association with the menses, often coupled with a state of hydration; and (d) diuresis at the peak of the attack or as the headache subsides.

The headache itself results from local vascular phenomena involving dilatation of the cranial arteries. That various types of vessels are involved, if not painfully, may be surmised from the blanching or flushing of the face, coldness of the hands, and sensations of chilliness which may accompany headache.

Studies were therefore undertaken to define the nature and magnitude of the fluid and electrolyte variations associated with vascular headache (Schottstaedt and Wolff, 1955).

Method. In order to study all phases of the attack of migraine headache, subjects were observed over periods of 7 to 18 days. They continued to perform their daily work, collecting all urine voided and pooling this into four specimens daily. The collection periods ended (a) upon arising in the morning, (b) before the noon meal, (c) before the evening meal, and (d) before retiring for the night. Records were kept of food and fluid ingested, of events and physical activities of the day, of behavior and emotional responses to these events and activities, and of the onset, duration, fluctuations in intensity, and termination of headache. Sodium and potassium determinations were performed in duplicate on all urine specimens. Creatinine determinations were made in

TABLE 4-3   24-Hr Fluid Intake and Output in Subject E.P.

Date	Morning Weight (lb.)	Fluid Intake (cc)	Urine Output (cc)	Comments
3/27	133	2190	1990	Birthday party for child; patient then relaxed
3/28	132	2010	1620	Landlord began work in apartment
3/29	132	1620	1440	Overslept; rushed to church—marginal headache
3/30	132	2400	1040	Tense day
3/31	132	2460	1740	Moderate headache in morning, gone in afternoon
4/1	132	2520	1580	Quiet day
4/2	132	3400	1164	Many difficulties: refrigerator broke down, sewing machine wouldn't work; had to go to hospital
4/3	133	3120	1695	Landlord painting; house a shambles
4/4	134	2280	1975	Continued painting and plastering
4/5	134	1710	1680	Severe headache began during Communion
4/6	134	1410	1155	Headache continued, began improving during the night
4/7	132	1200	1775	Awoke improved; brief, blinding headache in morning, with subsidence during afternoon
4/8	132	—	1260	No headache

duplicate. Ten subjects, experiencing 28 headaches, were studied.

Results. Observation 1. Mrs. E. P., a 25-year-old housewife with two children, was studied for two weeks, between 3/27 and 4/8/53. She had recurrent vascular headaches of the migraine type, which had first occurred during adolescence and which were becoming increasingly frequent and severe. Excretion rates for all substances studied were low prior to the onset of headache and high during the period of subsidence.

Though her daily fluid intake increased from 2400 to 3400 cc, there was a slight decrease in the 24-hr output and she gained 2 lb. in weight. She retired late 4/4, "worn out" but satisfied, knowing that the apartment repairs and redecorations were complete, the house in order again, and all the Easter preparations accomplished. Easter Sunday, 4/5, while at Communion, she developed a severe, throbbing headache. A striking decrease in creatinine excretion occurred during the brief period of "blinding" headache. A summary of fluid intake and life situations is given in Table 4-3. A mild, transitory headache and a moderately severe headache of short duration were observed in this patient following short periods of increased work and responsibilities associated with feelings of tension. These two headaches were not accompanied by fluctuations in weight. The first was too brief for study. The second was preceded by low excretion rates of water, sodium, potassium, and creatinine and was followed by high excretion rates of these substances. A third headache, of high intensity and lasting three days,

occurred after three days of domestic disarray, disorganization, and disrupted routine. Weight gain occurred during the few days immediately preceding headache, and weight loss accompanied subsidence of headache. Excretion rates of water, sodium, potassium, and creatinine were low prior to headache and high during the phase of subsidence of headache.

Observation 2. M. S., a 28-year-old housewife and physician, was studied for 50 days.

A mild headache occurred in this subject after prolonged feelings of tension and depression. A transient subsidence of headache occurred with mobilization for work. This was accompanied by a slight increase in creatinine excretion and by a considerable increase in potassium excretion. With "let-down," headache recurred, to disappear the following day during a period of relaxation associated with water diuresis. See Table 4-4.

Other studies demonstrate that the fluid, electrolyte, and renal circulation changes described above are most likely linked with the altered adaptive patterns. These include a variety of behavior patterns, attitudes, and feelings in reaction to stressful life circumstances, sometimes linked with headache and other disorders, but not specifically or causally related.

A concept of the disturbance in salt and water metabolism in subjects attempting a variety of adaptive arrangements and including

TABLE 4-4 Fluid and Electrolyte Excretion in Subject M. S.

Phase	H_2O (cc/min)	S. D.	Na (μeq/min)	S. D.	K (μEQ./MIN.) Day	Night	S. D.	Creatinine (mg/min)
Average of 47 asymptomatic days ...	0.76	±0.17	96	±20	54		±5	...
Two days before headache	0.45	...	31	...	23	18	...	0.920
Two days with subsiding headache ..	1.48	...	130	...	72	...	...	1.014

Each recurrence of headache was accompanied by decreased rates of excretion of water, sodium, potassium, and creatinine; and each subsidence of headache, by increased rates of excretion of water, sodium, and potassium, with creatinine excretion returning to average levels.

The data for the 26 headaches included in this report are shown in Table 4.5.

TABLE 4-5 Summary of Fluid and Electrolyte Excretion for 26 Headaches

	H_2O (CC/MIN)	Na (μEQ/MIN)	K (μEQ/MIN)	CREATININE (μG/MIN)
Before or early in headache	0.47	47	26	0.738
Subsiding headache	1.44	133	68	1.044

those persons with vascular headache of the migraine type is formulated as follows (Schottstaedt and Wolff, 1955).

In the maintenance of a constant environment within the human organism, stores of fluid and salt are of paramount importance. When in response to situations, persons were prepared for short, violent action, as for fight or flight, or during situations evoking tempestuous and aggressive behavior with attitudes and feelings of excitement, intense anger, and apprehension, sodium and water loss occurred. Reactions featured by listless behavior, reduced activity, slowed and decreased speech, with attitudes and feelings of despair, hopelessness, and depression, were associated with retention of fluid and electrolytes. Retention of fluid and electrolytes accompanied responses of fright in terrorizing situations and reactions to severe noxious stimulation and pain. When persons were faced with threatening situations eliciting restless behavior, increased alertness, readiness for action, with mixed feelings of confidence, uneasiness, and tension, renal excretion of water and sodium was decreased and body weight was increased.

Situations evoking similar behavior and feelings, yet featured by unusual constraint, were sometimes associated with retention of potassium as well. Diuresis of water and salt with resultant weight loss occurred with ending of such periods of threat.

These patterns suggest the responses in man to the threatening situations created by the invasion of microorganisms: retention during the phase of consolidation in pneumonia, diuresis during resolution of consolidation. During protracted efforts to remain alert, on guard, and ready for action, water and salt are conserved. With the ending of the period of threat, diuresis rids the body of excess water and salt. Both patterns are presumably mediated by neurohumoral devices.

SUMMARY AND CONCLUSIONS

Studies of persons subject to vascular headache of the migraine type, made before, during, and after headache attacks, gave the following results:

1. Decreased rates of excretion of water, sodium, potassium, and creatinine were usu-

ally observed prior to and during the early phases of vascular headache of the migraine type.

2. Increased rates of excretion of water, sodium, and potassium were usual with subsidence of the headache attacks.

3. Creatinine excretion returned to "normal" values during subsidence of headache, with exceptions. On these latter occasions potassium excretion was high.

4. Weight gain prior to the headache attack was common but not invariable. It sometimes occurred well in advance (7 to 10 days) of the onset of headache. (This phenomenon is discussed in detail in the following pages.)

5. Weight loss with subsidence of headache was usual. However, it was sometimes delayed 24–48 hr.

THE SIGNIFICANCE OF TWO VARIETIES OF FLUID ACCUMULATION IN MIGRAINE PATIENTS

Two kinds of edema have thus been observed in patients subject to vascular headache of the migraine type. One was a localized fluid accumulation that developed during the headache and occurred primarily in those scalp areas in which headache was experienced. This was featured by tenderness and slight-to-moderate pitting.

The second was a more generalized fluid accumulation that commonly developed before the headache, involved many parts of the body, and was demonstrable by weight gain and pitting of dependent body areas. Data on this type, analyzed by Schottstaedt and Wolff (1955) were presented above.

The following studies were undertaken to determine the frequency, magnitude, genesis, and natural history of these two sets of phenomena and their possible relevance to the pathophysiology of headache (Ostfeld et al., 1955).

Local Edema

Observations were made during more than 200 vascular headaches of the migraine type. Significant local alteration of tissue turgor and slight-to-moderate edema very frequently oc-

curred in the area of headache. While the presence of such local edema was not noted to precede the headache attack, it became more pronounced the longer the headache persisted and often outlasted the headache. In such edematous scalp areas, tenderness and a lowering of deep pain thresholds were predictably noted. When, as a result of administration of vasoconstrictor agents, the intensity of headache subsided, the deep pain thresholds returned to normal levels and edema was reduced. These changes occurred more promptly as a result of administration of vasoconstrictor agents than when the headache ended spontaneously. The behavior of the small cranial vessels of the bulbar conjunctiva before and during migraine attacks is described in detail above.

During periods of conjunctival dilatation there was haziness of the conjunctival tissue and an indistinctness of the vascular structures which was compatible with and probably due to local edema. At such times subjects complained of a burning sensation in the eye. Usually within 15 to 20 min after the start of a norepinephrine infusion, the haziness and blurred outlines attributable to edema began to be reduced, and ultimately they were eliminated. Together with these changes there was a dwindling intensity of headache and reduction of the burning sensation in the eye.

Widespread Fluid Retention

The phenomenon of widespread fluid retention was studied in 134 patients with vascular headache of the migraine type. The clinical manifestations of the widespread fluid retention were complaints about the sudden gain in weight, "tightness of rings on fingers," "clothes don't fit," etc. The subjects even complained that the skin "feels thicker." This variety of edema, in contrast to the localized edema in the region of the headache, was nontender, and reached a maximum just before the onset of headache.

Sixty-three of the 134 patients affirmed that they had experienced one or more of the above symptoms in association with headache. Daily weight measurements were made by 51 of

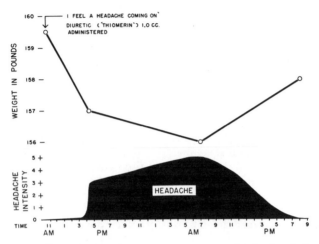

FIG. 4-16. Failure of induced diuresis to prevent a migraine headache attack.

these patients through at least one headache attack. In 31 there was a gain of approximately 2 lb.; 16 gained 3 to 5 lb.; and a weight gain of 17 lb. was noted in one subject. Six subjects who weighed themselves twice daily observed that the weight gain was manifested before the onset of headache in periods ranging from four hours to six days.

The time of occurrence of diuresis was less predictable. It commonly occurred during the periods of dwindling headache intensity, but it was also observed before or immediately after the onset of the headache. Less frequently, two and in one case even three headaches were experienced and terminated during a period of sustained weight gain, with diuresis occurring only on elimination of the second or third headache.

Studies were undertaken to ascertain the relevance of this generalized fluid retention to the genesis, frequency, and severity of headache.

Series 1. On four occasions, three patients subject to the migraine type of vascular headache were observed during a period of weight gain. When these patients, because of various premonitory head sensations, were anticipating headaches, they were given 1 to 2 cc of a mercurial diuretic. A diuresis was produced on three of the four occasions, but the usual vascular headache in each instance began at the

anticipated time. On two occasions the headache began during the induced diuresis, and once, three hours later. The intensity and duration of pain were about the same as in previous attacks. A typical instance of the failure of induced diuresis to prevent headache is shown in Fig. 4-16.

Series 2. Various agents were used to prevent fluid accumulation, and the effect on the frequency and intensity of headache was noted. Three patients were studied in the following manner. Daily body weight and occurrence and intensity of headache in each patient were recorded for one month, during which time no diuretics were taken. Acetazoleamide (Diamox), a carbonic anhydrase inhibitor type of diuretic, was then given in 250-mg amounts orally twice daily for another month to each of the three patients. Again, the body weight each day and the incidence and severity of headache were recorded. During the administration of the diuretic agent weight fluctuations were minimized, but the frequency and severity of headache were not altered, as shown in Fig. 4-17. Also, two subjects were given a low-salt (approximately 2 gm daily) diet for two weeks and two were given sodium-removing carboresins for one to two weeks. During the low-salt regimen the variations in body weight were not strikingly altered and headache incidence and severity were unchanged as compared with the control period.

Series 3. Attempts to precipitate headache by inducing a state of overhydration through the use of hormones were made. Three patients subject to the migraine type of vascular headache were given daily injections of 5 units of vasopressin (Pitressin) tannate

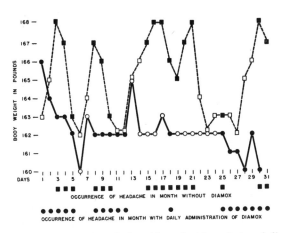

FIG. 4-17. Occurrence of headache with and without induced diuresis.

in oil and drank 2500 cc of fluid daily for two to three days. A weight gain of as much as 6 to 9 lb. was effected, accompanied by nausea, abdominal cramps, and malaise, but no headache resulted (Fig. 4-18). Likewise, in two patients, the intramuscular injection of 20 mg desoxycorticosterone acetate (DOCA) and the ingestion of 20 gm salt daily were attended with moderate weight gain but no headache was experienced.

Comment. The foregoing data indicate that weight gain and widespread fluid retention are phenomena which are concomitant but not causally related to headache, since (a) weight gain did not invariably occur with headache; (b) weight gain was prevented without preventing the occurrence or altering the severity of headache in patients subject to migraine

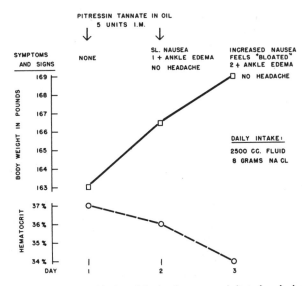

FIG. 4-18. Failure of induced hydration to precipitate headache.

headache; (c) weight gain was induced without inducing headache in patients subject to them.

It is possible that the alteration in retention and excretion of sodium, potassium, water, and corticosteroids is not causally related to headache, but is part of a nonspecific alteration of fluid metabolism and urinary excretion which may accompany vascular headache.

Schottstaedt and Wolff (1955) have shown that the behavior pattern in response to situations perceived as threatening is accompanied by a reduced urinary excretion of sodium, potassium and water, and is followed by a diuresis of all these substances during subsequent relaxation. The occurrence of headaches in those subject to them in such a setting has also been well documented. It is likely, therefore, that headache and overhydration are consequences of parallel body dysfunctions which occur independently as parts of a response to a threatening life situation. The pathophysiology of the generalized fluid retention remains unclear.

Series 4. In order to demonstrate further the lack of relationship between the nonlocalized edema and localized edema, daily observations on both were made on three subjects. Alteration in body weight was taken as an index of widespread fluid retention and edema. The degree of scalp edema was taken as an index of localized edema and was readily estimated from the depth of depression remaining after a standard measured pressure had been applied to the relevant area of the scalp. Two of the patients showed local scalp edema during three headache episodes without appreciable changes in body weight. The third subject was observed during two headaches and experienced successively, gain in weight, diuresis with loss of weight, and then local scalp edema. When body weight was maximal, local scalp edema had not yet occurred; and when local scalp edema was most notable, diuresis had already lowered body weight to its initial level (Fig. 4-19). It is therefore evident that these two phenomena may be separated in time and result from the operation of different mechanisms.

Attempts to Induce Headache with Blister Fluid

Armstrong, Keele *et al.* (1953, 1957) have shown that blister fluid has the capacity to induce pain on an exposed blister base. This capacity they attributed first to a substance having some of the features of serotonin and later to an agent akin to a polypeptide, bradykinin (Armstrong *et al.*, 1954). Since Goodell, Bigelow, and Harrison had shown that blister fluid injection into the skin also lowered pain thresholds, the effect of this naturally occurring substance was assayed in respect to its capacity to induce headache.

On ten occasions five male subjects, three who were subject to headache, and two who were not, were immersed up to the neck in a tub of water 109° to 110° F until bilateral temporal artery dilatation was evident. No headache was present at this time. Fluid was then removed from a blister, which had been prepared by burning the forearm of the same subject with radiant heat two to four days previously. The usual volume of blister fluid obtainable was approximately 0.2 cc. It was allowed to remain in contact with the glass syringe for at least seven minutes, the time required to activate bradykinin in the opinion of Armstrong and Keele (1954). The fluid was then injected subcutaneously into the scalp within a few millimeters of one dilated temporal artery and an injection of sterile isotonic salt was made in the scalp alongside a similar dilated temporal artery on the opposite side of the head. The injections were made by a third experimenter who was handed two syringes labeled A and B by the person who had aspirated the blister fluid. This second person did not reveal the identity of the contents of syringes A and B until 24 hr later. The subject remained in the water for another 10–15 min after the injection, during which time no headache occurred. In all instances, however, 20 to 60 min after the injection, headache indistinguishable from the migraine type of headache occurred at the site of the blister fluid injection and persisted from 1–12 hr. No headache occurred in the opposite control sides injected with sterile saline; nor did headache occur following injection of blister fluid in the absence of induced vasodilatation.

Comment. That a combination of temporal artery dilatation and a naturally occurring pain-threshold-lowering agent can produce headache is significant. The latency of 20–60 min between injection and headache indicates a dissimilarity between this contrived situation and true migraine headache, for in the latter, pain thresholds are lowered at the same time as

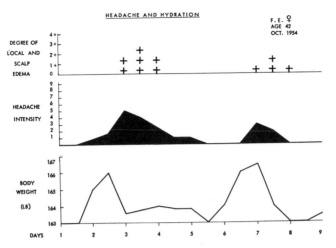

FIG. 4-19. Note the disparity in time between the occurrence of local edema and general accumulation of fluid.

the extracranial dilatation appears and headache begins.

Assay of Local Tissue Fluid Collected from Subsurface Tissues at Migraine Site

A series of experiments aimed at delineating the pain-threshold-lowering capacity and the physical and chemical nature of the local edema fluid in headache were undertaken.

ASSAY OF PAIN-THRESHOLD-LOWERING PROPERTIES OF FLUID ASPIRATED FROM AREAS OF HEADACHE

At the time of the occurrence of headache of the migraine type in two subjects, 2 cc of sterile isotonic saline were injected into the area of headache and the headache-free area of the opposite side, and as much of the fluid was withdrawn as possible. Approximately 0.1 to 0.2 cc could be drawn back with the syringe. This withdrawn fluid was injected intradermally in the forearm immediately contiguous to the sites whose thresholds had been previously determined, and threshold determinations repeated.

The fluid from the headache side was injected into one forearm and that from the headache-free side into the other. In both pa-

tients there was erythema in both sites, but more erythema about the site of headache fluid injection. In the latter site there was a lowering of pain threshold of 20 to 30 millicalories; this was about 10 to 15% more lowering than on the opposite control arm at the site of fluid injection.

ASSAY OF PAIN-THRESHOLD-LOWERING PROPERTIES OF URTICARIAL FLUID

In a subject with "cold allergy" an ice bag placed on one side of his head was followed within a few minutes by the appearance of a large edematous area, and with the subject's report that he experienced a "disagreeable pounding sensation" in that side of his head. Similar studies to those described using fluid from headache areas were then carried out with fluid obtained from such urticarial wheals in this subject with cold allergy. After the pain threshold in both forearms had been measured, lively urticaria was induced in this subject by immersing one hand in ice water. Then 5 cc of sterile isotonic saline were injected into the urticarial area and into the dorsum of the other hand and approximately 0.2 cc of fluid withdrawn from each site. The fluid from the urticarial area was injected intradermally into one forearm very near the site whose

TABLE 4-6   Artery Electrolytes

	Na (mEq. 100 gm dry tissue)					K (mEq. 100 gm dry tissue)				
	1	2	3	4	5	1	2	3	4	5
"Headache" arteries	53.3	49.3	47.0	37.1	50.2	21.3	18.6	16.0	11.2	20.7
"Normal" arteries	50.0	46.0	49.2	51.8	. . .	17.0	15.1	21.9	22.1	. . .

thresholds had been previously determined, and the fluid from the normal area similarly injected into the other forearm. The urticarial fluid induced a threshold lowering of 60 millicalories, which was about 30% more lowering than occurred near the injection site of saline in the other forearm.

Comment. These differences, while small in magnitude, support the inference that there is an agent at the site of subsurface tissue fluid accumulations in headache and hives that promotes lowering of pain thresholds and local vasodilatation, and that this agent is present to a lesser degree, or not at all, in headache-free areas.

CHEMICAL AND MICROSCOPIC ANALYSIS OF SECTIONS FROM SUPERFICIAL TEMPORAL ARTERIES

On 12 occasions, sections of superficial temporal arteries were removed under general anesthesia during migraine headache attacks involving them. In addition, sections of six temporal arteries were taken from subjects who seldom if ever experienced headache, and who were undergoing craniotomy for other reasons. A portion of each vessel was embedded in paraffin, sectioned, and stained with hematoxylin and eosin and with Weigert's stain. Another portion was stripped of adventitia, dried to constant weight, dissolved in concentrated sulfuric acid, diluted appropriately, and its sodium and potassium concentrations were determined by means of the Barclay flame photometer.

Microscopic sections of the vessels removed during headache revealed only pallor and homogeneity of staining of the perivascular tissue and its spaces, a finding compatible with edema. "Headache" vessels exhibited neither collagen swelling with necrosis nor cellular infiltration and, aside from the manifestations of edema, differed in no way from the "nonheadache" vessels. For example, the temporal artery of one subject who had had about 2000 headache attacks involving this vessel showed no evidence of irreversible damage, such as collagen deposit, fibrosis, athermatous, or arteriosclerotic changes. Furthermore, the concentrations of sodium and potassium calculated on a dry-weight basis were not significantly different in the two groups of vessels (Table 4-6).

Comment. The highly circumscribed and often sharply unilateral localization, and the predictability of the site of involvement in vascular headache of the migraine type, strongly suggests that the effects produced in the tissue, as well as in both large and small vessels, are neurogenic.

Recently, biopsies of temporal arteries made during attacks of migraine have shown the vessels to be histologically and histochemically normal, but substantial amounts of catecholamines are bound by the tunica adventitia of migrainous arteries, while no such binding occurs in controls. The significance of this observation awaits further study.

ACETYLCHOLINE IN MIGRAINE HEADACHE

In 1959, Kunkle seriously investigated the possibility that acetylcholine might be implicated in the mechanism of migraine headache. In his search he used spinal fluid.

His incentives for implicating acetylcholine were certain accessory symptoms and signs which accompany migraine headache in some patients. These clues, he noted, often so trivial as to be overlooked, suggest a centrally integrated neural discharge over parasympathetic pathways. Commonest are nasal congestion and excessive lacrimation, probably resulting from impulses over the greater superficial petrosal branch of the facial nerve. Rare, but no less significant, are miosis, more marked on the side of the pain when the headache is unilateral, and bradycardia, presumably mediated by the oculomotor and vagus nerves, respectively.

The route of vasodilator nerves to superficial head vessels is unknown. That to intracranial arteries is not fully charted, but may be via small branches of the facial nerve to the sheath of the internal carotid artery just as it enters the middle fossa.

If acetylcholine is released in the walls of certain cranial arteries in the migraine attack, a portion may enter the bloodstream. Here it is undoubtedly soon destroyed by the ample supply of circulating cholinesterases. The chances are slight, therefore, that it could be detected, even early in the headache.

Kunkle argued that another and more direct approach to this biochemical problem is one aimed at the vicinity of the dilated arteries. Facial and scalp vessels are accessible, but an attempt to demonstrate a release of acetylcholine into these tissues would present formidable technical difficulties. The intracranial arteries, however, are bathed in cerebrospinal fluid, a sample of which can readily be obtained by lumbar puncture. In addition is the advantage that in man this fluid normally contains no detectable acetylcholine and exhibits very little cholinesterase activity.

Accordingly, Kunkle's study was focused upon patients in whom headache of migraine type appeared to arise in part at least from intracranial arteries. This kind of headache is identified by the following characteristics: distinct accentuation anteriorly on mild or moderate rotary head jolt, absence of change during manual compression of scalp arteries, mild improvement during the latter portion of a 10-sec period of straining (the Valsalva maneuver), and, of particular diagnostic value, sharp accentuation beginning 1-2 sec after release of the strain and lasting for several seconds. Also of aid in separating intracranial from extracranial vascular pain is the resistance of intracranial headache to a therapeutic trial of parenterally administered ergotamine tartrate. In some patients the responses to these maneuvers may suggest that both intra- and extracranial arteries are at fault. Occasionally, the reports made by the patient are inconclusive, but in most instances a tenable anatomic inference can be made.

For this projected study cluster headache was of particular value. This migraine varient, high in intensity and relatively brief in duration, usually occurs in bouts of headache in rapid succession, once or more each 24 hr. Once a series of headaches has begun, the patient is uniquely accessible to study. Furthermore, the pain is in some patients intracranial and in others, extracranial, and the accessory features of parasympathetic overflow listed above are found more frequently than in other types of migraine. For these reasons, the disorders were especially appropriate for physiologic analysis.

Kunkle pointed out that his project arose from a chain of hypotheses: (1) that some forms of migraine headache are attributable to painful dilatation of intracranial arteries; (2) that the vasodilatation is neurogenic and employs, as the end-organ mediator, acetylcholine; and (3) that acetylcholine, thus released in intracranial arterial walls, may diffuse sufficiently through the surrounding cerebrospinal fluid to be detected in the lumbar sac. The outcome of the search for acetylcholine hinges upon the validity of these assumptions, some of which clearly remain open to question and modifications.

In the group of 37 patients with diseases other than headache, no acetylcholine was found in the cerebrospinal fluid samples except for those from two patients with grand mal seizures. In one patient the most recent convulsion was 25 hr before lumbar puncture; in the other, 10 days; acetylcholine-like effects equivalent, respectively, to 0.004 and 0.005 μg/ml of cerebrospinal fluid were recorded.

In none of the patients with headaches diagnosed as nonvascular was an acetylcholine-like reaction found. Among the 22 with headache diagnosed as vascular, however, the assays demonstrated an acetylcholine-like substance in five, all male. In amount, it was equivalent to 0.004 to 0.06 μg of acetylcholine per milliliter of cerebrospinal fluid. In four of these patients the headache appeared to be intracranial in origin, and in one, both intracranial and extracranial. In each case, headache was present at the time of lumbar puncture—in three for ten to 48 hr, and in two for 15 to 30 min.

Kunkle (1959) argued that his results lend considerable support to the basic hypothesis that acetylcholine participates in the mechanism of migraine headache.

Possible explanations for the negative assays in one-half of the patients with intracranial vascular headaches include release of the vasodilator substance in amounts too small to be detected, unduly rapid breakdown of the substance at site of its action, limited diffusion across vessel walls and through the subarachnoid spaces, or the concomitant presence in some cerebrospinal fluid specimens of agents such as serotonin, with opposing effects upon the clam heart.

PROTEOLYTIC ENZYMES IN CEREBROSPINAL FLUID DURING SEVERE MIGRAINE HEADACHE WITH EVIDENCE OF INTRACRANIAL DYSFUNCTION

As mentioned above, a study of tissue fluid removed from regions of local tenderness in the scalp during vascular headache of the migraine type indicated that this fluid contained a

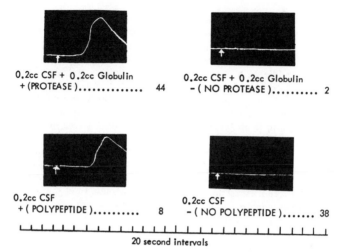

0.2cc CSF + 0.2cc Globulin
  + (PROTEASE).............. 44

0.2cc CSF + 0.2cc Globulin
  − (NO PROTEASE).......... 2

0.2cc CSF
  + (POLYPEPTIDE).......... 8

0.2cc CSF
  − (NO POLYPEPTIDE)....... 38

20 second intervals

FIG. 4-20. Rat uterus bioassay of cerebrospinal fluid collected from 46 subjects with active disease of the central nervous system.

pain-threshold-lowering substance (Chapman et al., 1960). It had many of the properties of vasodilator polypeptides derived from plasma proteins. Armstrong et al. (1957) demonstrated that such polypeptides were present in blister fluid, in fluid collected from painful joints, and in inflammatory pleural fluid. The properties of the polypeptide correspond closely to those of bradykinin, the name given by Rocha e Silva, Beraldo, and Rosenfeld (1949) to the substance or substances produced on incubation of snake venom or trypsin with serum, plasma, or plasma globulins.

It has been postulated that vascular headache of the migraine type is an epiphenomenon arising as a sequel of the excessive operation of the normal mechanism for functional vasodilatation in the head. The painful dilatation, chiefly of some of the branches of the external carotid artery, is viewed as incidental to dilatation of the branches of the internal carotid artery (usually nonpainful), perhaps because of the common innervation of these vessels. Since the fluid in the tissues surrounding the branches of the external carotid artery contained vasodilator polypeptides of the bradykinin type, (Ostfeld et al., 1957) the possibility that a vasodilator polypeptide system (protease and polypeptide) also was implicated in functional vasodilatation

within the central nervous system seemed worthy of exploration. Furthermore, it seemed pertinent to ask whether excessive amounts of these substances were present in pathologic states within the central nervous system (Chapman and Wolff, 1959).

Attempts have been made to ascertain whether and under what circumstances such an enzyme and vasodilator system is present in the central nervous system. To this end cerebrospinal fluid was collected from subjects with (1) active disease of the central nervous system; (2) inactive, nonprogressive, or no disease of the central nervous system; (3) vascular headache of the migraine type; (4) sustained nervous stimulation and pain arising from disorders of the legs or pelvic organs; and (5) disease syndromes classified as chronic schizophrenia. Specimens were either assayed at once or immediately frozen in solid carbon dioxide.

Method for Assaying Protease and Vasodilator Polypeptides with a Smooth Muscle Preparation

The assay method is described in detail elsewhere. Freshly collected or thawed cerebrospinal fluid (0.2 cc) was added to the 3-cc chamber. If contractions were observed, the specimen was recorded as inducing a polypep-

TABLE 4-7   41 Subjects with Inactive, Nonprogressive, or No Disease of the
Central Nervous System

Subject No.	Disease Category	Cerebrospinal Fluid Total Protein (MG %)		Protease	Polypeptide	Negative
		Range	Mean			
10	Cerebrovascular accident (old, small, or vascular insuf.)	20–42	34	0	0	10
4	Myasthenia gravis	28–64	40	0	0	4
4	Seizure disorder (idio., not freq., or recent)	24–41	33	0	0	4
3	Progressive muscular dystrophy	19–38	38	0	0	3
2	Pituitary adenoma	20 & 37	29	0	0	2
2	Primary lateral sclerosis (old)	39 & 45	42	0	0	2
2	Bell's palsy	20 & 40	30	0	0	2
2	Myelopathy (old, post. sp. anaes., idio.)	48 & 56	52	0	0	2
2	Cerebral dysplasia	16 & 24	20	0	0	2
2	Occl. vasc. dis. (periph. neuropathy)	36 & 45	40	0	0	2
6	Syringomyelia, old polio. and misc.	32–46	39	0	0	6
1	Dietary insuf. (senile osteoporosis)		32	1	0	0
1	Hypert. vas. dis. (cerv. osteoarthritis)		40	1	0	0
41		41 specimens		2	0	36

tide reaction. If no contractions were observed, 0.2 cc of the specimen was incubated with 0.2 cc of an 8% solution of bovine globulin (fraction II) for 3 min at 29°C. If the resultant mixture induced contractions, the specimen was recorded as inducing a protease reaction. If no contractions were observed, the specimen was recorded as negative.

It was inferred that the specimens which gave protease reactions contained detectable amounts of a proteolytic enzyme capable of acting on plasma proteins (globulin) to form polypeptides of the bradykinin type and that specimens which gave polypeptide reactions contained detectable amounts not only of the enzyme but of the products of proteolytic activity, presumably polypeptides (see Fig. 4-20).

Subjects with Inactive, Nonprogressive, or No Disease of Central Nervous System

Cerebrospinal fluid specimens from subjects with inactive, nonprogressive, or no disease of the nervous system only rarely induced contractions of the rat uterus under the conditions

of the assay (2 of 41 specimens studied). (Table 4-7).

Subjects with Migraine Headache

Eighteen specimens of cerebrospinal fluid were collected from subjects (Table 4-8) during or one day after vascular headache of the migraine type. Protease reactions were observed in 15 of these specimens. Polypeptide reactions were induced by three. All the latter were collected from subjects with involvement of both intracranial and extracranial tissues. Eight specimens were collected in the headache-free interval (more than seven days after a migraine attack). Seven of these resulted in negative reactions. One specimen, collected eight days after the cessation of pain but during a continued but transient oculomotor palsy (ophthalmoplegic migraine), gave a polypeptide reaction.

Comment. These observations indicated that increased protease concentration in the cerebrospinal fluid occurs during vascular headache of the migraine type. Further, a

TABLE 4-8   19 Subjects with Migraine Headache

| | Cerebrospinal Fluid Total Protein (mg %) | | | | |
Observations	Range	Mean	Protease	Polypeptide	Negative
In subjects with pain mainly from extracranial tissue					
14 during headache	22–60	36	13	0	1
2 one day after headache	24 & 78		2	0	0
7 one week after headache	22–49	37	0	0	7
In subjects with pain also from intracranial tissue					
2* during headache	23 & 41		0	2	0
1† 8 days after headache	88		0	1	0
26 observations			15	3	8

*One had transient hemiplegia and aphasia.
†Ophthalmoplegic migraine.

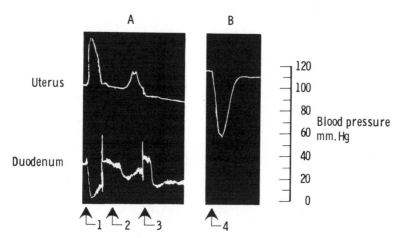

FIG. 4-21. Action of "headache stuff" (A) on isolated rat uterus and rat duodenum (suspended in a single 3-cc chamber containing low-calcium Ringer-Locke solution at 29°C.) and (B) on the blood pressure of a rat (weight 150-200 gm; cannulae in the carotid artery for recording of pressure, and in the jugular vein for injection of specimens); 1 = 20 milliunits bradykinin (as defined by Rocha e Silva), 2 = 10 milliunits bradykinin, 3 and 4 = 0.015 cc subcutaneous perfusate from the head collected during severe vascular headache of the migraine type. Note that this special low-calcium solution (0.02 gm $CaCl_1/1$) permits discrimination of "headache stuff" from bradykinin, since the uterus remains sensitive to bradykinin but does not respond to "headache stuff." The duodenum continues to respond to both. (The ratio of activity of "headache stuff" to bradykinin in this solution is duodenum 1, uterus 0.08-0.10.) In solutions containing higher concentrations of calcium (0.06 gm $CaCl_2/1$) the uterus is more sensitive to "headache stuff" (ratio duodenum 1, uterus 0.30-0.50). Also, the rat blood pressure is much more sensitive to "headache stuff" than the bradykinin (ratio duodenum 1, blood pressure 35-50).

smooth-muscle-contracting substance is present in the cerebrospinal fluid in subjects with such headache in which intracranial as well as extracranial tissues are implicated. Since vasodilatation of the intracranial vessels is associated with vascular headache of the migraine type, the demonstration of protease and polypeptide in the cerebrospinal fluid supports the hypothesis that the protease-polypeptide system is implicated in local vasomotor control of the intracranial vessels. The intracranial vasodilatation during a migraine attack, however, rarely is painful; the pain stems chiefly from the branches of the external carotid artery. In those instances in which there is pain from noxious stimulation of intracranial vessels, it is inferred that a pain-threshold-lowering substance is present in relatively high concentrations in the pain-sensitive regions within the cranium, particularly about the vessels at the base of the brain.

Its presence may be relevant to local edema formation in the cerebrum as well as intracranial vascular structures. Such edema, of the uncus for instance, might cause pressure on the third cranial nerve. It might also be relevant to transient hemiplegias in some patients during and after headache attacks.

TABLE 4-9   "Headache Stuff"

---

1. Present in subsurface tissue of the head in aching and tender sites during and shortly after vascular headache of the migraine type
2. When introduced into the human skin it
    (a) Induces vasodilatation
    (b) Lowers pain threshold
    (c) Increases capillary permeability
    (d) Increases vulnerability of tissue to injury
3. Relaxes rat duodenum
4. Contracts rat uterus
5. Depresses rat blood pressure
6. Its action on rat blood pressure is diminished by
    (a) Incubation with chymotrypsin (destruction of polypeptide)
    (b) Boiling (destruction of proteolytic enzyme)
    Its action on rat blood pressure is eliminated by a Plus b (incubation with chymotrypsin, followed by boiling)
7. Its activity diminishes rapidly when it is allowed to stand at room temperature.
8. Its properties are those of a mixture of a polypeptide and a proteolytic enzyme

---

FURTHER DEFINITION OF A BIOCHEMICAL AGENT IMPLICATED IN MIGRAINE HEADACHE

As shown above, during the painful phase of attacks of vascular headache of the migraine type there is dilatation of the large and small blood vessels of the head both intra- and extracranially, often more on one side than the other. In most attacks, however, the pain stems chiefly from the large subsurface cranial arteries and their branches. Aching pain is experienced when these vessels are distended, pulled upon, or displaced. Yet dilatation of these vessels, for instance that induced by immersion of the body in hot water, is not usually painful and does not induce other focal features of the migraine attack, i.e., edema, tenderness on pressure, and heightened vulnerability of tissue to injury. These observations led to the hypothesis that in addition to vasodilatation, a local sterile inflammation occurs. Also a substance (or substances) accumulates in the walls of the arteries and in the adjacent perivascular, areolar, and supporting tissues as well that lowers pain thresholds, increases capillary permeability, and heightens vulnerability to injury.

Method

The observations of Keele and his associates (1957) demonstrating that the pain-producing substance in blister fluid had many of the properties of the group of vasodilator polypeptides referred to as bradykinin, kallidin, or plasma kinins, led us to assay on the isolated rat uterus specimens of subsurface tissue fluid collected during headache. The rat uterus contracts in the presence of minute amounts of these polypeptides. Preliminary analysis demonstrated that specimens collected during headache contracted the rat uterus. To characterize the active substance, the rat uterus, rat duodenum, and rat blood pressure were used for quantitative assay.

Specimens were collected (a) from the tender regions of the head during headaches of a wide range of intensity (15 subjects, 23 specimens), (b) from tender regions of the head following headache attacks of ten persons, (c) from nontender regions of the heads of four persons subject to headache but during headache-free periods, and (d) from 18 persons not subject to headache attacks. For comparison, specimens were also drawn at the same time

TABLE 4-10 "Headache Stuff"

1. Its properties are not those of epinephrine, norepinephrine, oxytocin, cerebrotonin, angiotonin (hypertensin), or pepsitensin.
2. Although some of the following may be present in small amounts in the stuff, it is not mainly acetylcholine, histamine, serotonin, adenosine, adenosine triphosphate (ATP), potassium, or isoproterenol (Isuprel).
3. It has certain features in common with, but can be differentiated from, other polypeptides and proteolytic enzymes: bradykinin, urinary kallikrein, urinary kallidin, plasma kallikrein, plasma kallidin, plasmin, wasp kinin, substance P, substance Z, and substance U.

from (e) the subcutaneous tissues of the forearm of each subject.

Results

It was found that specimens collected from the head during the headache attacks contained a substance that could be distinguished from serotonin, potassium, ATP, substance P, acetylcholine, and histamine, although these and other substances may also have been present. The active substance relaxed the isolated rat duodenum, contracted the rat uterus, and depressed the blood pressure of the rat (Fig. 4-21, Tables 4-9 and 4-10). A constant ratio of activity on these several assay preparations among several specimens of tissue fluid indicated that the observed activity of the specimens was due to a single substance.

The activity of the specimens dwindled when they were allowed to stand at room temperature, but the specimens could be stabilized by boiling with alcohol. Incubation with chymotrypsin inactivated the stabilized specimens indicating that the active substance remaining after stabilization is a polypeptide (Fig. 4-22). The heat-stabilized substance had many of the properties of bradykinin, kallidin, or plasma kinin. However, when analyzed quantitatively with several assay procedures it was evident that the substance is not identical with any of these, although it closely resembles them and is a polypeptide of the same type. This substance has been labeled "neurokinin" and has been found in the laboratory to be released during neuronal excitation. It is released into tissue fluid of the skin of man during dorsal root stimulation and during axon reflex flare. It is not the result of vasodilatation alone, since it is

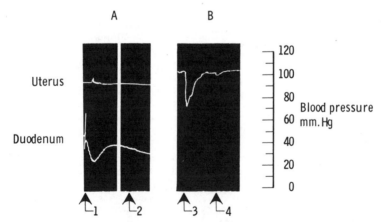

FIG. 4-22. The effect of boiling and of incubation with chymotrypsin on "headache stuff." Subcutaneous perfusate was collected from the head during a severe migraine headache. The total specimen was placed in a boiling water bath for 5 min. One-half of the specimen was then incubated with 1 mg chymotrypsin for 5 min; 1 and 3 = 0.01 cc perfusate after boiling; 2 and 4 = 0.01 cc after boiling followed by incubation with chymotrypsin. Note again that in this low-calcium solution the uterus does not respond to "headache stuff" in this amount.

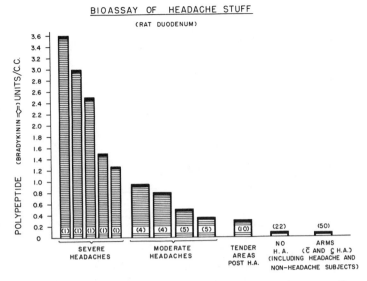

FIG. 4-23. Results of bioassay of subcutaneous perfusates grouped according to the intensity of pain.

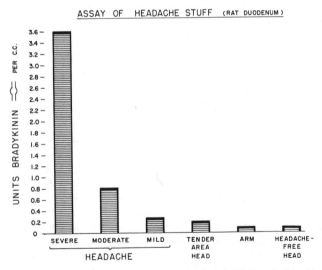

FIG. 4-24. Bioassay of specimens of subcutaneous perfusate from a single subject collected during severe, moderate, and mild headache attacks and during a headache-free period 24 hr after the termination of a severe headache, while the region perfused was still "tender" to pressure.

not released during reactive hypermia (Chapman *et al.*, 1960). It has also been found in the cerebrospinal fluid of patients during severe and long-lasting vascular headache of the migraine type. Small or trace amounts of this polypeptide were found in the following groups of specimens: those collected from the arms of persons subject to migraine attacks both during headache and headache-free periods, those from the heads of these subjects

ASSAY OF HEADACHE STUFF (RAT DUODENUM)

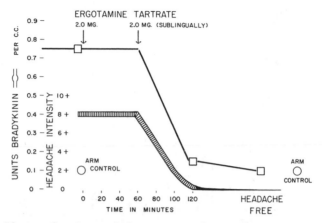

FIG. 4-25. Bioassay of specimens of subcutaneous perfusate collected from a single subject (a) during a severe headache, (b) after the administration of ergotamine tartrate when the pain had diminished almost entirely, and (c) one week after the headache attack during a headache-free period.

during headache-free periods, and those from the heads and arms of persons not subject to headache attacks. On the other hand, the polypeptide content of specimens collected from the heads of patients during headache was large, averaging eight times as much, and in rare instances 35 times as much as control values (Fig. 4-23). Specimens collected shortly after termination of the headache also contained increased amounts of the substance. The amount of active agent found in the specimens was closely related to the intensity of the headache attack (Fig. 4-24). Following administration of ergotamine tartrate in subjects with headache, the intensity of headache, amplitude of cranial artery pulsations, local tenderness, and polypeptide content all decreased concurrently (Fig. 4-25).

Comparison of activity of specimens before and after heat stabilization demonstrated that the depressor action on the blood pressure was substantially reduced by boiling (destruction of a heat-labile proteolytic enzyme?). The observations suggest, therefore, that in addition to the polypeptide, headache fluid contains a proteolytic enzyme capable of forming neurokinin (presumably by cleavage of a plasma globulin present in subsurface extracellular fluid). This enzyme has been termed neurokinin-forming enzyme (NFE) (Table 4-11).

In other experiments, headache fluid has been shown to lower pain threshold, to induce vasodilatation, to increase capillary permeability, and to increase tissue vulnerability to injury (see Table 4-12).

Comment. The increased content of polypeptide (neurokinin) and protease (NFE) found locally could account for many of the features of vascular headache of the migraine type. Neurokinin is an extremely powerful vasodilator. When injected intradermally, tissue fluids containing mixtures of neurokinin and NFE induce pain, lower pain threshold, and increase capillary permeability.

The release or activation of neurokinin-forming enzyme and subsequent formation of neurokinin has been observed during neuronal excitation in man in a variety of circumstances. The potent hypotensive and vasodilator action of eurokinin and its formation during neuronal excitation suggest strongly that it serves in local vasomotor control for the nervous system. Migraine headache attacks are linked to activity of the central nervous system, since they often occur after long periods of alertness, striving, extraordinary effort, or

TABLE 4-11   Tissue Fluids Containing
Neurokinin-Forming Enzyme and Neurokinin

1. Induce vasodilatation
2. Lower pain threshold
3. Increase capillary permeability
4. Increase vulnerability of tissue to injury

Neurokinin-Forming Enzyme (NFE)	Neurokinin
1. No action on rat uterus	1. Contracts rat uterus
2. No action on rat duodenum	2. Relaxes rat duodenum
3. Depresses rat blood pressure	3. Depresses rat blood pressure
4. Boiling destroys depressor action	4. Action on rat uterus, duodenum, and blood pressure is stabilized by boiling (destruction of peptidase)
5. Not inhibited by trypsin inhibitors (pancreactic soy bean)	5. Destroyed by chymotrypsin

major frustration. The painful local reaction in the extracranial vessels may thus be an epiphenomenon of the excessive operation of the normal mechanisms for functional vasodilatation within the central nervous system. A common innervation of the branches of the external and internal carotid arteries could lead to a simultaneous release of vasodilator substances both intracranially and extracranially.

CONCLUSION

The pain of vascular headache of the migraine type can be seen as the outcome of the combined effects of large artery dilatation plus the action of pain-threshold-lowering substances accumulating in the blood vessel walls and perivascular tissue. Two such substances have been defined as a vasodilator polypeptide (neurokinin) and a proteolytic enzyme (neurokinin-forming enzyme), both implicated in local vasomotor control. The result is a sterile inflammatory reaction, neurogenically induced.

TABLE 4-12   Comparison of Properties (Relatively Well Established)

	BLISTER FLUID	SEROTONIN	BRADYKININ	HEADACHE SUBSTANCE	NEUROKININ
Molecular weight approximately	1000	177	1089	?	?
Pain initiated (superficial and deep)	+	+	+	+	+
Pain duration	Prolonged	Prolonged	Prolonged	Prolonged	Prolonged
Vasodilatation	+	+	+	+	+
Increases permeability	+	+	+	+	+
Lowers pain threshold: superficial deep	+	+	+	+	+
Increases tissue vulnerability	+	+	+	+	+
Soluble in water	+	+	+	+	+
Contracts rat uterus	+	+	+	+	+
Antagonized by atropine	0	0	0	0	0
Antagonized by antihistamine	0	0	0	0	0
Relaxes rat duodenum	+	0	+	+	+
Contracts guinea pig ileum	+	+	+	0	0
Depresses rat blood pressure in amounts close to threshold for rat uterus or duodenum	0	0	0	+	+
Destroyed by chymotrypsin	+	0	+	+	+

PROLONGED BUT REVERSIBLE BRAIN IMPAIRMENT OCCURRING WITH MIGRAINE
Complicated Migraine

The term "complicated migraine" is usually employed when the neurological manifestations which characterize migraine persist beyond the immediate headache period. Such neurological complications include hemiparesis, hemisensory defects, occlusion of the retinal artery, ophthalmoplegia, and related signs and symptoms. Most of these conditions are assumed to be due to prolonged vasoconstriction or vasodilatation occurring as a part of the migraine syndrome. If the brain becomes ischemic enough during this vasoactive process, permanent damage may ensue, or cerebral infraction may occur. Death has been reported in this situation, though probably this is a rare occurrence (Guest and Woolf, 1964).

A related condition is basilar artery migraine, as reported by Bickerstaff (1961). This symptom complex often occurs in young women and is characterized by loss of vision, dysarthria, ataxia, vertigo, and tinnitus. The symptoms are often bilateral and may progress to loss of consciousness.

The incidence of complicated migraine is uncertain. The best study, by Heyck and Krayenbuhl (1969) reports on 980 patients with migraine, in whom they found an incidence of unilateral sensory signs of 3.8% and unilateral motor signs in 1.2%. These figures suggest that complicated migraine is a rare phenomenon. However, given the relative incidence of migraine in the general population, one may assume that complicated migraine will be found by those alert to its existence in figures higher than those previously reported.

Hemiplegic Migraine

Hemiplegic migraine illuminates the basic nature of the intracranial accompaniments of the vascular headache of the migraine type. This variety of attack is accompanied by motor and sensory defects. Recovery is usually not prompt, and indeed the hemiplegic signs and symptoms may persist for days or weeks, although complete recovery is usual. Such periods of motor and sensory defects may recur many times in the life span of the patient. Sometimes the symptom complex occurs in families with a strangely monotomous duplication of the clinical defects from person to person and in succeeding generations. This variety of attack may alternate with the more usual type of migraine beginning with visual aura or simply with hemicrania and vomiting. Between attacks there are no signs of impairment.

Whitty (1953) has assembled the facts on reported cases of hemiplegic migraine. He cites a report of Jelliffe (1906) of a patient who had had attacks since childhood. The onset was with visual symptoms which proceeded to a right hemiparesis with sensory loss. Headache was severe, though described as mainly right-sided. All symptoms subsided completely in three to four days, and he was able to return to his normal routine. In 1910 Clarke published the history of a family of which three generations had suffered from the complaint. The attacks had a striking similarity from case to case. He gave details of six cases, though no less than 11 persons amongst 23 siblings were known to be affected. In all six the onset was with visual symptoms which proceeded to a hemiplegia with some degree of hemianesthesia, and was followed in a few hours by severe hemicrania and vomiting when the neurological signs were right-sided with aphasia, though in two cases attacks on the other side were mentioned. The attacks lasted two to three days and recovery was complete. They had occurred since childhood with a tendency to be less frequent as age advanced, his oldest patient being 54 years at his death from pneumonia. This description illustrates two points which are common in hemiplegic migraine: its strong familial tendency and the similarity in the pattern of attack within the family tree. Dynes (1939) also described the condition in a mother and daughter. Here the hemiparesis was either right- or left-sided, and again the course of the attack was the same in each case: signs would begin in the hand (and speech in right-sided attacks), proceed to a hemiparesis with some anesthesia, but visual signs occurred relatively late. Symonds (1952) has added two further cases. In both there was a family history of similar attacks. In one, where the family history showed three generations affected, the patient had had a carotid angiogram done during the height of an attack. This showed no abnormality. The electroencephalogram gave evidence of marked electrical abnormality throughout the right hemisphere. (The paresis was on the left.) The cerebrospinal fluid contained three polymorphonuclear leukocytes per cubic millimeter, but was otherwise normal, though late in a previous attack there had been 185 polymorphonuclear cells per cubic millimeter. An air encephalogram done shortly after this had been normal. The case is of special interest as the first record of cerebral angiography done during an attack. As Symonds remarks, the evidence of its normality must exclude arterial spasm in any but the smallest arteries.

Whitty (1953) reported five additional patients with hemiplegic migraine, in three of whom there was clearly stated evidence for its familial occurrence, although migraine attacks occurred in other members of all five families.

Ophthalmoplegic Migraine

Elliot (1940), in reviewing the subject, quoted Charcot's definition of ophthalmoplegic migraine as migraine associated with a third or other ocular nerve palsy, which is transient at first, but later may become permanent. The syndrome occurs in persons of all ages. Patients as young as three and as old as 70 years of age have been described.

Ophthalmoplegic symptoms, according to Riley (1932) may develop in a patient who has had migraine headaches for many years; and 50 years may intervene between the occurrence of the first migraine headache attack and the paralysis of the eye muscles.

The ache of ophthalmoplegic migraine is experienced behind or over the eye. It is usually confined to one side of the head and on the same side as the ophthalmoplegia. Occasionally the headache is bilateral. When the duration of the headache is prolonged, or when the pain is very intense, nausea and vomiting occur. Vertigo may be associated with the headache. In addition to the headache, the usual preheadache visual disturbances of migraine may occur, including spots before the eyes and homonymous field defects; but these are not relevant to this discussion.

The headache usually precedes the extraocular paralysis, the latter appearing 6–10 hr after the onset of the headache, or with the subsidence of the attack. More rarely, from one to ten days may elapse between the onset of a long-lasting headache and the palsy. The third, fourth, sixth, or portions of the fifth cranial nerves may be involved. Occasionally all of them may be involved, presenting a complete external ophthalmoplegia. In partial third nerve palsy the internal musculature of the eye

alone may be involved, resulting in difference in size of the pupils, loss of accommodation, and defects in convergence and divergence.

In patients who have repeated attacks, it is usual for the paralysis to be transient in the earlier ones, with complete recovery; but later the paralysis may persist for a few days to many months, with certain palsies ultimately becoming permanent.

When a patient is seen with an ocular palsy for the first time, it is difficult to choose between intracranial aneurysm and ophthalmoplegic migraine. When such palsies are numerous, short-lived, and recurrent over a period of years, there need be no such difficulty.

The evidence from postmortem examination, concerning the cause of such palsies, is inconclusive. The reported lesions have included gray granulations on the roots of the oculomotor nerve, a fibrochondroma of the nerve, a neurofibroma, and a ruptured aneurysm of the posterior communicating artery. Thrombosis of the central retinal artery has occurred occasionally in connection with ophthalmoplegic migraine. In the light of more recent experience with subarachnoid hemorrhage, it would appear that at least some of the patients described as having ophthalmoplegic migraine had cerebral aneurysms pressing on the third, and perhaps other, cranial nerves. (With an aneurysm, the pupil on the affected side is *almost always* dilated and fixed, whereas only a third of those with ophthalmoplegic migraine and third nerve palsy have a dilated and fixed pupil.)

It was suggested in the first edition of this book (1948) that transient dilatation and thickening or edema of the cerebral arterial walls and their adjacent tissues, such as probably occurs during migraine attacks, is responsible for the palsy of the cranial nerves. The third cranial nerve closely approximates the posterior cerebral artery and the posterior communicating artery. Also, the third, fourth, fifth, and sixth cranial nerves are in close approximation to the internal carotid and the anterior and middle cerebral arteries.

Thus it is likely that ophthalmoplegic migraine is the result of pressure exerted by greatly dilated, thickened, edematous arterial walls, or edema of other tissues involved in migraine headache attacks.

Headache with Labyrinthine Syndrome ('Ménière's Syndrome')

Sir Charles Symonds (1952) has called attention to the frequent occurrence of headache as a symptom in Ménière's syndrome, together with loss of hearing, tinnitus, and vertigo. The tinnitus and defects in hearing may be present in such patients most of the time for years. But during attacks these symptoms are augmented and the vertigo becomes conspicuous. It is during the attack and sometimes outlasting it that the headache is featured. Two areas are commonly involved. One is postauricular or suboccipital on the side of the tinnitus and hearing defect, and may be described as a throbbing or pulsating ache, though sometimes as a steady ache. The second is a sustained sensation of tightness, pressure, and ache of wider distribution, chiefly in the back of the head and neck. The latter may be associated with head tilting and may follow sustained contraction of skeletal muscle. The sustained tinnitus and loss of hearing, the "dead cheek" phenomenon with hypoesthesia in the lateral aspect of the face and about the ear found in some patients with Ménière's syndrome with prolonged headache probably also represents the effects of pressure of distended and edematous posterior fossa arteries on afferent fibers contained in the fifth, seventh, eighth, ninth, and tenth cranial nerves. These phenomena, with their unfortunate longer-lasting effects, are in many ways similar to those linked with ophthalmoplegic migraine, the edematous process in this instance, however, involving mainly the contents of the posterior fossa.

Bickerstaff (1961) studied 34 patients whose clinical symptoms also suggested involvement of the basilar system. All were under the age of 35; all but two were under 23. Twenty-six were adolescent girls. A history of migraine in close relatives was obtained in 28 cases.

The first symptom was usually visual; in some, this consisted of total loss of vision, and in others of simple visual images throughout both visual fields, usually so intense as to obscure vision. This was followed by vertigo, ataxia of gait, dysarthria, and occasionally tinnitus—not necessarily in that order, and the ataxia was not necessarily associated with vertigo. Sensory manifestations consisted of tingling or numbness in both hands and feet, and sometimes around both lips and on both sides of the tongue. These symptoms lasted from 2 min to a maximum of 45 and then subsided rapidly, though if there had been complete loss of vision, this dwindled more gradually (5 min) through a period of graying of vision. In each instance the premonitory symptoms were followed by severe throbbing headache, usually in the occipital region, and often accompanied by vomiting. The headache finally ended when the patient slept. These attacks were infrequent, but in the girls commonly occurred with menstruation. Between attacks many patients had more usual attacks of vascular headache of the migraine type. Over the years the more bizarre features described above no longer occurred.

Swanson and Vick (1978) have reported their experience with 12 patients considered to have basilar artery migraine. They find this to be a distinctive disorder characterized by symptoms referable to dysfunction of brainstem structures in conjunction with more typical migraine phenomena. They describe in detail one patient in whom an attack of basilar artery migraine was captured by the electroencephalogram and appeared as a typical photoconvulsive episode. This patient on several occasions became unconscious without warning. She had two attacks in a brightly lit environment while she was standing at the foot of an upward moving escalator. In each episode she suddenly lost vision and then quickly became unconscious for about 3 min, slumping in an akinetic fashion to the floor. Subsequently, during photic stimulation and electroencephalographic recording, she had an attack similar to those described above. The investigators make the point that approximately half of their patients with basilar artery migraine responded to anticonvulsant drugs. They discussed the possible relationships between basilar artery migraine and epilepsy but have drawn no specific conclusions.

Peripheral Vasomotor Reactions and Migraine

Appenzeller has reviewed vasomotor function in scalp and finger vessels in ten patients with classic migraine during periods free of headache (1969). After ten minutes of heating his patients' chests, he observed normal vasodilatation in the scalp in only two patients. In eight of the ten patients with classical migraine, no vasodilatation in the hand vessels was observed during 40 seconds' heating of the chest, and in some patients marked alterations in blood flow were observed during the heating period. A significant vasodilatation was produced in all control subjects, but in only two of the ten migrainous subjects. On the basis of his studies, Appenzeller suggests the following hypothesis. First, in patients with migraine the blood vessels are continuously constricted because of abnormal neurogenic influences. Second, the vessels dilate and thereafter become painful because of local elaboration of vasoactive substances which are either endogenous or exogenous.

Heyck (1960) has accumulated evidence which, he feels, relates the opening of arteriovenous shunts to the signs and symptoms of migraine. He suggests that a short circuit of blood in the regional circulation has consequences which include arterialization of venous blood in the discharging veins, hemodynamic changes at the site of the migraine attack, and marked reduction and resistance in the arteriovenous circuit. He infers that these vascular changes, together with tissue hypoxia and acidosis which lowers the pain threshold, can be the cause of migraine pain which is experienced in a peripheral section of a vessel. Perivascular edema is then explained on the basis of transudation, the result of increased filtration pressure in arterioles and bridge vessels located in the shunt circuit. However, a histologic description of these cerebral arteriovenous vessels and their demonstration during a true episode of migraine remains to be accomplished.

Brain Dysfunction and Cerebrospinal Fluid Abnormalities in Patients with Ophthalmoplegic Migraine

The walls of the cerebral blood vessels seem to be in an unusual state at the time of, or shortly after, migraine attacks. Accidents such as hemiplegia and aphasia lasting some days or weeks after performing angiograms have occurred in four such instances in the experience of H. G. Wolff at the New York Hospital and resulted in the policy of avoiding such procedures on patients suffering from migraine who have recently had attacks. The spinal fluid showed minor changes in color, protein content, and cells. It was assumed on the basis of these severe reactions that in some instances the walls of the cerebral blood vessels have become unusually sensitive to the presence of the radio-opaque material, resulting in an alteration in their permeability. The evidence supporting the view that with the migraine attack a sterile inflammatory reaction occurs, suggests that the ordinarily innocuous radio-opaque material has become a traumatizing agent.

ELECTROENCEPHALOGRAPHIC ABNORMALITIES IN PATIENTS WITH MIGRAINE

When electroencephalography is performed in patients who are examined for the complaint of headache, without reference to the types of headache, the number of abnormal records is not different from that found in a similar group of headache-free individuals.

However, the incidence of abnormal electroencephalographic records increases significantly when patients with vascular headache of the migraine type are studied.

Townsend (1967) observes that more abnormalities are seen to occur in the electroencephalograms of migraine patients than in the electroencephalograms of a comparable control population. He further notes that the difference is only statistically significant and is not of diagnostic importance, though the electroencephalogram is "one of the physical signs in the syndrome of dysrhythmic migraine." He suggests also that there is accumulating evidence of a peculiarity in the electroencephalographic response of patients with migraine to rhythmic light stimuli, the so-called "H-response." Smyth and Winter (1964) associate this response with instability of the control system relating vascular tone to cortical activity.

Nonfocal Abnormalities

Selby and Lance (1960) studied the electroencephalograms of 459 patients with migraine and allied vascular headache. All records were taken during the headache-free period. Of the 459 records, 139, about one-third, were considered to be abnormal. Activity of 4 to 7 cps occurring persistently or in runs, accounted for 122 of the abnormalities. Wave and spike paroxysms were seen in two cases. In another, diffuse 3 cps activity was the abnormality.

Heyck (1969) reported the electroencephalographic study of 62 patients with migraine. Nonspecific, diffuse, slow-wave dysrhythmias were seen in 13 patients. An additional five patients had focal abnormalities making a total of 18 (29%) with abnormal electroencephalograms.

In 1952 Weil reported studies on 31 patients with migraine headache. The electroencephalogram was clearly abnormal in eight (26%). Runs of high-amplitude slow activity were seen in four records and random or paroxysmal theta activity occurred in the other four. Seven of the eight cases had had, during their attacks, either aphasia, syncope, hemimotor or hemisensory abnormality, or ophthalmoplegia. The headaches of none of the eight were modified by ergotamine, but all patients reported considerable improvement or were made free of symptoms when phenobarbital and dilantin were administered. Weil classified these headaches associated with these electroencephalographic abnormalities as dysrhythmic migraine, and suggested that this special group be treated with anticonvulsant medication.

Goldensohn (1976) has reviewed the incidence of abnormal electroencephalograms in patients with headache. Of 200 patients with recurrent headache and negative neurological examinations who were seen over a two-year period 27% had abnormal records. Those with muscle contraction and post-traumatic headache in which there was no associated neurological defect had the lowest incidence of EEG abnormality at 12 and 13%, respectively. Of those with vascular headaches, 32% did show EEG abnormalities.

Although EEG abnormalities are common in headache, Goldensohn finds that the nature of these abnormalities is different when structural lesions exist. Patients with migraine characteristically show a preponderance of paroxysmal features and exaggerated photic sensitivity as well as nonspecific features. However, polymorphic slow-wave foci occur infrequently in migraine, and when such a slow-wave focus, or severe diffuse abnormalities, is seen, the question of intracranial pathology would certainly be raised and further investigation would be indicated. Polymorphic slow-wave foci are especially liable to occur in complicated migraine, often disappearing after an interval of several months if the patients are carefully followed. In brief, Goldensohn finds the EEG useful in the interpretation and investigation of migraine patients, but seldom conclusive in itself.

Some EEG changes are said to have a special relationship with episodic headache although they are probably normal variants and should not be accorded special significance. Among these are 14 and 6/sec positive spikes, midtemporal 6–12 cps waves, and small sharp spikes.

Hockaday (1978) has reported on the late outcome of childhood-onset migraine and factors affecting the outcome, with particular reference to electroencephalographic changes. She found that only one-quarter of patients diagnosed as having migraine at age 20 years or under were free of migraine 8–25 years later. The clinical types most likely to terminate are basilar attacks in females and all forms of vascular headache in males. Hockaday notes further that abnormal electroencephalograms often occur—most frequently in classical migraine.

Focal Abnormalities

Abnormal electroencephalograms between attacks are seen more frequently in those patients who have focal motor, sensory, or mental symptoms as part of the migraine attack. Unfortunately, there are few series selected on this basis alone, so that an accurate incidence cannot be determined.

In the series studied by Selby and Lance (1960), 74 patients had impairment of consciousness during an attack. Excluding 18 of these who were considered as possibly having an associated seizure disorder, 41% of the remaining had abnormal electroencephalograms in the headache-free period. Whitty (1953) describes five cases of familial hemiplegic migraine. In three the electroencephalograms showed diffuse slow activity over both hemispheres between attacks.

Because of the importance of the duration of electroencephalographic abnormalities in understanding the underlying mechanisms giving rise to these abnormalities, this category will be subdivided into three separate groups.

1. TRANSIENT FOCAL ABNORMALITIES LASTING MINUTES

Some patients exhibit focal electroencephalographic changes that appear only very briefly during the occurrence of a focal neurological sign, and then disappear almost simultaneously with the dwindling of the neurological defect.

In 1945, while studying the effects of decompression in pilots making simulated high-altitude flights, Engel *et al.* (1953) became aware of a phenomenon in which scintillating scotomata appeared in one or both homonymous visual fields, and as the scotomata began to disappear, a unilateral throbbing headache appeared on the side opposite the visual disturbance. This headache was usually associated with nausea, vomiting, and abdominal cramps. In two patients electroencephalograms were recorded simultaneously with the appearance of the scotomata. The records showed 4 to 7 cps activity over the occipital lobe corresponding to the visual defect. The focal electroencephalographic abnormality disappeared simultaneously with the resolution of the scotomata.

Engel, in 1945, reported three patients with recurrent unilateral headaches of the migraine type which were preceded by homonymous visual field disturbances. In all three patients slow waves appeared in the occipital area opposite the field defect, once the patients became aware of the scotomata. The electroencephalographic changes were transient, and all abnormal waves disappeared soon after the visual disturbance cleared. In one patient the scotomata remained for several minutes, actually fluctuating in size several times before disappearance. The appearance and disappearance of slow waves over the occipital area relevant to the visual field defects could be closely correlated with the increasing and decreasing size of the scotomata, respectively.

2. TRANSIENT FOCAL ABNORMALITIES LASTING HOURS OR DAYS

These are exemplified by hemiparesis accompanying and sometimes outlasting the migraine attack.

Symonds (1952) reported his notes of a patient who developed a left hemiparesis during the pre-headache phase of migraine and had a normal arteriogram at the height of the hemiparesis. The electroencephalogram showed slow activity over the right hemisphere. The hemiparesis gradually diminished over the period of several days and finally the electroencephalogram became normal.

In one of Whitty's (1953) patients with hemiplegic migraine, the electroencephalogram was made while the patient was hemiparetic on the left with a left hemihypesthesia and a left homonymous hemianopsia. The record showed paroxysms of high-amplitude 2 to 3 cps waves over both temporal areas, a little more marked over the right side. Three days later there was a recurrence of the symptoms, and this time more severe than the first. The electroencephalogram at this time showed one cps wave over the entire right hemisphere. The tracing and neurological findings gradually became normal over the next eight days.

Engel in 1953 reported two more patients with migraine who had electroencephalographic changes during their attacks. The first was a 26-year-old Negro male who had had a normal tracing between attacks of transient left-sided symptoms. On the particular occasion that prompted hospital admission, there was a left hemiplegia and left homonymous hemianopsia. An electroencephalogram taken 6 hr after the onset of the left-sided symptoms showed high-amplitude 1 to 2 cps waves predominantly over the right frontal area, and to a lesser degree over the right parietal and occipital areas. The left-sided motor and visual defects did not dwindle rapidly as they had in the past and actually persisted for several weeks. Two weeks after admission the only abnormality seen electroencephalographically was some 5 to 7 cps activity in the right occipital region. Four months later the neurological examination and electroencephalogram were normal.

The following reports from the New York Hospital are of patients who had vascular headache of the migraine type with focal motor, sensory, or mental abnormalities occurring as a part of their attacks, and transient focal electroencephalographic abnormalities lasting for days. The first patient was a young woman with familial hemiplegic migraine.

P. C., a 20-year-old white woman, on the morning of 11/20/60 while leaving Mass, suddenly experienced hazy vision. Within a few minutes she became aware of numbness of the right arm, and within a few more minutes, the right leg and face became numb. As the sensory disturbance evolved she developed aphasia. Both the aphasia and sensory disturbance reached their maximal degree of severity within 30 min. Almost simultaneously with the onset of nausea

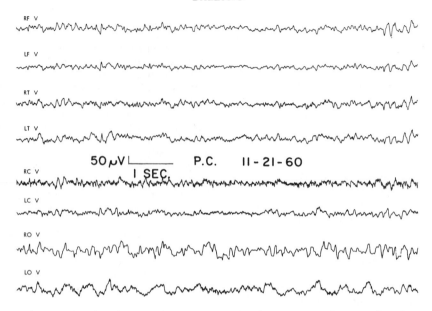

FIG. 4-26. The electroencephalogram taken 24 hr after the onset of sensory disturbance and headache. The 2 to 5 cps activity can be seen to occur independently on the left and on the right, the maximal defect being in the occipital areas.

and vomiting at that time she began having a severe nonthrobbing bilateral supra-orbital headache. She was brought to New York Hospital where she was admitted, in an obtunded state.

Examination revealed her to be irritable, agitated, and at times combative, and she had difficulty expressing herself. She reacted slowly to commands but would not attempt to read or write. There was no obvious visual field defect. She reacted to noxious stimulation bilaterally. There was no gross palsy of arms or legs; however, skilled acts with the right hand were performed awkwardly and with difficulty. The tendon reflexes were slightly more active on the left side; however, the superficial abdominal reflexes were present and equal bilaterally and plantar responses were flexor. Pulse, blood pressure, and respiration were normal, but oral temperature was 38.4°C. A hematocrit reading of 38, and a white-cell count of 17,000 with 84% neutrophils were revealed. A lumbar puncture yielded a clear and colorless cerebrospinal fluid, with an initial pressure of 260 mm, no cells and protein of 12 mg %.

During the first 24 hr she slept much of the time, but vomited frequently and was irritable and uncooperative when awake. She continued to have difficulty in thinking and in expressing herself and was poorly oriented as to time and place. This cloudy mental state cleared within 48 hr, as did the

headache, and the feelings of numbness on the right side.

Examination at that time revealed no abnormality except for swelling and erythema of the right eyelid associated with a slightly dilated right pupil, and slightly more active deep-tendon reflexes on the left than on the right. Visual fields were normal.

An electroencephalogram taken 24 hr after the onset of her symptoms revealed two separate foci of slow activity, i.e., high-amplitude, sometimes sharp 2 to 5 cps activity occurring (1) over the left hemisphere and (2) in the right occipital areas (Fig. 4-26). Although the maximal defect occurred in the left occipital area, the abnormal electrical activity on the right frequently appeared independently of that on the left. An electroencephalogram taken five days after the initial episode revealed only a small amount of 3 to 5 cps activity in the left occipital area. There was still a moderate amount of 3 to 6 cps activity in the right occipital area (Fig. 4-27). Two weeks after the beginning of the headache attack only a very small amount of 5 to 7 cps activity was present in the right and occasionally in the left occipital area, the records showing a well-formed 8 to 9 cps activity in other areas (Fig. 4-28). The tendon reflex asymmetry, the left being slightly more active than the right, was the only abnormality found on examination after two weeks of hospitalization. The final

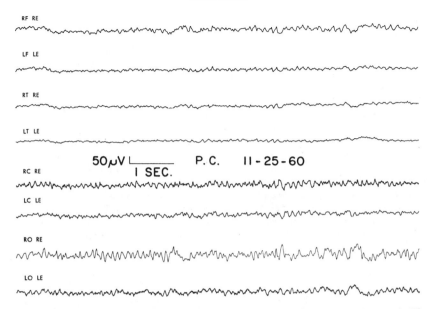

FIG. 4-27. The electroencephalogram taken five days after the onset of the attack. The record shows considerable improvement, but 3 to 5 cps activity is still present in the right occipital area, with some synchronous slow activity in the left occipital area.

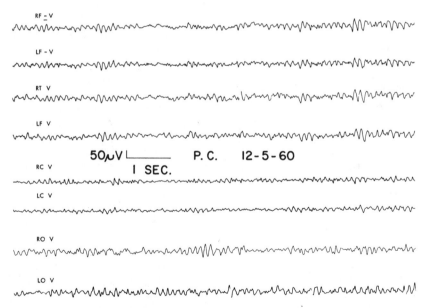

FIG. 4-28. The electroencephalogram taken two weeks after the initial episode shows only a small amount of 5 to 7 cps activity in the occipital areas. This activity was no longer present five days later.

electroencephalogram taken on a day before discharge, 20 days after admission, revealed a well-formed 8 to 9 cps activity in all areas. The previously noted 5 to 7 cps activity no longer was present.

The patient's past history revealed that she had had many attacks of unexplained fever and vomiting as a child. At the age of 12, in the setting of a stressful home situation, she had her first episode of severe headache preceded by a unilateral sensory disturbance. She continued to have similar attacks four to five times every year. Although the onset of an attack was always frightening to her, she rarely sought medical treatment, usually preferring to go to bed at home and remain there until the episode ended. It was only because of her escort's alarm that she was brought to the hospital at the onset of the most recent attack. The sensory disturbance occurred most frequently on the right side, but on many occasions involved the left side alone. The right leg was slightly weaker than the left when the right-sided sensory disturbance was most striking. She found that she usually had considerable difficulty holding objects, and might drop them unless they were kept in view. Hypalgesia and hypesthesia were common, but analgesia never occurred. Aphasia and mental cloudiness were frequent occurrences. The duration of these symptoms varied from a few minutes to 24 hr. The headache was never unilateral, and when severe usually lasted 18 to 24 hr. Photophobia, fever, nausea, vomiting, and puffiness of the eyelids either on the right or left frequently occurred with the attacks.

The patient's mother had been studied in the New York Hospital in 1940 for evaluation of recurrent headache attacks associated with unilateral sensory disturbance, and mental depression with weeping, nausea, and vomiting. The episodes and symptoms were almost identical with those experienced by her daughter. She had had several of these attacks every year since the age of 20. She died at the age of 43 due to a generalized peritonitis secondary to pelvic disease. An autopsy revealed no abnormality of the brain. A maternal aunt also had vascular headache of the migraine type.

3. PERSISTENT FOCAL ABNORMALITIES

Persistent focal slow activity seen in the headache-free intervals accounts for only a small percentage of the electroencephalographic changes in patients with vascular headache of the migraine type when this group is studied without further subdivision.

In Selby and Lance's (1960) report, only 15 of 139 abnormal records showed lateralizing defects. No mention is made concerning the clinical course of these 15 patients. Focal abnormalities occurred in 5 of 18 abnormal records reported by Heyck (1969). However, Heyck mentioned that all five patients had focal symptoms at the time of the migraine attack. In the 51 patients studied by Dow and Whitty (1947) localized unilateral electroencephalographic abnormalities were seen in four patients, all of whom had focal clinical signs occurring as part of their headache attack. Ventriculography was performed and found to be normal in three of these four patients. Neither Heyck nor Dow and Whitty indicate whether the electrical abnormality was on the side opposite the focal clinical signs, and there is no mention regarding the presence or absence of permanent focal motor, sensory, or mental defects.

Comment. Patients having focal motor, sensory, or mental disturbances during one phase of a migraine attack may have focal electroencephalographic abnormalities. These abnormalities are usually localized in the hemisphere or area of that hemisphere relevant to the clinical findings. Either delta or theta activity may make up the electrical focus. The duration of the electrical abnormality coupled with the change in focal neurological signs gives some insight into the underlying mechanisms which lead to cerebral dysfunction in these patients.

When electroencephalographic abnormalities develop simultaneously with the appearance of focal motor, sensory, or mental symptoms and within a few minutes disappear promptly with the resolution of these clinical symptoms, the cerebral dysfunction is probably due to a very brief period of ischemia. Since vasoconstriction of extracranial and intracranial vessels has been established as a part of the preheadache phenomena occurring in migraine attacks, it seems reasonable to assume that ischemia ensues. The three patients studied by Engel *et al.* (1945) would seem to exemplify this process. All had transient lateralized neurological defects lasting only minutes associated with an electroencephalogram showing focal slow activity over the hemisphere opposite the side of visual impairment, and all showed complete and prompt return of the electroencephalogram to normal.

When focal neurological and electroencephalographic signs develop during the early phase of a migraine attack and persist for several hours or even days, then completely resolve, another pathological process must be implicated. In his notes (already cited) Symonds indicated that the neurological and electroencephalographic changes in his patient could not be linked to occlusion of the larger cerebral vessels because of a normal arteriogram. He indicated that the process is cerebral edema. If one postulates prolonged ischemia, either as the result of vasoconstriction or small-vessel occlusion in this instance, edema is an expected occurrence.

A more attractive postulate for the development of intracranial edema follows. Local edema in the painful region on the outside of the head of patients with severe vascular headache of the migraine type is a common manifestation. This usually becomes more conspicuous as such intense headache persists. It is unlikely that the ischemia which initiated the attack some hours before is solely responsible for this progressive accumulation of fluid. Indeed there is much to show that such extracranial edema is the result of a separate neurogenic activity linked with vasodilatation. Granting that ischemia could increase cerebral-blood-vessel permeability directly, it follows from what occurs on the outside of the cranium that a similar neurogenic factor is also implicated in the development of intracranial edema.

The slow resolution of such edema, in the absence of significant tissue destruction, would account for the prolonged neurological and electroencephalographic abnormalities, yet be compatible with complete return of both to normal.

When persistent focal electroencephalographic abnormalities are encountered in patients having focal clinical signs as part of their migraine attack, these abnormalities are the result of permanent tissue damage. This is of even more importance if the electrical abnormality is over the area of the brain relevant to the clinical motor, sensory, or mental findings. Cerebral infarction is probably the pathological process. Cerebral vascular accidents, i.e., thrombosis or hemorrhage with resultant cerebral infarction, are known to occur occasionally during the preheadache phase of migraine.

Dunning in 1942 reported his notes of a patient who had had cerebral hemorrhage which occurred during an attack of migraine, leaving the patient with residual neurological defects. He also reviewed six similar cases previously reported in the literature.

The electroencephalographic abnormalities that occur in patients with vascular headache of the migraine type fall into two broad categories:

A. In this category are the electroencephalograms taken during the headache-free period that show a persistent nonfocal abnormality. These records predictably show paroxysmally diffusely occurring 4 to 7 cps activity in excessive amounts. The genesis of these disturbances is not known, but a relationship to epileptic phenomena has been suggested by some.

B. In this category are the electroencephalograms showing focal abnormalities. It is further subdivided into three groups:

1. Electroencephalograms that are altered very briefly during an attack of vascular headache of the migraine type with fleeting focal motor or sensory defects. (Short-lived ischemia due to vasoconstriction is probably the initiating event.)

2. Electroencephalographic abnormalities that develop during an attack of vascular headache of the migraine type associated with defects in motor, sensory, or mental function, and that disappear within hours or days, concurrently with the resolution of the clinical signs. (Local brain edema is the likely pathogenic process.)

3. Electroencephalograms taken during the headache-free period that show a persistent focal abnormality occurring most frequently in patients having conspicuous motor, sensory, or mental abnormalities during one or another phase of the migraine attack. (It is suggested

that cerebral infarction is the precipitating accident.)

MIGRAINE AND ORAL CONTRACEPTIVE AGENTS

In recent years an increase in cerebral vascular accidents in young women given oral contraceptives has been reported. Not infrequently, increasingly severe vascular headaches or a change in the migraine pattern has been described as a harbinger of an impending stroke, Whitty *et al.* studied 25 migraine patients who were taking oral contraceptives and noted that there was an increase in the intensity and in the frequency of their migraine attacks (1966). In addition, in five patients, typical attacks of migraine were precipitated by these contraceptive agents. The risk of a stroke in a young woman using oral contraceptives is enhanced by a history of migraine. Salmon and his colleagues have reviewed their records of 129 young women with migraine of whom 100 developed neurologic and ophthalmic diseases while employing oral contraceptives (1968). In roughly 26% of the stroke patients, the area of the brain involved was supplied by the vertebral basilar system. More than half of their patients with serious neurological sequelae had a significant history of migraine that preceded the vascular accident. Patients with hypertension, vascular disease, migraine, facial paralysis, and endometriosis were particularly predisposed to neurologic difficulties while taking the contraceptive pill. Transient ischemic attacks which appeared during therapy with oral contraceptives invariably resulted in strokes. Our own experience based on five patients personally surveyed is that the risk of thrombosis with permanent damage to the nervous system in young women taking oral contraceptives is enhanced by the presence of amigrainous diathesis.

Based on the evidence mentioned above, there seems little doubt that oral contraceptives will increase not only the frequency but also the severity of attacks of migraine, and particularly attacks of complicated migraine. Oral contraceptives may precipitate typical migrainous headaches in those who have never experienced this form of headache prior to therapy. Patients whose migraine attacks are aggravated by oral contraceptives should probably have these agents withdrawn before permanent damage to the nervous system ensues. Some neurologists consider migraine as a relative contraindication to the dispensing of oral contraceptives in spite of other good indications for their use.

HEADACHE IN CHILDHOOD (TABLE 4-13)

Though the symptom of headache in childhood is a relatively common one, the literature on this subject is rather sparse, and the incidence of headache in childhood is unknown (Rothner, 1978). In part this may be related to difficulties with communication. In the preverbal child, headache may manifest itself primarily as irritability, poor food habits, and torpor. As a general rule, it may be stated that the younger the child, the less likely will the headache be related to psychosomatic problems, the eyes, or to migraine. Children with headache in the preverbal and toddler groups may be found to have an increased intracranial pressure or an intracranial infection.

Migraine in children usually occurs in the context of a family history of that disease. Juvenile migraine differs from adult migraine in several ways. Gastrointestinal distress is common and may be the sole manifestation of the syndrome. Cyclic vomiting of childhood is considered to be a migraine equivalent which often disappears by age five to eight, with the appearance thereafter of a more classical headache pattern. Usually the juvenile migraine episode is of short duration, and prodromata are not striking.

Sillanpaa (1976) reported on the prevalence of headache in Finnish children starting school. In the two Finnish cities of Tampere and Turku, there were 4825 children, aged 7 years, who started their primary school in the autumn of 1974. At the first clinical examination performed by school doctors, 87.8% of the pupils and their mothers were interviewed to detect the occurrence of headache. The overall prevalence of headache proved to be 37.7%. Occasional headache, which was considered to

TABLE 4-13   Headache in Children

	VASCULAR (MIGRAINE)	MUSCLE CONTRACTION	TRACTION AND INFLAMMATORY (INCREASED INTRACRANIAL PRESSURE)
Sex	Males 2:1	Females 3:1	No sex differential
Age of onset	4 to 10 years	6 to 12 years	At any time
Prodromata	Scotomata, pallor, abdominal complaints, malaise, irritability	None	None
Associated findings	Nausea, vomiting, hyperemesis, confusional state	Avoids school or other stress situations	Vomiting, lethargy, positive neurologic signs, progressive head pain
Family history	Positive for migraine	Disturbed relationships	None
Therapy	Phenobarbital, diphenylhydantoin, cyproheptadine, rarely ergot Propranolol	Environmental manipulation, psychotherapy	As required by the lesion (surgery, radiotherapy, etc.)

be significant, was found in 31.7%. More frequent headache, occurring once a month or more, was found in 6.0% of cases. The prevalence of migraine was 3%. This compares with the study Bille performed in Upsala in 1962 of 9000 school children, where 39% were found to have headache. Sillanpaa showed a two-fold higher frequency of migraine (3%) than Bille found (1.4%).

Juvenile Head Trauma and Migraine

It is important to realize that juvenile head trauma syndromes may be related to migraine and that migraine may occur after head trauma, particularly after trauma sustained in sporting activities such as football and baseball. Haas and his associates (1969, 1975) describe a clinical spectrum of juvenile head traumas in an analysis of 50 attacks in 25 patients. Attacks were grouped into four clinical types: (1) hemiparetic, (2) somnolent, (3) blindness and (4) brainstem signs. They suggest that these four types of juvenile head trauma syndromes are different manifestations of a common underlying process. All attacks followed mild head trauma after a latent interval, generally of 1 to 10 min. Forty of the 50 attacks occurred in patients under 14 years of age. Full recovery occurred after a variable period of time in all but one patient who demonstrated an occlu-

sion of the branch of the middle cerebral artery on angiography. In their clinical and laboratory features, these juvenile head trauma syndromes resemble classical migraine and presumably have a similar underlying mechanism.

In many of these children the migraine process probably involves the basilar artery. Symptoms include sudden onset of transient bilateral visual disturbances, gait ataxia, vertigo, pulsatile occipital headache with vomiting, and dysarthrias of varying forms. In young women the attacks may be related to menstruation. As patients age, basilar artery migraine is often supplanted by more characteristic forms of vascular headache. Pediatric patients in whom there is a clinical picture of confusion related to basilar artery migraine and who have a family history of migraine and transient electroencephalographic changes may not require neurodiagnostic study, if the syndrome is recognized.

Muscle Contraction

Muscle contraction headache is common in children. The pain is described as diffuse, sometimes bandlike, and is not usually associated with nausea and vomiting. The pain may be relieved by simple analgesic agents. It is often associated with muscle spasm and complaints of neck tenderness. The headaches are almost always related to stress situations at school, or play, or to disturbed family relationships.

Traction and Inflammatory Headache

Headache associated with traction or inflammation of pain-sensitive structures of the head also appears in children. When associated with fever, meningitis or encephalitis should be suspected. Cranial arteritis does not occur in children, nor do the major neuralgias. If increased intracranial pressure occurs, the head pain is described as diffuse, often beginning in the occiput initially, but radiating thereafter to the frontal and temporal areas. Tumors involving the pituitary may produce a well-localized vertex head pain. With brain tumors, the same observations apply as described for adults. In addition, the pain is often present upon awakening and may be increased after exercise or head jolts. The pain becomes progressively more severe and is accompanied by obvious neurologic signs including increasing head size, ataxia, and papilledema.

Planning the Work-up

Successful treatment of the child with headache depends upon the establishment of a specific diagnosis. A careful history and physical examination should be done. Measurement of the head is essential. Fontanelles and suture lines should be palpated. Fundoscopy should be performed and attempts should be made to outline the visual fields. Skull films and an electroencephalogram are almost always ordered if the complaint is severe or chronic. If a tumor is suspected, a CAT scan should be done. Films of the cervical spine should be obtained if the pain is occipital in character. Children may be susceptible to occipital neuralgia, particularly after trauma to this region. If further neurologic work-up is indicated, the child should be hospitalized.

Therapy of Headache in Children

It is best to avoid using ergot and methysergide in childhood migraine in all but the most

unusual circumstances. If the child responds to nothing else and ergot must be used, a rectal suppository can be employed, using half the adult dose if the child is age 6 or older. If the migraine episodes occur rarely, no specific therapy is indicated. If they occur frequently, perhaps weekly, we suggest therapy with anticonvulsant agents. Phenobarbital is frequently employed in a dose of 5 mg/kg, or in older children, 30 mg, t.i.d., providing somnolence is not severe. Occasionally, diphenylhydantoin is added or used alone, if somnolence does become a problem. Cyproheptadine hydrochloride, 4 mg at bedtime, is helpful as headache prophylaxis in frequent episodes. If the electroencephalogram is dysrhythmic, the physician may feel more strongly about using anticonvulsant agents in the situation of recurrent headaches. If drug therapy is employed, careful and repeated examinations should be done.

Ludvigsson (1973) has described the use of propranolol in the prophylaxis of migraine in children. Thirty-two children between the ages of 7 and 16 years were included in a double-blind single-crossover study. Each child received propranolol and placebo for periods of three months, the preparations being allocated at random. It was demonstrated that propranolol has a good prophylactic effect on migraine in school children. The drug did not seem to cause noticeable side effects if certain categories of patients were excluded from treatment, particularly those with asthma, cardiac decompensation, or cardiac arrhythmias. Begin with small doses, e.g., 10–20 mg/day. Bille of Sweden has also described his experiences with prophylaxis of migraine in children. He advised that, initially, measures for maintaining sound biologic rhythms in terms of life, work, rest, meals, and sleep should be followed, and sometimes prophylaxis with a mild sedative may be all that is required. If symptoms persist, it is important to try to counteract those trigger mechanisms which are suspected to provoke the migraine attacks, including dietary factors. Cyproheptadine and propranolol may be employed together in the prophylaxis of migraine in children.

Treatment of muscle contraction headache

in children rarely requires the use of medication. Counseling should be provided. The patient and the parents should be interviewed separately and together. If there is no resolution of the problem, a psychiatric consultation should be obtained. Sometimes, simple behavioral and especially environmental manipulations will suffice to relieve the situation and formal psychotherapy will not be necessary. But if the headache is only one part of an obvious disorder of mood, thought, or behavior, the patient should be referred quickly for formal psychotherapy. Depression can occur in children and these cases can be responsive to the tricyclic compounds such as amitriptyline (Elavil).

In those unusual circumstances where muscle spasm and neck pain have produced chronic headache, use of simple measures of physical therapy and a Thomas' collar may prove helpful.

Sometimes, despite all efforts, attempts to diagnose and to treat the headaches which appear in childhood may be unsuccessful. In this situation, the wise physician resorts to periodic examinations and observation. Most frequently, the headache will be found to be a self-limited problem and will resolve spontaneously.

Gascon and Barlow (1970) described acute confusional migraine in four children, ages eight to sixteen years, who had episodes of confusion and agitation much resembling toxic metabolic psychosis. Only one confusional episode occurred in each of these reports, but at other times the children had typical symptoms of migraine. Their electroencephalograms after the attack (generally within one day) showed generalized disorganization of the background activity with focal slowing in the posterior regions of either the right or left hemisphere. The electroencephalograms subsequently returned to normal.

Emery (1977) has also reported four children, ages five to fifteen years, with a similar problem. Ehyai and Fenichel (1978) have observed five such cases in 100 successive children with migraine and advise that the syndrome may be considerably more common than has been appreciated in the past. Of their

cases, the acute confusional state was the initial manifestation of migraine in one situation, and in three of the eight children reported previously. The diagnosis may be difficult in the absence of a history of migraine but a positive family history for the disorder is an important clue.

In their original report, Gascon and Barlow suggested that the confusional state was secondary to focal edema, perhaps associated with vasoconstriction in the carotid system. The frequent finding of unilateral, temporal, and occipital slowing also suggests hemispheric ischemia as the primary pathologic process, perhaps eventually producing edema related to anoxia.

In general, no specific therapy is required for acute confusional migraine beyond reassurance of the family and patient of the benign nature of the attacks and its relationship to the migraine process. Ergot compounds are not necessarily helpful since many of the complaints are thought to be related to intracranial vasoconstriction.

"MIGRAINE EQUIVALENTS"

Occasionally, in a patient who has had migraine headache and associated phenomena for many years, the headache attacks may end temporarily or permanently and be replaced by the periodic recurrence of other bodily disturbances which then become the basis of the dominant complaint. Often these disturbances are painful, sometimes not. Chest, abdominal, and extremity pains are instances of the former, whereas recurring attacks of vomiting, diarrhea, transient mood disorder, and fever are instances of nonpainful disturbances.

These equivalents are paroxysmal, recurrent symptom complexes, occurring in patients with a previous history or family history of migraine, an absence of symptoms between attacks, or a replacement of headaches by the equivalent syndrome; they may be relieved with appropriate therapy, often similar to that used to abort the headache attack itself. Migraine equivalents may take many forms, and involve the abdomen, chest, pelvis, eye, cerebral cortex (hemiplegic), and perhaps other organs. It has been estimated that migraine equivalents may occur in approximately 20% of subjects with migraine.

A NEUROGENIC THEORY OF MIGRAINE HEADACHE

A concept that embraces most of the facts about the mechanism of vascular headache of the migraine type can now be formulated, although important steps in the argument still lack experimental confirmation. Let us begin with a consideration of some basic aspects of the blood supply of the brain. One striking fact about the cerebral circulation is the predictable and major vasodilatation that occurs with even the slightest increase in blood CO_2. Indeed, this vasodilatation occurs before any change in the CO_2 content or the slightest change in the pH of the blood can be measured, and is even more important in its effect than pure hypoxia. Any of the variety of factors that induce acidosis has a similar effect. Almost equally striking is the effect of hypoglycemia. When the sugar content of the circulating blood is reduced by insulin or other means, conspicuous cerebral vasodilatation results. Such humoral alterations are extremely sensitive indications of danger for the organism.

Extreme augmentation of functional activity of the brain, as after strychnine administration to curarized animals, results in striking vasodilatation of cerebral arteries and increased cerebral blood flow. The local increase in functional activity within the occipital lobes or stimulation of the retina induces local cerebral vasodilatation.

A sudden fall in systemic arterial blood pressure, ischemia due to exsanguinating hemorrhage, a fall in cardiac output due to asystole or inefficient tachycardia, the pooling of venous blood with faulty return to the right side of the heart, the sudden interruption of carotid blood flow by pressure or ligation—all, if sufficiently severe, induce cerebral vasodilatation.

Factors that slow the intracranial circulation, such as increased intracranial pressure due to intracranial masses or major obstruction to the venous outflow from the head, also induce intracranial vasodilatation. Such compensation

as is achieved by cerebral vasodilatation begins long before the systemic arterial pressure begins to rise. Indeed, the latter compensating device set off by asphyxia, CO_2 accumulation, or impaired venous outflow, is a tardy one to come into action.

Noxious agents, such as carbon monoxide, that replace oxyhemoglobin, or drugs, such as the coal-tar derivatives that lead to sulf- and methemoglobin formation, that endanger the abundant supply of oxygenated blood to the brain, induce cerebral vasodilatation.

In short, any agent or process that endangers the continuous and abundant supply to the brain of blood rich in oxygen and glucose and poor in CO_2 results in the prompt and major dilatation of the cerebral blood vessels.

Moreover, noxious stimuli originating within the cranial cavity due to sterile inflammation, as from subarachnoid hemorrhage, or from infections (bacterial or viral meningitis), induce cerebral vasodilatation. Probably noxious stimuli arising from displacement and traction of pain-sensitive intracranial structures has a similar effect.

Some persons who have recurrent headache attacks may, after lumbar puncture, experience a headache that is eliminated by ergotamine tartrate. This suggests that cranial vasodilatation may indirectly result from the noxious stimulation of intracranial structures.

If one now turns to another body of evidence, it is notable that processes or procedures that threaten the brain seriously, such as sleep loss, hunger, exhaustion, and sustained conflict also induce cranial vasodilatation and headache. Many persons experience headache with motion sickness. This suggests that the effects of vestibular and retinal stimulation, along with other vasomotor and sensory effects resulting from spread of excitation, may induce cranial vasodilatation. It is conceivable that afferent impulses from a sustained source of noxious stimulation in the eyes and ears, the cervical spine, the muscles of the neck or the nasal structures, may in some instances result in vascular headache. But whether such a vasomotor reaction is an indirect effect of sustained duress, as from continuous noxious experience, or an actual reflex effect from noxious stimulation, must remain for the moment unresolved.

It has been demonstrated in laboratory animals that cerebral vasoconstriction and vasodilatation can both be induced neurogenically. It has also been shown in man that the extracranial vessels vary their tone quickly and frequently, especially in those persons who are subject to vascular headache of the migraine type. Moreover, the sudden hydrostatic changes resulting from headstanding are followed by prompt reflex vasoconstriction, both within and outside the cranium.

In short, according to the neurogenic concept of vascular headache of the migraine type, any noxious factor within the brain that threatens survival of the cerebrum may induce cerebral vasodilatation. If this be sufficiently great, the cranial arteries on the outside of the head dilate. With the liberation of chemical factors such as proteases and polypeptides, edema and a lowering of the pain threshold are engendered. Tenderness and headache ensue. Thus, almost simultaneously, the same changes would be occurring inside and outside the cranial cavity. It is conceivable that the initial event within the head is vasoconstriction, resulting in ischemia, more striking in one region than in others, and especially in some persons. But other noxious factors may also initiate events.

Migraine is thus viewed as a form of relatively benign cerebral vasospasm, an episodic disorder of an integrative nature produced by the interaction of the central vasomotor centers, the extra- and intracranial blood vessels, and the microcirculation. It involves both the central and the peripheral vasomotor mechanisms, as well as a sterile inflammatory reaction, evoked by activity of the nervous system, with the eventual production of the clinical syndrome as it is appreciated by the patient.

SUMMARY

1. The outstanding feature of the migraine syndrome is periodic severe headache, usually unilateral in onset, but which may become generalized. The headaches are associated with irritability and nausea, and often with photophobia, vomiting, constipation, or diarrhea. Not infrequently the attacks are ushered in by scotomata, hemianopia, unilateral paresthesia, and speech disorders. The pain is commonly limited to the head but it may include the face. Often there is a familial history of the disease.

2. Evidence has been presented which suggests that the preheadache phenomena of migraine are associated with cerebral vasoconstriction.

3. The headache phase of migraine is associated with increased pulsation and vasodilatation of the cranial arteries, chiefly the external carotid arteries. Intracranial vasodilatation may also occur.

4. The distribution of these vascular changes does not always correlate well with the clinical features of the episode of migraine. Painless preheadache phenomena imply focal cerebral anoxia, but in actuality the reduction in cerebral blood flow may be hemispheric. Further, the reduction in cerebral blood flow may outlast the relatively brief aural timespan. Similarly, the distribution of increased cerebral blood flow may not correlate well with the locale of the headache. Frequently the intracranial vasodilatation may be hemispheric while the headache is sharply localized. The increased blood flow may even be bilateral with a hemispheric headache. These newest findings regarding the vasomotor activity of the extracranial and intracranial blood vessels suggest a profound alteration in blood vessel regulation in migraine, a continuing instability of vasomotor regulatory mechanisms which may persist far beyond the headache episode.

5. Two varieties of edema occur in the body as a part of the migraine syndrome. Local edema may appear at the site of headache. Generalized weight gain and fluid retention may also occur.

6. The sensitivity of minute vessels in the bulbar conjunctival sac to the vasoconstrictor agent norepinephrine is increased during the preheadache phase of migraine and is reduced during the headache itself.

7. Local accumulation of a vasodilator polypeptide, neurokinin, related to bradykinin,

has been found in the subsurface tissues of patients with migraine.

8. Tyramine, a pressor amine present in certain foods, can evoke migraine in susceptible subjects.

9. Complicated migraine is a term employed when the neurological manifestations which characterize migraine persist beyond the immediate headache period. Included in this group are hemiplegic and ophthalmoplegic migraine.

10. EEG changes of several types may occur in patients with migraine, depending in part on the severity of the episode.

11. Migraine may appear during or be exacerbated by the ingestion of oral contraceptives in women. Increasing migraine during the period of oral contraceptive use is a harbinger of more serious intracranial disease and a relative contraindication to the continued use of these drugs.

12. Biochemical changes which may be relevant to the migraine process are reviewed. Plasma levels of serotonin fall suddenly at the onset of migraine.

13. It is proposed that histamine, serotonin, the plasma kinins, and other vasoactive substances participate in the sterile inflammatory reactions involving painful and distended blood vessels. They are considered as an integral but peripheral part of the migraine process, but are important primarily in that part of the migraine episode wherein an increase in vascular permeability occurs.

14. A neurogenic therapy of migraine is proposed. Migraine is viewed as a form of relatively benign cerebral vasospasm, an episodic disorder of an integrative nature produced by the interaction of the central vasomotor centers, the extracranial and intracranial blood vessels, and the microcirculation. It involves both central and peripheral vasomotor mechanisms, as well as a sterile inflammatory reaction, evoked by the activity of the nervous system.

REFERENCES

Adams, C. G. M., C. C. Orton, and K. J. Zilkha (1967). Catecholamines and enzyme histochemistry in migrainous arteries. *Background to Migraine,* Second Migraine Symposium, pp. 19–29. William Heinemann, London.

Alpers, B. J., and H. E. Yaskin (1951). Pathogenesis of ophthalmoplegic migraine. *Arch. Ophthalmol. 45,* 555.

Altschuler, J. A., R. A. McLaughlin, and K. T. Neusburger (1968). Neurological catastrophe related to oral contraceptives. *Arch. Neurol. 19,* 264.

Alvarez, W. C. (1934). The present day treatment of migraine. *Proc. Mayo Clin. 9,* 22.

Anthony, M. (1976). Plasma-free fatty acids and prostaglandin E, in migraine and stress. *Headache 16,* 58.

Anthony, M., H. Hinterberger, and J. W. Lance (1967). Plasma serotonin in migraine and stress. *Arch. Neurol. 16,* 544.

Anthony, M., and J. W. Lance (1971). Histamine and serotonin in cluster headache. *Arch. Neurol. 25,* 225.

Appenzeller, O. (1969). Vasomotor function in migraine. *Headache 9,* 147.

Armstrong, D. et al. (1952). Pain-producing substances in blister fluid and in serum. *J. Physiol. 117,* 4P.

Armstrong, D. et al. (1954). Development of pain-producing substance in human plasma. *Nature 174,* 791.

Armstrong, D., R. M. L. Dry, C. A. Keele, and J. W. Markham (1953). Observations on chemical excitants of cutaneous pain in man. *J. Physiol. 120,* 326.

Armstrong, D., C. A. Keele, J. B. Jepson, and J. W. Stewart (1957). Pain-producing substances in human inflammatory exudates and plasma. *J. Physiol. 135,* 350.

Armstrong, H. G., and J. W. Heim (1938). The effect of acceleration on the living organism. *J. Aviat. Med. 9,* 199.

Batson, O. V. (1944). Anatomical problems concerned in the study of cerebral blood flow. *Fed. Proc. 3,* 139.

Bickerstaff, E. R. (1961). Basilar artery migraine. *Lancet 1,* 15.

Bille, B. (1962). Migraine in school children. *Acta Paediatr. Scand. (Suppl.) 51, Suppl. 136,* 1–151.

Boisen, E. (1975). Strokes in migraine: report on seven strokes associated with severe migraine attacks. *Dan. Med. Bull. 22,* 100–106.

Camp, W. A., and H. G. Wolff (1961). Studies on headache; electroencephalographic abnormalities in patients with vascular headache of the migraine type. *Arch. Neurol. 4,* 475.

Carlsen, L. A., L. G. Eklund, and L. Oro (1968). Clinical and metabolic effects of prostaglandin E1 in man. *Acta Med. Scand. 183,* 423–430.

Chapman, L. F., H. Goodell, and H. G. Wolff (1959). Increased inflammatory reaction induced by central nervous system activity. *Trans. Assoc. Am. Physicians 72,* 84.

Chapman, L. F., H. Goodell, and H. G. Wolff (1959). Neurohumoral features of the axon reflex. *Fed. Proc. 18,* 95.

Chapman, L. F., A. O. Ramos, H. Goodell, G. Silverman, and H. G. Wolff (1960). A humoral agent implicated in vascular headache of the migraine type. *Arch. Neurol. 3*, 223.

Chapman, L. F., A. O. Ramos, H. Goodell, and H. G. Wolff (1960). Neurokinin; a polypeptide formed during neuronal activity in man. *Trans. Am. Neurol. Assoc. 85*, 42.

Chapman, L. F., A. O. Ramos, H. Goodell, and H. G. Wolff (1961). Neurohumoral features of afferent fibers in man. *Arch. Neurol. 4*, 617.

Chapman, L. F., and H. G. Wolff (1958). A property of cerebrospinal fluid indicating disturbed metabolism within the central nervous system. *Trans. Assoc. Am. Physicians 71*, 210.

Chapman, L. F., and H. G. Wolff (1959). Studies of proteolytic enzymes in cerebrospinal fluid: capacity of incubated mixtures of cerebrospinal fluid and plasma proteins to form vasodilator substances that contract the isolated rat uterus. *Arch. Intern. Med. 103*, 86.

Charcot, J. M., cited by R. L. Rea (1938). *Neuro-Ophthalmology*. C. V. Mosby, St. Louis.

Clark, D., H. B. Hough, and H. G. Wolff (1936). Experimental studies on headache: observations on histamine headache. *Assoc. Res. Nerv. Dis. Proc. 15*, 417.

Clarke, J. M. (1910). On recurrent motor paralysis in migraine: with report of a family in which recurrent hemiplegia accompanied the attacks. *Brit. Med. J. 1*, 1534.

Cochrane, C. G. (1971). Initiating events in immune complex injury. In *Progress in Immunology*, p. 146. Academic Press, New York.

Cole, M. (1967). Strokes in young women using oral contraceptives. *Arch. Intern. Med. 120*, 551.

Couch, J. R., and R. S. Hassanein (1976). Platelet aggregability in migraine and relation of aggregability to clinical aspects of migraine. *Neurol. 26*, 348.

Couch, J. R., and R. S. Hassanein (1977). Platelet aggregability in migraine. *Neurol. 27*, 843–848.

Curzon, G., P. Theaker, and B. J. Phillips (1966). Excretion of 5-hydroxy-indole acetic acid in migraine. *J. Neurol. Neurosurg. Psychiatry 29*, 85.

Dalessio, D. J. (1972). Dietary migraine. *Am. Fam. Physician 6*, 60.

Dalessio, D. J. (1976). The relationship of vasoactive substances to vascular permeability and their role in migraine. *Research and Clinical Studies in Headache*. Vol. IV, pp. 76–84. S. Karger, Basle.

Dalessio, D. J., W. A. Camp, H. Goodell, and H. G. Wolff (1961). Studies on headache. The mode of action of UML-491 and its relevance to the nature of vascular headache of the migraine type. *Arch. Neurol. 4*, 235.

Dalessio, D. J., L. F. Chapman, T. Zileli, McK. Cattell, R. Ehrlich, F. Fortuin, H. Goodell, and H. G. Wolff (1961). Studies on headache: the responses of the bulbar conjunctival blood vessels during

induced oliguria and diuresis and their modification by UML-491. *Arch. Neurol. 5*, 590.

Dalessio, D. J., W. A. Camp, H. Goodell, L. F. Chapman, T. Zileli, A. O. Ramos, R. Ehrlich, F. Fortuin, McK. Cattell, and H. G. Wolff (1962). Studies on headache. The relevance of the prophylactic action of UML-491 in vascular headache of the migraine type to the pathophysiology of this syndrome. *World Neurol. 3*, 66.

Dalessio, D. J., S. Otis, and R. Smith (1978). Vasomotor phenomena, platelet antagonism, and migraine therapy. In *Research and Clinical Studies in Headache*. Vol 6, pp. 34–41. S. Karger, New York.

Deshmukh, S. V., and J. S. Meyer (1976). Platelet dysfunction in migraine and effect of self-medication with aspirin. *Stroke 7*, 11.

Deshmukh, S. V., and J. S. Meyer (1977). Cyclic changes in platelet dynamics and the pathogenesis and prophylaxis of migraine. *Headache 17*, 101–107.

Dexter, J. D., J. Roberts, and J. A. Byer (1978). The five-hour glucose tolerance test and migraine. *Headache 18*, 91–95.

Dow, D. J., and C. W. M. Whitty (1947). Electroencephalographic changes in migraine. *Lancet 2*, 52.

Dunning, H. S. (1942). Intracranial and extracranial vascular accidents in migraine. *Arch. Neurol. Psychiat. 48*, 396.

Dynes, J. B. (1939). Alternating hemiparetic migraine syndrome. *Brit. Med. J. 2*, 446.

Edmeads, J. (1977). Cerebral blood flow in migraine. *Headache 17*, 148–162.

Edmund, J. (1952). Unilateral headache following histamine injected into the temporal region. *Acta Psychiat. Scand. 27*, 261.

Ehyai, A., and G. M. Fenichel (1978). The natural history of acute confusional migraine. *Arch. Neurol. 35*, 368–369.

Ekbom, K. (1969). Prophylactic treatment of cluster headache with a new serotonin antagonist, BC-105. *Acta Neurol. Scand. 4*, 601.

Ekbom, K. (1970). *Studies on Cluster Headache*. Stockholm.

Elliot, A. J. (1940). Ophthalmoplegic migraine (with report of a case). *Can. Med. Assoc. J. 43*, 242.

Emery, E. S. (1977). Acute confusional state in children with migraine. *Pediatrics 60*, 110–114.

Engel, G. L., E. B. Ferris, and J. Romano (1945). Focal electroencephalographic changes during the scotomas of migraine. *Am. J. Med. Sci. 200*, 650.

Engel, G. L., W. W. Hamburger, M. Reiser, and J. Plunkett (1953). Electroencephalographic and psychological studies of a case of migraine with severe pre-headache phenomena. *Psychosom. Med. 15*, 337.

Engel, G. L., J. P. Webb, E. B. Ferris, J. Romano, H. Ryder, and M. A. Blankenhorn (1944). A migraine-like syndrome complicating decompression sickness. *War. Med. 5*, 304.

Franks, W. R., W. K. Kerr, and B. Rose (1945a).

Some effects of centrifugal force on the cardiovascular system of man. *J. Physiol. 104*, 9P.

Franks, W. R., W. K. Kerr, and B. Rose (1945b). Some neurological signs and symptoms produced by centrifugal force in man. *J. Physiol. 104*, 10P.

Froelich, W. A., C. C. Carter, J. L. O'Leary, and H. E. Rosenbaum (1960). Headache in childhood; electroencephalographic evaluation of 500 cases. *Neurology 10*, 639.

Gascon, G., and C. Barlow (1970). Juvenile migraine presenting as an acute confusional state. *Pediatrics 45*, 628-635.

Gell, P. G. H., and R. R. A. Coombs (1968). *Clinical Aspects of Immunology*, 2nd ed., p. 575. Davis, Philadelphia.

Goldensohn, E. S. (1976). Paroxysmal and other features of the electroencephalogram in migraine. In *Research and Clinical Studies in Headache* (A. P. Friedman, and M. Granger, eds.), pp. 118-128. S. Karger, New York.

Graham, J., H. I. Suby, P. M. LeCompte, and N. L. Sadowsky (1967). Inflammatory fibrosis associated with methsergide therapy. *Research and Clinical Studies in Headache*, Vol. I, pp. 123-164. Karger, Basel/New York.

Graham, J. R., and H. G. Wolff (1938). Mechanism of migraine headache and action of ergotamine tartrate. *Arch. Neurol. Psychiatry 39*, 737-763.

Gronvall, H. (1938). On changes in the fundus oculi and persisting injuries to the eye in migraine. *Acta Ophthalmol. 16*, 602.

Guest, I. A., and A. L. Woolf (1964). Fatal infarction of the brain in migraine. *Brit. Med. J. 1*, 225.

Haas, D. C., G. S. Pineda, and H. Lourie (1975). Juvenile head trauma syndromes and their relationship to migraine. *Arch. Neurol. 32*, 727.

Haas, D. C., and R. D. Sovner (1969). Migraine attacks triggered by mild head trauma, and their relation to certain post-traumatic disorders of childhood. *J. Neurol. Neurosurg. Psychiatry 32*, 548.

Hanington, E., and A. M. Harper (1968). The role of tyramine in the etiology of migraine, and related studies on the cerebral and extracerebral circulations. *Headache 8*, 84.

Harrington, D. O., and M. Flocks (1953). Ophthalmoplegic migraine: pathogenesis; report of pathological findings in a case of recurrent oculomotor paralysis. *Arch. Ophthalmol. 49*, 643.

Heyck, H. (1969). Pathogenesis of migraine. *Research and Clinical Studies on Headache*, Vol. II, pp. 1-28. Karger, Basel/New York.

Heyck, H., and H. Krayenbuhl (1964). *Der Kopfschmerz*. Berlin, George Thieme/Verlag.

Hockaday, J. M. (1978). Late outcome of childhood onset migraine and factors affecting outcome, with particular reference to early and late EEG findings. In *Current Concepts in Migraine Research* (R. Greene, ed.), pp. 41-48. Raven Press, New York.

Horranen, E., O. Waltimo, and T. Kallanranta (1978). Toxic effects of ergotamine used for migraine. *Headache 18*, 95-98.

Hunt, J. R. (1915). A contribution to the paralytic and other persistent sequelae of migraine. *Am. J. Med. Sci. 150*, 313.

Jasper, H. H., and A. J. Cipriani (1945). Physiological studies on animals subjected to positive G. *J. Physiol. 104*, 6P.

Jacobson, E. (1938). *Progressive Relaxation*. University of Chicago Press, Chicago.

Kalendovsky, Z., and J. H. Austin (1975). Complicated migraine; its association with increased platelet aggregability and abnormal coagulation factors. *Headache 15*, 18.

Kaneko, Z., J. Shiraishi, H. Inaoka, T. Furukawa, and M. Sekiyama (1978). Intra- and extracerebral hemodynamics of migrainous headache. In *Current Concepts of Migraine Research* (R. Greene, ed.), pp. 17-24. Raven Press, New York.

Kety, S. S., and C. F. Schmidt (1946). Effects of alterations in the arterial tension of carbon dioxide and oxygen on cerebral blood flow and cerebral oxygen consumption of normal young men. *Fed. Proc. 5*, 55.

Kudrow, L. (1975). The relationship of headache frequency to hormone use in migraine. *Headache 15*, 37-40.

Kunkle, E. C. (1959). Acetylcholine in the mechanism of headaches of the migraine type. *Arch. Neurol. Psychiat. 81*, 135.

Kunkle, E. C., R. F. Kibler, G. C. Armistead, and H. Goodell (1949). Central sensory excitation, and inhibition in response to induced pain. *Trans. Am. Neurol. Assoc. 74*, 64.

Kunkle, E. C., D. W. Lund, and P. J. Maher (1948). Studies on headache: analysis of vascular mechanisms in headache by use of the human centrifuge. *Arch. Neurol. Psychiat. 60*, 253.

Lance, J. W., and M. Anthony (1966). Some clinical aspects of migraine. *Arch. Neurol. 15*, 356-361.

Lance, J. W., M. Anthony, and A. Gonski (1967). Serotonin, the carotid body, and cranial vessels in migraine. *Arch. Neurol. 16*, 553.

Lashley, K. S. (1941). Patterns of cerebral integration indicated by scotomas of migraine. *Arch. Neurol. Psychiat. 46*, 331.

Lennox, W. G., E. L. Gibbs, and F. A. Gibbs (1935). Effect of ergotamine tartrate on the cerebral circulation of man. *J. Pharmacol. Exp. Ther. 53*, 113.

Lennox, W. G., and M. A. Lennox (1960). Borderlands of epilepsy. *Epilepsy and Related Disorders*. Little, Brown, Boston.

Lennox, W. G., and H. C. Leonhardt (1937). The flow and concentration of blood as influenced by ergot alkaloids and as influencing migraine. *Ann. Intern. Med. 11*, 663.

Lewis, T. (1938). Suggestions relating to the study of somatic pain. *Br. Med. J. 1*, 321.

Livingston, P. C. (1939). The problem of blackout in aviation (amaurosis fugax). *Brit. J. Surg. 26*, 749.

Lord, G. D. A., and J. W. Duckworth (1977). Immunoglobulin and complement studies in migraine. *Headache 17*, 163–168.

Ludvigsson, J. (1973). Propranolol used in prophylaxis of migraine in children. *Lancet 2*, 779.

Majerus, P. W. (1976). Why aspirin? *Circulation 54*, 357–359.

Marcussen, R. M., and H. G. Wolff (1949). Therapy of migraine. *JAMA 139*, 198.

Marcussen, R. M., and H. G. Wolff (1950). Studies on headache: (1) effects of carbon dioxide-oxygen mixtures given during preheadache phase of the migraine attack; (2) further analysis of the pain mechanisms in headache. *Arch. Neurol. Psychiat. 63*, 42.

Mathew, N. T. (1978). 5-hydroxytryptophane in the prophylaxis of migraine. *Headache 18*, 111.

Mathew, N. T., F. Hrastnick, and J. S. Meyer (1976). Regional cerebral blood flow in the diagnosis of vascular headache. *Headache 15*, 252.

Matthews, W. B. (1972). Footballer's migraine. *Brit. Med. J. 2*, 326–327.

McCulloch, J., and A. M. Harper (1978). Phenylethylamine and cerebral circulation. In *Current Concepts in Migraine Research* (R. Greene, ed.), pp. 85–95. Raven Press, New York.

McNaughton, F. L. (1937). Discussion of mechanism of migraine headache and action of ergotamine tartrate. *Assoc. Res. Nerv. Dis. Proc. 18*, 664.

Medina, J. L., and S. Diamond (1976). Migraine and atopy. *Headache 15*, 271–274.

Medina, J. L., and S. Diamond (1978). The role of diet in migraine. *Headache 18*, 31–35.

Mustard, J. F., R. L. Kinlough-Rathbone, and C. S. Jenkins (1972). Modification of platelet function. *Ann. N.Y. Acad. Sci. 201*, 343–359.

O'Brien, M. D. (1967). Cerebral cortex perfusion rates in migraine. *Lancet 1*, 1036.

O'Brien, M. D. (1971). Cerebral blood changes in migraine. *Headache 10*, 139–143.

Ostfeld, A. M., L. F. Chapman, H. Goodell, and H. G. Wolff (1957). A summary of evidence concerning a noxious agent active locally during migraine type. *Arch. Intern. Med. 96*, 142.

Ostfeld, A. M., D. J. Reis, H. Goodell, and H. G. Wolff (1955). Headache and hydration: the significance of two varieties of fluid accumulation in patients with vascular headache of the migraine type. *Arch. Intern. Med. 96*, 142.

Ostfeld, A. M., D. J. Reis, and H. G. Wolff (1957). Studies in headache: bulbar conjunctival ischemia and muscle contraction headache. *Arch. Neurol. Psychiat. 77*, 113.

Ostfeld, A. M., and H. G. Wolff (1955). Studies on headache: arterenol (norepinephrine) and vascular headache of the migraine type. *Arch. Neurol. Psychiat. 74*, 131.

Ostfeld, A. M., and H. G. Wolff (1957). Studies on headache: participation of ocular structures in the migraine syndrome. *Mod. Probl. Ophthalmol. (Basel) 1*, 634.

Ostfeld, A. M., and H. G. Wolff (1958). Identifica-

tion mechanisms, and management of the migraine syndrome. *Med. Clin. North Am. 42*, 1497.

Patrikios, J. S. (1950). Ophthalmoplegic migraine. *Arch. Neurol. Psychiatry 63*, 843.

Pfeiffer, J. B., and E. C. Kunkle (1951). Fluctuations in cranial arterial tone as measured by histamine "responsiveness". *Trans. Am. Neurol. Assoc. 76*, 244.

Pool, J. L., T. J. C. vonStorch, and W. G. Lennox (1936). The effect of ergotamine tartrate on pressure of cerebrospinal fluid and blood during migraine headache. *Arch. Intern. Med. 57*, 32.

Reif, Lehrer, L. (1976). Possible significance of adverse reactions to glutamate in humans. *Fed. Proc. 35*, 2205–2212.

Riley, H. A. (1932). Migraine. *Bull. Neurol. Inst. N.Y. 2*, 429.

Rocha e Silva, M., W. T. Beraldo, and G. Rosenfeld (1949). Bradykinin, a hypotensive and smooth muscle stimulating factor released from plasma globulin by snake venoms and by trypsin. *Am. J. Physiol. 156*, 261.

Rothner, A. D. (1978). Headaches in children. A review. *Headache 18*, 169–175.

Sakai, F., and J. J. Meyer (1978). Regional cerebral hemodynamics during migraine and cluster headaches measured by the 133 Xe inhalation method. *Headache 18*, 122–133.

Salmon, M. L., J. Z. Winkelman, and A. J. Gay (1961). Neuro-ophthalmic sequelae in users of oral contraceptives. *JAMA 206*, 85.

Sandler, M. (1975). Monoamines and migraine: a path through the wood? In *Vasoactive Substances Relevant to Migraine* (S. Diamond, D. J. Dalessio, J. R. Graham, and J. L. Medina, eds.), p. 3. C. C. Thomas, Springfield, Ill.

Sandler, M., M. B. H., and E. Hanington (1974). A phenylethylamine oxidizing defect in migraine. *Nature 250*, 335.

Saxena, P. R. (1972). The effects of anti-migraine drugs on the vascular response by 5-hydroxytryptamine and related biogenic substances on the carotid bed of dogs. *Headache 12*, 44.

Schottstaedt, W. W., and H. G. Wolff (1955). Variations in fluid and electrolyte excretion in association with vascular headache of the migraine type. *Arch. Neurol. Psychiat. 73*, 158.

Schumacher, G. A., and H. G. Wolff (1941). Experimental studies on headache: contrast of histamine headache with headache of migraine and that associated with hypertension. *Arch. Neurol. Psychiat. 45*, 199.

Selby, G., and J. W. Lance (1960). Observations on 500 cases of migraine and allied vascular headache. *J. Neurol. Neurosurg. Psychiat. 23*, 23.

Sicuteri, F. (1966). Vasoneuractive substances in migraine. *Headache 6*, 109.

Sicuteri, F., B. Anselmi, and M. Fanciullacci (1974). The serotonin theory of migraine. *Adv. Neurol. 4*, 383–399.

Sicuteri, F., F. Buffoni, B. Anselmi, and P. L. De-lBianco (1972). An enzyme (MAO) defect on the platelets in migraine. *Res. Clin. Study Headache 3*, 245.

Sillanpaa, M. (1976). Prevalence of migraine and other headache in Finnish children starting school. *Headache 15*, 288–290.

Simons, D. J., E. Day, H. Goodell, and H. G. Wolff (1943). Experimental studies on headache: muscles of the scalp and neck as sources of pain. *Assoc. Res. Nerv. Dis. Proc. 23*, 228.

Skinhoj, E. (1973). Hemodynamic studies within the brain during migraine. *Arch. Neurol. 29*, 95–98.

Skinhoj, E., and O. B. Paulson (1969). Regional blood flow in internal carotid distribution during migraine attack. *Brit. Med. J. 3*, 569–570.

Smith, I., A. H. Kellow, and E. Hanington (1970). Clinical and biochemical correlation between tyramine and migraine headache. *Headache 10*, 43.

Smyth, V. O. G., and A. L. Winter (1964). The EEG in migraine. *Electroencephalogr. Clin. Neurophysiol. 16*, 194.

Somerville, B. W. (1972). The role of estradiol withdrawal in the etiology of menstrual migraine. *Neurol. 22*, 824–828.

Spira, P. J., E. J. Mylecharane, J. Misbach, J. Duckworth, and J. W. Lance (1978). Internal and external carotid vascular responses to vasoactive agents in the monkey. *Neurol. 28*, 162–174.

Stevenson, D., and D. J. Dalessio (1978). The relationship of the allergic state to headache. *Sandorama 11*, 10–13.

Stewart, W. K. (1945). Some observations on the effect of centrifugal force in man. *J. Neurol. Neurosurg. Psychiat. 8*, 24.

Swanson, J. W., and N. Vick (1978). Basilar artery migraine. *Neurol. 28*, 782–786.

Symonds, C. P. (1952). Migrainous variants, the annual oration. *Trans. Med. Soc. Lond. 67*, 237.

Torda, C., and H. G. Wolff (1945). Experimental studies on headache: transient thickening of walls of cranial arteries in relation to certain phenomena of migraine headache and action of ergotamine tartrate on thickened vessels. *Arch. Neurol. Psychiat. 53*, 329.

Townsend, H. R. A. (1967). The EEG in migraine. *Background to Migraine*, Vol. 1, pp. 15–21. Springer-Verlag, New York.

Tunis, M. M., R. G. Clark, R. Lee, and H. G. Wolff (1951). Studies on headache: further observations on cranial and conjunctival vessels during and between vascular headache attacks. *Trans. Am. Neurol. Assoc. 76*, 67.

Tunis, M. M., H. Goodell, and H. G. Wolff (1953). Studies on headache: evidence of tissue damage and changes in pain sensitivity in subjects with vascular headaches of the migraine type. *Trans. Assoc. Am. Physicians 66*, 332.

Tunis, M. M., and H. G. Wolff (1952). Analysis of cranial artery pulse waves in patients with vascular headache of the migraine type. *Am. J. Med. Sci. 224*, 565.

Tunis, M. M., and H. G. Wolff (1953). Studies on headache; long-term observations of the reactivity of the cranial arteries in subjects with vascular headache of the migraine type. *Arch. Neurol. Psychiat. 70*, 551.

Tunis, M. M., and H. G. Wolff (1954). Studies on headache: cranial artery vasoconstriction and muscle contraction headache. *Arch. Neurol. Psychiat. 71*, 425.

Verstraete, M. (1976). Are agents affecting platelet functions clinically useful? *Am. J. Med. 61*, 897–914.

von Euler, U. S. (1951). Nature of adrenergic nerve mediators. *Pharmacol. Rev. 3*, 247.

Weil, A. (1952). Observations on dysrhythmic migraine. *J. Nerv. Ment. Dis. 134*, 277.

Weiss, H. J. (1975). Platelets: physiology and abnormalities of function. *New Eng. J. Med. 293*, 531–541.

Weiss, H. J. (1978). Antiplatelet therapy. *New Eng. J. Med. 298*, 1344–1346 and 1403–1406.

Welch, K. M. A., E. Chabi, J. H. Nell, K. Bartosh, A. N. C. Chee, N. Mathew, and V. Achar (1976) Biochemical comparison of migraine and stroke. *Headache 16*, 160.

Whitty, C. W. M. (1953). Familial hemiplegic migraine. *J. Neurol. Neurosurg. Psychiat. 16*, 172.

Whitty, C. W. M., J. M. Hockaday, and M. M. Whitty (1966). The effect of oral contraceptives in migraine. *Lancet 1*, 856.

Wolff, H. G. (1961). Man's nervous system and disease. *Arch. Neurol. 5*, 235.

Wolff, H. G. (1962a). A concept of disease in man. *Psychosom. Med. 24*, 25.

Wolff, H. G. (1962b). Dormant human potential (editorial). *Arch. Neurol. 6*, 261.

Wolff, H. G., A. M. Ostfeld, D. J. Reis, and H. Goodell (1955). Significance of the two varieties of fluid accumulation in patients with vascular headaches of the migraine type. *Trans. Assoc. Am. Physicians 68*, 255.

Wolff, H. G., and M. M. Tunis (1952). Analysis of cranial artery pressure pulse waves in patients with vascular headache of the migraine type. *Trans. Assoc. Am. Physicians 65*, 240.

Wolff, H. G., M. M. Tunis, and H. Goodell (1953). Evidence of tissue damage and changes in pain sensitivity in subjects with vascular headaches of the migraine type. *Arch. Intern. Med. 92*, 478.

Wood, E. H., E. H. Lambert, E. J. Baldes, and C. F. Code (1946). Effects of acceleration in relation to aviation. *Fed. Proc. 5*, 327.

Ziegler, D. K., R. Hassanein, and K. Hassanein (1972). Headache syndromes suggested by factor analysis of symptom variables in a headache-prone population. *J. Chronic Dis. 25*, 353.

5

MIGRAINE THERAPY

REVISED BY DONALD J. DALESSIO

MANAGEMENT OF THE MIGRAINE ATTACK

Attention has centered on two types of procedures: those designed to end the headache attacks, and those aimed at their prevention. Broadly speaking, the headache attack may be managed in three ways: by procedures or agents that act primarily at the site of the pain; by the use of agents that raise the threshold to pain; and by the use of agents that modulate a variety of functions of the central nervous system.

Procedures or Agents That Act Primarily at the Site of Production of Pain

1. MISCELLANEOUS AGENTS

Since vasodilatation of the cranial arteries has been shown to be the cause of the pain during the migraine attack, it follows that any agent or procedure that reduces this dilatation will reduce the intensity of the headache. It is for this reason that pituitrin, ephedrine, benzedrine, epinephrine, caffeine, and possibly hypertonic salt solutions have sometimes been found useful. In fact, when they succeed in reducing the amplitude of pulsations by 40 to 50%, headache is eliminated. Similarly, pressing the finger against the common carotid artery or certain of the branches of the external carotid artery, such as the temporal, occipital, or supraorbital arteries, will afford relief. Also, an ice cap placed over these vessels has been found useful both through raising the threshold of pain, as does any cold stimulus,

and through direct vasoconstrictor action of the cold. The breathing of 100% oxygen has a vasoconstrictor effect on cerebral vessels, and is reported to be of use in terminating migraine headache attacks (Alvarez, 1934, 1939). All these agents have but a variable and short-lived influence, or unpredictable effects, on patients, and cannot be counted upon for therapeutic use. There is, however, one vasoconstrictor agent, namely, ergotamine tartrate, that is so constant in effect and duration as to give it a most important place in the management of the headache attack.

2. ERGOTAMINE TARTRATE

(a) Its Use in Termination of the Acute Attack. The administration of fluid extract of ergot has been known for at least half a century to terminate migraine headache attacks. However, the elaboration of ergotamine tartrate has introduced a more convenient means of administration of the active principle.

Ergotamine tartrate is best administered intramuscularly in doses of 0.25 to 0.50 mg. It is a wise precaution never to administer it more often than twice daily. Headache is usually relieved within an hour in more than 90% of instances (Friedman and Merritt, 1957).

The drug should be administered early in the course of the headache. While the drug is being absorbed and before it begins to act, some subjects prefer to sit upright in a chair, since lying down makes the headache worse. Patients can be taught how to give themselves intramuscular injections of the drug, but this is less desirable than administration by a physician. In the first place, the patient should never be allowed to feel that termination of a headache with ergotamine is proper treatment of the migraine state. Furthermore, as will be discussed later, the physician's aim should be to lengthen the interval between headaches. This is possible in most instances through consideration of the attitudes and life situation of the patient.

Ergotamine tartrate when taken by mouth is not always predictably effective. Here, too, the danger through abuse by self-administration must be recognized. Furthermore, vomiting may begin before the headache has been abolished, and the physician desirous of giving ergotamine intramuscularly will be at a loss to know how much of the ingested agent has actually been absorbed. If, however, it is necessary to use the oral method, 2 to 4 mg can be taken sublingually, or swallowed at the onset of the headache, followed by 2 mg each hour until the headache is gone, or until a total not exceeding 6 mg has been taken (Diamond and Baltes, 1972).

Patients should be informed of the probable side effects of ergotamine tartrate, the most unpleasant of which are nausea and vomiting. It must be emphasized, however, that vomiting is not essential for the relief of headache, and it is desirable to administer only sufficient drug to stop the headache without inducing emesis.

The abuse of ergotamine tartrate by some patients with migraine occurs, but apparently is not widespread. Also, the occurrence of ergotism in those with migraine attacks who are otherwise healthy is fortunately infrequent.

Certain persons may take ergotamine tartrate excessively without apparent harm. This has been demonstrated by several patients with migraine headaches who have inadvertently taken ergotamine tartrate too frequently. Several women reported that they had taken 0.25 mg intramuscularly daily for four years, and one patient for seven years.

Several careful observers have called attention to unreported instances of ergotism. Also Cleveland and King (1961) discussed the occurrence of gangrene in a patient with migraine following the improper use of ergotamine tartrate. This patient for approximately two weeks had been given an injection of 0.25 mg of ergotamine tartrate every 4 to 6 hr, night and day.

With the passage of time more reports of undesirable effects following the administration of ergotamine tartrate have accumulated. Thus, Carter (1958) describes three patients who after their first ingestion of ergotamine tartrate (two 1-mg tablets) developed serious thrombophlebitis. The occurrence of occlusive vascular disease after repeated administration has now been observed several times. Ask-Upmark (1960) reports on the danger of producing cardiac arrest by injection of ergotamine tartrate in patients who have bradycardia as part of their attacks. Goldfischer (1960) reports the experience of a 35-year-old woman with an 18-year history of vascular headache of the migraine type. She had been taking ergotamine tartrate for eight years with complete elimination of each headache attack and without adverse side effects. Twenty minutes after the intramuscular administration of 0.5 mg of ergotamine tartrate given for a severe migraine attack which had proved refractory to the previous oral administration of 2 mg of ergotamine tartrate, she developed severe substernal pain, a rise in temperature to 38.5°C, leukocytosis, rise of erythrocyte sedimentation rate and of the serum glutamic oxalacetic transaminase level to 76 units. Electrocardiographic evidence included inverted T-waves.

Fuchs and Blumenthal (1950) reported two patients with serious sequelae of ergotamine tartrate administration. The first patient, 30 to 40 min after the ingestion of two Cafergot tablets (containing 2 mg. of ergotamine tartrate) developed massive emesis, precordial pain, palpitations, numbness of the extremities, and cramps in both thighs. The nail beds were cyanotic, pulses barely obtainable, and the extremities cold. She recovered 24-hr later. The second patient, following administration of 1 cc of dihydroergotamine subcutaneously developed substernal pain. The electrocardiogram indicated evidence of coronary occlusion.

In addition to nausea and vomiting, the most commonly observed side effects from ergotamine tartrate are numbness and tingling of the hands and feet, muscle pains and stiffness of the thighs, and tightness of the muscles about the neck. A feeling of sleepiness or exhaustion is probably in part a manifestation of the migraine state of which the subject is not aware as long as the headache persists. However, ergotamine itself produces prostration in many patients.

If these side effects disappear within 24 hr, there is no contraindication to the further use of the drug. The patient should remain in bed as long as any symptoms persist, especially if there has been pain and inflammation in varicose veins. If any of these symptoms persist for longer than 24 hr, ergotamine tartrate should be given again only with misgivings.

Abuse of ergotamine tartrate by patients with migraine may occur. Ergotism in such patients is uncommon, but the physician should be familiar with the syndrome. The clinical picture of ergotism is dramatic and terrifying. First there is vigorous vomiting, then the extremities, usually the feet, become pulseless, and swell with congestion and cyanosis. Ultimately gangrene develops. Jaundice may also occur. The convulsions which rarely accompany ergotism are probably not due to ergot but to vitamin and other essential deficiencies.

Ergonovine qualitatively resembles ergotamine tartrate in its effect on the cranial vessels and on headache. However, the usual therapeutic dose (ergotrate, 0.2 mg intramuscularly) is only about half as successful in terminating headaches. Fewer gastric symptoms result from its use than from ergotamine, but in view of its limited effectiveness, the absence of gastric symptoms is not sufficient recommendation for the regular use of this drug. The failure of ergonovine to be constantly effective demonstrates that it is not the oxytoxic agent in ergot that is responsible for the termination of headache attacks, but rather that fraction which contracts arterial walls found especially in ergotamine. Ergonovine, because of its strong oxytoxic properties, should never be given to patients during pregnancy. D.H.E. 45 (dihydroergotamine), another derivative of ergot, but less predictable in its effect, may reduce or abolish the headache when given in 1-mg amounts intramuscularly, without inducing nausea and vomiting.

Proprietary preparations are available, usually containing 1 mg of ergotamine tartrate and 100 mg of caffeine alkaloid. They are alleged to have superior therapeutic effectiveness when taken by mouth in two to four, with a maximum of six tablet amounts, early in the course of the headache and preferably in the prodromal stage. Results to date indicate that these preparations have a therapeutic effect, but do not justify the conclusion that they are significantly superior to ergotamine tartrate alone when taken by mouth; both are inferior to ergotamine tartrate administered intramuscularly in 0.5-mg amounts, especially when the headache is severe and has persisted for some hours.

Still other agents have been mixed with ergotamine tartrate, such as acetophenetidin and belladonna, but the superiority of these mixtures over the ergot preparation alone is unproven. Ergotamine tartrate either alone or with caffeine alkaloids is prepared also for sublingual use to hasten absorption. Patients who are extremely nauseated or vomiting may find it convenient and effective to use a suppository with the same ingredients. If, for one reason or another, the medium used for making the suppositories dries out or hardens, the preparation is of little value.

Ergotamine tartrate may also be administered by using an aerosol device. This will deliver .36 mg of ergotamine tartrate into the oral cavity so that it may be absorbed from the lungs.

(b) *Abortion of Attacks.* If a patient awakes in the morning with the discomfort that is known by him to merge into intense hemicrania, it is sometimes possible to abort the impending attack by the following measures. (1) The patient should remain in bed, relaxed, in a darkened room. (2) In addition to bed rest, further relaxation is induced by a prolonged warm bath. (3) Two milligrams of ergotamine tartrate may be taken under the tongue, or in some alternate manner.

Practical Considerations in Therapy

Prescription drugs used to abort migraine headache are most commonly ergot derivatives and their varied formulations (see Tables 5-1, 5-2). A few contain only ergotamine tartrate. Several are a combination of ergotamine with caffeine and other materials, such as anti-

TABLE 5-1 Common Pharmaceutical Products Useful in Migraine, Abortive Therapy

ROUTE	DRUG	DOSAGE
Oral	Ergotamine tartrate (Gynergen) Ergotamine, caffeine, phenacetin, belladonna (Wigraine)	1 tablet immediately—repeat every 1/2 hr if necessary, to a minimum of 6 tablets per attack
	Ergotamine and caffeine (Cafergot) Ergotamine tartrate, cyclizine and caffeine (Migral)	2 stat—repeat 1 every 1/2 hr to a maximum of 10 per week 2 tablets at onset. May repeat 1 tablet every 1/2 hr up to 6 per day, 10 per week
	Isometheptene mucate, dichloralphenazone and acetaminophen (Midrin)	2 capsules at once, followed by 1 capsule every hour until relieved, up to 5 capsules in a 12-hr period
Sublingual	Ergotamine (Ergomar), (Ergostat)	1 tablet immediately, under the tongue—repeat at 1/2-hr intervals if necessary, but not more than 3 tablets in any 24-hr period
Inhalation	Ergotamine (Medihaler-Ergotamine)	One dose immediately—repeat every 5 min to a maximum of 6 per day, if necessary
Intramuscular	Ergotamine tartrate (Gynergen)	1/2 to 1 cc immediately and no more than 3 cc per week
	Dihydroergotamine (DHE-45)	1 cc at hourly intervals, up to 3 cc per day, if necessary
Rectal	Ergotamine and caffeine (Cafergot, Cafergot-PB) Ergotamine, caffeine, phenacetin and belladonna (Wigraine)	Insert 1 suppository in rectum immediately—repeat in 1 hr, if necessary

spasmodics and sedatives. Almost all routes of administration are available with these. With Cafergot, Migral, or Wigraine, two tablets should be administered at the onset of the headache, followed by one tablet every ½ hr, up to a maximum of six tablets if no relief is obtained. Rectal suppositories should be administered at the onset of the attack and repeated in one hour if necessary. Ergotamine (Ergomar, Ergostat) should be placed under the tongue at the first sign of a headache and should be repeated at ½ hr intervals if necessary, but not more than three tablets in any 24-hr period. Ergotamine may also be inhaled by means of a metered-dose device (Medihaler-Ergotamine) at the onset of the aura or pain; it can be repeated as necessary every 5 min, up to six doses. The most rapid relief of migraine headaches can be achieved by

parenteral administration of the ergotamine preparations.

A compound containing isometheptene mucate, dichloralphenazone, and acetaminophen (Midrin) may be effective in aborting migraine. It is especially useful for those who cannot tolerate ergotamine. During an attack, sedatives and pain-relieving drugs are often used to help the patient's symptoms. Phenothiazines, such as chlorpromazine (Thorazine), given as rectal suppositories, may help the nausea and vomiting that accompany an acute attack. Hydroxyzene (Vistaril) is especially useful. When a migraine headache lasts for more than 24 hr, there is often a sterile inflammation around the enlarged vessel. The use of steroids, for example dexamethasone (Decadron-LA), 16 mg intramuscularly, will sometimes hasten the end of a prolonged migraine.

TABLE 5-2 Common Pharmaceutical Products
Useful in Migraine, Prophylactic Therapy
(Oral Route)

DRUG	DOSAGE
Ergotamine tartrate (Gynergen)	1 mg twice daily—skip 1 day a week
Ergotamine, pheno-barbital, and belladonna Bellergal Spacetabs Bellergal	1 tablet twice daily 1 tablet four times daily
Methysergide maleate (Sansert)	2 mg three times daily
MAO Inhibitors Phenelzine sulfate (Nardil) Isocarboxazid (Marplan)	15 mg three times daily —reduce 10 mg four times daily— reduce to main-tenance dose in one month
Cyproheptadine (Periactin)	4–16 mg daily as tolerated
Propranolol (Inderal)	20 mg t.i.d. and increase as required
Amitriptyline (Elavil)	50–100 mg h.s.
Clonidine (Catapres)	0.1 mg t.i.d.
Platelet inhibitors (see pp. 147–148)	

MIGRAINE HEADACHE, CRANIAL ARTERIES, AND ERGOTAMINE TARTRATE

The significance of cranial vessels in the migraine headache has long been known; see reviews by Riley (1931) and Bassoe (1933). Such suggestions arose from the observations that: (1) the intensity of the headache during a migraine attack is diminished when the common carotid artery on the affected side is pressed upon—Parry and Möllendorf, cited by Liveing (1873); (2) the headache is found to diminish in intensity locally when the particular artery which supplies the affected region is pressed upon; (3) striking dilatation of the temporal arteries and veins may often be seen during the attack of migraine headache.

The relation between the amplitude of pulsations and the headache induced experimentally by histamine is considered elsewhere (Chapter 9). It seems likely from these studies that there is an analogous relation between the amplitude of pulsations and headache in the migraine attack. Thus, the amplitude of pulsations of the superficial branches of the external carotid artery closely parallels the intensity of the headache, and reduction in the intensity of the headache is intimately associated with decrease in the amplitude of pulsations. In fact, headache ends when the amplitude of pulsations of these arteries is sufficiently decreased, whether by means of ergotamine, epinephrine, or pressure. The properties of these agents differ widely; yet they have in common a capacity to decrease the amplitude of pulsations of cranial arteries. It is reasonable to postulate that their ability to reduce headache is dependent on the one property they possess in common.

It has long been known (Dale, 1906) that preparations of ergot in relatively large amounts diminish the responses of smooth muscle to epinephrine and adrenergic nerve stimulation. It was emphasized early, however, that ergot derivatives are used in the clinic in amounts so small that they could not produce the aforementioned paralytic effects. Nevertheless, it was on the basis of such effects that ergotamine was introduced into the therapy of migraine. It was assumed that the attack of migraine headache resulted from spasm of the cranial arteries following excessive autonomic nerve excitation and that the ergotamine caused relaxation of these blood vessels. Such an explanation of the headache-terminating action of ergotamine has been discarded, since it is easy to demonstrate that responses via the cranial sympathetic pathways, such as dilatation of the pupils on pinching the skin of the neck, are not disturbed by the amounts of ergotamine that terminate severe headache.

Central vs. Peripheral Action of Ergotamine Tartrate and Its Relevance to Migraine Therapy

The question was raised whether the effectiveness of ergotamine tartrate is due to a direct vasoconstrictor action on peripheral blood vessels or whether vasoconstriction occurs secondarily to a central action of the agent (Pichler *et al.*, 1956).

That ergotamine tartrate has significant central effects, as well as peripheral vasoconstrictor effects, in man and animals, has been demonstrated (Barcroft *et al.*, 1951; Dale, 1906). Its capacity to potentiate the analgesic action of certain agents and the sedative effect of the barbiturates has also been reported. Ergotamine tartrate diminishes the pressor reflex in the cat, and the carotid sinus reflex is inhibited by ergotamine tartrate in amounts of 0.25 mg/kg in cats. In the observations of von Euler and Schmiterlow (1944) ergotamine tartrate administered to cats in amounts of 0.1 mg/kg of body weight inhibited selectively the carotid sinus pressor reflex elicited by lowering the intracarotid pressure, whereas the reflex could still be noted in response to chemical stimuli.

Experiments were designed to ascertain whether ergotamine tartrate in the amounts usually given to migraine headache patients has a significant central effect in blocking or diminishing vasomotor reflexes, by Wolff and his colleagues.

Eleven healthy young men and, in addition, two patients, one with cervical sympathectomy and the other with stellate ganglion ectomy served as subjects.

Procedure and Results: Because the peripheral vasoconstriction and elevation of the blood pressure following immersion of a hand in ice water is mediated through central autonomic nervous activity, the cold pressor response was used to test the alleged central effects of ergotamine tartrate in five subjects. In each of them there was a rise in blood pressure equivalent in magnitude to that effected by the cold before the administration of the ergotamine tartrate. Thus, ergotamine tartrate failed to eliminate or diminish the "cold" pressor effect.

After the administration of 0.5 mg of ergotamine tartrate, when the vasoconstrictor effect on the temporal artery had become evident in decreased amplitude of pulsations and when the subjects were experiencing nausea, carotid sinus pressure evoked responses identical with those elicited before the administration of the agent. The slowing of the pulse rate as recorded electrocardiographically was evident mainly in the first five heart beats during pressure on the carotid sinus.

Hydergine is an equiproportional mixture of 0.1 mg of each of the methanesulfonates of three dihydrogenated ergot alkaloids, dihydroergocornine, di-

hydroergokryptine, and dihydroergocristine, and was used in combination with ergotamine tartrate for the following reasons: hydergine inhibits the vasomotor center, and, it has a peripheral vasodilator action, as demonstrated by Barcroft, Konzett, and Swan (1951), and is without notable effect on the intensity of migraine headache.

The administration of 0.3 mg of hydergine did not significantly change the amplitude of temporal artery pulsations, either before or after ergotamine tartrate. Also, it did not alter the effectiveness of ergotamine tartrate in diminishing the amplitude of temporal artery pulsations or the feelings of nausea, nor did it alter the magnitude of the carotid sinus reflex. All these results indicate that the peripheral vasoconstrictor action of ergotamine tartrate on the temporal artery occurs independently of any demonstrable central action on the vasomotor centers.

When norepinephrine is administered intravenously in amounts sufficient to elevate the blood pressure, there is mediated through the carotid and aortic pressor receptors, medullary cardioinhibitor centers, and the vagi, a significant slowing of the pulse.

A 4-cc solution of 0.1% norepinephrine in 500 cc of 5% dextrose in water (norepinephrine, 0.008 mg/cc) was infused intravenously for 5 min at a rate of 10 to 15 drops per minute, sufficient to raise the systolic blood pressure 20 to 30 mm Hg, and to slow the pulse rate by approximately 10 to 20 beats per min. The infusion was repeated 15 min and 50 min after the intravenous administration of 0.5 mg of ergotamine tartrate. However, the electrocardiograms recorded throughout the experiment showed no significant difference between the bradycardia elicited by norepinephrine during control periods and that elicited during the periods of effective action of ergotamine tartrate (see Fig. 5-1).

The persistence of the peripheral vasoconstrictor effect of ergotamine tartrate following cervical sympathectomy was demonstrated in three experiments on two patients.

The first subject was a woman age 54. On 1/20/54, right cervical sympathectomy, and on 2/9/54, left stellate ganglionectomy, had been performed (at the New York Hospital, by Dr. Bronson Ray). After each of these procedures a Horner syndrome appeared on the involved side and the hand on this side was warm. The Horner syndrome was clearly in evidence when these observations were made, on 8/30/55, and a starch-iodine test showed absence of facial sweating on the left, whereas profuse sweating occurred over the rest of the face and body.

In the first observation pulsations were recorded from the left temporal artery, i.e. from the side of the

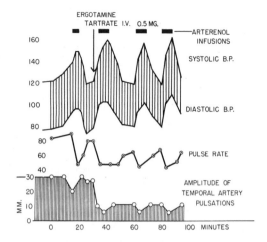

FIG. 5-1. Demonstration of the ineffectiveness of ergotamine tartrate in blocking norepinephrine-induced bradycardia.

stellate ganglionectomy. One week later, in a second observation, pulsations were recorded from the right temporal artery, i.e. on the side of the cervical sympathectomy. Following intravenous administration of ergotamine tartrate (0.5 mg), records of temporal artery pulsations were made at 1 to 2 min intervals for an hour.

Similar studies were made in another woman, aged 36, who had undergone a bilateral stellate ganglionectomy (10/6/52, on the right side and 10/8/52, on the left side). A bilateral Horner syndrome was evident on the day of this experiment, in September 1955.

The decrease in amplitude of pulsations of the temporal artery following ergotamine tartrate was neither retarded nor diminished as compared with its effects in intact subjects. Thus, in these two subjects with ostensibly sympathectomized extracranial arteries, the vasoconstrictor action of ergotamine tartrate was as effective as in intact control subjects.

It may be concluded that the effective action of ergotamine tartrate is peripheral, and that the therapeutic effect depends on its ability to produce a prolonged and powerful vasoconstriction.

Agents That Act by Raising the Threshold to Pain

In this category may be placed acetanilid, acetylsalicylic acid, amidopyrine, acetophen-etidine, codeine, and morphine. Allied to these agents, though less effective in relieving pain than in reducing restlessness, nausea, and vomiting, are the bromides, barbiturates, and chloral hydrate.

Based on long clinical experience with the use of analgesic drugs in alleviating migraine headaches of varying degrees of severity, the following classification of their effectiveness may be made. (1) For the alleviation of a mild headache of the "dull aching" variety, acetanilid, acetophenetidin, or acetylsalicylic acid, each in 0.3- to 0.6-gm amounts, or in various combinations have been used. (2) For the alleviation of a moderately severe headache, codeine phosphate in 60-mg amounts is used. (3) For the termination of a very severe headache, morphine sulfate in 15-mg amounts is used. The following data have been obtained from experiments designed to evaluate analgesic effects quantitatively (Wolff et al., 1941). They lend support to the above inferences.

Acetylsalicylic acid in 0.3-gm amounts raises the threshold to head pain about 33%, a peak effect that lasts approximately 10 min. The threshold remains elevated 20–25% for about 1½ hr. Larger amounts of the drug (0.9–1.8 gm) raise the threshold no further, although the effects last longer with the threshold raised over 20% for 2½ hr. Acetanilidid or acetophenetidin in 0.3-gm. amounts have an affect that really differs little from that of a similar amount of acetylsalicylic acid. Their use is not recommended. Furthermore, it is to be emphasized that if 0.3 to 0.6 gm of acetylsalicylic acid does not abolish the pain, no additional amounts will. Brief headache attacks of high intensity (15–30 min) may be diminished or eliminated by inhalation of 1 cc trichlorethylene.

Combinations of agents that both induce relaxation and raise the pain threshold are still popular, although their superiority is difficult to establish. For example, two tablets or capsules, taken at four-hour intervals, each containing a combination of a barbiturate (isobutyl-allyl-barbituric acid, 45 mg) acetophenetidin (120 mg), acetylsalicylic acid (180 mg), and caffeine (40 mg) are effective and widely used for headaches of mild to moderate intensity and especially for those with muscle contraction as the dominant source of pain. It should be appreciated, however, that such a combination constitutes a sizable amount of medicament, and when taken frequently, leads to a chronic dullness, lethargy, and possibly addiction.

Ergotamine tartrate is so dramatic and predictable in its results that it has generally replaced codeine in the management of the most severe headaches. But there is still a place for codeine especially in those migraine attacks in which nausea and vomiting are outstanding features. The distressing nausea created by ergotamine in some persons is reason enough to avoid its use if possible. The physician may therefore try either 60-mg doses of codeine or 0.25- to 0.50-mg doses of ergotamine, both intramuscularly, and on the basis of its effectiveness give either one or the other drug during subsequent attacks. Codeine, like ergotamine, preferably should not be given to those who cannot lie down for a few hours, since there is a slight danger of syncope in persons with violent nausea, vomiting, and abdominal discomfort.

Rarely, during status migrainus when ergotamine has been recently given and therefore may not be used again, morphine sulfate in 15-mg amounts may be injected once. Morphine sulfate should greatly reduce the intensity of the most severe headache. The administration of morphine sulfate is to be avoided, however, because of the repetitive nature of migraine headaches.

Agents That Act Primarily by Lowering the Blood Pressure

Nitroglycerin and erythrol tetranitrate, also acetylcholine and mecholine (Brock *et al.*, 1934) have been used to stop migraine headache attacks, although these agents in themselves induce headaches and can be shown to make a migraine headache worse. It is conceivable, if given in small enough doses, that they may lower the systemic blood pressure sufficiently to reduce the amplitude of pulsations of cranial arteries, resulting in less severe headache. This is an undesirable as well as ineffective method of dealing with headache and should not be used.

It is to be remembered in evaluating any of the above therapeutic procedures that all migraine headaches stop spontaneously if enough time elapses.

PREVENTION OF MIGRAINE ATTACKS

The migraine attack is a relatively innocuous sign that the organism is under stress. It should be heeded, for unlike other signs such as those of peptic ulcer which are ominous and less reversible, the migraine syndrome touches with a light hand. In a sense, the painful episode is a benefaction, since it imposes rest upon those who unwittingly tax themselves dangerously.

Perhaps even more numerous than the varieties of treatment of the acute headache have been the methods suggested for the prevention of these attacks. Many of these preventive measures have in the past been based on unsubstantiated concepts of the nature of the migraine headache. In general, preventive procedures may be divided into seven classes: (1) procedures that produce effects through "shock" and prolonged rest; (2) surgical procedures that aim to eliminate the source of pain in headache or interrupt afferent pain pathways; (3) chemical agents that induce relaxation and improve sleep; (4) agents or procedures that act by inducing feelings of security through suggestion, reassurance, and confidence in the well-planned regimen imposed by sanitarium or physician; (5) procedures that relieve anxiety and induce relaxation by improving the attitudes, habits, and life situation of the patient; (6) agents or procedures that induce vasoconstriction; and (7) agents or procedures that reduce the reactivity of the vasomotor center. The last three of these preventive measures are the most effective.

Agents or Procedures That Induce Vasoconstriction

Ergotamine tartrate, in amounts of 1 to 2 mg, or even twice this much, when taken by mouth daily, shortly before retiring time, may terminate a series of vascular headaches of the cluster type. This is more likely to happen if the patient has already been suffering from several attacks each night during a period of one or two months, i.e. if the series is spontaneously approaching its termination. Furthermore, the daily use of ergotamine tartrate in this manner is far more likely to be effective in those suffering with cluster headaches if the physician interests himself in and gives close attention to the problems and circumstances that confront the patient and are relevant to the current period of duress.

It is important that the daily administration of ergot be sharply limited by the physician.

Agents or Procedures That Reduce the Reactivity of the Vasomotor Centers

Methysergide (Sansert) may be helpful in preventing or reducing the intensity and frequency of vascular headaches in patients whose headaches are severe and cannot be controlled by other means. The usual adult dose of this medication is 4 to 8 mg daily. There should be a medication-free interval of three to four weeks after every six-month course of treatment. No pediatric dosage has been established.

About two out of three persons with intractable or severe headaches have fewer and less intense headaches or have their headaches eliminated during the period of the administration of methysergide. Its chief effect is in preventing the headache attack itself, whether the headache be exclusively unilateral, generalized, or of the cluster type. If the headache episode does not respond to methysergide, then the diagnosis of recurrent migraine should be considered to be in doubt.

There are serious and significant side effects which may occur in patients receiving methysergide, which are discussed elsewhere. All patients receiving this medication should remain under the supervision of their physician and should be examined regularly for the development of fibrotic or vascular complications.

The Actions of Methysergide and Their Relevance to the Migraine Syndrome

Earlier studies established that the capacity of ergotamine tartrate and related agents to terminate vascular headaches of the migraine type stems from their property of inducing constriction of painfully dilated cranial arteries.

It has been reported by a number of investigators that methysergide (1-methyl-D-lysergic acid butanolamide bimaleate), while lacking the capacity to terminate an existing headache, is often effective in reducing the number and severity of attacks for longer or shorter periods when the agent is maintained at adequate levels in the blood by daily intake (Doepfner and Cerletti, 1958; Friedman, 1960). In the hope that the later phenomenon would shed further light on the pathophysiology of vascular headache of the migraine type, investigations were undertaken to define the relevant pharmacodynamic properties of methysergide.

ANTISEROTONIN ACTION

As just mentioned, methysergide is a potent antagonist to many of the pharmacodynamic actions of serotonin, and the possibility has been reviewed that its antiserotonin action may be relevant to its prophylactic effects in migraine (Dalessio *et al.*, 1961).

VASOCONSTRICTOR ACTION

Methysergide does not immediately induce significant vasoconstriction in most subjects. Intravenous administration in the anesthetized cat or rat of 0.5 to 2.0 mg/kg results in a moderate fall in blood pressure and does not significantly alter the vascular tonus of the perfused hind limb of the cat. Observations of the bulbar conjunctiva of patients receiving large amounts of methysergide for several days indicated that the vascular tonus of the vessels of the conjunctiva was not altered. In a few subjects, however, severe peripheral vascular insufficiency (St. Anthony's fire) and/or myocardial ischemia occurred several days after beginning methysergide therapy and subsided rapidly when the drug therapy was discontinued. The mechanism by which ergot derivatives induce severe peripheral vascular insufficiency of this type is poorly understood. Possibly these reactions are atypical responses in hypersensitive individuals not necessarily related to the vasoconstrictor action of many of the ergot derivatives. However, the possibility cannot be excluded that the episodes of vascular insufficiency in these patients receiving methysergide result from an exceptionally active conversion, perhaps by demethylation, of methysergide to a vasoconstrictor agent (Dalessio et al., 1961). Loss of the methyl group at the 1 position from methysergide results in the formation of lysergic acid butanolamide. Intravenous administration of this latter agent in amounts of 0.5 mg/kg raises the blood pressure of the rat.

Although methysergide does not induce vasoconstriction directly, it does potentiate the pressor action of norepinephrine. Less concentrated solutions of norepinephrine were required to induce vasoconstriction when applied to the surface of the bulbar conjunctiva when methysergide was instilled into the bulbar conjunctival sac or when methysergic 8 to 16 mg/day was administered orally for several days. In the cat, the pressor response to intravenous injection of norepinephrine was potentiated by infusion of methysergide in amounts of 1 mg/kg hr. The responses of the nictitating membrane of the cat to both norepinephrine and cervical sympathetic stimulation are strikingly augmented by the administration of methysergide. The elevation of blood pressure of human subjects induced by constant intravenous infusion of morepinephrine was potentiated by the intravenous administration of methysergide in amounts of 0.03 mg/kg.

In summary, it is unlikely that methysergide exerts its prophylactic action in migraine headache solely by inducing a persisting vasoconstrictor state, despite the fact that occasional individuals react to the agent by developing severe peripheral vascular insufficiency. The possibility that the capacity of methyser-

gide to potentiate other vasoconstrictor agents including norepinephrine may be relevant to its prophylactic action in patients with migraine headache must be considered (Dalessio et al., 1962).

ANTIINFLAMMATORY ACTION

Other investigators demonstrated that methysergide is effective in reducing edema formation induced by injection of serotonin in the rat's paw. To investigate the possibility that this phenomenon was not specific to inflammation induced by serotonin, the area of flare induced by intradermal injection of manganese butyrate was determined before and seven days after administration of methysergide (8 mg/day) (Dalessio et al., 1961).

The flare reactions induced after treatment with methysergide were significantly smaller than those induced in the control periods (see Fig. 5-2). Also, the volume of inflammatory exudate in croton oil pouches in the rat was significantly reduced when the animal received methysergide (5 mg/kg/day) beginning seven days before the croton oil was injected.

The possibility that the nonspecific, antiinflammatory action of methysergide is mediated by the release of adrenal steroids was not supported by studies of the plasma and urine of patients receiving methysergide 8 to 16 mg/day.

Many features of vascular headache of the migraine type suggest that it is due to a local sterile inflammatory reaction. The antiinflammatory action of methysergide, linked with the capacity to promote vasoconstriction, may contribute to its prophylactic action in migraine.

INHIBITION OF VASOMOTOR REFLEXES

Damping of the pressor reaction to carotid occlusion is a well-recognized property of many of the ergot alkaloids. Approximately ten times more methysergide than ergotamine tartrate is required to inhibit the pressor response in the cat produced by unilateral carotid artery occlusion. In the anesthetized cat, this pressor response can be abolished by

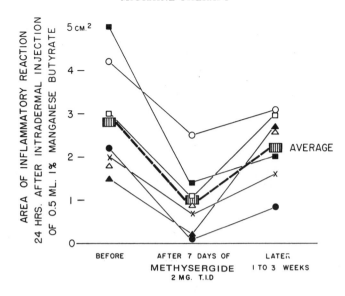

FIG. 5-2. The anti-inflammatory action of methysergide in seven human subjects.

infusion of methysergide at a rate of 1 mg/kg/hr. Moreover, the pressor response resulting from direct electrical stimution of the hindbrain of the cat can be reduced by more than a third after the administration of 1 mg of methysergide intravenously.

The depressor reflex induced by stimulation of the control end of the vagus nerve in the cat is inhibited only slightly by methysergide, and the heart rate is not altered. The depressor response to intravenous acetylcholine is not altered by infusion of methysergide at this rate. These results suggest that methysergide in this amount has a moderate depressing action on the vasomotor centers, thus damping vasoconstrictor reflexes. Although the amounts of the agent required to abolish these reflexes in the cat is approximately 100 times more than the amounts that are effective in the prevention of migraine attacks, it is possible that damping of vasoconstrictor reflexes is a feature of the prophylactic actions of methysergide in patients with migraine.

Further evidence of the relevance of the action of methysergide on vasomotor centers to the prevention of headache is afforded by a study of a series of persons subject to vascular headaches of the migraine type as regards the effect of this alkaloid on the carotid sinus reflex, the cold pressor reflex, and the breath-holding reflex (Dalessio *et al.*, 1962). These were selected as samples of vasomotor reflexes that could be tested in man, although it is recognized that they represent different reactions from those implicated in the vascular headache of the migraine type. The magnitude of these reflexes was studied before, during, and in some instances after the daily administration of four to six 2-mg amounts of methysergide. It was observed that those subjects experiencing the most striking reduction or elimination of headache also exhibited the greatest inhibitory effect on their vascular reactions to noxious and painful stimulation.

Although many subjects with vascular headache of the migraine type taking 1-methyl-D-lysergic acid butanolamide bimaleate daily showed slight slowing of the rate of the heart, and some had less variation of rate and less bradycardia following carotid sinus stimulation, the predictable effect of the agent as regards vasomotor responses was in the pressor reaction to noxious and painful stimulation administered under uniform conditions. No pressor reactions of pathologic magnitude were found in the subjects studied, yet in all instances in which the agent had a therapeutic effect as regards headache, there was concurrently a slight lowering of the initial level of the blood pressure and a progressive reduction in the blood pressure response to painful stimulation (see Fig. 5-3). Subjects who reacted in this hypodynamic way mentioned that the pain though undiminished in intensity, did not have the same significance as before. They also said that they were less adversely affected by those many circumstances in their daily lives that had previously much disturbed them. In instances of recurrence of headache while taking this agent, the former higher level of pressor response to noxious stimulation was once more evident. It thus appears that the reactions to noxious symbols or threats as well as to noxious stimuli were reduced, an observation in keeping with the effects in experimental animals.

Rats were trained to climb a pole in response to an acoustic signal in order to avoid an electric shock (a conditioned escape response). The reaction of the rats to this stress was measured by the defecation rate, or the number of fecal pellets excreted within 10 min. After control observations, the agent was given one hour before the test. In amounts of 2 mg/kg subcutaneously which did not interfere with the escape response, the effect of the agent in reducing the reaction to this threatening situation as expressed by the defecation rate was about one-third of the control level. This reduced response was shown not to be due to a direct inhibition of peristaltic activity (Cerletti *et al.*, 1960).

The effective therapeutic action of the agent is thus linked with effects on patterns integrated at a high level as well as on brain stem vasomotor reactions. These observations further support the view that the subject with vascular headache of the migraine type is one whose periods of extra alertness or general over-responsiveness are coupled with a proclivity to implicate vasomotor responses and especially those involving cranial vascular beds in his adaptive reactions.

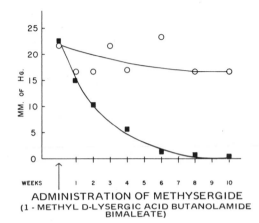

CHANGE IN PEAK PRESSOR RESPONSE

ADMINISTRATION OF METHYSERGIDE
(1 - METHYL D-LYSERGIC ACID BUTANOLAMIDE BIMALEATE)

FIG. 5-3. A curvilinear representation of the fall in pressor response to noxious stimulation, being a composite of data from nine subjects with migraine headache of the vascular type, who were significantly benefited by administration of methysergide (lower curve). Over a period of 10 weeks and especially during the first few weeks, the peak pressor response following immersion of the hand in ice water for 5 min gradually decreased. The total decrease was approximately 25 mm Hg. The upper curve is data from seven patients who were not benefited by the agent and who showed no such reduction in response to noxious stimulation.

ACTION ON HIGHEST INTEGRATIVE FUNCTIONS

From several hours to several days after the administration of methysergide had been initiated, many subjects noted slight anorexia, nausea, "foggy" feelings, mild euphoria, feelings of relaxation, and difficulty in rapid problem solving. Some reported a general slowing of activity, difficulty in focusing the eyes, and disturbances in gait and equilibrium. These changes were most apparent in those who attempted to continue difficult tasks, maintain schedules, and demand excessive output of energy of themselves. This central action of methysergide makes it likely that the pattern of striving and excessive output of effort, so commonly seen in individuals who have migraine headache attacks, will be abandoned.

The demethylated derivative of methysergide (lysergic acid butanolamide) when administered to unanesthetized cats in amounts of 2 mg/kg resulted in behavioral changes resembling those induced by LSD-25, whereas similar amounts of methysergide had no such effect.

INHIBITION OF CHANGES IN RESPONSIVITY OF CRANIAL VESSELS ASSOCIATED WITH SHIFTS OF BODY FLUID

Since fluid retention and diuresis are part of the migraine attack, reactivity of the bulbar conjuctival blood vessels during such periods of fluid shifts and the effects of methysergide on these changes were studied (Dalessio *et al.*, 1961, 1962). Thirty-two separate experiments on 17 subjects were performed, as follows. A standard water load of 1000 cc was inbibed within 10 min and the urine output in cubic centimeters per minute was measured. Urine volumes were replaced each 15 min in order to maintain the overhydration. When a satisfactory urine flow was obtained, the subject was required to smoke one cigarette deeply and rapidly. Reactivity of the bulbar conjunctival blood vessels to serial dilutions of norepinephrine was assayed (*a*) before water drinking, (*b*) during the initial diuresis prompted by water loading, (*c*) during the oliguric phase produced by the diencephalic response to nicotine stimulus, (*d*) during the diuretic phase after spontaneous termination of oliguria. Nicotine has been shown to be a potent stimulus to the neurohypophysis, and since cigarette smoking has proved to be as satisfactory as the administration of the pure alkaloid, this method of inducing oliguria was used. The procedure has the further advantage of inducing an antidiuresis by making use of the subject's endogenous hormonal substances. Those patients in whom nicotine produced predictable fluid shifts and who then exhibited alterations in vascular responsivity were used to assay the effect of methysergide. The effects of intravenous administration of cortisol during the diuretic phase were also noted.

The results were as outlined below; also, see Fig. 5-4.

1. In overhydrated subjects in whom oliguria is induced, the conjunctival blood vessels become dilated and the response of these vessels to serial dilutions of norepinephrine is diminished (from Ca 1:200,000 to Ca 1:50,000).

2. During the spontaneous diuresis which follows induced oliguria, the dilated conjunctival blood vessels become slightly constricted, and the response of these vessels to serial dilu-

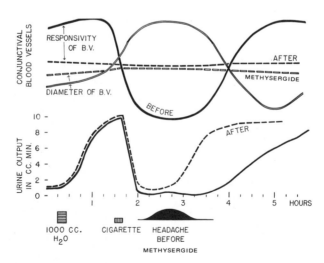

FIG. 5-4. Schema of damping effect of methysergide on blood vessel responsivity.

tions of norepinephrine is returned to the pre-oliguria status.

3. These changes in vascular diameter and responsivity to vasoconstrictor agents are related to the duration and degree of the induced oliguria and subsequent diuresis, being more profound in those patients in whom the fluid shifts were most striking.

4. The prior administration of methysergide reduced the degree of vasodilatation and the magnitude of these vascular responses during oliguria, and also the degree and duration of the latter.

5. The intravenous administration of cortisol given during the oliguric phase shortened the period of oliguria, increased the urine flow, and increased the sensitivity of the bulbar conjunctival blood vessels to serial dilutions of norepinephrine.

6. Headache occurred in seven patients during the oliguric period and diminished with the onset of diuresis. After prior administration of methysergide, no headaches occurred in these same circumstances.

It is suggested by these experiments that during the stage of fluid retention in patients with vascular headache of the migraine type, the cranial blood vessels, besides being dilated and edematous, are relatively less responsive to endogenous substances. The increased responsivity of the cranial blood vessels during the phase of diuresis possibly corresponds to the gradually reduced intensity of the headache phase associated with the onset of diuresis.

Were local vascular muscle tone the only factor involved, the opposite reaction would be more likely. Thus, according to Zweifach and Metz (1955) (direct observations made on the mesenteric blood vessels of the otherwise intact rat), vasoconstriction in response to a vasoconstrictor agent is usually pronounced and prolonged when initially the vascular bed is moderately dilated. Inversely, vasodilatation in response to a vasodilator agent is likely to be striking and prolonged when initially the blood vessels are moderately or occlusively constricted. An exaggerated response thus seems to be the usual one when the initial contractile state of the blood vessel walls is definitely of the

opposite order to that induced by a just-applied vasoconstrictor or vasodilator agent.

Many of these observations also suggest that one of the initiating factors in vascular headache of the migraine type may be the stimulation of the neurohypophysis with subsequent elaboration of the antidiuretic hormone and consequent overhydration. This may be another form of inappropriate antidiuretic hormone secretion as distinguished from the "cerebral salt-wasting syndromes" (hyponatremia with supranormal extracellular fluid volumes associated with cerebral injury) accompanied by abnormal antidiuretic hormone secretion.

SIDE EFFECTS

Inflammatory fibrosis associated with methysergide therapy represents a potentially serious side effect which drastically alters the applications of this drug. Graham and his associates (1967) have investigated 27 patients who developed a syndrome resembling retroperitoneal fibrosis while taking methysergide as a treatment for headache. Of these 27 patients, 14 were operated upon and the diagnosis was confirmed at operation. In the remaining 13, the syndrome regressed markedly upon withdrawal of the drug. Exacerbations and remissions of the disease occurred concurrently with administration and cessation of methysergide therapy. A causal relationship between the drug and this disease is therefore obvious. Also, suggestive evidence relating methysergide therapy to the development of valvular heart disease and to pleural-pulmonary fibrosis has been presented by Graham. Pathologic examination of tissues of patients taking methysergide showed essentially the same findings as those found in idiopathic cases of retroperitoneal fibrosis. The method by which methysergide produces fibrotic reactions is unknown.

Saxena (1972) also investigated the mechanism of action of methysergide in vascular headache in a study employing the external carotid artery of dogs. He found that methysergide caused a dose-dependent decrease in blood flow almost exclusively in the common and internal carotid arteries. Blood pressure was not appreciably changed by the drug, and thus vascular resistance in the carotid region was increased. There was no alteration in vascular resistance in other areas including the femoral, superior mesenteric, renal, and vertebral arteries. Evidence was also found for the depression of central vasomotor loci by methysergide in the higher dose ranges.

Methysergide was not effective in antagonizing the vasoconstrictor action of serotonin in the carotid vessels. Saxena suggested that selective carotid vasoconstriction, and not peripheral antiserotonin action, was most relevant to the antimigraine action of the drug.

CONCLUSIONS

The migraine attack is characterized by initial vasoconstriction followed by vasodilatation. Methysergide, when effective, prevents both the preheadache or vasoconstrictor phase and the headache or vasodilator phase. Of its two actions, i.e., inhibition of central vasomotor reflex effects and augmentation of peripheral vasoconstriction produced by catecholamines, the former could be significant in inhibiting the initial vasoconstrictor phase of the attack, and the latter in minimizing the subsequent painful dilatation of the vasodilator phase. On the other hand, it is conceivable that the prevention of the initial vasoconstriction makes the subsequent vasodilatation unlikely to occur, and that in the prophylaxis of vascular headache of the migraine type the peripheral actions of methysergide on cranial blood vessels are significantly supplemented by its effects on the nervous system. The magnitude of cranial vascular responsivity is reduced, thereby preventing crises of vasoconstriction and vasodilatation that characterize the migraine attack. These observations further support the thesis that the migraine attack is the symptomatic manifestation of a recurrent heightened reactivity of cranial blood vessels.

Moreover, the concurrent reduction during administration of methysergide in intensity and frequency of headaches, and in magnitude of vasomotor reflexes adds further support to the inference that unstable cranial vasomotor functions are a prime factor in the pathophysiology of this variety of headache.

BC-105 and Migraine Prophylaxis

Sicuteri and his associates (1967) have conducted clinical trials on BC-105, a powerful antagonist of serotonin and histamine, and a weak acetylcholine antagonist. It is related to cyproheptadine. The drug proved an effective prophylactic agent in migraine headache and had "a curative effect in chronic migraine." The drug should be used especially in those patients who do not respond to ergotamine or when the latter agent, for various reasons, is contraindicated.

Clonidine, Periactin, and Migraine Prophylaxis

Clonidine is an imidazoline derivative which has been used in the treatment of hypertension. Its main pharmacologic effect is a significant decrease in the responsiveness of blood vessels to vasoconstrictor or vasodilator drugs. Zaimis and Hanington (1969) showed that, in animals given repeated doses of clonidine, both vasoconstrictor and vasodilator responses to norepinephrine and epinephrine were abolished. They suggested that clonidine was able to induce a change in the vascular smooth muscle, making it less capable of responding to vasoconstrictor or vasodilator drugs. This effect on blood vessels led them to suggest that clonidine might be of value in migraine. See also Kallanranta et al. (1977).

Cyproheptadine (Periactin), an antihistaminic with mild-to-moderate antiserotonin activity, also affords headache prophylaxis. The usual oral dosage is 4 mg four times a day, although this may be increased as required to a maximum divided daily dose of 32 mg. No fibrosis has been reported after the use of this drug, but the patient may experience dry mouth (xerostomia), drowsiness, and appetite stimulation.

Beta Blockers in Migraine

The beta-adrenergic receptors of the nervous system are found throughout the body and are responsible for altering a variety of body activities. There are two types of beta receptors, Beta 1 (B1) receptors which are found primarily in the heart, and Beta 2 (B2) receptors which are found especially in the smooth muscles of the bronchioles and in the arterioles. When the sympathetic nervous system is stimulated, there is excitation of Beta 1 receptors causing cardiac effects including increased heart rate and contractility. Stimulation of the Beta 2 receptors causes relaxation of the smooth muscle. Generally this is associated with vasodilatation. Until this year propranolol (Inderal) has been the only Beta receptor blocker available in the United States. It is a nonselective blocker which competitively blocks both Beta 1 and Beta 2 receptors. Since the painful stage of migraine is associated with vasodilatation of the intracranial and extracranial arterioles, the suggestion has been made that Beta blockers would prevent this dilatation and hence enhance migraine prophylaxis. Multiple controlled studies have been done since the original suggestion was made by Weber and Reinmuth (1972). Often a starting dose of 20 mg is given two or three times daily, increasing by 20–40 mg every third or fourth day until control is achieved. Peak plasma levels of propranolol are reached approximately 90 min after oral intake. Some investigators have suggested that large doses of the drug need to be employed, in the range used in some cardiac conditions, such as 200 to 400 mg in two or three divided doses. They do not report serious side-effects, but the experienced clinician will recognize that this drug does, in fact, have widespread cardiac effects and should be employed with caution in migraine patients with cardiac disease, particularly those with conduction defects, congestive heart failure, and also in those atopic individuals who may be predisposed to bronchial asthma. One can monitor the effect of propranolol by observing the pulse rate. In general, the pulse rate should not be significantly depressed below 60 beats/min in a healthy individual with migraine.

Our studies on the physiologic effects of training techniques, such as biofeedback, suggest that they may work by altering sympathetic tone, as one retrains the autonomic nervous system. In this respect they produce a response similar to that evoked by propranolol, reducing sympathetic tonus in patients with migraine.

Agents Which Relieve Depression

Antidepressant medications may be helpful in the treatment of migraine. They are especially useful therapy for patients with frequent and severe attacks of migraine which do not respond to other medication. Both tricyclic antidepressants and monoamine oxidase inhibitors may be used.

Couch, Ziegler, and Hassanein (1976) demonstrated that amitriptyline would produce a better than 50% improvement in migraine in 72% of patients, and a better than 80% improvement in 57% of patients. Depression was absent in 40 patients, borderline in 53, and moderate to severe in 17. Overall depression ratings improved minimally with therapy and there was a weak relationship between improvement in depression and improvement in migraine. Their study suggests that amitriptyline is effective in migraine prophylaxis and it appears to have a primary effect on migraine that is relatively independent of its antidepressant action.

Lance (1969) has shown that the long-term treatment of patients with intractable migraine with the monoamine oxidase (MAO) inhibitor, phenelyzine sulfate (Nardil), reduces the severity and frequency of the attacks to less than half the original number. Patients are given an oral regimen of 15 mg phenelzine or 10 mg isocarboxazid (Marplan) three times a day. After 10 to 14 days, this is reduced to a maintenance dose.

Hypertensive crises have sometimes occurred in those taking monoamine oxidase inhibitors after ingestion of certain foods, particularly those with a high tyramine content. In general, patients with migraine who employ monoamine oxidase inhibitors for headache prophylaxis should avoid protein foods in which aging or protein breakdown is used to increase flavor. In particular, patients should be instructed not to take foods such as cheese (especially strong or aged varieties), sour cream, Chianti wine, sherry, beer, pickled herring, liver, or canned figs; raisins, bananas, or avocados (particularly if over-ripe); chocolate, soy sauce, or the pods of broad beans such as fava beans; yeast extracts; or meats prepared with tenderizers.

Platelet Antagonists and Migraine Prophylaxis

If one accepts the premise that vasoactive materials are important in the vascular permeability which characterizes migraine, then obviously the role of the platelets is critical to the cascade schema of sterile inflammation which accompanies the migraine attack. Recent published studies suggest that there is chronic aggregation of platelets in migraine patients which may be unrelated to the type or severity of the migraine attack (Deshmukh and Meyer, 1977). There is also a significant increase in platelet adhesiveness during the headache phase of migraine and this parallels the increase in plasma serotonin levels during the headache prodromata, and the subsequent decrease in serotonin levels during the headache phase. It is suggested that alterations in platelet aggregation are responsible for the observed changes in plasma serotonin levels since, at least in humans, platelets contain virtually all of the plasma serotonin. Platelet antagonists currently employed in the treatment of ischemic vascular disease may also be useful in migraine.

These include particularly aspirin, sulfinpyrazone (Anturane), fenoprofen (Nalfon), and dipyridamole (Persantine). Generally these drugs lengthen the survival time of platelets, and inhibit their adherence to various materials such as collagen *in vitro*. Therapeutic doses are aspirin, one tablet twice daily; sulfinpyrazone 200 mg 2-4 times daily; fenoprofen 300 mg 3 times daily; and dipyridamole 100–400 mg daily, in divided doses.

Our preliminary studies on the effects of platelet antagonists in the treatment of migraine suggest that sulfinpyrazone and fenoprofen may be particularly effective in reducing the intensity and frequency of headache attacks. These compounds have been prescribed differently. Sulfinpyrazone is used for headache prophylaxis, while fenoprofen is employed in the treatment of the acute attack itself. When compared to oral ergotamine tartrate in standard dose, the drugs appear to have a similar spectrum of action in terms of pain relief (See Tables 5-3 and 5-4).

We recognize that such open trials are subject to many methodologic variables since methods for grading pain and pain relief are nonspecific and difficult to employ. The placebo effect of the study situation and the institution in which treatment was given cannot be eliminated. Nonetheless, it seems evident that substances which interfere with platelet aggregation offer yet another therapy for recurrent vascular headaches, not only for treatment of the acute episode, but for prophylaxis as well.

S. V. Deshmukh, and J. S. Meyer (1977), investigated the pathophysiologic role of platelets in the pathogenesis of migraine. Twenty-seven patients with migraine were studied while off medication during a headache-free period. The migraineurs showed a higher platelet aggregation response to adenosine diphosphate (ADP) ($p > 0.025$) when compared to 35 normals. Platelet function tests were performed in 14 migraine pa-

TABLE 5-3   Fenoprofen and Sulfinpyrazone Compared with Ergotamine

DRUG	NUMBER OF PATIENTS	INTENSITY OF TREATED MIGRAINE (NUMBERS OF PATIENTS)				SIDE EFFECTS
		Complete Relief	Minimal Pain	Moderate Pain	Maximal Pain	
Ergot	10	3	4	3	—	4
Sulfinpyrazone	15	4	6	5	—	1
Fenoprofen	15	5	4	6	—	3

TABLE 5-4   Frequency of Migraine Episodes During Treatment

| | | | INTENSITY OF MIGRAINE (NUMBER OF ATTACKS) | | |
DRUG	NUMBER OF PATIENTS	Complete Relief	Minimal Pain	Moderate Pain	Maximal Pain
Ergotamine	10	24	30	17	
*Sulfinpyrazone	15	—	24	14	3
Fenoprofen	15	28	40	12	5

*Used prophylactically.

tients during the headache-free period and repeated subsequently in 11 patients during the prodrome and in the headache phase. Platelet adhesiveness to glass beads and aggregation response to ADP, epinephrine, thrombin, and serotonin increased during prodrome. During the headache phase, adhesiveness increased further, but aggregation in response to ADP and epinephrine decreased. The increase in platelet aggregation during the prodrome and decrease during the headache phase parallels the reported increase in plasma serotonin level during the prodrome and subsequent decrease during the headache phase. Since platelets contain virtually all the serotonin present in blood and release it during aggregation, it is possible that changes in plasma serotonin levels in migraine are secondary to changes in platelet aggregation. Given the above findings, pharmacologic inhibition of platelet aggregation is a rational form of prophylaxis of migraine and other vascular headaches.

Chemical Agents That Induce Relaxation and Improve Sleep

Among the first of the chemical agents used to achieve these ends in patients with migraine, with the aim of preventing attacks, were the bromide salts. Since the introduction of the barbiturates and acetanilid, antipyrine, phenacetin, and more recently the "tranquilizers," the bromides have been replaced. When sole dependence is placed upon sedative agents to prevent headaches they are unsatisfactory, first of all because they lead to addiction and other toxic drug effects, and secondly because they fail to influence the underlying basis of conflict and tension. However, in conjunction with other more fundamental means of inducing relaxation they are useful.

Agents or Procedures That Act by Inducing Feelings of Security through Suggestion, Reassurance, and Confidence

1. DIETARY FACTORS IN MIGRAINE

Foods which contain tyramine may precipitate headaches, particularly in patients who are treated with monoamine oxidase inhibitors (Hanington and Harper, 1968). Tyramine is found in significant amounts in cheese, fish, beans, and dairy produce. Tyramine is a sympathomimetic amine which acts both directly and through the release of norepinephrine. Hanington and Harper (1968) postulate that the release of norepinephrine from the tissues could give rise to a selective cerebral vasoconstriction. When the tissue stores of norepinephrine then became exhausted, a rebound dilatation effecting mainly the extracerebral vessels could occur, resulting thereafter in headache.

From time to time carbohydrates or the mineral constituents of the diet have been prohibited because of their alleged etiologic significance in migraine. Dietetic regimens have been designed to reduce the supposedly increased intracranial pressure by preventing the retention of fluids. To be sure, the migraine subject may feel more comfortable on this or that diet; but food per se either through its effect on intestinal stasis, fluid retention, or by virtue of allergic or sensitivity effects, is probably of little importance, except as noted above.

Patients most spectacularly cured by the removal of offending articles of food again became subject to headache as soon as tension and worry came upon them. Furthermore, food, per se, can hardly be blamed in these patients when headache comes at long intervals and then only at the menstrual period or after some unusual excitement or stress (Medina and Diamond, 1978).

Hyslop (1934) cites the case of a migraine subject who occasionally had migraine headache attacks some hours after eating pork. He was found to be sensitive to many articles of food by skin tests. He could, however, eat pork without unpleasant sequelae if he was in good condition but he was sure to have an attack if he ate pork when tired or under emotional stress.

It is Balyeat's (1933) opinion that the migraine headache is due to localized edema in the pia or cortex of the brain or in both. The postulated edema is, according to him, probably due to an increase in capillary permeability in these localized areas and this in turn to hypersensitivity to one or more foods. His results of treatment in 350 cases seen during four years are: excellent (from 80 to 100% relief) 30%; good (from 60 to 80% relief) 30%; fair (from 40 to 60% relief) 20%; poor 20%. These results would be more impressive were it not for the fact that similar results have been obtained, as will be shown later, without interfering with dietary habits.

No well-controlled clinical study has yet been reported to support the contention that migraine headache is an allergic reaction, or to prove that the benefit from prescribed diets is specifically due to elimination of offending allergens. It is conceivable that food sensitivity does occasionally induce a headache. It is pointed out that the mucous membranes of the nasal and paranasal structures exhibit vasomotor changes as a part of the reaction to allergens, and may give rise to headache. But in the case of the nose reaction associated with migraine headaches, the assumption that the allergens are responsible for the headache must be closely questioned in any given case until proven valid. Allergy, nasal disease, and headache are the topics of discussion in Chapter 12. Migraine and allergy are also discussed in Chapter 4.

To illuminate further this matter of food allergy, the following experiment was performed. Four able physicians, experienced in experimental methods, and themselves migraine patients, were the subjects. These four physicians, who were of the opinion that they could predictably produce migraine headache in themselves by eating chocolate in any form and in minimal amounts, were each given a set of lettered, sealed envelopes, with the key to the contents held in the laboratory, and unknown to the subject. Each envelope contained either 8 gm powdered chocolate or 8 gm lactose, in eight black capsules. The two sets of capsules were indistinguishable in appearance. Two subjects ingested the contents of an envelope at convenient intervals. One subject ingested the contents of an envelope at regular intervals, three times a week. The fourth subject who commonly awoke on Saturday mornings with a migraine headache attack after eating chocolate on Friday evening, ingested his capsules on Friday evenings for a period of four months. All were instructed to include no chocolate in their regular diet. Careful records were kept by each subject, including the following data: the letter on the envelope; the date and time of ingestion of the contents; the date and time of onset of all headaches experienced during the experimental period.

It was found in these subjects that headaches sometimes followed the chocolate, sometimes the lactose, but most commonly attacks occurred without reference to the ingestion of capsules. Migraine headaches followed the ingestion of lactose just as frequently as they followed the ingestion of chocolate. The data thus accumulated indicate that in these individuals who considered themselves "allergic" to chocolate even in minimal amounts, the occurrence of their headaches was no more related to the ingestion of chocolate than it was to the ingestion of lactose.

5-HYDROXYTRYPTOPHANE IN THE PROPHYLAXIS OF MIGRAINE

N. T. Mathew (1978) has investigated the proposed abnormalities in serotonin metabolism demonstrated in patients with migraine. It has been suggested that migraine may result from reduced brain serotonin turnover and that a decrease in the frequency of migraine attacks could be achieved after the administration of L-tryptophane, a precursor of serotonin.

In order to test the effectiveness of 5-hydroxytryptophane (5-HTP), which is an immediate precursor of serotonin (5-hydroxytryptamine) (5-HT) in the prophylaxis of migraine, Mathew performed a double-blind study. Twelve patients with migraine, six with classical, and six with common migraine, were assigned randomly to one of two groups in a double-blind crossover design. One group was given 5-HTP for the first week, and then placebo for the second week. The other group received the placebo first and then 5-HTP. The dose of 5-HTP was 300 mg per day. The efficacy of the treatment was evaluated by using a Headache Index, emphasizing headache frequency and intensity as compared with previous experience. The drug's safety was monitored by recording side effects and changes in vital signs. Analysis of Mathew's data showed that 5-HTP was not superior to placebo in preventing migraine attacks in the amount employed. Slight drowsiness and mild diarrhea were the most common side effects.

SLEEP RATIONING

It has long been known that vascular headache of the migraine type often begins in the early hours of the morning on awakening from a deep sleep. It is also well known that the unusually long sleep on Sunday mornings may be followed by vascular headache. Some patients complain that an attack is often preceded by even a short period of very deep sleep taken during the afternoon of a nonworking day. Whether the especially deep sleep is in itself an aspect of the beginning of the attack or whether it initiates the attack, is as yet uncertain. It has been suggested that deep sleep with its slow respiration may result in a mild asphyxia that precipitates the attack.

T. Dalsgaard-Nielsen (1957) cognizant of the relation between sleep and onset of vascular headache, has introduced additional therapeutic measures. He suggests raising the head end of the bed 20 cm, reducing the number of hours of sleep, and in some instances administering ergotamine tartrate, 1 mg, by mouth before retirement.

THE WELL-DIRECTED THERAPEUTIC REGIMEN

In short, many patients have been helped by one or another of the aforementioned procedures, but it is not to be forgotten that through such means the patient's relation to his environment changes from a state of helplessness, insecurity, or anxiety to a position of being looked after and encouraged through planned treatment. It is an error to attribute success to any regimen without evaluating the change in attitude created in the patient. When purely chemical or physical means appear to have been helpful to a patient in the prevention of migraine it is essential to look further for another aspect of treatment that has, wittingly or unwittingly, been imposed by the physician (Diethelm, 1936, 1938). This consists commonly of rest or removal from disturbing influences, reassurance by the physician, restoration of self-confidence, and supportive influence of a sympathetic and well-directed therapeutic regimen.

Imputing to a drug or diet effects that are actually produced by the feeling of security, confidence, and reassurance engendered by the physician and the situation he creates is not the only mistake of which the physician may be guilty. Thus, physician and patient may erroneously accord to specious "psychologic" explanations, good effects which actually arise from feelings of security and confidence, or from changes in habit and attitude to life situations.

RESULTS AND PROGNOSIS

The prognosis of a patient with migraine should be viewed somewhat as that of a patient with peptic ulcer. Migraine headache attacks may be terminated, or the interval between episodes greatly prolonged, but unless the subject has discovered a suitable pattern of life and is able to adhere to it, headache will recur. Just as peptic ulcer may recur after years of quiescence, so it is reasonable to anticipate that headaches will recur during a major crisis and periods of great stress when the organism is taxed to the limit. The subject should be acquainted with these possibilities, since return of the symptom may otherwise cause unwarranted alarm and discouragement. At such times therapy should be resumed for a short period.

It must not be assumed that personality and situational readjustments can always be achieved. Therapeutically, even searching psychoanalysis may sometimes founder on the unresolvable difficulties created by certain fixed personalities and situations. But given more plastic material good results may be anticipated. Fromm-Reichman (1937) analyzed eight patients with migraine, of whom five became practically headache-free, two got decided relief as to the number and intensity of their attacks, and one remained unchanged.

It may be pointed out that success in treatment is determined not only by the ability of the physician but by the patient's attitude toward his physician, and the respect and security engendered by his reputation or that of the institution he represents. Some patients cannot be helped by any physician; also a physician, despite his great usefulness to one individual, may be quite unsuitable for another.

Critchley (1936) points out that Europeans with migraine are adversely affected by tropical climates. It has been possible to confirm this observation in those who are especially unable to adapt themselves to new situations. It is probable that the climate makes it more difficult to 'get things done' in the time that would be usual in the temperate zone. Driving, energetic people are irritated by the laissez faire attitude prevailing in tropical regions.

According to Captain C. S. Mullin (1959) headache was a frequent complaint of personnel in isolated Antarctic bases. It was the basis of 50% of sick call entries in a given study. The headaches could not be attributed to eye stress, the cold, poor ventilation, sinus, or other infections, or constipation. The headaches were mainly of the vascular type, but muscle-contraction type headache also occurred. According to the physician in charge, the headache was related to the strongly felt need for careful control of aggression under circumstances of enforced close personal associa-tions. The headaches occurred more frequently in the sophisticated civilian and officer groups than in the enlisted groups, allegedly because of the more rigidly self-imposed restraint. Also such leaders were more constrained from using common means for dispelling aggression that were available to the enlisted groups. These included violent swearing, vigorous horseplay, loud, but good-natured, complaining, and the exchange of frank and fearful insult mutually recognized as a method of dealing with the situation.

The occupation of the individual is important in prognosis, since certain jobs entail responsibilities, decisions, and pace which may be excessive and which permit of little modification, e.g., high-pressure salesmanship, auctioneering, or work that requires rapid fire decisions or constant alertness.

For the woman with migraine the period of pregnancy may be relatively free of headache. If during the pregnancy she accepts the limitations and reduction in energy imposed by her changed state; if she is nourished and satisfied by the personal and social implications of her state, pregnancy becomes a period of well-being. On the other hand, if her pregnancy is unacceptable for the above or other reasons, headache may be even more frequent and severe.

Prolonged illness, advancing age, the loss of mobility, vision, or hearing may decrease the frequency and severity of attacks, as also may major surgical operations, skull fractures, or other severe injuries when subjects are able to accept such states as legitimate reasons for relaxation and withdrawal from competition. The frequency and intensity of attacks, however, may be augmented if these changes or accidents are met with resentment, fear, or struggle. Here, as elsewhere, the signs of a poor prognosis are fixed attitudes in the face of unalterable situations.

In the main, a better prognosis can be offered to patients who have had the migraine syndrome but a short time as compared with those who have had headaches since childhood. Migraine, as is commonly known, disappears usually at the menopause in women and in men at the age of 45 or 50 years. The important aspect of the improvement may be that this age period brings with it declining drive, resignation, or spontaneous adjustment of major conflicts. For rigid persons, however, middle life may bring with it increasing difficulty with adjustment, and their migraine may become worse instead of better. Moreover, when migraine begins during the age period between 40 and 50 the prognosis is poor. This is clearly seen in those with hemmed-in lives, circumscribed by family, poor finances, and many responsibilities, for whom the menopause or age of 45 means life failure with no further opportunity for success.

Wolff and colleagues found the application of the principles that have been outlined to be of value in the prevention of migraine attacks, as can be seen in Table 5-5. To be sure, the physician is not the only factor in the improvement, since with the passage of time many life situations spontaneously resolved themselves. Improved circumstances, however, coupled with understanding by the patient brought about better adjustments.

Correlations of migraine attacks and personality features, emotional reactions, and situations became apparent when life experiences were viewed in terms of a long time span. Both the frequency and intensity of attacks in these subjects were reduced through better understanding of themselves and management of their situations. Moreover, even though patients were unable to eradicate headaches immediately or completely, they experienced increasingly greater security when they appreciated that the situation was in their hands.

BIOFEEDBACK AS THERAPY

Introduction

Training migraineurs to volitionally induce vasodilatation in their fingers often leads to a reduction in the incidence and intensity of migraine attacks. The phenomenon was discovered incidentally at the Menninger Clinic where the possibility of volitionally influencing certain autonomic nervous functions has been studied (Sargent et al., 1973). A subject was provided with a feedback of her finger temperature and instructed to increase it using autosuggestion. Being coincidentally a migraine sufferer, the subject, having noticed symptoms of an imminent attack, found it possible to abort it by applying the newly acquired method. This empirical observation led to its rapid integration into the therapy of migraine (Wickramasekera, 1973; Sargent et al., 1973; Mitch et al., 1976).

An often surmised physiological rationale of the phenomenon is based on the assumption that migraineurs generally have a persistent peripheral vasoconstriction, which, at the time of an attack, increases, coinciding with vasodilatation in the carotid arterial beds. (Appenzeller, 1969). Induced vasodilatation in hands should somehow prevent or reduce carotid vasodilatation.

This rationale does not necessarily have to be correct. It does not follow that clinical improvement which correlates with the modification of a single autonomic response proves that response to be the cause of the improvement, rather than one of the many factors of a migraine's complex pathophysiology. External carotid vasodilatation and resulting throbbing

TABLE 5-5

Total number of patients in series	64
Male	17
Female	47
Duration	1–50 yrs.
Time since beginning of treatment	3 mos.–5 yrs.
Number of patients with no recurrence of headache, or on rare occasions	18 (28%)
Number of patients with headaches that are much less frequent and less intense	23 (36%)
Number of patients still having headaches that they have to some extent controlled	10 (16%)
Number of patients with transient episodes of freedom from headache but with recurrent severe attacks	6 (10%)
Number of patients who failed to improve	7 (10%)

pain in migraine are only incidental effects of migraine syndrome, which is a complex cascade of pathological events.

Sovak *et al.* (1978) proposed to study, in normal subjects and migraineurs, the effects of vasodilatation in hands as induced by heat or by volition (using feedback training) on the segments of the carotid vasculature accessible to examination by noninvasive techniques.

METHODS

Five normal, healthy volunteers 26–37 years of age, two males and three females, and 12 female migraineurs from the patient population of the Scripps Medical Institute were subjects of the study. Migraineurs had a complete neuro- and psychological workup; the diagnosis of vascular headache was established and subject's motivation for feedback therapy ascertained. Subjects were taken off all medication. They were instructed to abstain from ethanol and caffeine for at least 6 hr preceding the training session. Forty-five-min sessions were conducted twice a week for four weeks in a dimly lighted room with the subjects seated in a reclining chair. During the introductory session the importance of the subject's involvement and responsibility for the training outcome was stressed. In migraineurs, in addition, we made every effort to heighten the subjects' expectation and to make them responsible for the therapy. We emphasized the importance of a personal commitment to a program of frequent daily practice in order to learn the technique and to be able to use it for preventing and/or alleviating the migraine headache (Sargent *et al.*, 1973).

All subjects were taught a relaxational technique. They received a taped version of the exercise instructing them to autogenically relax in a stepwise fashion all muscle groups to produce "a strong pulse in the fingertips" and to feel "warm hand, warm fingers." The tape's autosuggestive effect was emphasized by consequently using the first person of the singular (*I* feel... *I* do, etc.). Further, subjects memorized and recorded on a cassette tape this instructional set in their own voice.

Temperature feedback was provided by an electrothermometer (Biotemp) using a thermistor probe taped to the volar aspect of the middle finger's third phalanx of the dominant hand in normals, or the hand of the headache side in migraineurs.

Subjects were instructed to relax but not to succumb to sleep, to stay alert, to observe the parameter display attentively, in a state of pleasant reverie rather than using forceful concentration, and to increase the temperature. Each subject was given the electrothermometer to use at home and practice as often as possible, but not less than twice a day.

The criterion for successful training was defined as the capability to volitionally raise hand temperature by at least 2°C within 15 min in the laboratory setting.

Following the training, subjects were brought into the same room in which they had been trained for a mock-up familiarizing session which, in addition to the usual procedure, included affixing various sensors for the collection of hemodynamic data. After we ascertained that the subjects could perform under these modified circumstances, the proper experimental sessions were scheduled.

Finger temperature was recorded as described above. Pulse volume changes of the same finger and of the frontotemporal region were determined by reflectance photoplethysmography (Ohmidge and Narco instruments). Sensors were placed superior to the foramen supraorbitale and over the area of palpable pulsations of the temporal ramus of the superficial temporal artery, posterior to the linea temporalis of the os frontale. All probes were attached by double-stick discs. Subjects were asked to refrain from relaxing and the baseline values were recorded. They were then instructed to apply the previously learned hand-warming technique. As they did so, the parameters were continuously recorded. These experimental sessions varied from 20 to 30 min, after which subjects were asked to stop relaxing and were engaged in a conversation until their temperature returned to baseline.

After an interval of approximately 15 min, a new baseline was registered and the hand contralateral to the training side was exposed to a current of hot air (85°C). The parameters were again recorded throughout the exposure which was continued until vasodilatation of at least 30% above the baseline value was achieved.

Average pulse volumes for each measurement were obtained from the average of the integrated areas under ten consecutive pulse peaks. The "test" pulse volume was determined at the time of maximum pulse amplitude increase. Changes relative to baseline values were expressed as percentages. Mean heart rate during a period of at least 60 sec was calculated from the pulse volume recordings. Statistical significance of observed changes within each individual was determined at 95% confidence level using Student's T test.

Clinical status of migraineurs was evaluated after three months by questionnaires based on a log of frequency and intensity of headaches and eventual intake of medication. The patients were rated "clinically improved" when at least two of these three factors showed at least a 50% reduction.

RESULTS AND DISCUSSION

All subjects with the exception of two migraineurs learned the technique. Out of ten successfully trained migraineurs, eight were clinically improved and two unimproved. The results of hemodynamic observations are summarized in Figures 5-5, 5-6, and 5-7.

It can be seen that with the *volitional exercise* in both normals and improved migraineurs, the average pulse volume increased in the finger while it decreased in that portion of the frontotemporal region supplied primarily by the supraorbital artery (SA). Three of eight improved migraineurs, however, have shown no change in pulse volume. Response from the area supplied primarily by the superficial temporal artery (TA) was variable both in normals and in migraineurs. There was a tendency toward moderate bradycardia in normals and improved migraineurs.

With *heat*, in all normal subjects pulse volumes of both SA and TA terminal vascular beds increased. In migraineurs, the degree and direction of the response varied greatly.

Tachycardia was elicited in all cases except in nonimproved migraineurs.

Temperature followed the increase in the finger pulse volume with a lag ranging from approximately 10 to 30 sec. It remained elevated for several minutes after the pulse volume had returned to the control levels. It is known that even with a completely arrested antebrachial circulation, hand skin temperature decreases very slowly (Greenfield, 1963).

In all instances when the finger pulse volume (F-PV) increased, it did so in stepwise, wavelike fashion: after an initial increase lasting approximately 20–60 sec, F-PV decreased transiently for a period varying from 1 to 3 min. Thereafter, it increased again, surpassing the previously reached volume. During experiments with heat this pattern was qualitatively paralleled in the frontotemporal region.

In volitional experiments, with finger vasodilatation progressing, the pulse volume of the frontotemporal region (FT-PV) decreased transiently at first. Even a brief decrease in F-PV elicited an immediate return of FT-PV to control levels. When F-PV increased substantially (i.e., when it more than doubled), FT-PV decreased and remained depressed for the duration of the extended hand vasodilatation. The magnitude of these changes proved to be statistically significant.

F-PV is representative of the skin blood perfusion; the skin blood flow, however, represents only about 10% of the total forearm-hand blood flow (Greenfield, 1963). Since an increase of the finger pulse volume could signify vasodilatation in the skin, or skin and muscle, we previously attempted to characterize it: using Doppler ultrasonography in experimental setup similar to the one described above, we found in the antebrachial arteries of normal subjects an increase of the mean blood flow velocity, simultaneously occurring with increase of pulse volume in the finger, induced either by volition or heat (Sovak *et al.*, 1976). This increase in both parameters indicates that the vasodilatation is total, i.e., encompassing both skin and muscle. This has been described as typical of general deep muscular relaxation (Langen, 1969).

Using Doppler ultrasonography we had

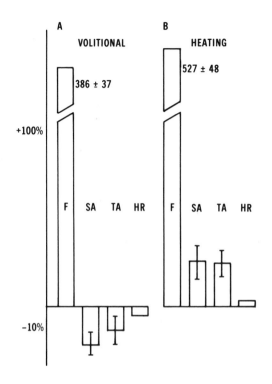

VOLITIONAL				
SUBJECT	F	SA	TA	HR
A.	280.3 ±32.2	−14.2±5.6	−14.6± 4.1	−2.7
B.	644.4 ±54.2	−27.1±7.4	N/A	0.0
C.	314.3 ±41.0	− 8.2±8.7NS	−14.3±15.2NS	−4.6
D.	521.0 ±48.2	−18.3±3.0	− 3.1± 1	−8.2
E.	170.2 ± 9.3	−17.0±4.8	− 9.2± 9.3NS	−5.0
Av.	386.04±36.98	−16.9±5.9	−10.3± 7.9	−4.1

HEATING				
SUBJECT	F	SA	TA	HR
A.	484.4±42	27.3± 7.2	32.7 ±12.1	+3.3
B.	680.4±64.3	18.2± 4.4	27.3 ± 6.3	+4.1
C.	468.7±48	32.2±12.2	18.1 ± 4.4	+3.9
D.	582.8±54.2	31.1±11.2	22.2 ± 7.3	+5.1
E.	420.2±33.1	24.2±10.1	28.0 ±11.0	+6.7
Av.	527.3±48.32	26.6± 9.02	25.66± 8.22	+4.62

N/A = Not available.
NS = Not statistically significant at 95% level of confidence.

FIG. 5.5. Average heart rate (HR) and pulse volumes in digital (F), supraorbital (SA), and superficial temporal (TA) arterial beds of five normal subjects measured at maximum peripheral digital vasodilatation produced by volition (A) or heat (B), and estimated as percent difference from baseline. Ten measurements in each group.

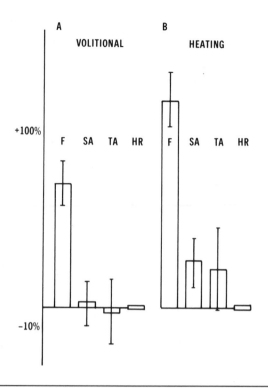

Volitional

Subject	F	SA	TA		HR
F.	300.426±48.105	−26.675 ±11.05	N/A	N/A	− 1.64
G.	140.370±15.680	−22.270 ± 7.92	N/A	N/A	−11.76
H.	77.61 ±23.39	−58.09 ±14.15	−13.51 NS±15.66NS		− 2.7
I.	10.15 ± 6.70	− 8.96 ± 8.43	18.56 ± 7.80		− 3.78
J.	67.15 ±15.09	+ 2.14 NS±13.30	—		− 2.51
K.	101.58 ±21.59	+11.42 NS±14.80	9.14 NS±11.08		− 1.82
L.	228.16 ± 4.84	+ 5.50 NS± 7.92	−19.27 ±14.64		0.00
M.	22.08 ±21.09	−11.42 NX±12.89	−48.06 ±11.49		− 8.65
Av.	117.82 ±19.561	−13.544 ±11.3075	−10.628NS±12.134		− 4.10

Heating

Subject	F	SA	TA		HR
F.	507.367±45.144	+23.077 ±14.115	N/A	N/A	+ 8.3
G.	121.700± 9.950	− 1.99 NS±14.76	− 4.36NS± 8.56		+ 3.0
H.	34.16 ±12.08	−28.56 ±14.710	− 4.69NS±11.38		+16.7
I.	18.23 ±18.98	−15.76 ± 9.73	−23.79 ±10.02		− 2.6
J.	72.21 ± 9.52	+ 4.08 NS±10.62	N/A	N/A	0.0
K.	61.92 ±13.41	−13.19 ± 9.05	−29.06 ± 9.92		+39.0
L.	98.30 ±19.12	− 2.87 NS± 6.49	.07NS±14.81		+ 6.4
M.	130.91 ±35.56	−12.09 ±10.42	+42.8 NS±11.82		+ 3.3
Av.	130.599±20.471	− 5.91 NS±11.237	− 3.18NS±11.085		+ 9.27

N/A = Not available.
NS = Not statistically significant at 95% level of confidence.

FIG. 5-6. Average heart rate (HR) and pulse volumes in digital (F), supraorbital (SA), and superficial temporal (TA) arterial beds of eight improved migraineurs measured at maximum peripheral digital vasodilatation produced by volition (A) or heat (B), and estimated as percent difference from baseline. Ten measurements in each group.

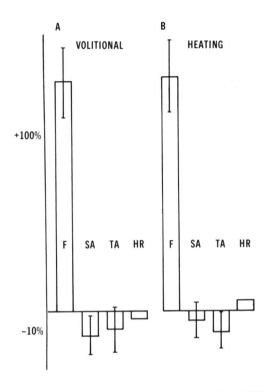

	VOLITIONAL			
SUBJECT	F	SA	TA	HR
N	71.95 ±10.94	−5.42NS±12.92	−12.94±10.34	0
O	52.82 ±12.53	8.85NS±13.57	7.75NS±22.66	0
Av.	62.385±11.745	1.7 NS±13.24	− 2.59NS±16.5	0

	HEATING			
SUBJECT	F	SA	TA	HR
N	39.92± 7.01N/A		N/A 5.65NS±11.01	0
O	80.81±15.33	29.68±15.42	20.12NS±28.56	0
Av.	60.37±11.17	29.68±15.42	12.89NS±19.79	0

N/A = Not available.
NS = Not statistically significant at 95% level of confidence.

FIG. 5-7. Average heart rate (HR) and pulse volumes in digital (F), supraorbital (SA), and superficial temporal (TA) arterial beds of two unimproved migraineurs measured at maximum peripheral digital vasodilatation produced by volition (A) or heat (B), and estimated as percent difference from baseline. Ten measurements in each group.

previously found in normal subjects that voli- tionally induced increase in the finger pulse volume coincided with decreased blood flow both in the supraorbital (SA) and superficial temporal (TA) arteries, while heating invar- iably increased the blood flow in these arteries (Sovak *et al.*, 1976).

Vasoconstriction in hand skin and simul- taneous dilatation in the skin of the forehead has been described previously as a correlate of a nonspecific arousal evoked by a novelty situ- ation, (the so-called "orienting reflex" of Pav- lov). However, vascular response was found to be variable: a stimulus of high intensity (stress) produced parallel vasoconstriction in both ar- terial beds (Vina, Vadova, 1961). Vasoconstriction in the forehead with simultaneous volitionally induced dilatation in fingers has not hitherto been described. The finding suggests that the mechanisms regulating the two arterial beds must be different.

The supraorbital artery (SA) is a branch of the ophthalmic artery and thus it reflects, to some extent, the internal carotid artery blood flow (Brisman *et al.*, 1970). Vasoconstriction of SA, however, does not necessarily have to re- flect reduction in cerebral parenchymal perfu- sion. Cerebral blood flow, being autoregu- lated, is known to remain remarkably stable under a variety of manipulation. This is be- cause the adrenergically innervated branches of the internal carotid artery, by changing their tone, protect the brain parenchyma against sudden perfusion changes (Olesen, 1972). Both ophthalmic and SA arteries belong to this system. At the onset of a migraine attack, the brain parenchymal perfusion decreases (Skinhoj and Paulson, 1969). It induces local anoxia and, as a result, the adrenergically in- nervated branches of the internal carotid sys- tem respond with vasodilatation.

It remains a matter of speculation whether constriction of these branches during the dila- tation phase could possibly interrupt the chain of events of a migrainous attack. In view of the variability seen in our migraineurs, even the occurrence of such constriction does not seem likely. Three out of eight improved patients have actually shown no change in SA pulse volume during the volitional exercise.

There is conflicting evidence for the efficacy and specificity of the hand-warming proce- dure for migraine therapy, and the observa- tion of the relationship of forehead-finger vas- cular beds also differ. Untrained migraineurs who in one session learned to dilate their hand arteries invariably showed dilatation in their external carotid arterial bed (Price and Tursky, 1976).

It has been argued that dilatation of external cranial arteries should abort migraine attacks, (Friar and Beatty, 1976), but improvement was reported by persons trained to constrict these arteries (Zamani, 1974; Turin and Johnson, 1976). Another study has reported a similar finding: migraineurs trained to cool their hand have, in spite of their positive therapeutic ex- pectation, remained unimproved (Mullinix *et al.*, 1978). In contradistinction, improvement in migraine has been reported, whether the subjects were given a true or false finger tem- perature feedback (Fahrien, 1977).

It seems to us that two factors mainly con- tribute to the general confusion of conflicting data and hypotheses:

1. Vascular responsiveness of migraineurs to a variety of exo- or endogenous stimuli is qual- itatively and quantitatively variable. Mi- graineurs exhibit excessive stress responses, marked by release of catecholamines and, thereof, resulting peripheral vasoconstriction. "Cooling" hands is therefore a correlate of stress experience, and not a "neutral" manipu- lation. Migraineurs also quickly learn to recog- nize any false feedback. No matter how "neut- ral" the instructions may be, true "control" conditions can hardly be achieved because of the subjects' expectation and popularization of feedback procedures.

2. Pathophysiological processes reflected by the vasomotoric states in vascular headaches are so variable that no single hemodynamic manipulation aimed at redistribution of the cardiac output could possibly be specifically active.

A redistribution of the cardiac output, as in the cases we observed, cannot alone serve as explanation of feedback therapy; otherwise, migraine could be treated by submerging hands into hot water. Interestingly, such treatment is known to be efficient, but only when learned as a part of a relaxation ceremonial (Sargent *et al.*, 1973). There is no apparent reason why incidence and intensity of migraine attacks should decrease in patients trained by feedback to occasionally manipulate their hemodynamics. What else should then be the cause of their improvement?

In both normal subjects and improved migraineurs, bradycardia occurred during volition experiments, although the subjects were awake. Therefore, it is apparent that in these subjects the general vegetative balance had changed. Since digital arterial beds have no significant parasympathetic innervation, (Greenfield, 1963) there could not be a preponderance of parasympatheticus. Since high sympathetic vasodilatation output would dilate the muscle but constrict the hand skin arteries (Lindgren and Urnas, 1953), the vasodilatation in finger could not be of sympathetic origin. Decreased sympathetic output, however, would produce vasodilatation in both muscle and skin. We have previously shown this to be the case (Soval *et al.*, 1976). In volition-induced vasodilatation in fingers the improvement does not appear to be a specific result of the feedback training, rather it only reflects a *general decrease* of the tonic sympathetic outflow.

During heat, vasodilatation in hands occurs as a result of local discharge of the cholinergic sympathetic nerves, leading to increase in sweat gland activity (Fox and Hilton, 1958). The concomitant tachycardia can be attributed to the sympathetic-mediated response to the stress of heating.

These findings cast doubt on the role of finger temperature feedback training as a method of operant conditioning of a specific autonomic response. Its salutary effects on migraine have established feedback as an effective therapeutic approach; its mode of action, however, should be reassessed. It is conceivable that feedback training belongs to the same realm as general relaxational procedures, desensitization, hypnosis, or autohypnosis (Andreychuk and Skriber, 1975). Comparisons of feedback procedures with these modalities are scarce and contradictory. It remains to be investigated whether feedback training, by reducing the tonic sympathetic outflow, induces more permanent changes in the psychophysiological background of migraineurs.

To summarize, responses of supraorbital (SA), superficial temporal (TA), and digital (F) arterial beds and the heart rate were studied in five normal subjects and ten migraineurs, when their hand temperature was increased by volition and/or by heat. Volitional digital arterial dilatation coincided in the normals with SA and TA vasoconstriction. Such correspondence varied in migraineurs. Bradycardia resulted in most subjects except in unimproved migraineurs. Heat-induced hand vasodilatation led to dilatation in SA and TA and to tachycardia. Eight migraineurs improved clinically; in these subjects the finger temperature feedback training apparently did not result in conditioning of a single autonomic response (i.e., digital vasodilatation), but in a general decrease of sympathetic tonic outflow.

SUMMARY

This chapter has reviewed the various drugs and other strategies used in migraine therapy.

1. The migraine headache attack itself is treated specifically by means of 0.25 to 0.5 mg ergotamine tartrate given intramuscularly. The use of this agent may be accompanied by nausea and vomiting. Though less effective, ergotamine tartrate may be given by mouth in 2 to 4 mg amounts, to be swallowed or placed under the tongue. This may be repeated again in 30 min, and a third time in another 30 min if the headache has not been eliminated. The amount so administered should not exceed 6.0 mg in any one day.

2. Much more important, though more difficult, is the prevention of attacks. Any procedure that enlists the interest or enthusiasm of the physician, or convinces the patient that he is being cared for, will modify for a time the frequency and intensity of attacks. Hence, the large variety of recommendations. This fact is a cue to the nature of the forces that operate to bring about headache attacks, and indicates what will prevent them. It becomes apparent that procedures aimed at a better understand-

ing of the patient, his life situation, and factors that constitute a threat can be of basic therapeutic importance. As mentioned above, patients with migraine headaches are tense, driving, perfectionistic, order-loving, rigid persons who during periods of threat or conflict become progressively more tense and fatigued. Management should include methods that reduce first of all the potency of the precipitating factors in the tension. The long-term aim of therapy should be that of helping the individual to understand the basis of his tension, the factors in his life that aggravate it, and to aid him in resolving his conflicts. About two patients out of three can be appreciably helped by such aid.

3. In the management of the patient with the migraine syndrome, it is desirable while engaging in the process of understanding the patient's life situations and attitudes, to be able to terminate headache attacks rapidly and induce a respite in the frequency of the attacks. By thus preventing the episodes the patient may be encouraged to explore the possibility of changing attitudes and behavior patterns. It is in this way that the ergot alkaloids are so useful; on the one hand the headache attack, if treated early, can be terminated by ergotamine tartrate given intramuscularly, and on the other, the daily ingestion of methysergide reduces the likelihood of attack in a manner superior to any other agent thus far studied. However, the fundamental problem of management of the migraine syndrome cannot be reduced to the administration of the ergot alkaloids in one form or another, although by their means suffering can be reduced and remissions facilitated. The key problem is still, and will remain, despite further pharmacological developments, the patient-physician relationship as it leads to a better understanding and the resolution of conflicts and frustrations.

4. Methysergide may be used in preventing or reducing the intensity and frequency of vascular headaches in patients who cannot be controlled by other means. The usual adult dose of this medication is 4 to 8 mg daily. There should be a medication-free interval of three to four weeks after every six-month course of treatment.

5. Cyproheptadine is a serotonin and histamine antagonist which may also be used for headache prophylaxis. Generally it is employed at bedtime, when 8 to 12 mg should be given; a smaller dose may be given in the morning. A combination of methysergide and cyproheptadine is sometimes effective in eliminating vascular headaches neither drug relieves when used individually.

6. Foods which contain tyramine and other vasoactive substances should be avoided in patients with migraine. During a period of recurrent migraine, avoidance of alcohol is also suggested.

7. Treatment with tricyclic antidepressants and/or sedative agents such as diazepam should be considered, especially where chronic migraine is evident, and where there are associated symptoms of anxiety and/or depression.

8. Propranolol is a useful medication in the prophylaxis of migraine. The usual adult starting dose is 20 mg twice or three times daily, but the medication should be titered to the patient's response. Large doses of propranolol may be necessary. The medicine should be employed with caution in patients with cardiac disease, congestive heart failure, and in those atopic individuals predisposed to bronchial asthma.

9. Using biofeedback training techniques, it has been possible to demonstrate increase in finger pulse volume blood flow coincident with decreased blood flow in supraorbital and superficial temporal arteries, with reduction in intensity and frequency of vascular headaches. It is unlikely that the feedback training results in conditioning of a single autonomic response such as digital vasodilatation, but rather in a generalized decrease of sympathetic tonic outflow.

References

Alvarez, W. C. (1934). The present day treatment of migraine. *Proc. Mayo Clinic 9*, 22.

Alvarez, W. C. (1939). The new oxygen treatment for migraine. *Am. J. Dig. Dis. 6*, 728.

Alvarez, W. C., and A. York Mason (1940). Results obtained in the treatment of headache with the inhalation of pure oxygen. *Proc. Mayo Clinic 15*, 616.

Andreychuk, P., and C. Skriber (1975). Hypnosis and biofeedback in the treatment of migraine headache. *Intern. Clin. Exp. Hypnosis 23*, 172.

Appenzeller, O. (1969). Vasomotor function in migraine. *Headache 9*, 147.

Ask-Upmark, E. (1960). Migraine. *Brit. Med. J. 2*, 823.

Balyeat, R. M. (1933). *Migraine: Diagnosis and Treatment.* J. B. Lippincott Co., Philadelphia and London.

Barcroft, H., H. Konzett, and H. J. C. Swan (1951). Observations on the action of the hydrogenated alkaloids of the ergotoxine group on the circulation in man. *J. Physiol. 112*, 273.

Bartschi-Rochaix, W. (1954). Zur physiopathologic der migranosen prodrome. *Schweiz. Med. Wschr. 84*, 51.

Bassoe, P. (1933). Migraine. *JAMA 101*, 599.

Brisman, R., B. L. Grossman, and J. W. Correll (1970). Accuracy of transcutaneous Doppler ultrasonics in evaluating extracranial vascular disease. *J. Neurosurg. 32*, 529.

Brock, S., M. E. O'Sullivan, and D. Young (1934). The effect of non-sedative drugs and other measures in migraine, with especial reference to ergotamine tartrate. *Am. J. Med. Sci. 188*, 253.

Carter, E. R. (1958). Bilateral thrombophlebitis after a single dose of ergotamine tartrate for migraine. *Brit. Med. J. 11*, 1453.

Cerletti, A., B. Berde, W. Doepfner, H. Emmenegger, H. Konzett, W. R. Schalch, M. Taeschler, and W. Weidman (1960). Effect of deseril (methysergide, UML-491) on a conditioned response. *Publication of Pharmacological Laboratories,* Sandoz, Ltd., Basel, Switzerland.

Cleveland, F. E., and R. L. King (1961). Gangrene following ergotamine tartrate therapy of migraine. *Bull. Mason Clinic 2*, 1.

Couch, J. R., D. K. Ziegler, and R. Hassanein (1976). Amitryptyline in the prophylaxis of migraine. *Neurol. 26*, 121.

Critchley, M. (1936). Prognosis in migraine. *Lancet 2*, 35.

Dale, H. H. (1906). On some physiological actions of ergot. *J. Physiol. 34*, 163.

Dalessio, D. J., W. A. Camp, H. Goodell, and H. G. Wolff (1961). Studies on headache. The mode of action of UML-491 and its relevance to the nature of vascular headache of the migraine type. *Arch. Neurol. 4*, 235.

Dalessio, D. J., W. A. Camp, H. Goodell, L. F. Chapman, T. Zileli, A. O. Ramos, R. Ehrlich, F. Fortuin, McK. Cattell, and H. G. Wolff (1962). Studies on headache. The relevance of the prophylactic action of UML-491 in vascular headache of the migraine type to the pathophysiology of this syndrome. *World Neurol. 3*, 66.

Dalessio, D. J., L. F. Chapman, T. Zileli, McK. Cattell, R. Ehrlich, F. Fortuin, H. Goodell, and H. G. Wolff (1961). Studies on headache: the responses of the bulbar conjunctival blood vessels during

induced oliguria and diuresis and their modification by UML-491. *Arch. Neurol. 5*, 590.

Dalsgaard-Nielsen, T. (1957). Hypnocephalaca clinostatica bei migrane-kranken. *Schweiz. Arch. Neurol. Psychiatry 79*, 313.

Deshmukh, S. V., and J. S. Meyer (1977). Cyclic changes in platelet dynamics and the pathogenesis and prophylaxis of migraine. *Headache 19*, 101–108.

Diamond, S. (1964). Depressive headaches. *Headache 4*, 255.

Diamond, S., and B. J. Baltes (1972). Management of headache by the family physician. *Am. Fam. Physician 14*, 68.

Diethelm, O. (1936). *Treatment in Psychiatry.* Macmillan, New York.

Diethelm, O. (1938). Treatment of psychoneuroses. *Conn. Med. J. 2*, 1.

Doepfner, W., and A. Cerletti (1958). Comparison of lysergic acid derivatives and antihistamines as inhibitor of the edema provoked in the rat's paw by serotonin. *Intern. Arch. Allergy 12*, 89.

Fahrien, S. L. (1977). Autogenic biofeedback training for migraine. *Mayo Clinic Proc. 52*, 776.

Fox, W. II, and S. M. Hilton (1958). Bradykinin formation in human skin as a factor in heat dilation. *J. Physiol. (Lond.) 142*, 219.

Friar, L. R., and J. Beatty (1976). Migraine: management by trained control of vasoconstriction. *J. Consult. Clin. Psychol. 44*, 1:46–53.

Friedman, A. P. (1960). Clinical observations with 1-methyl-d-lysergic acid butanolamide bimaleate (UML-491) in vascular headache. *Angiology 11*, 364.

Friedman, A. P., and S. Losin (1961). Evaluation of UML-491 in treatment of vascular headaches. *Arch. Neurol. 4*, 241.

Friedman, A. P., and H. H. Merritt (1957). Treatment of headache. *JAMA 163*, 1111.

Fromm-Reichman, F. (1937). Contributions to the psychogenesis of migraine. *Psychoanal. Rev. 24*, 26.

Fuchs, M., and L. S. Blumenthal (1950). Use of ergot preparations in migraine. *JAMA 143*, 1462.

Goldfischer, J. D. (1960). Acute myocardial infarction secondary to ergot therapy. *N. Engl. J. Med. 262*, 860.

Graham, J., H. I. Suby, P. M. LeCompte, and N. L. Sadowsky (1967). Inflammatory fibrosis associated with methysergide therapy. *Research and Clinical Studies in Headache,* Vol. I, pp. 123–164. Karger, Basel/New York.

Greenfield, A. D. (1963). The circulation through the skin. *Handbook on Physiology,* Vol. II. Am. Phys. Soc., Washington.

Hanington, E., and A. M. Harper (1968). The role of tyramine in the etiology of migraine, and related studies on the cerebral and extracerebral circulations. *Headache 8*, 84.

Harding, H. G. (1961). Hypnosis and migraine or vice versa. *Northwest Med. 60*, 168.

Hyslop, G. H. (1934). Migraine: suggestions for its treatment. *Med. Clin. North Am. 18*, 827.

Kallanranta, T., H. Hakkarainen, E. Hokkanen, and T. Tuovinen (1977). Clonidine in migraine prophylaxis. *Headache 17*, 169–172.

Lance, J. W. (1969). *The Mechanism and Management of Headache*. Butterworth, London.

Langen, D. (1969). Peripheral changes in blood circulation during autogenic training and hypnosis. In *Psychophysiological Mechanism of Hypnosis* (L. Chertok, ed.), Springer Verlag, New York.

Lindgren, P., and B. Urnas (1953). Activation of sympathetic vasodilator and vasoconstrictor neurons by electrical stimulation in medulla of dog and cat. *Circ. Res. 1*, 479.

Liveing, E. (1873). *On Megrim, Sick Headache and Some Allied Disorders*. J. and A. Churchill, London.

Mathew, N. T. (1978). 5-hydroxytryptophane in the prophylaxis of migraine. *Headache 18*, 111.

Medina, J. L., and S. Diamond (1978). The role of diet in migraine. *Headache 18*, 31–35.

Mitch, P. S., A. McGrady, and A. Iannone (1976). Autogenic feedback training in migraine. A treatment report. *Headache 15*, 267.

Mitchell, K. R., and D. M. Mitchell (1971). Migraine: an exploratory treatment application of programmed behavior therapy techniques. *J. Psychosom Res. 15*, 137.

Mullin, C. S., Jr. (1959). Headache in the Antarctic. *JAMA 179*, 101.

Mullinix, I. U., B. I. Norton, S. Hack, and M. A. Fishman (1978). Skin temperature biofeedback and migraine. *Headache 17*, 242.

Oleson, J. (1972). The effect of intracarotid epinephrine, norepinephrine, and angiotensin on the regional cerebral blood flow in man. *Neurol. 22*, 978.

O'Sullivan, M. E. (1936). Termination of one thousand attacks of migraine with ergotamine tartrate. *JAMA 107*, 1208.

Pichler, E., A. M. Ostfeld, H. Goodell, and H. G. Wolff (1956). Studies on headache: central versus peripheral action of ergotamine tartrate and its relevance to the therapy of migraine headache. *Arch. Neurol. Psychiatry 76*, 571.

Price, K. P., and B. Tursky (1976). Vascular reactivity of migraineurs and non-migraineurs: a comparison of responses to self-control procedures. *Headache 16*, 210.

Riley, H. A. (1931). Migraine. *Bull. Neurol. Inst. N.Y. 2*, 429.

Sargent, J. D., E. E. Green, and E. D. Walters (1973a). Preliminary report on the use of autogenic feedback training in the treatment of migraine and tension headaches. *Psychosom. Med. 35*, 120–135.

Sargent, J. D., E. C. Walters, and E. E. Green (1973b). Psychosomatic self-regulation of migraine headaches. *Seminars in Psychiatry 5*, 415–428.

Saxena, P. R. (1972). The effects of antimigraine drugs on the vascular responses evoked by 5-hydroxytriptamine and related biogenic substances on the external carotid bed of dogs: possible pharmacological implications to their antimigraine action. *Headache 12*, 44.

Sicuteri, F., G. Franchi, and P. L. DelBianco (1967). An anti-aminic drug, BC-105, in the prophylaxis of migraine. *Intern. Arch. Allergy Appl. Immunol. 31*, 78.

Skinhoj, E., and O. B. Paulson (1969). Regional blood flow in internal carotid distribution during migraine attacks. *Brit. Med. J. 3*, 569.

Sovak, M., A. Fronek, R. Doyle, and D. R. Helland (1976). Some hemodynamic observations during biofeedback vosomotor training. *Proceedings San Diego Biomedical Symposium, 1976*. Academic Press, New York.

Sovak, R. M., M. Kunzel, R. Sternbach, and D. J. Dalessio (1978). Is volitional manipulation of hemodynamics a valid rationale for biofeedback therapy of migraine? *Headache 18*, 197–202.

Stroebel, C. F., and B. C. Glueck (1976). Psychophysiological rationale for the application of biofeedback in the alleviation of pain. In *Pain* (M. Weisenberg and B. Tursky, eds.). Plenum Press, New York.

Vinojvadova, O. S. (1961). The orienting reflex and its neurophysiological mechanisms. *Moscow Acd. Ped. Nauk.*, RSFSR.

von Euler, U. S., and C. G. Schmiterlow (1944). The action of ergotamine on the chemical and mechanical reflexes from the carotid sinus region. *Acta Physiol. Scand. 8*, 122.

Weber, R. B., and O. M. Reinmuth (1972). The treatment of migraine with propranolol. *Neurol. 22*, 366.

Wickramasekera, I. (1973). Temperature feedback for the control of migraine. *J. Behav. Therapy Exp. Psychiat. 4*, 343.

Wolff, H. G., J. D. Hardy, and H. Goodell (1941). Measurement of the effect on the pain threshold of acetylsalicylic acid, acetanilid, acetophenetidin, aminopyrine, ethyl alcohol, trichlorethylene, a barbiturate, quinine, ergotamine tartrate and caffeine: an analysis of their relation to the pain experience. *J. Clin. Invest. 20*, 63.

Zaimis, E., and E. Hanington (1969). A possible pharmacological approach to migraine. *Lancet 2*, 298.

Zamani, R. (1974). Treatment of migraine headache through operant conditioning of vasoconstriction of the extracranial temporal artery (biofeedback) and through deep muscle relaxation. *Ph.D. thesis, Univ. of Michigan, Ann Arbor, Michigan*. University microfilm #26,259.

Zweifach, B. W., and D. B. Metz (1955). Relation of blood-borne agents acting on mesenteric vascular bed to general circulatory reactions. *J. Clin. Invest. 34*, 653.

6

CLUSTER HEADACHE

REVISED BY DONALD J. DALESSIO

One variety of vascular headache has features special enough to justify separate description. It is unilaterial, anterior, intense, brief, and many attacks occur in quick succession, sometimes several in a 24-hr period; hence the name, cluster headache. It is almost always on the same side, with unilateral redness and swelling of the cheek and conjunctiva, and rhinorrhea. It was originally termed by Harris (1926, 1936) migrainous neualgia; later by Horton histaminic cephalagia; and more recently, cluster headache by Kunkle *et al.* (1952).

CLINICAL FEATURES

Cluster headache is a "specific unilateral type of headache." The pain occurs in attacks, is constant, of high intensity, burning, and "boring" in character. It involves the region of the eye, the temples, the neck, and often the face, and may extend into the shoulder on the involved side. It may spread to the upper teeth and occasionally to the lower teeth. Attacks often begin after middle age. Generally the attacks last less than one hour, commence, and often terminate, suddenly, and often awaken the patient at night. The pain is so severe that the patient frequently jumps out of bed before he is fully awake.

This pain is associated with certain other characteristic manifestations that appear on the affected side. These are profuse watering and "congestion" of the conjunctiva, rhinorrhea and nasal obstruction, increased perspiration, and frequently evidence of vaso-

dilatation in the skin. Swelling of the temporal vessels may be noted. So severe and frequent are the attacks of pain—they may occur regularly, day and night, for a period of months—that almost every patient has contemplated suicide. During and after the attacks, marked tenderness is frequently found when pressure is applied over the branches of the external and common carotid arteries. The pain is not confined to the distribution of any cranial nerve but conforms to the ramifications of the external carotid artery.

Cluster headache may be distinguished from trigeminal neuralgia because trigger zones are invariably absent in the former and the pain does not follow the distribution of the fifth nerve. It is different from migraine because nausea, vomiting, and scotomata are invariably absent, and the attack usually lasts less than an hour.

Kunkle, making a careful analysis of 30 instances of this disorder in 1952, pointed to the unique tempo of its recurrence as a striking feature. (By 1960 he had studied 90 patients so afflicted, generally confirming his earlier observations.)

Of the 30 patients, 24 were males. The illness began between the ages of 17 and 40 in nine-tenths of the group and between 21 and 25 in one-half. It was right-sided in 19, left-sided in seven, and either right- or left-sided in four. In one individual the headache was on a few occasions bilateral.

In two-thirds of the patients the attacks always or commonly began during sleep. The usual duration in all but one patient was under

2 hr and often under 30 min, but the headache lasted in some attacks up to 7 hr. A peculiar feature in 24 patients was the occurence of the headaches in recurrent clusters of one to five per 24 hrs for several days or weeks, with symptom-free intermissions lasting two months to two years, or occasionally longer. A regular periodicity in the occurrence of the individual headaches or the clusters was noted in only a few patients.

PATHOPHYSIOLOGY

The pathophysiology of the pain was analyzed by history in each case and by observation of the attacks in six patients. Opportunities to examine a patient during his headache were limited by the brevity and unpredictable occurrence of the attacks. In a few the pain was eased during compression of the ipsilateral temporal artery (visibly enlarged in one instance) and was unaffected by brisk rotary head jolt. In four patients an attack was rapidly terminated by the intravenous injection of ergotamine tartrate. In two of these four, a trial was made of controlled elevation of intracranial pressure by the intrathecal injection of normal saline, a procedure known to ease only headache associated with dilatation of intracranial arteries. The pain was unaffected by this procedure.

The disorder has been attributed by Horton to a unique form of histamine sensitivity. Evidence for this has been cited as follows: a headache apparently identical with that of a spontaneous attack could be precipitated in some patients by the hypodermic administration of histamine in small amounts, usually 0.35 mg histamine base; gastric acidity was found to rise during an attack, and the attacks often subsided after histamine "desensitization" over an extended period of time. These observations, however, can be reinterpreted in different fashion. The headache, as Horton was the first to describe, can sometimes be reproduced not only by histamine but also by the ingestion of alcohol, indicating perhaps merely an increased suceptibility of cranial arteries in these patients to diverse vasodilator agents. Finally, improvement in the headaches after an elaborate program of histamine injections has not been shown, by controlled experiments, to be due to a desensitizing effect of this agent. The characteristic feature of the headache to occur in clusters of unpredictable length, followed by short or long spontaneous remissions, represents a major obstacle in the evaluation of any prophylactic regimen. Among the patients here reported, a series of histamine injections had been given elsewhere in 11 of them without significant benefit.

Precipitating factors for the attacks could not be identified with certainty, although in seven patients the headache clusters tended to follow or accompany periods of increased tension and conflict. Brief personality study yielded evidence of chronic tension in 16; of these only a few were compulsive and driving by temperament. In one-third of the group a history was obtained of periodic headache in one or more close relatives, but in only one instance was such headache of the "cluster" type.

This disorder warrants close comparison with migraine headache. It clearly differs from typical migraine, most conspicuously in the absence of visual or other prodromes, the rarity of nausea and vomiting, and the brevity and unusual tempo of the attacks. It is also unlike migraine in certain minor features: its predilection for males and its tendency to strike consistently on the same side of the head in all attacks.

The common accompaniments of cluster headache are conjunctival injection and increased lacrimation on the side of the pain. Kunkle points out that these, together with ipsilateral nasal congestion and bradycardia (rare), suggest parasympathetic discharge over the seventh and, in a few, the tenth cranial nerves. The detection of an acetylcholine-like substance in the cerebrospinal fluid during an attack supports this view.

Some patients will exhibit one or more signs of Horner's syndrome during an attack. Ptosis and meiosis may be noted. Often the face is pale, with contrasting injection of the conjunctiva, nasal congestion and/or rhinorrhea. However, these signs do not have to be present for a diagnosis of cluster headache to be made. The attacks tend to appear in groups or clusters, with each cluster lasting several weeks to several months. Provocative factors which may precipitate attacks include ingestion of alcohol or other vasodilating substances such as nitroglycerin. Graham (1972) has described the peculiar facial characteristics associated with cluster headache. Patients may have thick furrows in their forehead, vertical creases accentuated at the glabella, telangiectases, coarse cheek skin ("peau d'orange"), a square, thickly upholstered chin with a sharp crease between it and a well-chiseled lower lip. Similar facial characteristics are sometimes present in women. Graham also observed that such a profile may be found in patients with a carcinoid syndrome, or in heavy smokers.

Ekbom's monograph on cluster headache provides a concise and clear description of this difficult problem (1970). Ekbom makes the point that two clinical forms can be distinguished, which he terms upper and lower syndromes. These differ with respect to the age of onset, as well as radiation of pain from the eye. He notes that in the upper syndrome the maximal pain has an orbital or supraorbital localization, radiating from the eye to the forehead and to the temple. The lower syndrome was characterized by an infraorbital radiation of pain, ipsilateral partial Horner syndrome, ipsilateral hyperhydrosis of the forehead, but absence of clinically visible swelling of the superficial temporal artery. Ekbom suggests that the upper syndrome is associated with dilatation of the external carotid artery and that the lower syndrome is characterized primarily by dilatation of the internal carotid artery.

He finds that nitroglycerin (1 mg sublingually) can by used as a provocative agent, and that this proved to be a simple and reliable diagnostic method, comparable to Horton's use of histamine as a provocative agent. Provoked attacks of cluster headache with nitroglycerin could be partially or entirely eliminated by physical exercise or by an intravenous infusion of norepinephrine. During induced attacks, the heart rate was significantly reduced and the systolic and diastolic blood pressures were significantly increased. Electrocardiograms were made and the changes were characteristic of increased vagal tone. Ekbom concludes that attacks of cluster headache are associated with both vagal and sympathetic stimulation and are blocked by procedures which produce cranial arterial constriction.

Ekbom also reports on carotid angiography in cluster headache, with observations made during an attack of headache. Four of eighteen patients had generalized ectasia of all cerebral arteries. In the remaining patients the findings on carotid angiography were essentially within normal limits. One patient was examined before and during an attack. Localized narrowing of the extradural part of the internal carotid artery was observed distal to its exit from the carotid canal. The ophthalmic artery was markedly dilated. When the headache had dimished, another injection of contrast medium was made. This showed that narrowing of the artery had spread to the upper portion of the carotid canal. It is suggested that edema with or without a spastic contraction of the arterial wall characterized the headache attack in this patient.

On the basis of a clinical comparison with 40 consecutive migraine patients, Ekbom made the following observations: Visual prodromes are invariably lacking in cluster headache patients, whereas they occur commonly in patients with migraine. The intensity and character of the pain in cluster headache is usually different from that described in migraine. There was a lower incidence of migraine among close relatives of patients with cluster headache compared to those of migraine subjects. Ekbom concludes that, from a clinical point of view, cluster headache is not merely a variant of migraine headache.

However, the pathophysiology of vasodilatation during cluster headache is probably similar to that during migraine headache attacks. It would appear that an agent liberated locally causes a circumscribed vasodilator reaction. The demonstrated presence of vasodilator polypeptides in painful regions during migraine headache strongly indicts them although histamine and acetylcholine, as well as other vasodilator agents, may also be involved. It may ultimately be demonstrated that one or more of these agents if the causative one. However, the fact that histamine is a convenient agent for the production of experimental headache and that it is possible to precipitate headache more readily in those with migraine and those with cluster headache through its use does not justify the inference that histamine is the responsible local vasodilator agent.

Cobb and Finesinger (1932) in collaboration with Chorobski and Penfield (1932) pointed out that the greater superficial petrosal nerve contains secretory fibers for the lacrimal glands and vasodilator fibers for the mucous membranes of the nasal cavity. They also showed that the nerves contained afferent fibers from the dura matter, internal carotid artery, and the sphenopalatine ganglion to the cells in the geniculate ganglion. Also, the greater superficial petrosal branch of the seventh cranial nerve conveys vasodilator fibers to the ipsilateral cerebral hemispheres. Gardner inferred, therefore, that parasympathetic impulses over the petrosal nerve cause unilateral lacrimation, unilateral swelling and secretion of the nasal mucosa, and unilateral head pain. Hence, section of this nerve was undertaken in a group of 26 patients with symptoms and signs of unilateral headache such as are found in cluster headache and in migraine. In some (about one-third) the headache was dramatically eliminated. In about another third some improvement for the patient ensued. Assuming that the nerve section had a specific therapeutic effect (which seems likely), it is clear that the superficial petrosal nerve is not the only efferent neural structure involved in cranial vasodilatation and unilateral headache.

Anthony *et al.* (1978) examined whole-blood histamine levels in 49 patients before, during, and after typical attacks of cluster headache. Nineteen of the headaches occurred spontaneously, five were precipitated by the ingestion of alcohol, and the rest were induced by the sublingual administration of 1 mg of nitroglycerin. A statistically significant rise in blood histamine occurred during headache. Histamine receptor blockade was studied by using several different forms of antihistamines to block both types of histamine receptors, H_1 and H_2, but the effect in terms of preventing headache was not particularly significant.

On the other hand, Sjaastad and Sjaastad (1977) studied urinary histamine excretion in migraine and cluster headache. They found that urinary excretion of histamine was increased on one or more occasions in 7 of 22 patients with cluster headache and the excretion was significantly higher on attack days than on attack-free days. With migraine, increased excretion was found in 5 of 31 patients

on days of an attack, whereas the corresponding figure for headache-free days was 7 of 24 patients. The authors suggest that the demonstrated changes in histamine excretion are more likely to be a consequence than a cause of an attack of cluster headache.

Sjaastad and Sjaastad (1977) further studied several parameters of histamine metabolism in cluster headache and migraine, including urinary excretion of radioactive C^{14} histamine and its metabolites, exhaled radioactive CO_2, and fecal radioactivity after oral as well as subcutaneous administration of radioactive histamine. They found no marked deviation from normal values except in one patient with a cluster headache variant, in whom an aberration in C^{14} histamine degradation was present. Sjaastad and Sjaastad concluded that the relationships of metabolic aberrations in histamine metabolism to cluster headache and migraine cannot be demonstrated to any significant degree.

Horven and Sjaastad (1977) also examined patients suffering from migraine, cluster headache, and atypical cluster headache, with respect to corneal temperature, intraocular pressure, and corneal indentation pulse amplitude changes during pain attacks. Significant increases in these three parameters were demonstrated during attacks of cluster headache. No significant changes were found in migraine. The authors interpret these studies to suggest that there are significant pathophysiological differences between migraine and cluster headache. Perhaps even more interesting is their finding that a marked increase in intraocular pressure could be measured shortly after the onset of pain, pointing strongly to intraocular vasodilatation as the mechanism behind the severely painful attacks which characterize cluster headache.

CHRONIC CLUSTER HEADACHE

While the episodic variety of cluster headache is well recognized by physicians, some of the clinical subtypes are not familiar to many and may lead to difficulty in diagnosis. Ekbom *et al.* (1971) were the first to recognize that cluster headache may become chronic. This was later confirmed by Kudrow (1977). In chronic cluster headache periods of remission between headache diminish and headache attacks become more frequent. As this occurs the physician will note diminished responsiveness to prophylactic medications, particularly ergotamine tartrate in its various forms, methysergide, and corticosteroids. The problem then becomes one of recurrent severe headache leading to incapacity, a tendency towards drug dependency and pain-centered behavior, which may require the admission of the patient to the hospital. It is in this situation that the prophylactic use of lithium is most helpful. Indeed, prophylactic lithium therapy should be reserved for those cases of chronic cluster headache which do not respond to ordinary medications. It should not be used as the primary form of treatment in ordinary cluster headache which is liable to be self-limited, no matter what the therapy.

Chronic Paroxysmal Hemicrania

Sjaastad and Dale (1971) have described another cluster headache variant, termed chronic paroxysmal hemicrania, a syndrome of strictly unilateral headache, always occurring on the same side of the head and unaccompanied by nausea or vomiting. The most characteristic clinical finding is the frequency of attacks, often short-lived, with 16 to 18 episodes occurring every 24 hr. These patients, admittedly rare, are often female, and respond strikingly to salicylates and to antiinflammatory medications, particularly indomethacin.

Hormonal Changes

Kudrow (1974) has investigated the alterations in plasma testosterone and luteinizing hormone (LH) in patients in the active phase of cluster headache. Under controlled conditions plasma testosterone and LH levels were obtained from five males with episodic cluster headache, during the active cluster and remission periods. In addition, plasma testosterone binding globulins (TBG) were determined. Plasma LH levels paralleled testosterone levels

in both remission and active periods. These hormones were significantly depressed during the active phase compared to the remission period, while TBG levels remained unchanged. These results suggest that a transient impairment in the hypothalamic–pituitary pathway occurs in cluster headache syndrome during the active phase.

THERAPY OF CLUSTER HEADACHE

Most patients with cluster headache will respond to vasoconstrictor agents. Short courses of methysergide or of ergotamine tartrate are invariably effective (see Tables 6-1 and 6-2). If the headaches occur primarily at night, then the emphasis should be on nocturnal medication given before bedtime. If the cluster paroxysm proves particularly difficult, then addition of cyproheptadine may be helpful. Ekbom has reported on the prophylactic treatment of cluster headache with the serotonin antagonist, BC-105, which is related chemically to cyproheptadine. Since neither cyproheptadine nor BC-105 are vasoconstrictor agents, but instead inhibit the effects of serotonin and histamine, one may assume that their beneficial effects in the prevention of cluster

TABLE 6-1   Cluster Therapy Treatment Chart, Prophylactic (Oral)

DRUG	DOSAGE
Methysergide maleate (Sansert)	2 mg three times daily
Triamcinolone (Aristocort)	4 mg four times daily 16 mg every other day
Methylprednisolone (Medrol Alternate Day Therapy Pac)	4 mg four times daily
Cyproheptadine (Periactin)	8 mg at bedtime
Ergotamine tartrate (Gynergen)	1 mg twice daily—skip one day a week
Ergotamine, phenobarbital and belladonna	
Bellergal Spacetabs	one tablet twice daily
Bellergal	one tablet 3–4 times daily
Lithium (Eskalith)	900 mg per day

TABLE 6-2   Cluster Therapy Treatment Chart, Abortive

ROUTE	ORAL	DOSAGE
Oral	Ergotamine tartrate (Gynergen)	one tablet immediately—repeat every ½ hr if necessary to a maximum of 6 tablets per day
	Ergotamine, caffeine, phenacetin, belladonna (Wigraine)	
	Ergotamine and caffeine (Cafergot)	2 stat—repeat one every ½ hr to a maximum of 6 per day
	Ergotamine tartrate, cyclizine, and caffeine (Migral)	2 tablets at onset. May repeat one tablet every ½ hr up to 6 per day.
Sublingual	Ergotamine (Ergomar, Ergostat)	one tablet immediately under the tongue—repeat at ½ hr intervals if necessary, but not more than 3 in any 24-hr period
Inhalation	Ergotamine (Medihaler-Ergotamine)	one dose immediately—repeat every 5 min to a maximum of 6 per day, if necessary
Intramuscular	Ergotamine tartrate (Gynergen)	½ to 1 cc immediately and no more than 3 cc per week
	Dihydroergotamine (DHE 45)	1 cc at hourly intervals, up to 3 cc per day, if necessary
Rectal	Ergotamine and caffeine (Cafergot, Cafergot-PB)	insert one suppository in rectum immediately—repeat in one hour, if necessary
	Ergotamine, caffeine, phenacetin, belladonna (Wigraine)	

headache are related to their powerful inhibitory properties against serotonin and histamine, and to a lesser extent against acetylcholine. Sicuteri *et al.* (1967) also observed that BC-105 potentiated the effect of ergotamine in cases of migraine. Consequently it may also be of value to combine the two preparations in some cases of cluster headache.

Prednisone

Couch (1978) studied a group of 15 patients (14 male, 1 female), ages 20–71 (mean 43.5), who had suffered from cluster headache for 1–50 years (mean 15.0), and who were treated with Prednisone only after ergot preparations and other analgesics failed to produce significant relief. Frequency of cluster headache at the time Prednisone therapy began was at least one per day in 11 patients, and at least one every other day in four patients. The peak Prednisone dose employed was 60–80 mg/day for eight patients, 40 mg/day for four, 30 mg/day for one, and 10 mg/day for two pa-

tients. The course of Prednisone lasted 10–30 days.

Overall, eight patients received excellent relief (complete cessation of headache, and two received very good relief (> 75% decrease in frequency of headache). Fair relief (50% decrease in frequency) was seen in three, and no relief in two patients. Of the eight patients who received 60–80 mg of Prednisone/day, six had very good or excellent results, while two had fair relief. Of the patients receiving 30–40 mg of Prednisone/day, three had excellent relief and two had none. Of those receiving 10 mg/day, one had excellent relief (but may have been at the end of a cycle of cluster headache), and one had fair relief.

Eleven patients were followed after therapy stopped and they showed fair or better response. Nine of these had received very good relief, and in seven the headache recurred as the Prednisone was tapered off or discontinued, while in two there was no recurrence. In two patients with fair response, there was recurrence of cluster headache with discontinuation of Prednisone. No serious side-effects were encountered.

Lithium

Ekbom (1974), Kudrow (1977), and Mathew (1978) have all reported on the efficacy of lithium in the prophylaxis of chronic cluster headache. Mathew's study, being the most recent, will be reported in detail. He proposed a clinical trial of lithium carbonate in 31 patients (20 men and 11 women) with cluster headache. Fourteen had episodic cluster headache and 17 had chronic cluster headache; 13 were primary and 4 secondary. Serum lithium levels were determined at regular intervals to monitor the therapeutic range. The average follow-up period for the chronic cluster headache patients was 16 weeks. Nine of 17 chronic cluster headache patients showed more than 90% improvement based on a headache index devised by Mathew. Two patients had 60–90% improvement and three had 25–60% improvement. Three patients derived no benefit from lithium treatment, one complaining of aggravation of the headache. Persistence of episodic autonomic symptoms without accompanying headache was noted in four patients during the initial weeks of therapy. Improvement for primary and secondary cluster headache patients was not significantly different. The response to treatment in the patients with episodic headache was assessed after two weeks of treatment. The usual length of cluster headache periods and the possibility of natural remission were taken into account in assessing the results of therapy. Eight of 14 had no further attacks after one week of therapy, and during the first week, therapy shortened the usual length of the cluster periods. One patient showed 75% improvement and two had less than 50% improvement with no effect on the length of cluster periods. Three patients derived no benefit from treatment.

Major side effects of lithium therapy were tremor, weakness, lethargy, and nausea. The tremor was relieved by concomitant use of propranolol in two patients. A self-rating depression scale (Zung) obtained during the initial office visit showed no significant depression in any of the 31 patients, indicating that beneficial effect of lithium in cluster headache is independent of its antidepressant action.

SUMMARY

1. Cluster headache is delineated from migraine by virtue of its unique clinical characteristics: it is consistently periodic, of short duration, often nocturnal, and may be associated with unilateral lacrimation and rhinorrhea. It more nearly resembles a paroxysmal disorder than any other form of migraine.

2. Two clinical forms of cluster headache can be distinguished, upper and lower syndromes, which differ in respect to the patient's age and onset, radiation of pain from the eye, and certain associated signs during attacks.

3. The pathophysiology of vasodilatation during cluster headache is presumably similar to that occurring in classical migraine. Clinical evidence points to a locally liberated vasodilator agent of some nature.

4. Therapy with vasoconstrictor agents and/or agents which interfere with the activities of vasoactive amines is frequently helpful.

5. Cluster headache may become chronic or in rare situations, it may never exhibit the typical pattern characterized by prolonged remission. In chronic cluster headache the pathophysiology is unchanged, but treatment may be extremely difficult. In this situation lithium prophylaxis may be effective.

6. A variant form of cluster headache, termed chronic paroxysmal hemicrania, is characterized by frequency of attacks with recurrent unilateral headache episodes appearing throughout the day. The pain is unilateral, never changes sides, and is unaccompanied by nausea or vomiting. The most characteristic clinical finding is the striking number of painful episodes; often six to eighteen attacks may occur in a single day.

REFERENCES

Anthony, M., J. W. Lance, and G. Lord (1978). Migrainous neuralgia—blood histamine levels and clinical response to H1 and H2 receptor blockade. In *Current Concepts in Migraine Research* (Raymond Greene, ed.), pp. 149–152. Raven Press, New York.

Chorobski, J., and W. Penfield (1932). Cerebral vasodilator nerves and their pathway from the medulla oblongata, with observations on the pial and intracerebral vascular plexus. *Arch. Neurol. Psychiat. 28*, 1257.

Cobb, S., and J. E. Finesinger (1932). The vagal pathway of the vasodilator impulses. *Arch. Neurol. Psychiat. 28*, 1243.

Couch, J. R., and Ziegler, D. K. (1978). Prednisone therapy for cluster headache. *Headache 18*, 219–222.

Ekbom, K. (1969). Prophylactic treatment of cluster headache with a new serotonin antagonist, BC-105. *Acta Neurol. Scand. 45*, 601.

Ekbom, K. (1970). *Studies on Cluster Headache.* Sundbyberg, Sweden. Selna Tryckeri A. B.

Ekbom, K. (1974). Litium vid kroniska symptom av cluster headache. *Opusc. Med.* 19, 148–156.

Ekbom, K., B. Olivarius, and B. deFine (1971). Chronic migrainous neuralgia—diagnostic and therapeutic aspects. *Headache 11*, 97–101.

Gardner, W. S., A. Stowell, and R. Dutlinger (1947). Resection of greater superficial petrosal nerve in the treatment of unilateral headache, *J. Neurosurg. 4:*105,

Graham, J. R. (1972). Cluster headache. *Headache 11*, 175.

Harris, W. (1926). *Neuritis and Neuralgia,* p. 418. Oxford Univ. Press, London.

Harris, W. (1936). Ciliary (migrainous) neuralgia and its treatment. *Brit. Med. J. 1*, 457.

Horton, B. T. (1956). Histaminic cephalgia: differential diagnosis and treatment. *Proc. Mayo Clin. 31*, 325.

Horven, I., and O. Sjaastad (1977). Cluster headache syndrome and migraine. Ophthalmologic support for two-entity theory. *Acta Ophthalmol. 55*, 35–51.

Kudrow, L. (1974). Physical and personality characteristics in cluster headache. *Headache 13*, 197–202.

Kudrow, L. (1977). Lithium prophylaxis for chronic cluster headache. *Headache 17*, 15–18.

Kunkle, E. C., J. B. Pfeiffer, Jr., W. M. Wilhoit, and L. W. Hamrick, Jr. (1952). Recurrent brief headache in "cluster" pattern. *Trans. Am. Neurol. Assoc. 77*, 240.

Mathew, N. (1978). Clinical subtypes of cluster headache and response to lithium therapy. *Headache 18*, 31–35.

Sicuteri, F., G. Franchi, and P. L. Del Bianco (1967). An antiaminic drug, BC-105, in the prophylaxis of migraine. *Intern. Arch. Allergy Appl. Immunol. 31*, 78.

Sjaastad, O., and O. V. Sjaastad (1977). Urinary histamine excretion in migraine and cluster headache. *J. Neurol. 216*, 91–104.

Sjaastad, O., and O. V. Sjaastad (1977). Histamine metabolism in cluster headache and migraine. *J. Neurol. 216*, 105–117.

Sjaastad, O., and I. Dale (1974). Evidence for a new treatable headache entity. *Headache 14*, 105–108.

7

THE CEREBRAL CIRCULATION, CEREBROVASCULAR DISEASE, AND SUBARACHNOID HEMORRHAGE

REVISED BY DONALD J. DALESSIO

To the peculiarities of the cerebral circulation is attributable the type of headache associated with cerebral aneurysm and subarachnoid hemorrhage.

Subarachnoid hemorrhage is responsible for 2% of sudden deaths. It comprises 7% of all cerebral vascular disease, approximating in frequency parenchymatous cerebral hemorrhage, which accounts for 8%. The most common cause of subarachnoid hemorrhage is rupture of intracranial arterial aneurysms. To provide a background for understanding the origin of this headache, and to bring together anatomic facts may prove useful in subsequent research, the anatomy of the cerebral circulation is surveyed, and data are presented that relate to aneurysm of the circle of Willis, the usual source of subarachnoid hemorrhage.

ANGIOARCHITECTURE—MACROSCOPIC

The cerebral arterial tree in man, unlike that of many organs, has no hilum from which the vessels plunge into the body of the structure. On the contrary, the internal carotid and vertebral arteries are united by the circle of Willis and its six large branches, which encircle the globoid hemispheres at the base of the brain. These six great trunks then divide into branches. A few enter the basal ganglia and choroid plexus, but for the most part they spread themselves like a net in finer and finer branches over the surface of the cortex. Smaller arteries at innumerable points dive deeply into the cortical and subcortical tissues where, through their capillaries, they anastomose with one another and

with others coming through the brain substance from the opposite surface of the hemisphere.

The cerebral veins are divided into two groups, the internal and external, with incomplete anastomeses between them. The internal group drains through the great cerebral vein of Galen, running back directly over the pineal body. The external veins emanate from the region of the insula. Because with growth there is anterior displacement of the frontal lobe and posterior development of the main mass of the hemispheres, the direction of the terminal portion of the great veins is altered; the anterior veins are thus directed posteriorly and the posterior veins course obliquely and anteriorly as they pass to the superior sagittal sinus. The large venous sinuses drain into channels at the base of the skull. The blood then flows from the cranial cavity like fluid from a flask with a gradually tapering neck.

ANGIOARCHITECTURE—MICROSCOPIC

The blood vessels of the brain differ in no histologic essential from vessels elsewhere, though there are minor differences. In the cerebral arteries the elastic fibers have a different arrangement and possibly are more numerous than in other parts of the body (Triepel, 1897; Cobb and Blain, 1922). Furthermore, the cerebral veins have, in relation to their large lumen, extremely thin walls, composed mainly of connectvie tissue with no uniform number of layers. Muscle fibers are present in the bigger superficial veins, but are few in number and may be readily overlooked. Also, in most of the deep veins muscle fibers are seen, though again they are not numerous. Myelinated and unmyelinated nerves and endings traverse the surface of the cerebral vessels in no unusual way.

If the cerebral arteries are considered more in detail, the following features present themselves for consideration. First, a well-developed inner elastic layer; second, a minimal development of elastic tissue in the circular layer of the muscles; third, a striking lack of longitudinal elastic fibers; and, fourth, absence of an external elastic membrane, and lack of elastic tissue in the poorly developed adventitia.

The inner elastic layer of the brain arteries is directly under the endothelium, and appears as a simple membrane, encircling the lumen of the vessel. The membrane is fenestrated, though these fenestrations are not gaps, but represent deposits of a substance perhaps of a collagen nature of derived remnants of embryonal nuclei. The separation into layers which gives rise to the lamellated or fenestrated appearance increases with age. Although the inner elastic layer varies in thickness, the thickness of the elastic membrane in relation to that of the muscle layer is in general greater in the brain arteries than it is in many other parts of the organism.

Beginning in middle life, the elastic fibers no longer multiply sufficiently to replace themselves. In contrast to the diminishing replacement capacity of the elastic tissue is the increase of the collagen connective tissue, which appears wherever there is space resulting from degeneration. Thus, septa occur between lamelli of the loosened elastic interna, and the wall elements necessary for specific functions are replaced by a tissue that cannot easily perform these functions. The splitting of the inner elastic membrane into two or more plates with advancing age progresses from the larger to the smaller arteries of the brain. In the later years this change in the larger arteries it is less evident. The changes of the intima in the brain arteries with age are also well defined, although less striking than are the changes in the arteries of the heart. Here the thickness of the intima approaches that of the media, but in the brain, the thickness of the intima only rarely approximates that of the media.

The media consists of one to 20 circular muscle layers. In both the inner and the outer portions single longitudinal fibers are scattered. The muscle fibers are separated by collagen. The elastic fibers are relatively scarce, and are almost without exception circular in arrangement. The muscle fibers lying next to the internal elastica send delicate processes in through the fenestrations in the elastic membrane, thus binding the layers together.

The transition of structure from that usual in extracranial arteries to that of the intracranial arteries is strikingly shown in the posterior fossa. In the transition there is an increase of the elastic tissue, and more especially an aggregation of the elastic tissue into the inner elastic membrane, which assumes a greater thickness as the arteries enter the skull. Also, the irregularly grouped elastic fibers disappear from the muscle layers.

Fang (1958) in a review of the microscopic structure of cranial arteries, epitomized the current position as follows: ". . . in regard to the basic similarities and differences in the histological details of intracranial and extracranial (systemic and peripheral) arteries . . . the early foundation was laid by Triepel in 1897. At that time he studied and came to the conclusion that there are only three basic morphologic differences between the intracranial and extracranial arteries: First, that there is the prominence of the internal elastic lamina in the intracranial (larger) arteries. Second, there is a relative paucity of elastic fibrils in the media coat of the intracranial arteries; and, third, there is very poor development to virtual absence of elastic fibrils in the adventitial coat. These main points do hold true today."

Both cerebral and dural arteries, in passing into the region protected from outside pressure, reduce the adventitia and, in man especially, the elastic longitudinal fibers are almost completely lost. We have, then, arteries that seem to be built to meet pressure requirements only from within. The intramural stretch imposed by the blood pressure seems to be adequately taken care of by the very strong internal elastic layer and by the media. It would seem possible that the elastic tissue increase of the intracranial vessels may meet a special pressure requirement, since nerve tissue would be most apt to be embarrassed by constant and excessive impacts of pulse waves.

It has been pointed out by Triepel that the elastic modulus of smooth muscle is much smaller than that of elastic tissue and may, in fact, be as low as one-thirtieth of the latter; or expressed differently, the amount of stretch to a given load in the case of smooth muscle may be as much as 30 times greater than that of elastic tissue. This indicates that elastic tissue is relatively rigid as compared with smooth muscle, and would add rigidity to a tubular vascular system. Such rigidity would be relatively slight if the elastic tissue were indifferently spread throughout the smooth muscle and adventitia, but would increase appreciably if most of the elastic tissue were assembled in one layer. Elastic tissue is segregated into a well-developed layer that is relatively rigid, and is surrounded by a smooth muscle layer, probably devoid of elastic tissue and relatively distensible. This in turn is surrounded by a sponge-like perivascular space that is also nonrigid. This arrangement contrasts with blood vessels in skeletal muscle, for example, where the elastic tissue is interspersed throughout blood vessel walls, which arrangement gives comparatively slight shock-absorbing quality. It therefore seems likely on physical grounds that the structure of cerebral arteries aids appreciably in dampening the impact resulting from a large quantity of blood being delivered at high pressure. Such a postulate does not preclude other purposes of such architectural development. Thus, the rigid walls may serve to assure to the capillaries an abundant blood supply at high pressure and speed, a matter of grave importance to the brain.

The walls of the veins of the brain are extremely thin in relation to the large lumen and are composed chiefly of connective tissue. The small veins that spring from the capillaries are not to be distinguished in their structure from the precapillary arterioles. In the larger veins that adjoin them there is an elastic membrane, but it is thin and, as the veins become increasingly larger, there is relatively less and less elastic layer. When the veins leave the parenchyma and enter the pia arachnoid, the elastic layer is reduced to a very thin line lying just external to the endothelium.

Since the pial arteries are figuratively the floodgates of the cerebral circulation, it is reasonable to infer that alterations in their caliber directly influence the cerebral circulation. These pial arteries give rise to smaller vessels forming different patterns, depending on whether they supply the neocortex of the paleocortex. In the neopallium the smaller arteries, after leaving the surface, give off a few capillaries in lamina I, and many more in laminas II, III, IV, and V, beneath which lamina VI is again less vascular. In the fiber tracts, the arterioles and venules roughly parallel the fibers, so that there is a linear pattern of vessels, the capillary net crossing between making many small irregular quadrangles.

Similarly, the cerebellum receives its blood from the pial arteries over its convexity. However, the blood vessels in the pia mater over the cerebellum do not follow the surface of the cortex and produce duplicates such as are found over the cerebrum, but send out from the arteries on the surface single vessels like combs and fringes, which dip down into the furrows supplying two opposed furrow walls. The smaller arteries penetrate into the molecular layer and pass through it, giving off capillaries which make large loops. In the granular layer, however, they give off many more capillaries and the loops are smaller and more rounded. Hence, when a thick section is examined with low-power magnification, a dense weave of capillary network appears as a dark band corresponding in position with this cellular layer.

The basal ganglia, being relatively centrally placed, have arteries that enter from all surfaces and penetrate toward the center of the cell mass, subdividing into finer branches. The capillary network forms a pattern of uneven rounded loops which, under magnification, have the appearance of finely spun nets drawn over the surface of transparent spheres. The capillary bed forming the net appears as a continuous anastomosis.

Finley (1936) pointed out that the substantia nigra receives its blood from four pial arteries, namely the basilar artery, posterior cerebral artery, posterior communicating artery, and the choroid artery. According to Finley the density of the capillary net in the brain parallels the density of the nerve cells in any given region. He points out that the capillary net in the cellular zone is more dense than in the reticular zone, but in those parts of the reticular zone where the nerve cells are grouped, there is also found a greater number of capillaries. He also points out that the second outstanding difference between the capillaries of the two regions is the short distance between the artery and the vein in the compact zone as compared with that distance in the reticular zone. In other words, there is a shorter capillary bed in the former than in the latter.

In the spinal cord the circulatory mechanism, although analogous to that seen in the brain, differs because of the relative position of the white matter which, lying outside the gray, causes the arterial arrangement to be reversed.

As in the brain, the gray matter has a richer blood supply than the white matter. The larger arteries lying in the subarachnoid space, commonly three in number, send branches through the white matter to the gray beneath. The surface arteries and their perforating branches thus supply the blood to the spinal cord. No vessels are found within the central canal. There is less anastomosis between the different segments of the cord than between different parts of the brain, although free anastomosis takes place between capillaries here, as in the brain (Cobb, 1932).

The arteries of the dura over the brain in man, like those of the (Pfeifer, 1930) scalp, are characteristically serpentine in their course. They resemble the brain arteries in structure as regards the arrangement of elastic tissue. They, too, have a well-developed inner elastic layer which, as in the brain vessels, tends to subdivide into laminas. The muscle layer contains a few thin elastic fibers. However, the externa on the side toward the brain differs from that toward the skull. On the brain side there are only a few thin circular elastic fibers. On the skull side there are numerous strong circular fibers. Longitudinal fibers, with the exception of a few on the dural side, are absent.

Intracranial blood vessels are supplied by both myelinated and unmyelinated nerves and endings. But few ganglion cells are observed along the vessels of the central nervous system, although peripheral nerve fibers may be traced along the vessels of the medulla, pons, mesencephalon, diencephalon, cortex, and the vessels of the pia and choroid plexus. From histologic studies no definite conclusions may be drawn as to the possible motor or sensory function of such nerves or endings.

CENTRAL NEUROGENIC CONTROL OF BLOOD FLOW

Observations made over much of the last decade have demonstrated that electrical stimulation of certain areas of the brainstem of certain animals, including the cat and the monkey, may produce significant increase in cerebral blood flow (Ingvar and Soderberg, 1958). Increase in the cerebral blood flow has also been accompanied by an increase in cerebral metabolism. The initial increase in cerebral blood flow associated with electrical stimulation was rapid and could not be produced by alterations in cerebral metabolism alone. In addition, it has been noted in man that epileptic discharges within the central vasomotor centers may result in neurogenic vasodilatation (Meyer et al, 1966). Large increases in cerebral blood flow may also occur during rapid eye movement sleep (Reivich et al., 1967).

Meyer et al. (1971) have studied cerebral blood flow and oxygen consumption measured during electrical stimulation of the brain stem in 25 monkeys. Increases in cerebral blood flow occurred rapidly when certain regions of the brainstem were stimulated. These increases occurred with and without electroencephalographic activation. The stimulated areas were located in the pons and midbrain reticular formations, thalamus and hypothalamus and were accompanied by temporary loss of autoregulation of blood flow. Meyer and his collaborators conclude that there appear to be centers within the brain which influence cerebral blood flow and metabolism, and they suggest that these centers may account for rapidly occurring increases in cerebral blood flow which are noted during epileptic seizures and REM sleep. Conversely, neurogenic loss of autoregulation which appears after head injury could also be related to decreased activity of these centers.

Anatomic studies of the cerebral blood vessels have shown that arterial vessels on the surface of the brain and in the depths of the brain are invested by nerve fibers (Falck et al., 1968). In particular, catecholamines have been demonstrated by fluorescence techniques to be present on the arteries at the base of the brain, though these cannot be demonstrated after cervical sympathectomy (Nielsen and Owman, 1967). Waltz and associates (1971) have measured the effects of stimulation of the cervical sympathetic nerves on cortical blood flow in vascular reactivity of the cat. They find that, after unilateral electrical stimulation of the cervical sympathetic trunk, there is a decrease in cerebral blood flow with associated arteriolar constriction. They conclude that stimulation of the cervical sympathetic trunk can cause alterations of the cerebral circulation and its regulatory mechanisms but do not suggest that the control of the cerebral blood flow and vascular caliber is one of the normal functions of the autonomic nervous system.

SUBARACHNOID HEMORRHAGE

The Genesis of Cerebral Aneurysm

The main cerebral blood supply derives from the basilar and internal carotid arteries, meeting in the polygonal arrangement known as the circle of Willis. The internal carotid arteries branch abruptly to give rise to the anterior cerebral and middle cerebral vessels, while a further abrupt branching, the anterior commissure, connects two of these, the anterior cerebrals. The paired vertebrals join to form the basilar, which forks at its anterior end into the posterior cerebrals, and these last are connected with the rest of the "circle" by still another abrupt bifurca-

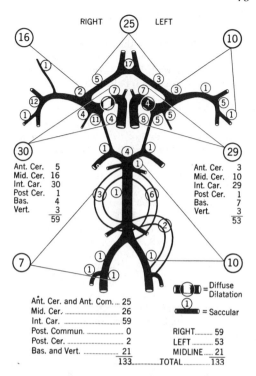

FIG. 7-2. Arteries involved in 133 aneurysms. There were 108 patients, but in 16 of these the aneurysms were multiple. The total number of aneurysms for each main area is shown in each of the large circles near the outer borders. (From Dandy (1944) *Intracranial Arterial Aneurysms.*)

tion, the posterior commissures, which join the internal carotid. A rapidly moving volume of blood is thus forced through a highly angular system of arteries.

The vessels composing the circle of Willis are characterized by a high frequency of aneurysm, particularly at or near the points of bifurcation. A major factor in the occurrence of such aneurysm is congenital weakness of the artery walls, and this appears to be closely related to the angularity of the circle. The relation of the architecture of the circle of Willis to the incidence of aneurysm is shown in Figures 7-1 and 7-2.

Bremer (1943) made a study of the origin of congenital aneurysms of the cerebral arteries. It is his conception that the aneurysms stem from two sources, the first having to do with bifurcations and wall defects. Thus the increase in width of each hemisphere and of the brain as a whole changes the

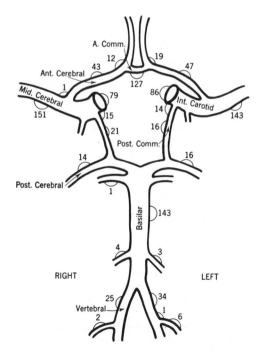

FIG. 7-1. Location of intracranial aneurysms in 1023 cases. (From McDonald and Korb, chart 1, p. 299, in "Intracranial Aneurysms" *Arch. Neurol. Psychiat.*, 42:289 (1939).

course of the cranial arteries, and with this the angle at which they leave the parent stem. The middle cerebral artery runs to the lateral surface of the hemisphere and the anterior cerebral artery to the mesial surface, while the growth of the corpus callosum is responsible for the anterior pull of the anterior cerebral artery.

Since the points of origin of these arteries from the internal carotid artery lie close to the base of the brain, growth in width of the hemisphere spreads them apart until the angle between them is almost 180 degrees. The two internal carotid arteries and the posterior communicating arteries are, by the expansion, merely moved laterally, but the angle of the junction of the posterior communicating arteries with the single median basilar is much increased. The angle between them at their divergence may again be as much as 180 degrees in the adult, whereas in the original pattern the angle between the two arterial trunks was very narrow. In contrast, the superior cerebellar arteries sprout from the two sides of the median basilar artery, accommodating to the increasing width of the hindbrain without essentially altering their angle of emergence.

Bremer notes also that the primary and secondary branches of all of the cerebral arteries are submitted to a peculiar type of disturbance. The enlargement of the hemisphere is not accomplished by addition to the two ends of the structure (as, for example, in the growth of the long bones) but by interstitial growth due to increase in the number of nerve cells and fibers. The growth of the hemisphere is most rapid in the early months of fetal life and is retarded later with the appearance of convolutions. The latter allow the cortex to continue its expansion without adding proportionately to the proportions of the hemisphere. Still later, however, the bulk is again increased because of the myelination of the nerve fibers. The middle and posterior cerebral arteries both approach the hemisphere from the center of its lesser curvature and their branches spread fanwise, directed at right angles to its length. As interstitial growth proceeds, these branches are spread further apart so that ultimately angles of 180 degrees result. All of the bifurcations described as showing angles expanding as a result of growth of the brain are occasional sites of aneurysms. The clinical importance of Bremer's observations is indicated in Fig. 7-2 where the arterial bifurcation is shown to be a common site of aneurysm. This is less striking in Fig. 7-1.

The second step in Bremer's explanation of these congenital defects is based upon the fact that structural defects occur at such wide angles of bifurcation. Vessels such as the cranial veins that rest immediately against the unyielding surface of the skull are devoid of most of their muscularis on the adjacent side. Apparently the muscularis develops only when the intima requires additional strenthening to withstand the increasing centrifugal force of pulsation, and indeed any support will serve. (Bremer has shown that the musculature of the embryonic left pulmonary aortic arch fails to develop where the vessel is partially encircled by the recurrent laryngeal nerve.) Thus, at an acute fork of a bifurcation of embryonal cerebral vessels the two adjacent walls are pressed against each other and support each other. No musculature will develop until the branches become spread so far apart that the elasticity of the intima will no longer allow the two walls to touch. From this point forward the strengthening musculature is necessary and usually grows into the gap. Sometimes the muscle develops further toward the apex on one branch than on the other or on a main trunk than on a branch. The naked intima will then obtain support from the outer surface of the other muscular sheet. Thus, in the spreading of a bifurcation or fork in which a defect is already present, the wall may remain naked or be strenghened by new growth of muscle from the sides. The latter is by far the more common end state.

Bremer's second class of aneurysms arises from the sides of the cerebral arteries, not at recognizable forks, and falls into a different category of origin from those just described. These aneurysms may be explained as resulting from derangements of some of the many minute arteries and precapillary vessels that remain as persistent members of the original capillary plexus. These vessels usually arise at right angles, directly from the main arteries, piercing the masculature as endothelial tubes and surrounded by a minimal amount of connective tissue. They often retain their plexiform character just outside the vessel wall. During early development many of the members of the net degenerate and are lost. Occasionally they remain small or even undergo later degeneration. If these vessels persist to adult life, an aneurysm may result with a narrow pedicle and two or three minute vessels branching from it at recurrent angles. The adventitia found in the wall of such structures probably represents the usual reaction of the surrounding connective tissue to any expanding structure, a type of capsule formation, the muscularis and elastica not having developed in the original capillary. A characteristic of true cerebral aneurysm is the absence of internal elastic membrane as well as of the muscularis.

Such congenital defects in the vascular structure may result in spontaneous aneurysm at any age, or may wait upon the further changes of arteriosclerosis to produce aneurysm.

There are two additional anatomic features which predispose the circle of Willis to aneurysm formation. The circle is suspended in the large fluid space at the base of the brain, and lacks the surrounding tissues which support vessels in other regions. Further, the arteries are especially thin walled, owing to a limited elastica and media.

Gross congenital anomaly of the circle of Willis is a fifth factor in the high frequency of cerebral aneurysm. The failure of the basilar artery to join the posterior cerebral and complete the circle is a common anomaly and has been explained as a failure of the normal sequence of embryonic connections between these vessels. The posterior communicating artery is relatively larger and more important during the early weeks of intrauterine life, when it represents the origin of the posterior cerebral from the internal carotid, than later, when the posterior cerebral is reinforced by anastomosis with the basilar, and the posterior communicating artery is no longer essential for the maintenance of the blood supply of the posterior part of the cerebrum.

Hassler (1961) has called attention to the clinical significance of minute aneurysms. Microdissections of the larger arteries of the circle of Willis have disclosed that such aneurysms are common: 29 were found in 25 of 140 so-called normal subjects (ca. 17%); eight were found in five of ten subjects with ruptured berry aneurysms. In all, 45 minute aneurysms have been examined. All but two were situated on or very near the distal ridge between two branches, the part of the presumably congenitally weak junction between main trunk and branch that probably is most exposed to hemodynamic stress. Most were situated on the middle cerebral artery and on or near the anterior communicating artery. The age of the subjects ranged from 31 to 80 years. Two minute aneurysms probably caused subarachnoid hemorrhage by rupture. One was found in a living patient during operation, and the other at necropsy. It is Hassler's thesis that minute and major aneurysms are connected in genesis. He suggests that "the general thickening of the muscular coat of the arterial wall that then sometimes seems to be present at the level of "cushions" may perhaps be in some way connected with the diminution of this layer at other parts of the wall at points of branching."

The Qualities and Temporal Features of the Headache Associated with Subarachnoid Hemorrhage

Headache is the most common symptom of subarachnoid hemorrhage and occurs in every conscious patient. It is unusually of very high intensity and of sudden onset. It is often described as "something snapping inside the head," followed by an intense throbbing ache. The ache at the start is commonly located in the occipital region, and then radiates down the neck and back. Less commonly it is first located in the frontal region, bilaterally or unilaterally, in the temporal region, at the vertex, or deep in the eye, but such headache soon radiates into the occipital region. When associated with neck rigidity the headache is made worse by flexure of the neck.

In over half the patients the attack of sudden intense pain is accompanied by vomiting and drowsiness, neck rigidity, and loss of consciousness. Convulsions occur after the onset of such a headache in approximately 10 to 15% of patients. In 10% of patients there are prodromes of a few hours' to several days' duration, such as low-intensity frontal or occipital headache, pain in the eye, pain in the back of the neck, backache, or pain in the hamstring muscles. Occasionally the severe headache is preceded by vertigo, photophobia, diplopia, and rarely by vomiting.

The high-intensity headache following subarachnoid hemorrhage persists with but little modification for approximately one week from its onset with subsequent complete elimination of pain within two months. Sustained, chronic, or recurrent headache persisting longer than two months following rupture of intracranial aneurysm with subarachnoid hemorrhage is rare in patients who have not had headaches before the accident.

There is a conflict in the evidence concerning the occurrence of headache as a sequel of subarachnoid hemorrhage. This conflict may, however, be explained by consideration of the prerupture headache histories of patients.

In Magee's series (1943) of 150 patients with subarachnoid hemorrhages, only 18 were known to have had recurrent headaches for varying periods of time before the rupture that preceded hospitalization. In 22 of his patients who recovered, concerning whom no statement about prerupture headache is made and whom he was able to follow for from six to 48 months, 14 had headaches following recovery from their hemorrhage. In the New York Hospital series of 46 patients, 41% had histories of migraine headache or recurrent headache attacks. Of the 30 of these 46 patients who survived a few months to nine years, 12 had had periodic recurrent headaches for many years previous to their hemorrhage, and ten of the latter had headaches afterward. Only two of the 18 patients with no headaches previous to hemorrhage had headaches after recovery from subarachnoid hemorrhage.

It is probable that the initial severe headache associated with sudden hemorrhage into the subarachnoid space about the base of the brain is due to traction, displacement, distention, and rupture of pain-sensitive blood vessels and the pia arachnoid. The headache of several days' duration is probably secondary to a sterile inflammatory reaction about the blood vessels and meninges.

Incidence of Subarachnoid Hemorrhage According to Age and Sex

Forty-six patients at the New York Hospital with subarachnoid hemorrhage were studied. Postmortem evidence of subarachnoid hemorrhage, operative visualization, or xanthochromic cerebrospinal fluid or blood demonstrated by lumbar puncture were the criteria for inclusion. Neonatal and traumatic hemorrhages have not been included, nor have aneurysms detected at operation and autopsy but not associated with subarachnoid hemorrhage.

There were 23 females and 23 males. The age distribution was as follows:

Age	Patients
Under 20	2
21–30	5
31–40	8
41–50	19
51–60	8
61–70	3
71–80	1

Precipitating and Predisposing Factors in Subarachnoid Hemorrhage

The majority of New York Hospital patients were engaged in ordinary activity when rupture took place. In two instances the hemorrhages occurred during sexual intercourse. Magee noted excessive activity to be associated with rupture only rarely.

One patient who died had cirrhosis of the liver with bleeding tendency, and two patients who lived had lues. No premonitory signs which could definitely be considered to precede bleeding were noted.

Five of the New York Hospital patients had elevated blood pressure, and at least three had definite hypertensive vascular disease.

Symptoms

The symptoms included sudden violent headache, dizziness and vertigo, vomiting, drowsiness, stupor and coma, stiff neck and pain in the back of the thighs and legs, tightness of these areas, sweats, and chills, Convulsions occurred in 17% of the New York Hospital patients, and in 12% of Magee's. Low back pain was a striking feature in three patients.

Headache was fronto-occipital, fronto-ocular, frontotemporal, occipital, and sometimes general. It was described as a feeling of a sudden snap in the head followed by intense throbbing ache. Sudden onset of an extreme high-intensity pain, chiefly in the back of the head was most common.

Signs

The signs were fever, occasionally coming on 24 hr or more after the accident and lasting for over a week, stiff neck, Kernig's sign, third nerve palsy, delirium, hemiparesis, other evidence of corticospinal tract disease, and fundal hemorrhage. No prognostic information could be gained from the signs. Many of the patients who fully recovered lost consciousness and had convulsions at the onset of the illness.

A diagnosis of subarachnoid hemorrhage may be made after examination of the cerebrospinal fluid. A bloody spinal fluid is not conclusive evidence of subarachnoid hemorrhage. Xanthochromia seen in the supernatant fluid of the specimen, is, on the other hand, conclusive evidence of subarachnoid bleeding. Such xanthochromia may appear within 12 hours after hemorrhage into the subarachnoid space, and will deepen in specimens drawn in the subsequent 24–48 hr. According to the work of Barrows et al., (1965) a positive benzidine test for blood on the supernatant fluid of a freshly drawn centrifuged specimen is conclusive evidence of subarachnoid hemorrhage.

The advent of computerized tomographic scanning has been a landmark in the assessment of subarachnoid hemorrhage. In the preoperative period, valuable information can be obtained, especially for planning angiography, by using this method. For example, the size of the hemorrhage can be assessed, and one can determine if a clot is present. If an intracranial clot is present, angiography can be performed immediately. Otherwise, it can be delayed until the angiographic team is ready, in the first 24 hr. CT scanning may reveal the presence of multiple aneurysms. It is also useful in assessing ventricular size and the development of hydrocephalus during a period of altered CSF dynamics, related to the bleeding episode.

Treatment

The modern treatment of subarachnoid hemorrhage is based on the patient's status on neurological examination, which remains the most sensitive index of prognosis. Over an 18-year period, Hunt and Kosnick (1974) have studied 421 patients with intracranial aneurysms and have classified them according to surgical risk (See Table 7-1). It has been their policy to operate upon Grade I and Grade II patients as soon as possible, preferably within 24 hr of admission. Operative mortality has been 4% for 105 patients classified as Grade I at the time of operation, and 15% for 124 Grade II patients, or 10% for the two groups combined. In contrast, 50% of patients in Grade III, 60% of patients in Grade IV, and 100% of patients in Grade V died. By delaying operation on Grade III patients until clinical improvement occurred to Grade II or I, Hunt and his colleagues were able to improve the operative mortality from 50% to 28%. Thus, they follow the general policy of operating on Grade I and Grade II patients as soon as possible, and delaying operation on patients in Grade III, IV, and V until clinical improvement has occurred.

Early operative intervention is thus justified in a small percentage of patients with sub-

TABLE 7-1 Classification of Patients with Intracranial Aneurysms According to Surgical Risk

GRADE	CRITERIA*
0	Unruptured aneurysm
I	Asymptomatic, or minimal headache and slight nuchal rigidity
IA	No acute meningeal or brain reaction, but with fixed neurological deficit
II	Moderate to severe headache, nuchal rigidity, no neurological deficit other than cranial nerve palsy
III	Drowsiness, confusion, or mild focal deficit
IV	Stupor, moderate to severe hemiparesis, possibly early decerebrate rigidity and vegetative disturbances
V	Deep coma, decerebrate rigidity, moribund appearance

*Serious systemic disease, such as hypertension, diabetes, severe atherosclerosis, chronic pulmonary disease, or severe intracranial arterial spasm seen on arteriography results in placement of the patient in the next less favorable grade.

arachnoid aneurysmal hemorrhage. These cases are characterized by an early diagnosis, emergency angiography demonstrating no vasospasm, a favorable location for the aneurysm, and the absence of significant neurological signs suggesting cerebral dysfunction. Jane et al. (1977) have studied the natural history of intracranial aneurysms with rebleeding rates during acute and long-term periods of observation. For a patient with an anterior communicating aneurysm seen on day one, the chance that he will rebleed within the first day is approximately 50%. For posterior communicating aneurysms, the expected chance of rebleeding on the first day is 60%. Thereafter, the rate rapidly diminishes for both aneurysms. By day 30, the chance of rebleeding during the first six months has dropped to less than 10%. The authors have also followed a group of 213 patients for up to 21 years; of these, 54 had another bleeding episode during the first ten years, and another seven patients rebled between the tenth and twentieth years. To summarize, the first decade following subarachnoid hemorrhage is characterized by rebleeding episodes at the rate of approximately 3% per year. Subsequent rebleeding occurs at the rate of 2% per year. In 67% of subsequent hemorrhages, death occurs. Jane and his colleagues make the point that subarachnoid hemorrhage secondary to aneurysms should be considered as a chronic disease with a "relentless rate of re-bleeding".

Cerebral vasospasm occurring in association with ruptured intracranial aneurysm may be defined arteriographically as narrowing in one or more of the intracranial arteries, not obviously due to atherosclerosis, stretching by mass lesions, or radiographic artifacts. The recognition of this type of cerebral spasm is aided by a subsequent arteriogram in the same patient showing a normal arterial caliber. Cerebral vasospasm after intracranial bleeding usually has a delayed onset with a peak incidence approximately one week after aneurysmal rupture. It may last from several days to a month after it appears.

The effect of cerebral vasospasm on morbidity and mortality is difficult to state categorically. Data from several investigations indicate that there is some correlation between intracranial arterial spasm and mortality and perhaps to a lesser extent between intracranial spasm and clinical manifestations. Patients with varying degrees of neurological dysfunction without vasospasm show decreased regional cerebral blood flow and cerebral oxygen metabolism. These changes are particularly striking in patients with vasospasm. Many neurosurgeons prefer to wait one to two weeks after aneurysmal rupture before operating, though this is by no means a universal opinion. For example, in 1975 Yasargil and Fox outlined their view that vasospasm has no clinical significance and should not cause a surgeon to delay an early operation if the patient is mentally alert and has no other serious medical or neurological problems.

Cerebral vasospasm probably represents a region of ischemic smooth muscle damaged from prolonged irritation, the elaboration of vasoactive substances, and persistent contraction. Various drugs have been tried for relief of vasospasm. These include isoproterenol and lidocaine hydrochloride, alpha and beta blocking agents, direct smooth muscle relaxers, magnesium sulfate, and reserpine. Unfortu-nately, the response of cerebral vasospasm following hemorrhage to any of these methods of treatment is capricious and none of them can be recommended with any degree of confidence. Sundt (1977) points out that surgical trauma in patients with severe edema aggravates spasm and that gentle hands, gentle retraction, or, if possible, no retraction at all and use of microdissection techniques are most important in the surgical treatment of these patients. Presumably, a good deal of spasm is directly related to the blood which dissects around the aneurysm and adjacent arterial wall.

To reduce the risk of recurrent bleeding, the antifibrinolytic agent, epsilon amino caproic acid (Amicar) is often given 24–36 gm/24 hr in a continuous intravenous drip. Other antifibrinolytics may also be employed. In maintaining fluid balance, intravenous fluid should be used sparingly and in proper electrolyte combinations in order to minimize the danger of brain edema. Some have suggested hypothermia for two to five days in the stage of acute hemorrhage, a procedure of uncertain efficacy.

Finally, hypertension should be controlled. Sedation can be achieved with phenobarbital 60 mg four times daily. Maintaining blood pressure at a systolic level of 100 mm Hg in normotensive patients, a reduction of 10–30% from their baseline blood pressures, with a wide variety of agents including alphamethyldopa and diuretics such as furosemide appears to be helpful.

PARENCHYMATOUS CEREBRAL HEMORRHAGE

Though it is theoretically possible for hemorrhage in the brain parenchyma to occur without pain, this almost never happens. Cerebral (or cerebellar) hemispheric bleeding of any significant magnitude is accompanied by excruciating headache and, usually, by disturbance of consciousness. The venerable term *apoplexy*, implying sudden paralysis with total or partial loss of consciousness and sensation is most appropriate in this situation. Usually the intrahemispheric blood will distend the brain, producing traction on pain-sensitive structures described in Chapter 3, and frequently it will rupture into the subarachnoid space, producing typical signs and symptoms associated with subarachnoid bleeding.

Certain signs and symptoms are common to all forms of intracranial bleeding. These include progressive headache, stiffness of the neck, disturbances of consciousness, nausea, and vomiting. Transient or progressive neurological signs and/or seizures should be anticipated. Severe headaches in hypertensive patients, particularly morning headaches, should be considered a warning symptom of a possible, impending cerebral hemorrhage. Hypertension of any etiology is by far the most frequent cause of parenchymatous cerebral hemorrhage. The rupture may occur from an artery or cerebral vein, but the most frequent source of bleeding is from an arteriole which has degenerated, related to the hypertensive atherosclerotic process. Persistent elevation of the blood pressure, particularly in acute situations of malignant hypertension, will produce necrosis of the smooth muscle and elastic laminae of the vessel wall, evoking Charcot-Bouchard aneurysms. These frequently rupture and are a common source of parenchymatous hemorrhage and brain destruction. These microaneurysms are particularly distributed in the lenticulostriate branches of the middle cerebral arteries supplying the internal capsule and the basal ganglia. They also occur in the brainstem, especially in the pons. Charcot-Bouchard aneurysms may be identified with arteriographic techniques or a magnified CAT scan.

Thus, parenchymatous cerebral hemorrhage usually occurs in the region of the internal capsule or the basal ganglia and pons. Approximately one-fifth occur in the brainstem and cerebellum. The remainder are found in the frontal and occipital lobes.

Work-up of the patient with intracranial hemorrhage should proceed rapidly. X-rays of the skull and echoencephalogram are useful and a CAT scan should be done as an emergency procedure. If there is a suspicion of increased intracranial pressure, a lumbar puncture should be delayed unless there is a possibility of infection, such as bacterial meningitis. Spinal puncture may hasten herniation. At times, and particularly if anticoagulants are to be used, a careful lumbar puncture is necessary. Emergency arteriography is indicated if a surgical procedure for clot evacuation is contemplated, particularly if acute cerebellar hemorrhage is suspected, where surgery may be life-saving.

Most of these patients have pre-existing hypertension, and many will have striking elevation of the blood pressure during the cerebral hemorrhage. Since there is evidence that elevated blood pressure will promote further hemorrhage and increasing cerebral edema, the hypertension should be treated.

Many methods are available. Constant intravenous sodium nitroprusside allows good control in the acute situation. If this drug is not available, then magnesium sulfate given intravenously in a 6% solution can be employed, although magnesium toxicity from cumulative doses will occur if the drug is used for more than 18–36 hr. Respiratory care requires attention since respiratory suppression may occur with intravenous magnesium sulfide; this drug can also be used in intramuscular doses of 2–4 ml of a 20% solution at 1–2 hr intervals. For less severe hypertension, furosemide will suffice. Occasionally reserpine (1 mg intramuscularly, three hourly doses) can be used.

Treatment of pain and agitation is important since both increase hypertension. Phenobarbital can be given from 50–100 mg at hourly intervals and then as required thereafter. Morphine sulfate usually should be avoided because of respiratory suppression, but meperidine (Demerol) is sometimes effective in making the patient restful without overly sedating him. Fluid and electrolyte control is important—excess fluid intake should be particularly avoided. A mild dehydration in the first few days of hospitalization is probably acceptable. This can be obtained using one liter of 5% dextrose in water and 500 ml of isotonic saline per 24 hr, plus correction of any unusual fluid losses.

Increased intracranial pressure can be treated with dexamethasone (Decadron) 16 mg intravenously and 4 mg every 4 hr. Hyperosmolar agents such as intravenous mannitol are less effective but may be employed. A test dose of 100 mg of 20% mannitol solution should be given intravenously over 5 min. This should increase urine output to approximately 50 ml/hr. Failure to demonstrate any increase in urinary output contraindicates the use of this drug. If it is used, a slow infusion of 30 ml/hr of a 15% solution for 10–12 hr is advisable. Some authors suggest using intravenous glycerol, 1.2 gm/kg of body weight, given as a 10% solution over a 4-hr interval.

Treatment of seizures is important. Repeated seizures are best interrupted by administering diazepam intravenously, slowly over 1 to 2 min, up to 10 mg. Respiration should be continuously monitored when this drug is given. This drug cannot be used for prolonged control of seizures and, accordingly, a 400–800 mg loading dose of diphenylhydantoin sodium (Dilantin) can be given slowly intravenously, followed by 100 mg every 6 hr. The latter drug should not be used by the intramuscular route.

SUMMARY

1. The headache of subarachnoid hemorrhage is of high intensity and of sudden onset, is commonly located in the occipital region, and in almost all patients is associated with neck rigidity. Vomiting and drowsiness are frequent symptoms, and 10 to 15% of patients have convulsions.

2. The headache of subarachnoid hemorrhage usually persists at a very high intensity for a few days, but seldom for as long as a week, and subsides thereafter, with complete elimination of pain within two months. The persistence of headache for longer periods following subarachnoid hemorrhage in patients who have had no previous headaches is rare.

3. It is probable that the initial headache of subarachnoid hemorrhage is due to traction, displacement, distention, and rupture of pain-sensitive blood vessels and the pia arachnoid. The headache of several days' duration is probably secondary to a sterile inflammatory reaction about the blood vessels and meninges.

4. Ruptured cerebral aneurysm based on a congenital defect with or without arteriosclerotic changes is responsible for the headache, stupor, coma, convulsions, and other disturbances in a high proportion of patients with subarachnoid hemorrhage. However, it is unlikely that periodic headaches of a few hours' duration recurring over many years, as in the case with some patients, could stem from the slowly developing structural changes in an aneurysm.

5. Ruptured subarachnoid hemorrhage is an extremely serious disease. Death occurs in approximately 45% of patients with each major bleeding episode and there is a significant risk of recurrence. Approximately one-third of those who succumb will do so in the first 48 hr after bleeding, another third within the next month, and the remainder from recurrent bleeding episodes thereafter.

6. A precise regimen for every case of subarachnoid hemorrhage cannot be recommended with certainty. Early intervention is justified in a small percentage of cases with aneurysmal hemorrhage characterized by prompt diagnosis, angiography showing no vasospasm, a favorable location, and the absence of serious neurological signs. Surgery can be delayed until the risk of cerebral vasospasm has passed, and often patients can be effectively managed until then through drug-induced hypotension and antifibrinolytic therapy to reduce the risk of recurrent hemorrhage. The time of the bleeding episode and the clinical condition (grade) at the time of initiating treatment are the major variables influencing the natural history of subarachnoid hemorrhage and the decision to operate. If significant vasospasm is present, it is best to delay surgery for ten days to two weeks after the initial bleeding episode.

7. Cerebral (or cerebellar) hemispheric bleeding that is of any significant magnitude is accompanied by excruciating headache and usually by disturbance of consciousness. Hypertension is the most frequent cause of parenchymatous cerebral hemorrhage. The hemorrhage usually occurs in the region of the internal capsule or the basal ganglia and pons, but one-fifth of such hemorrhages occur in the brainstem and cerebellum.

REFERENCES

Barrows, L. J., F. T. Hunter, and B. Q. Banker (1955). The nature and clinical significance of pigments in the cerebral spinal fluid. *Brain 78,* 59.

Bremer, J. L. (1943). Congenital aneurysms of the cerebral arteries. *Arch. Pathol.* 35, 819.

Cobb, S. (1932). *The Cerebrospinal Blood Vessels. Cytology and Cellular Pathology of the Nervous System* (W. Penfield, ed.), Vol. 2, p. 575. Paul B. Hoeber, New York.

Cobb, S., and D. Blain (1933). *Arteriosclerosis of the Brain and Spinal Cord. Arteriosclerosis: A Survey of the Problem* (E. V. Cowdry, ed.), Chap. 4, p. 397. Macmillan, New York.

Dandy, W. E. (1944). *Intracranial Arterial Aneurysms.* Comstock Publishing, Ithaca, N.Y.

Falck, B., K. C. Nielsen, and C. Owman (1968). Adrenergic enervation of the pial circulation. *Scand. J. Clin. Lab. Invest.* 22, Suppl. 102, 6:B.

Fang, H. C. H. (1958). Pathology of cerebral vascular diseases: (A) comparison of blood vessels of the brain and peripheral vessels. *Cerebral Vascular Diseases, 2nd Conference* (I. S. Wright and C. H. Millikan, eds.), p. 17. Grune and Stratton, New York.

Finley, K. H. (1936). Angio-architecture of the substantia nigra and its pathogenic significance. *Arch. Neurol. Psychiat.* 36, 118.

Hassler, O. (1961). Morphological studies on the large cerebral arteries. With reference to the etiology of subarachnoid hemorrhage. *Acta Psychiat.* Suppl. 154, Vol. 36.

Hunt, W. E., and E. J. Kosnik (1974). Timing and periorbital care in intracranial aneurysm surgery. *Clin. Neurosurg.* 21, 79–89.

Ingvar, D. H., and U. Soderberg (1958). Cortical blood flow related to EEG patterns evoked by stimulation of the brainstem. *Acta Physiologica Scand.* 42, 130.

Jane, J. A., H. R. Winn, and A. E. Richardson (1977). The natural history of intracranial aneurysms: re-bleeding rates during the actue and long-term period and implication for surgical management. *Clin. Neurosurg.* 24, 176–184.

Kobayashi, S., A. G. Waltz, and A. L. Rhoton (1971). Effects of stimulation of cervical sympathetic nerves on cortical blood flow and vascular reactivity. *Neurol.* 21, 297.

Magee, C. G. (1943). Spontaneous subarachnoid hemorrhage. *Lancet* 23.

McDonald, C., and M. Korb (1939). Intracranial aneurysms. *Arch. Neurol. Psychiat.* 42, 289.

Meyer, J. S., F. Gotoh, and E. Favale (1966). Cerebral metabolism during epileptic seizures in man. *Electroenceph. Clin. Neurophysiol.* 21, 10.

Meyer, J. S., T. Teraura, K. Sakamoto, and A. Kondo (1971). Central neurogenic control of cerebral blood flow. *Neurol.* 21, 247.

Nielsen, K. C., and C. Owman (1967). Adrenergic enervation of pial arteries related to the circle of Willis in the cat. *Brain Res.* 6, 773.

Pfiefer, R. A. (1935). Grundlegende Untersuchungen fur die Angio-architektonik des Menschlichen Gehirns. Verlag Julius Springer, Berlin.

Reivich, M., G. Isaacs, and E. Evarts (1967). Regional cerebral blood flow during REM and slow wave sleep. *Trans. Am. Neurol. Assoc.* 92, 70.

Sundt, T. (1977). Cerebral vasospasm following subarachnoid hemorrhage: evolution, management and relationship to timing of surgery. *Clin. Neurosurg.* 24, 228–239.

Symonds, C. P. (1923). Contribution to the clinical study of intracranial aneurysms. *Guy's Hosp. Rep.* 73, 139.

Triepel, H. (1897). Das elastische Gewebe in der Wand der Arterien der Schadelhohle. *Anat. Hefte* 7, 189.

Yasargil, M. G., and J. L. Fox (1975). The microsurgical approach to intracranial aneurysms. *Surg. Neurol.* 3, 7–14.

8

HEADACHE AND ARTERIAL HYPERTENSION

REVISED BY DONALD J. DALESSIO

Three categories of headache are found in subjects with elevation in systemic arterial blood pressure.

The first category includes those headaches that occur with sudden major elevation of blood pressure and that result mainly from the dilatation of intracranial arteries. The sudden rise of blood pressure during violent exercise, sexual excitement, or great anger; the dramatic rise in blood pressure when a pheochromocytoma is massaged or pressed upon; the prompt rise in blood pressure with noxious stimulation of bladder or rectum in those with mid-thoracic spinal transections are examples.

The second category includes the headache associated with essential hypertension but not particularly induced by the elevation of blood pressure. The nature of the headache and the factors involved make them much like the vascular headache of the migraine type. The intracranial arteries are mainly responsible for the headache. Sustained contraction of neck and scalp muscles adds an additional component to the headache associated with essential hypertension.

The third category of headache linked with hypertension is found in those patients with renal failure, azotemia, and increased intracranial pressure. The mechanism of headache in this category is related to traction and displacement of pain-sensitive intracranial structures.

HEADACHE AND ESSENTIAL HYPERTENSION

These headaches are of a dull, diffuse, deep-aching nature, usually intermittent but occasionally continuous. They characteristically throb, especially at the onset. They may be generalized, unilateral, or occipital, and are commonly worse in the early hours of the morning, beginning sometime between midnight and 4 A.M. and reaching their peak intensity about daybreak or shortly before getting-up time. They usually awaken the patient in the early hours of the morning and commonly diminish in intensity after arising, the taking of a cup of hot coffee, and the assumption of the duties of the day. Patients often discover after the onset of the headache that they are more comfortable in the sitting position, and a few have the notion that sleeping in the 'head up' position minimizes the headache, and perhaps even prevents it. The headache is increased in intensity by bodily effort, stooping over, and coughing, and, as will be demonstrated, closely resembles migraine headache in other ways.

There is another variety of headache often coexistent with the syndrome described above, but sometimes occurring independently. It too occurs in the night and early hours of the morning and consists of a severe ache in the nape of the neck, in the occiput, and as high as the vertex. It is usually associated with neck rigidity, persistent torticollis, or elevation of the shoulders. The patient may complain that his head feels as though it were in a vise or clamp, or as though there were a steel band or tight cap about his head, sensations which have given the headache the colorful name of *douleur en casque*. The muscles of the necks and back of the head are tight and tender, and often small nodules are palpable which are exceedingly tender. This variety of headache is identical with the headache resulting from sustained muscle contraction, which will be described in detail in Chapter 19 where also are given facts about its management.

Pathophysiology of Headache

The following considerations are focused on the first of the headache described above. The term "hypertensive headache" is misleading, since it implies that the frequency and severity of the headache are directly related to the level of the blood pressure. As a matter of fact, it is a common clinical observation that the headache associated with hypertension yields to rest in bed or other methods of relaxation without a material change in the blood pressure level.

Almost all the patients with hypertension and associated headaches had headaches for many years (Sutherland and Wolff, 1940). In numerous instances the headache was known to precede the onset of the hypertension and changed in some patients only in intensity with the rise in blood pressure.

Observations. For three and four days, hourly determinations of the systolic and diastolic blood pressures were made on four patients suffering from headache associated with hypertension. No relation between either the incidence or the severity of the headache and the immediate level of the systolic or the diastolic blood pressure could be demonstrated. The headache might be present or absent when the pressure was high or moderate, or indeed even relatively low (Fig. 8–1).

Digital compression of the common carotid or the temporal artery resulted in decrease in the intensity of the headache on that side. When the effect of ergotamine tartrate on the headache of hypertension was tested (in the manner employed in the study of migraine headache), it was found that, despite sharp rises in blood pressure due to the ergotamine, there was a decrease in the amplitude of pulsations of extracranial arteries (Fig. 8-2). In other words, factors that constricted the cranial arteries diminished the intensity of the headache associated with hypertension.

High intracranial pressure has no part in the headache, since the cerebrospinal fluid pressure was shown to be normal during an attack.

During the headache the pressure of the cerebrospinal fluid was not unusual (from 80 to 170 mm of water), and there was no increase in the amplitude of pulsations of intracranial arteries. Moreover, the amplitude of pulsations of these arteries did not become less as the headache diminished in intensity.

The effect of increasing the pressure of the cerebrospinal fluid was tested on the headache associated

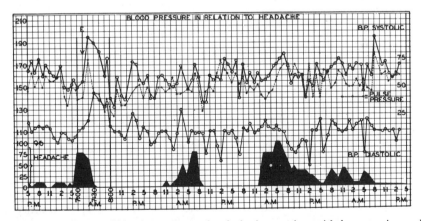

FIG. 8-1. Relation of blood pressure to headache in a patient with hypertension and associated headache. The fluctuations of the blood pressure, and the incidence and severity of the headache vary independently. Thus, headache occurred with a blood pressure of 140 systolic and 75 diastolic on one occasion, whereas headache disappeared as the blood pressure rose from 145 systolic and 90 diastolic to 195 systolic and 110 diastolic at another time. At E, to the left of the chart, is shown the record of a headache terminated by ergotamine tartrate.

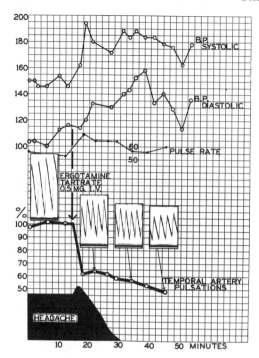

FIG. 8-2. Effect of ergotamine tartrate on headache associated with hypertension. The decrease in the intensity of the headache paralleled the decrease in amplitude of pulsations of the temporal artery. The fact that the headache is not causally dependent on the immediate level of the blood pressure is demonstrated here, for the blood pressure actually rose precipitously as the headache was abolished.

with hypertension. Increasing the cerebrospinal fluid pressure as high as 900 mm of water by means of a manometer attached to a needle in the lumbar subarachnoid space did not diminish the intensity of the headache (Schumacher and Wolff, 1941).

The effects of digital compression upon the common carotid and temporal arteries, and of ergotamine, as described above, indicate that the dural and superficial branches of the external carotid artery contribute significantly to the headache of hypertension.

Janeway (1913) found that a surprisingly large number of these (hypertensive) patients have been subject to migraine throughout life... The headache is one which appears on awakening or wakes the patient in the early morning hours, has its greatest intensity before arising and passes away either immediately after breakfast or during the course of the morning to reappear in the same manner day after day for considerable periods. The intensity of the pain and its location have varied somewhat, the most severe being similar to bad migraine, and in a few cases it is attended by nausea, and vomiting.

Gardner, Mountain, and Hines (1940) similarly found that a high percentage of patients with headaches in association with arterial hypertension had migraine, often of many years' duration. They inferred that of all individuals who develop high blood pressure, those who previously had migraine are far more likely to experience headache as one symptom of their hypertension than those not so affected.

A further similarity of the headache associated with hypertension to that of migraine is suggested by a consideration of the location, quality, and outstanding features of the headaches in Robey's (1931) series of patients with hypertension. Thus, most of the patients had frontal, orbital, frontotemporal, or temporal headache. The next most common site was the occiput, at which headache occurred one-half as frequently as at the former sites. Generalized headache occurred about one-fifth as frequently as did frontotemporal headache and half as frequently as occipital. Unilateral headache occurred in about 10% of the patients. The headaches were commonly throbbing, and were worse in the morning.

That the hypertension does not bear a direct relation to headache associated with it is further supported by the data of Robey. He found, among 448 patients with hypertension, 218 who never had headache; in short, half the patients with hypertension, 50 had headaches as a chief or major symptom, but these persons had practically the same level of systolic and diastolic blood pressure and of pulse pressure as did 150 patients who never had headaches.

The medical records of 5785 patients in Walker's (1959) general practice were examined for a history of migraine. The incidence was estimated as 5%. Of these patients, 55% gave a family history of migraine, and 79% were women. Observing that 52% of a group of hypertensives also suffered from migraine, Walker investigated the incidence of hypertension in 150 subjects with migraine, comparing the blood pressure with that of 150 controls of the same age and sex distribution suffering from other conditions.

The difference between the mean systolic pressures and between the mean diastolic pressures of the patients, age for age, with migraine and the controls was 10 mm Hg. The incidence of migraine and hypertension in those over 40 years of age was then determined. It was found that the incidence of migraine was greater in those with the higher levels of blood pressure.

The fact that the high level of blood pressure among hypertensive subjects is not a sufficient condition for headache does not justify the assumption that these phenomena are unrelated. Indeed, this, too, would be contradicted by the facts of common experience, since some persons with hypertension never had headache until the hypertension became established. It seems reasonable to postulate that a cranial artery only slightly relaxed for whatever reason would not distend so much, and possibly not to the point of producing pain, if the blood pressure were low. If, however, the sustained level were raised, distention would be greater and therefore pain might readily follow. In other words, a degree of relaxation in the contractile state of the arterial wall, compatible with comfort when blood pressure is average, would cause pain when the blood pressure is elevated.

It is clear that sudden rises in systemic arterial pressure may produce headache in individuals who are unaccustomed to having headache attacks, and that this headache may involve the intracranial vessels. This can be demonstrated in those who exhibit vigorous pressore responses following the administration of epinephrine and norepinephrine intravenously.

Ostfeld and Wolff (1958) re-examined the problem of headache in hypertensive states in a heterogeneous group of 80 hypertensive subjects and a "control" group of patients with normal blood pressure. Both groups were similar in age, race, sex, social background, and occupation. The incidence and severity of headache did not differ significantly in the two populations. Vascular headache of the migraine type and skeletal muscle-contraction headache together made up the great majority of headaches in both. A third type of headache among the hypertensive patients was limited almost entirely to hypertensive subjects with grade III or IV retinopathy. This headache was occipital in location, deep, and of moderate severity, either steady or faintly throbbing in quality, worse on lying down, and predictably had its onset on waking from sleep, commonly terminating an hour or so after waking. The vascular headache of the migraine type and muscle-contraction headache occurred more often among the relatively milder hypertensives; the third type of headache was more common among the severely hypertensive subjects. In patients experiencing the latter type of headache, it was common for blood pressure to fall by as much as 50 mm systolic and 30 mm Hg diastolic during sleep and to return suddenly to the usual levels on waking. This sudden rise in pressure impinging upon the relaxed intracranial vessel walls may be partly responsible for such headache. Also, CO_2 retention during deep sleep and slowed respiration in some individuals is of sufficient magnitude to reduce the tone of the cerebral blood vessels, and perhaps even to dilate them. Such accumulations of CO_2 are eliminated soon after waking.

For example, a subject with arterial hypertension had a blood pressure averaging during the waking state 220/125. During sleep her blood pressure averaged 165/105. On awaking in the morning after several hours of sleep the blood pressure suddenly rose 55 mm of Hg systolic, and 20 mm diastolic. This was associated with the onset of a headache which lasted about an hour and dwindled as the patient became active with her day's work (see Fig 8-3).

Such headaches associated with elevation in blood pressure on awaking after a deep sleep also occur occasionally in normotensive subjects who have fever or other evidence of infection.

Therefore the conception that a slack state of the arterial wall, compatible with comfort when the blood pressure is low or average, would cause pain when the blood pressure is relatively elevated, is supported by analogy with experimental evidence on headache induced by histamine. The headache and maximal distention of the cranial arteries occur not immediately after the injection of histamine, when the effect on the contractile state of these vessels is

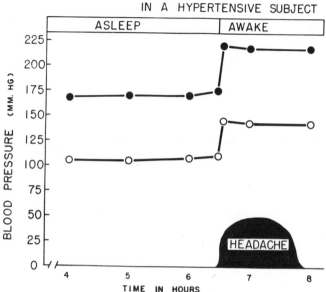

FIG. 8-3. Headache on awakening in a hypertensive subject.

greatest, but some time later, when the blood pressure returns to its initial level. It is at this time that the walls of the cranial artery react to the mounting pressure, and headache becomes associated with a level of blood pressure which is ordinarily accompanied by comfort. The relaxation of cranial arterial walls is thus seen to be one necessary factor in the production of headache induced by histamine, and the level of the blood pressure the other. The analogy to the circumstances in hypertension is close. During an average or normal contractile state of the arterial walls, distention does not occur and, correspondingly, there is no headache; but should this contractile state be impaired (low muscle tonus) through the effect of stress, fatigue, or other condition, distention and headache follow. In brief, high blood pressure is a necessary but not a sufficient condition for this type of headache. There is, however, a significant relation between headache associated with essential hypertension and the contractile state of the cranial arteries.

Fisher (1958) notes that of 100 patients receiving lumbodorsal sympathectomy for hypertension, 90% of 56 women, and 75% of 44 men had severe headaches, indicating that the presence of headache was one criterion for selection for surgery. In 54 cases, the location of the headache was primarily in the occipital region.

The relationship between hypertension and headache was assessed retrospectively by Traub and Korczyn (1978) among 241 patients attending a hypertension clinic. Headache was common (45.6%), particularly among women (68%). Patients with systolic blood pressure higher than 170 mm Hg and/or diastolic blood pressure higher than 110 mm had nocturnal and/or early morning headaches frequently. Fifty-four subjects became headache-free after antihypertensive therapy was given. Their blood pressure decrease was significantly greater than the blood pressure fall of those whose headache did not disappear with treatment.

Waters (1971) selected 1800 members of a community and polled them by questionnaire regarding headache. His responders were divided into four groups; three with various forms of headache and one without any head pain for a year prior to the study. He then measured blood pressure levels in these persons. He could find no significant differences in blood pressure levels among the four groups. Waters concluded that headache frequency is not related to blood pressure levels.

Headache in Association with Sudden Elevation of Systemic Arterial Blood Pressure

HEADACHE INDUCED BY DISTENTION OF BLADDER AND RECTUM IN SUBJECTS WITH SPINAL CORD INJURIES

Head and Riddoch (1917), in their classic experiments on patients with gross spinal cord injuries, found facilitation of spinal reflexes in that part of the cord below the level of the lesion and without suprasegmental control. It was shown that a sufficient stimulus to any receptive surface whose afferent fibers entered the distal stump of the cord was liable to evoke a massive response which overflowed widely into regions of the spinal cord normally associated with other reflexes (assuming that recovery from spinal cord "shock" and resumption of reflex activity of the distal stump of the spinal cord were not prevented by such complications as general infection and toxemia).

Especially investigated were abnormal autonomic reflex effects due to afferent impulses from bladder and bowel distention, both those of spontaneous occurrence due to urinary obstruction or flatulence and those artificially induced by inflation of the bladder or by enemas. Outbursts of intense and profuse sweating, especially of the head and neck, and sensations of "fullness" in the head were described as manifestations of such bladder or bowel distention. Though other precipitating stimuli evoked bursts of sweating, abnormal conditions of tension in the bladder were the most frequent and potent cause of spontaneous hyperhydrosis in these patients with transverse lesions of the spinal cord.

Analysis of the distribution of reflex sweating in relation to the level of the lesion showed a correlation with Langley's (1903) reported levels of sympathetic outflow from thoracolumbar segments to the upper parts of the body. When the lesion was high enough that the upper thoracic segments were included in the distal stump of the cord, profuse sweating occurred in the head and neck, which derive their sympathetic innervation from the upper thoracic segments. Somewhat lower lesions (down to the sixth thoracic segment) resulted in reflex sweating only of the arms and upper portion of the trunk, since the impulses for the head and neck arising from levels of the cord above the lesion were no longer reflexly activated by afferent impulses from the bladder. It was concluded that excessive sweating due to bladder distention (even in the head and neck) represented that activity of the nervous system below the level of the lesion of the spinal cord.

Since these classic studies, numerous other investigations of reflex autonomic responses occurring in spinal man have been carried out. The most detailed report of these phenomena, by Guttmann and Whitteridge (1946) included further analysis of reflex sweating and observations on other effects derived from bladder distention, such as vasoconstriction and diminished skin temperature in the extremities, flushing of the neck and face, nasal congestion, headache, hypertension, and bradycardia. Though vasoconstriction of the toes and fingers and a very large rise in blood pressure occurred during bladder distention when the complete lesion was at or above the fifth thoracic level, these investigators emphasized that in the neck, face, and nasal mucosa vasodilatation occurred. The seeming paradox of vasodilatation in the face and neck, on the one hand, concomitant with sweating in the face and neck and with vasoconstriction and sweating in the upper limbs, on the other (the last-mentioned responses all being manifestations of sympathetic activity in these parts), was explained on the basis of an adaptive pattern. Flushing of the head and the nasal congestion were interpreted as due to passive dilatation of vessels secondary to increased blood pressure. Headache was believed to be related to a sudden rise in intracranial blood flow. Since it was shown that arteries of the head did not participate in the vasoconstriction occurring in the extremities and visceral bed, it may be assumed that they were passively dialted by the heightened intravascular tension brought about by vasoconstriction elsewhere.

Thompson and Witham (1948), in their clinical observations on patients with complete lesions of the cord, have also described the occurrence of spontaneous paroxysms of hypertension and headache. They confirmed the observation of reflex autonomic discharges due to bladder obstruction in cases of high lesions of the cord and demonstrated the abolition or prevention of these reflex effects by the injection of tetraethylammonium chloride. They emphasized the clinical importance of the vasomotor and sudomotor reflexes as a source of intermittent symptoms (sweating, headache) in paraplegic patients and discussed methods of management to prevent their occurrence.

Schumacher and Guthrie (1951), undertook the following study to confirm the occurrence of headache during bladder or rectal distention in patients with high transverse lesions of the cord and to investigate the pathophysiology of such head pain. It has been shown that experimentally induced histamine headache can be eliminated by raising the intracranial pressure, thereby suppressing the pulsations of the painfully distended intracranial arteries. An old clinical observation is the transient reduction or abolition of the pain of migraine headache by compression of the carotid artery in the neck. It was thought worth while, therefore, to employ such manipulations in the study of 'bladder' headache, especially in view of the adaptive pattern proposed by Guttmann and Whitteridge.

METHODS

Bladder Distention Experiments. Bladder filling was carried out, in stages and at a variable rate of flow, through a Foley indwelling catheter from a reservoir of sterile saline solution, elevated 100 cm above the symphysis pubis and attached to the catheter by an intervening rubber tube with Murphy drip container and clamp. A Lewis recording cystometer, attached by a T tube to a catheter, provided a continuous ink-recorded graph of changes in intravesical pressure correlated with time. Usually is was possible to control leakage by slight traction on the catheter, bringing the Foley bag into closer apposition to the bladder neck.

Rectal Distention Experiments. A large (no. 26) Foley catheter with a distensible rubber retention bag was inserted into the rectum. Tap water was introduced into the bag in 50-cc increments by means of a large syringe. The bag was connected by a T tube and rubber tubing to the Lewis recording cystometer, permitting continuous pressure records.

Manipulative Procedures Designed to Modify Headache. Elevation of cerebrospinal pressure was studied. Spinal puncture was done with the patient in the lateral-recumbent position. Initially, bilateral compression of the jugular vein was carried out to ascertain the presence of free communication between the intracranial and spinal subarachnoid spaces and the manometer. After headache was induced by bladder distention, the cerebrospinal fluid pressure was increased by connecting with the lumbar subarachnoid space a flask of sterile fluid elevated 800 to 1000 mm above the spinal canal. The spinal needle and reservoir were connected by a three-way stopcock and an intervening spinal fluid manometer. A clamp was released from the connecting tube when it was desired to increase the cerebrospinal fluid pressure rapidly and reapplied when further increase in pressure was no longer desired. To reduce pressure rapidly, the clamped tube was disconnected and the fluid allowed to flow freely from the subarachnoid space. Pressure readings were taken at intervals by means of the glass manometer.

Digital compression of the neck: The effect on the induced headache of part of the neck was studied. Pressure was applied to the point of complete obliteration of palpable pulsations. A 10- to 20-sec period of compression was maintained. Control observations on the effects of digital compression on the posterior part of the neck and mastoid bones were carried out.

Intravenous injection of tetraethylammonium chloride: In subjects experiencing maximum effects from bladder distention, including marked hypertension and severe headache, tetraethylammonium chloride was injected intravenously in doses of 100 to 300 mg. Observations on sweating, pulse, blood pressure, headache intensity, bladder pressure, and cerebrospinal fluid pressure, already in progress prior to the injection, were continued.

RESULTS

In eight patients, all with lesions at or above the seventh thoracic level, bladder distention resulted in sweating, pilomotor reaction, slow pulse, significant hypertension, and severe headache. In seven of these, there developed severe hypertension, the maximum diastolic from 115 to 195 mm Hg (average, 140 mm); one of the eight had only moderate hypertension. This patient, with a lesion at the fifth thoracic level, had a large capacity, hypotonic bladder with considerable leakage around the catheter during experimental bladder filling. Six of the seven with severe hypertension experienced excruciating headache, of 9 plus to 10 plus intensity (in 1 to 10 plus minimal-maximal scale), associated with peak levels of blood pressure; the other patient had only moderately severe (6 plus) headache. The eighth, in whom only moderate hypertension was induced, also experienced headache of moderate intensity (5 plus). In each patient headache intensity waxed and

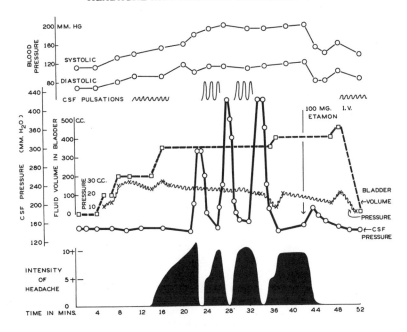

FIG. 8-4. Results of bladder distention in a subject with a complete transverse lesion of the cord at the eighth cervical level, showing effects both of increasing the subarachnoid pressure and of injecting tetraethylammonium chloride intravenously in abolishing the headache induced by bladder distention.

waned in close association with the rise and fall of blood pressure during the phases of bladder distention and deflation. In one of these eight subjects, identical effects, including extreme rise in blood pressure and agonizing headache, developed when the bladder distention experiment was repeated on another occasion (three months later) in connection with a different manipulative procedure, aimed at modifying the headache so induced.

Of two patients with lesions at the eighth and tenth thoracic levels, respectively, a moderate rise of blood pressure in the first and no rise in the second, and no headache in either, occurred with bladder distention.

In four patients without spinal subarachnoid block, in whom severe headaches were induced by bladder distention, raising the intracranial pressure to 500 mm of water by means of intrathecal injection of saline solution abolished headache completely, though all other factors remained constant, including volume and pressure of bladder fluid, elevated blood pressure, bradycardia, and sweating (Fig. 8-4). Such headaches could be repeatedly reinduced in full intensity (during the course of sustained bladder distention and hypertension) by reduction of the cerebrospinal fluid pressure to normal. These pa-

tients had lesions at the fifth, sixth, and eighth cervical and the seventh thoracic levels respectively. In two additional patients, in whom complete spinal subarachnoid block was demonstrated by compression of the jugular veins, procedures identical with those leading to induced rise in intracranial pressure in the four preceding subjects led to no reduction in intensity of headache.

In two of three patients in whom bladder volume and pressure were maintained at high levels, headache was completely and immediately abolished by the intravenous injection of 100 mg of tetraethylammonium chloride, with simultaneous reduction of blood pressure to average, or slightly above average, levels (Fig. 8-4). In one of these patients headache and hypertension returned again to their former high level with the waning of the effect of the drug. In the third patient, headache was diminished in intensity, but not abolished, in association with a slighter reduction in blood pressure. In all three patients sweating and pilomotor reactions ceased. Bladder volume and pressure were not affected by the administration of the drug.

In two patients, bilateral compression of the carotid artery to the point of obliteration of palpable pulsations resulted in the complete elimination of

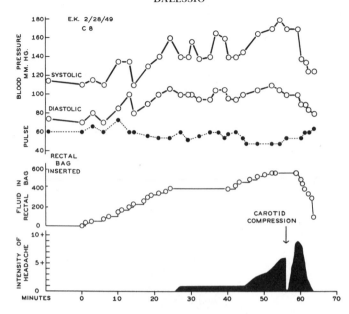

FIG. 8-5. Results of rectal distention (same subject as in Fig. 8-4) with complete transverse lesion of the cord at the eighth cervical level. As in the case of bladder distention, maximal rise in blood presssure and peak intensity of headache were assocatied with maximal rectal distention, all effects disappearing with rectal deflation. The effect of bilateral digital compression of the carotid arteries in eliminating headache is shown other factors remaining constant. Return of blood pressure to average levels and associated disappearance of headache following immediately on deflation of the rectal bag are shown.

headache in each of five trials, its diminution in three trials, and no effect in two trials. Systemic hypertension remained unaltered during compression of the carotid artery.

Of four patients, rectal distention in two (both with lesions of the cervical portion of the cord) led to effects identical with those resulting from bladder distention in the same patients, In one (Fig. 8-5), compression of the carotid artery completely eliminated headache transiently in each of two trials (only one trial shown), without alteration in systemic hypertension. In the other, the intravenous injection of tetraethylammonium chloride (300 mg) resulted in the same train of effects, including fall of blood pressure and elimination of headache, as that described with previous injections of this drug. During both procedures in which headache was eliminated, volume and pressure of the intrarectal fluid remained constant.

Two patients did not experience headache with rectal distention. In one, with a lesion of the cervical portion of the cord, moderate rise in blood pressure (to 160/106 mm Hg), bradycardia, profuse sweating, and pilomotor reaction developed. In a previous

bladder distention experiment on this patient headache developed, but in association with a higher rise in blood pressure (215/195 mm Hg, maximal). In the other patient, with a lesion at the tenth thoracic level, only slight rise in blood pressure (140/100), and no other autonomic effects, developed.

Comment. In these experiments, when the lesion of the cord was at a high enough level, the introduction of fluid into the bladder at a rate more rapid than that at which urine normally accumulates resulted very soon in changes in pulse and blood pressure, sweating and, later, headache, all of which became maximal at the point of maximal filling, but not invariably at the point of maximal pressure. Save for the fact that distention of the bladder and increase in the intravesical pressure led to these effects, there was no intimate correlation between either bladder volume or bladder pressure, on the one hand, and the resulting effects, on the other.

The peripheral and central pathways by which afferent impulses from the bladder ultimately reach effector organs may be analyzed on the basis of available evidence. It has been assumed, since the work of Head and Riddoch (1917), that the area of integration for such reflex effects lies within the segments of the distal stump of the spinal cord. The question may be raised whether afferent impulses from the bladder, via either the sacral roots or the hypogastric plexus, do not pass to the cells of the paravertebral sympathetic ganglia directly to excite postganglionic sympathetic neurons, with resultant sudomotor, pilomotor, and vasoconstrictor effects. This would seem highly unlikely in view of the participation of skeletal muscle contraction in the "mass reflex" of Head and Riddoch. In these experiments powerful muscle spasms of the lower extremities and trunk occurred repeatedly in association with bladder distention, thus indicating reflex excitation of anterior horn cells in cord segments. In addition, as Head and Riddoch have pointed out, stimulation of other receptor surfaces, such as the skin of the lower extremities, leads to a similar mass discharge. Such afferent impulses undoubtedly enter the spinal cord via somatic nerves and posterior roots to produce reflex effects. Lastly, direct synaptic connections between visceral afferent fibers and postganglionic cells in paravertebral sympathetic ganglia have not been proved to exist (when experiments were carried out with unquestionably decentralized ganglia).

Further clinical evidence supporting the concept that the intact segments of the distal stump of the spinal cord are the areas of central integration for the reflex effects initiated by bladder or rectal distention is the failure of occurrence of these effects with rectal distention in a subject who had had ascending myelitis, becoming finally stationary at the first thoracic level. It was evident that the distal, involved portion of the cord in this patient was destroyed during the course of the ascending inflammatory process.

The peripheral route of afferent impulses from the stretched bladder wall was considered by Guttmann and Whitteridge to be in the small unmyelinated fibers of the hypogastric nerves, since it had been previously found that impulses in these fibers continue as long as steady pressure is maintained in the bladder. Since the bladder has a double afferent innervation, an alternate possible pathway is the pelvic nerve entering the cord via the posterior roots of the second, third, and fourth sacral segments. Thompson and Witham found that relatively small amounts of procaine injected into the lumbar subarachnoid space prevented the reflex effects of bladder distention, whereas bilateral lumbar sympathetic block did not. These data support the concept that afferent impulses are conveyed by sacral roots to the sacral portion of the spinal cord with cephalad spread of the excitation process within the intact distal stump to autonomic effector neurons (preganglionic) in the lateral horn of the thoracolumbar segments, resulting in a mass outflow from these segments. As has already been suggested by previous authors, such mass discharges are undoubtedly made possible by the loss of inhibiting influences from higher centers (Berlin *et al,* 1954).

Though the lower limit of lesions of the neuraxis permitting reflex vasoconstriction and hypertension as a result of afferent impulses from the viscera seems roughly established, the upper limit of lesions permitting such abnormal reflexes has not been defined. It has been assumed, since such reflexes have not previously been demonstrated when the neuraxis was intact, that inhibitory impulses from suprasegmental areas prevent them. Whether such centers lie in the intracranial neuraxis, i.e., the brainstem, or in the region of the diencephalon (thalamus, hypothalamus) and basal ganglia, or at still higher (cortical) levels, is not known. In the data presented above, patients were not studied whose lesions were above the cervical level of the spinal cord. Though in spinal cats, just as in spinal man, the blood pressure rises with distention of the alimentary canal, it has been reported that in decerebrate cats the blood pressure falls (Irving *et al.,* 1937).

An opportunity to study the results of bladder distention in decerebrate man presented itself to Wolff and colleagues in a white man aged 24. After a severe craniocerebral injury seven months prior to the experiment, the subject had been under observation in the hospital, presenting a picture of total amentia and incontinence of urine and feces; he required daily tube feedings. He appeared totally unaware of, and unresponsive to, his surroundings. All four limbs exhibited fluctuating extensor rigidity with periodic brief tonic seizures. Fragmentary tonic neck (Magnus-de Klijn) reflexes could be demonstrated. Pronounced pupillary and oculomotor abnormalities indicated a severe lesion of the midbrain. Pneumoencephalography confirmed the presence of cerebral atrophy.

Bladder filling to a capacity of 470 cc and a pressure of 85 mm Hg resulted in a rise in blood pressure from 150/82 to 192/120 mm Hg, an increase in pulse rate from 100 to 130/min, and profuse sweating over the head, neck, and arms. Emptying the bladder led to disappearance of all effects. Thus, abnormal spinal reflexes resulting from bladder distention were not inhibited when the lesion was as high as the midbrain, indicating that the inhibitory centers preventing such effects in the intact subject lie above the level of the midbrain.

The close correlation between induced hypertension and the development of headache in patients with lesions of the cord, along with the occurrence of superficial vasodilatation in the head (skin and nasal mucosa), suggests that the mechanism of such headache is the distention of pain-sensitive cranial arteries. Such distention would appear to be due to the heightened intravascular tension caused by reflex vasoconstriction elsewhere (limbs and visceral bed). The transitory complete or partial elimination of the headache attendant on compression of the internal carotid arteries in the majority of trials supports this concept. The complete elimination of the headache by artificially raising the intracranial pressure in all trials in all subjects when the presence of subarachnoid block did not preclude this procedure further substantiates the proposed mechanism of production of head pain and suggests that intracranial (pial) arteries are the chief site of painful dilatation. The immediate fall in blood pressure and concomitant cessation of headache resulting from the injection of tetraethylammonium chloride would indicate that obstruction of the vasoconstrictor reflex with a drop in blood pressure permits reduction in the degree of distention of the cranial arteries to below pain threshold levels.

Headache with Pheochromocytoma

A 36-year old man, about five years before admission in 1949 to the New York hospital, first experienced episodes described as follows. After eating breakfast and riding to work in the subway the patient became aware of a thumping sensation in the abdomen, following which there would be a dull pain radiating from the mid-epigastrium to the lower part of the sternum. Gradually the abdominal sensation would subside and this would be followed by a blanching of the face and hands and profuse sweating lasting about 2 min, and therewith the onset of a bitemporal headache, which persisted for five minutes. The whole attack was encompassed within 15 min. These attacks would occur three to four times a day, and would be precipitated by exertion such as lifting, bending over, straining at stool, eating heavy meals, twisting and turning the body in a "certain way." They seldom occurred at night. Not all attacks were associated with headache. This symptom was so severe as to justify in the mind of his physician the taking of pills for the headache during the past three years. The headache attacks when severe would involve the occipital areas and sometimes would persist

for hours. A series of daily blood pressure measurements, taken from the right arm, were made from 8/2/49 to 8/17/49 in the lying, sitting, and standing positions. In the lying position the pressure ranged from 130/98 to 100/70; in the sitting from 126/104 to 104/78; and in the standing from 122/104 to 94/68. The patient was observed during one of his attacks, considered a mild one, during which the right-arm blood pressure rose to 200/120. Blood pressure readings at 1-min intervals showed that the level fell to 140/85 about 5 min after the attack. During the early phase of the attack the pulse was slow and irregular: 50–55, rising to about 72 and becoming more regular as the attack subsided. The resting level of the right-arm blood pressure after the patient had been lying quietly in bed for some hours was 140/85. An attack could then be precipitated with tetraethylammonium chloride, and headache along with the other described phenomena recurred for 50–60 min. During this period the blood pressure fluctuated widely, reading as high as 200 mm systolic and as low as zero. This was followed by a long period of hypotension of the systolic pressure below 100 for 4½ hr. At surgical operation an encapsulated pheochromocytoma of the left adrenal gland was extirpated by Dr. Bronson Ray on 8/18/49.

The patient was discharged on 8/28/49. During the subsequent months the blood pressure averaged 125/90 to 120/80. He had no further headache attacks and was free of complaints until May of 1953, when he had a few headaches. These were not associated with alteration in blood pressure. When last seen in April 1959 he was still free of headaches and his blood pressure was 90/60.

Lance and Hinterberger (1976) report significant vascular headaches in 80% of patients with pheochromocytoma. The headache is characteristically rapid in onset, bilateral and throbbing, and almost always associated with paroxysms of hypertension and elaboration of catecholamines. It is presumably related to a sudden rise in blood pressure, as are headaches associated with sexual excitement, fear, and unusual and prolonged exercise. Lance and Hinterberger could not relate distinctive symptoms to the various forms of catecholamine secretion which may occur with pheochromocytoma. Headache occurred in patients exposed to sudden release of norepinephrine, epinephrine, or both substances from mixed secreting tumors.

Severe Headache Associated With Orgasm

In 1974 Paulson and Klawans called attention to a peculiar variety of severe headache which appears to occur in association with orgasm. They described 14 patients seen over the course of several years who had severe head pain, either immediately during or after orgasm. The headache was often behind the eyes, bilateral or occipital, and of varying intensity, though usually rather short-lived. The pain was almost always throbbing. Paulson and Klawans divided the patients into two groups on the basis of the presumed pathophysiology of the headache. Three patients were thought to have low spinal fluid pressure, which was documented in two patients, perhaps due to a tear in the subarachnoid membranes that occurred or was widened during the physiologic stress of coitus. The relationship of posture to pain in these patients was identical to that seen in patients with headache following lumbar puncture, that is, pain with standing relieved by recumbency. In 11 other patients Paulson and Klawans suggested that vascular factors were of pathophysiologic significance. The point of their paper was that the benign course of the 14 patients differed from the usual impression that headaches associated with intercourse result from rupture or expansion of a vascular malformation or aneurysm.

In reply to this report, Lundberg and Osterman (1974) presented a brief study on the benign and malignant forms of headache associated with orgasm. They agreed with Paulson and Klawans that there is a benign but sometimes very troublesome and usually recurring type of vascular headache starting at the climax of sexual intercourse, and mentioned a number of such cases which had been followed for several years at the University of Uppsala. They emphasized, however, that bleeding associated with subarachnoid hemorrhage may in fact occur at the time of intercourse, and described 6 patients out of 50 with headache at orgasm in whom that had occurred. They emphasized that the occurrence of vomiting, disturbance of consciousness, stiff neck, and residual pain the day after the incident characterized the headache caused by subarachnoid hemorrhage and distinguished it from that of benign orgasmic cephalgia.

In reviewing the literature, Fisher (1968) described 66 representative cases of subarachnoid hemorrhage caused by the rupture of saccular aneurysms and in three of these persons the hemorrhage was associated with intercourse.

Thus, it seems evident that there are benign and malignant forms of headache associated with intercourse or, in formal terms, orgasmic cephalgia. In most cases, this is a benign syndrome. However, the alert clinician will be aware that bleeding may occur at the time of intercourse due to rupture of a saccular aneurysm, producing a severe and disabling headache. The subsequent course of the patient should differentiate the benign from the malignant forms of head pain. Where there is doubt, however, further neurological studies are certainly indicated, particularly spinal puncture and/or contrast studies, and a CAT scan.

HEADACHE ASSOCIATED WITH RENAL FAILURE AND HYPERTENSION

Patients with headaches like those described and analyzed may with the passage of time change their clinical state and develop another type of headache in association with their hypertension. Thus, when the patient develops evidence of renal failure, diffuse vascular disease, and azotemia, with failing vision and retinal hemorrhage, the headache may become almost continuous, generalized, and no longer reduced in intensity by getting out of bed, sitting up, or with the performance of routine duties. On the other hand, patients with severe renal disease and headaches may have been free of headaches earlier in the course of the hypertensive disease. Patients with hypertensive encephalopathy constitute a separate group.

In support of the notion that brain edema in some form produces the headache associated with hypertensive encephalopathy is the observation that the intravenous injection of osmotically active agents such as mannitol will reduce its intensity. Oral glycerol is also effective. It is assumed that the headache is reduced in intensity because with the relative dehydration of the brain produced after the administration of mannitol and glycerol, traction and displacement of pain sensitive structures are reduced.

The neurological signs associated with hypertensive encephalopathy are probably related to cerebral vasospasm, which may thereafter produce cerebral ischemia and cerebral edema. The primary therapeutic aim in hypertensive encephalopathy is to reduce the blood pressure, which is the only effective way to relieve the symptoms. Treatment of this condition is discussed in Chapter 7.

Graham (1976) makes the point that headache associated with hypertension frequently appears when the blood pressure is waning rather than at its zenith, so that it often occurs when a person arises in the morning or it wakes him from sleep. He relates this headache to vasodilatation which has been initiated by sudden changes in arterial blood pressure. Presumably the renin-angiotensin system is activated at the peak of blood pressure elevations, and vasodilating prostaglandins may be released into the circulation then, producing the headache. Graham suggests that the management of hypertensive headaches should include the avoidance of unusual fluctuations of blood pressure and the avoidance of hypotensive drugs such as hydralazine which may produce vasodilatation.

Graham and his group have conducted a fruitful long-term study of headache associated with end-stage renal disease which may occur as a course of dialysis concludes (1976). Graham has noted that nephrectomy and/or renal transplant will frequently cure this kind of headache unless the transplant is rejected and dialysis is resumed. In patients with dialysis headache, the head pain is proportional to their hypertension and to the fall in blood pressure occurring during dialysis, as well as the drop in serum sodium and osmolality which are induced by dialysis. As a consequence of these changes, Graham has found low circulating renin and aldosterone levels in patients with dialysis headache.

SUMMARY

1. In headache associated with essential hypertension, the high systemic arterial blood pressure is an important, but not a sufficient condition for the headache. There is, however, a close relationship between the headache and the contractile state of the cranial arteries, mainly those on the outside of the head. When for any reason the smooth muscle tone of the cranial artery walls is low, headache readily results, especially if the blood pressure is elevated. Conversely, when the tone of the cranial artery walls is high, headache is unlikely to occur, regardless of the high level of the systemic arterial blood pressure. The state of smooth muscle tone of the cranial arteries and the level of systemic blood pressure are not closely related. As regards pathophysiology and management, the headache associated with essential hypertension resembles that of the migraine syndrome stemming chiefly from the arteries on the outside of the head.

2. Another variety of headache resulting from sustained contraction of the skeletal muscles of the head and neck often occurs in patients with essential hypertension. It may occur independently of or together with the headache of vascular origin.

3. Sudden major elevations of blood pressure may induce headache in normotensive and hypertensive subjects. These headaches result mainly from dilatation of intracranial arteries. Such may occur in patients with pheochromocytomata, and in normotensive subjects after rapid intravenous administration of norepinephrine.

4. The headaches associated with arterial hypertension in those patients with renal failure, azotemia, brain edema, and increased intracranial pressure result from traction and displacement of pain-sensitive intracranial structures.

REFERENCES

Berlin, L., T. C. Guthrie, H. Goodell, and H. G. Wolff (1954). Studies on central excitatory state. 1. Factors responsible for the variability of the motor response to cutaneous stimulation in human subjects with isolated spinal cords. *Arch. Neurol. Psychiat.* 72, 764.

Fisher, C. M. (1968). Headache and cerebral vascular disease. *Handbook of Clinical Neurology*, Vol. V, p. 124. North Holland, Amsterdam.

Gardner, J. W., G. E. Mountain, and E. A. Hines (1940). The relationship of migraine to hypertension headaches. *Am. J. Med. Sci.* 200, 50.

Graham, J. R. (1976). Headache related to a variety of medical disorders. In *Pathogenesis and Treatment of Headache* (O. Appenzeller, ed.), pp. 49–67. Spectrum Publications, New York.

Guttmann, L., and D. Whitteridge (1946). Physiological disturbances produced by distention of the bladder. *Proc. Roy. Soc. Med.* 40, 229.

Head, H., and G. Riddoch (1917). The automatic bladder, excessive sweating, and some other reflex conditions in gross injuries of the spinal cord. *Brain* 40 (Pts. 2 and 3) 9, 188.

Irving, J. T., B. A. McSwiney, and S. F. Suffolk (1937). Afferent fibres from stomach and small intestine. *J. Physiol.* 89, 407.

Janeway, T. C. (1913). A clinical study of hypertensive cardiovascular disease. *Arch. Intern. Med.* 12, 755.

Lance, J. W., and H. Hinterberger (1976). Symptoms of pheochromocytoma with particular reference to headache, correlated with catecholamine production. *Arch. Neurol.* 33, 281–288.

Langley, J. N. (1902). The autonomic nervous system. *Brain* 26, 1.

Lundberg, P. O., and P. O. Osterman (1974). The benign and malignant forms of orgasmic cephalgia. *Headache* 14, 164.

Ostfeld, A. M., and H. G. Wolff (1958). Identification, mechanisms, and management of the migraine syndrome. *Med. Clin. N. A.* 42, 1497.

Paulson, G. W., and H. L. Klawans (1974). Benign orgasmic cephalgia. *Headache* 13, 181.

Robey, W. H. (1931). *Headache.* Lippincott, Philadelphia.

Schumacher, G. A., and H. G. Wolff (1941). Experimental studies on headache: contrast of histamine headache with headache of migraine and that associated with hypertension. *Arch. Neurol. Psychiat.* 45, 199.

Schumacher, G. A., and T. C. Guthrie (1951). Mechanism of headache and observations on other effects induced by distention of bladder and rectum in subjects with spinal cord injuries. *Arch. Neurol. Psychiat.* 65, 568.

Sutherland, A. M., and H. G. Wolff (1940). Experimental studies on headache: further analysis of the mechanism of headache in migraine, hypertension and fever. *Arch. Neurol. Psychiat.* 44, 929.

Thompson, C. E., and A. C. Witham (1948). Paroxysmal hypertension in spinal cord injuries. *New Engl. J. Med.* 239, 291.

Traub, Y. M., and A. D. Korczyn (1978). Headache in patients with hypertension. *Headache* 16, 245–247.

Walker, C. H. (1959). Migraine and its relationship to hypertension. *Brit. Med. J.* 2, 1430.

Waters, W. E. (1971). Headache and blood pressure in the community. *Brit. Med. J.* 1, 142.

9

TOXIC VASCULAR HEADACHE

REVISED BY DONALD J. DALESSIO

This headache category includes all conditions which produce vascular headache as a part of their symptom complex. The most common nonmigrainous vascular headache is that which is evoked by fever. Generalized vasodilatation may occur as a consequence of any significant fever, usually becoming more intense as the fever rises. In addition, nonmigrainous vascular headache is also associated with an entire series of miscellaneous disorders including such diverse entities as hangover, hypoglycemia, hypoxia, and reaction to medications.

The response of the vascular system to histamine, and the significant production of headache by histamine, is a model for toxic vascular headache, and this subject will be discussed in detail below. An analysis of toxic vascular headache was made possible through the observation that a chemical agent, histamine often given for testing gastric function, produces headache, especially if some of it happens to enter a vein. It has also been noted that in human brains during surgical procedures, and in experimental animals, histamine has the effect of dilating the cerebral arteries. It was postulated, therefore, that there was some relation between this fact and the headache. The headache resulting from such experimental introduction of histamine into the bloodstream is short-lived, intense, and predictable.

THE EFFECT OF HISTAMINE UPON THE VASCULAR SYSTEM

To ascertain experimentally the role of the blood vessels in headache, the agent used to produce pain must not only regularly produce headache in man but must be otherwise completely innocuous; its effects must be short-lived and at least one component of its action measurable. Histamine fulfills these requirements, since its effects on the intracranial blood vessels are predictable, the induced headache is equally predictable, and its effect on the blood pressure and the cerebrospinal fluid pressure is measurable.

Furthermore, it has been observed that after injection of histamine there is an increase in the amplitude of the intracranial pulsations (Pickering and Hess, 1933; Weiss *et al.*, 1932). If this increase represents an increased effect of cardiac systole on dilated cerebral arterial walls, then simultaneous measurement of cerebral blood flow and amplitude of intracranial pulsations should show a relationship. In other words, after the injection of histamine there should be first a decreased cerebral blood flow with but slight change in the amplitude of pulsation, followed by an increased cerebral blood flow and a great increase in the amplitude of the intracranial pulsations. Preliminary experiments on cats demonstrated this relationship.

A needle inserted into the cisterna magna was connected with a Frank capsule. Moving bromide paper in a camera recorded the waves made by a beam of light reflected from the capsule. Through a hole in the parietal portion of the skull a thermocouple was submerged beneath the surface of the brain. A stopper snugly fitting about the connections of the thermocouple sealed the hole in the skull.

It was observed that shortly after the injection of

histamine and coincident with the fall in systemic arterial blood pressure there was a decrease in cerebral blood flow with but little change or a slight fall in the amplitude of the intracranial pulsations. However, with the restoration of the blood pressure there was an increase in cerebral blood flow. Moreover, the amplitude of the intracranial pulsations considerably exceeded their original height.

It may be concluded, therefore, that the increased amplitude of intracranial pulsations after injections of histamine actually represents an increase in stretch of dilated intracranial vessels with each cardiac systole, and that dilatation itself is not sufficient to increase the amplitude and blood flow if there is at the same time a fall in blood pressure. However, vasodilatation plus a normal systemic arterial pressure will cause both increased cerebral blood flow and increased amplitude of intracranial pulsations. These considerations become particularly significant when it is recalled that the dural vessels, the dural sinuses, and the larger pial vessels are important pain-sensitive structures.

The Headache Experimentally Induced by Histamine

Since the increase in amplitude of intracranial pulsations is an expression of changes in pressure in the intracranial and intraspinal arteries, it seemed reasonable to use it as a means of studying the relation of cerebral vessels to headache produced by an experimental agent such as histamine. Information about this relationship has been obtained in human experiments in which, by means of a needle in the lumbar sac, the amplitude of the intracranial pulsations was ascertained and its relation to headache produced by histamine analyzed in the following manner (Clark *et al*, 1936).

Method. The subjects of these observations were patients on whom it was necessary to perform lumbar puncture for diagnostic purposes and several healthy volunteer adults. The results in the former differed in no wise from those in the latter. With the subject lying on his left side, a lumbar puncture was made and the needle connected with a Frank capsule by means of a column of sterile physiologic solution of sodium chloride contained in metal and heavy

rubber tubing. For comparison and in order to obtain a record of actual changes in arterial pulsations, simultaneous photographs were taken of the changes in the pulsations in the temporal artery. For this purpose another Frank capsule was connected with a tambour on the temporal pulse by an air system. The two capsules were arranged so as to reflect horizontal beams of light into the camera, which contained a moving strip of bromide paper. In this way changes in pressure within the subarachnoid space were recorded simultaneously with changes in the amplitude of the temporal pulse. Cerebrospinal fluid pressure was taken frequently by a manometer which could be connected or disconnected from the system by a stopcock. A device recording time at 0.2-sec intervals also made a record directly on the moving paper. Readings for blood pressure were made at frequent intervals.

The camera was started and a record taken of the resting stage in each subject. Histamine acid phosphate (0.1 cc of a 1:1000 solution) was then injected into the median basilic vein of the left arm. The exact moment of the injection as well as the moment of each reading of the blood pressure and each sensation experienced by the subject was signaled directly on the photographic record by tapping the time recorder. The camera was run continuously from the initial resting stage through the administration of the injection and the beginning of the headache and until the headache had completely disappeared. The recorded pulsations representing the changes in pressure in the subarachnoid space produced by intracranial and intraspinal pulsations will, for the sake of brevity, be referred to throughout as "intracranial pulsations."

In 19 subjects the effects of the injection of histamine were investigated. Sixteen technically satisfactory experiments were obtained on 11 subjects, and 14 technically satisfactory single injections of histamine in 9 subjects.

Figure 9-1 shows a series of sections taken from the record of a typical experiment. In I the temporal pulsations and the intracranial pulsations as recorded from the pulsatile expansions in the lumbar arachnoid space are minimal in the resting stage; in II the intracranial and temporal pulsations are at their greatest amplitude and the headache is maximal, while the arterial pressure after a fall has returned to slightly above the original resting level; in III the brain and temporal pulses are subsiding and the headache is growing less intense, while the arterial pressure remains at about the same level; in IV the pulsations are once more minimal and the headache has entirely disappeared.

In Fig. 9-2 are shown the results of continuous

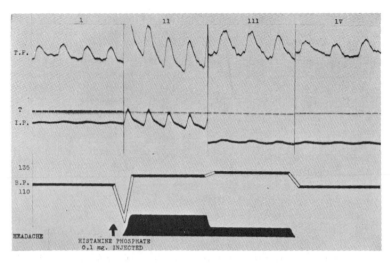

FIG. 9-1. Representative sections from a photographic record of the temporal pulse and intracranial pulsations during headache produced by histamine in a subject, with the duration of the headache, the variations in blood pressure, and the injection of histamine indicated diagrammatically. The time was recorded in this instance on the same line as the temporal pulse.

infusion of histamine. At I is shown the height of the intracranial pulsations before injections of histamine while at II and III are seen the pulsations after the infusion of histamine has started (0.1 mg of histamine acid phosphate per min). It is to be noted that the amplitude of the intracranial pulsations is but slightly increased during the period of infusion of histamine; the blood pressure falls and continues at a low level. The small intracranial pulsations and low blood pressure continue as long as the intravenous infusion persists. At IV, with the cessation of the infusion and the rise in blood pressure, the intracranial pulsations increase in magnitude and the headache begins. It reaches its maximum at V and persists for the usual length of time after histamine has been injected. At VI the headache is disappearing; at VII it is gone.

Great increase in intracranial pressure played no part in the production of the headache following injection of histamine. In fact, the pressure of the cerebrospinal fluid was in no case elevated to more than 300 mm of water, and the peak pressure usually occurred from 10 to 20 sec before the onset of the headache. When the headache was of maximum intensity and the intracranial pulsations were maximal, the cerebrospinal fluid pressure was falling toward the resting level or had reached it. Pickering and Hess (1933) made similar observations and inferences.

The effect of increased intracranial pressure on the headache produced by histamine was ascertained in four experiments on 1 of the 19 subjects by the procedure of raising the cerebrospinal fluid pressure to 500 or 600 mm of water by injection of physiologic solution of sodium chloride into the lumbar arachnboid space. Pickering and Hess's observation that the headache was relieved by this procedure was confirmed, but the relation of the improvement to the amplitude of the intracranial pulsations could not be satisfactorily determined with our technique.

In 3 of the 19 subjects the effect of another important cerebral vasodilator which seldom produces headache was ascertained, namely, carbon dioxide. In one subject, the change in the height of the amplitude of the intracranial pulsations after breathing 5% carbon dioxide and 95% oxygen was in one instance from 3.3 to 4.4 mm (+33%) and in another from 2.9 to 4.6 mm (+57%). There was a sensation of fullness in the head but not true headache or pain. In this same subject, however, histamine produced an increase of amplitude of 100% and at this point definite (although moderate) headache was experienced. With the administration of 10% carbon dioxide and 90% oxygen, the change in the magnitude of the intracranial pulsations was in another subject from 3.9 to 9.3 mm (+141%), in another from 3.4 to 9.4 mm (+170%), in a third from 3.9 to 10.3 mm. (+164%). The feeling of fullness in the head was more pronounced, but headache was

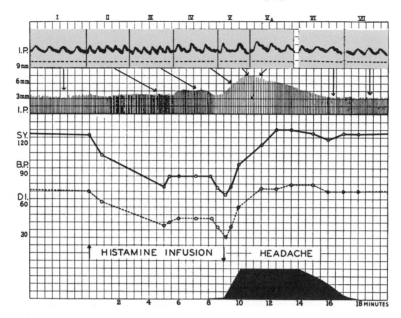

FIG. 9-2. Diagrammatic and photographic representation of the course of events in the experiment in which histamine acid phosphate (0.1 mg/min) was infused continuously during 9 min. Systolic blood pressure is indicated by the heavy black line SY. and diastolic pressure by the broken line DI. At I.P. the variations in rate and amplitude of the intracranial pulsation are represented and the top line I.P. is made up of approximately corresponding sections from the photographic record of the intracranial pulsation. Arrows point from the photographed intracranial pulsation to the corresponding pulsation represented diagrammatically. It should be noted that the slow rate of pulsation during the height of the headache and at the maximum amplitude of oscillation is exceptional to this case. The pulse rate is usually more rapid during the height of the headache.

not experienced. Histamine was not used on this subject.

Clearly the threshold for headache in the first subject (who experienced headache with an increase of 100%) was much lower than that in the second (who had no headache with an increase of 170%). But of paramount importance is the fact that headache did not occur in the first subject with an increase of 57% (carbon dioxide) but did occur when the increase reached 100% (histamine).

Comment. The results reported demonstrate that the intensity of the headache produced by histamine is proportional to the degree of dilatation and stretch of the intracranial vessels and the perivascular tissue. The evidence at hand does not indicate that stretch of the meninges as the result of great increase in intracranial pressure was an important factor in the production of the headache. Pickering

and Hess (1933) drew similar inferences from their experiments and supported this view by showing that raising the arterial pressure or lowering the cerebrospinal fluid pressure during the headache intensified the pain. Conversely, lowering arterial pressure or raising cerebrospinal fluid pressure decreased it; these facts of observation were confirmed by us.

The following explanation of these effects is offered. During the usual state of contraction of the walls of intracranial blood vessels, cardiac systole is reflected as a minor change in the intracranial pressure: the elastic contracted muscle resists pressure changes and absorbs the impact. It has been shown in other vascular beds and can be postulated here that under these circumstances a certain number of afferent impulses arise from the vessel walls with each systole. When, however, as after injection of histamine, the vessels are distended, the number of impulses arising from their walls greatly increases, accentuated with each systole (Bronk, 1935). Moreover, the ability of the now hypotonic walls of the vessels to absorb changes in pressure is much reduced and the variations in pressure within the vessels are thus more directly transmitted to sensory end-organs in and about their walls and to the subarachnoid space. The resulting unusual flood of afferent impulses causes pain.

CRANIAL ARTERIES CHIEFLY INVOLVED IN EXPERIMENTALLY INDUCED HISTAMINE HEADACHE

That the headache experimentally induced by histamine is linked with changes in intracranial circulation follows from the previous comment, but the vascular branches chiefly involved must now be defined. Pickering and Hess (1933) suggested, on the basis of their carefully conceived and conducted experiments, that "the disturbance producing the histamine headache arises in the dura matter" and that "the vessels concerned would be the meningeal arteries." Evidence from the experiments to be presented below would make it seem unlikely that the dural arteries are primarily responsible for the histamine headache. Pickering (1939) seems subsequently to have accepted the view that the distention of pial arteries was responsible for the headache.

In order to obtain further information concerning the contribution to pain made by specific cranial arteries in headache and concerning the nerve pathways that conduct these impulses, the following analysis was reported by Schumacher et al. (1940).

SERIES I

SUPERFICIAL TISSUES OF THE SCALP

The following procedure was performed on 15 patients. All afferent nerves from the scalp on one side were blocked from the midfrontal to the postparietal region with a 1% solution of procaine. This was done by infiltrating the tissues with procaine hydrochloride in a line extending from the middle forehead and temple, extending to the vertex.

Experiment 1. Four subjects received intravenous injections of histamine phosphate, 0.1 mg, immediately after the local analgesia had been produced. The subsequent histamine headache was severe, generalized, and of equal intensity and distribution on the two sides of the head.

Experiment 2. In 11 subjects subsequent injection of air into the subarachnoid space of the lumbar region for encephalographic study was accompanied by headache, which was of the same distribution and intensity on the two sides of the head. The unilateral analgesia had no appreciable influence on the headache of the corresponding side.

These observations indicate that the headache resulting from histamine and from injection of air into the subarachnoid space does not depend on the integrity of superficial sensation.

Temporal, Frontal, and Supraorbital Arteries

EFFECT OF A TIGHT HEAD BANDAGE

Pickering and Hess (1933) reported that in their series a tight bandage about the head, interfering with the circulation to the scalp, did not alter the intensity or quality of the histamine headache. Experiments done in the laboratory of the New York Hospital, however, indicate that some modification in the intensity and the distribution of the headache may occur as a result of this procedure.

Experiment. A sphygmomanometer cuff with a firm bandage fitted over it was applied about the head of three subjects. Histamine phosphate was then injected intravenously, and when the headache had made itself manifest, the cuff was inflated to well above the systolic blood pressure (200 mm Hg). The then tight and uncomfortable cuff caused the histamine headache to be imperceptible, considerably diminished, or indistinguishable from the discomfort produced by the tight band. With release of the pressure of air in the cuff the histamine headache again became apparent and seemed to have its former intensity.

In the light of the hypothesis advanced by Hardy, Wolff, and Goodell (1940) that the threshold of sensation to a given pain is raised by the introduction of a second pain, these data may not be interpreted as signifying that the diminution of headache by a tight bandage is due to the obstruction of scalp arteries, which thus prevents painful dilatation. It was demonstrated by these investigators in experiments on three subjects that if a painful stimulus produced by the concentrated thermal radiation from a 1000-watt lamp was allowed to fall on the forehead during the histamine headache it was possible by increasing the intensity of the secondarily induced pain to reach a level that made the underlying headache imperceptible. In short, a secondarily induced pain of graduated intensity approximating that of the histamine headache diminished the intensity of the latter. This will be alluded to later in discussing which arteries are chiefly responsible for the intensity of histamine headache.

The effect of a tight bandage may thus have two explanations: (1) painful dilatation of scalp arteries is prevented, and (2) what is more likely, the threshold of pain is raised by application of the tight and slightly painful bandage.

DIRECT MANIPULATION OF ARTERIES OF THE SCALP

In order to learn more about the role of the superficial arteries in headache produced by histamine, further experiments were performed as follows.

Experiment 1. In five subjects the effect of manual obliteration of the temporal artery on the histamine headache was investigated. In two subjects the obliteration seemed to reduce the intensity of the headache on that side; in three subjects it had little or no effect. Pressure on the nearby structures had no effect.

Experiment 2. In one subject, the entire frontal, temporal, and parietal areas on the right side of the scalp were thoroughly infiltrated with a 1% solution of procaine hydrochloride, the frontal, temporal, and supraorbital arteries themselves being thus surrounded with the analgesic. This resulted in analgesia over the entire left side of the head in an area bounded by the nose, the ear, and the vertex. Subsequent intravenous injections of 0.1 mg of histamine phosphate produced severe headache in the frontotemporal region, bilaterally, with no perceptible difference on the two sides.

Experiment 3. In four patients ligation of the superficial temporal artery on one side did not alter the quality of the histamine headache on the two sides of the head (see following section on middle meningeal arteries).

Experiment 4. Histamine phosphate was injected directly into the temporal artery in two subjects. In the first subject the agent was injected into the artery through the intact skin; in the other the right temporal artery was surgically exposed and the his-

tamine injected directly into its lumen. The results by the two methods were identical. The observations on the second subject follow.

The right temporal artery, after surgical exposure, was suitably held by means of a ligature placed about it. Manipulation of the artery was painful. Pulling the artery from below upward, while it was being immobilized in preparation for insertion of the needle, caused pain in the upper teeth. When the artery was pulled down from the temple the pain was felt in the temple, deep behind, and in the eye. Inserting the needle into the artery was very painful. The pain that resulted from spreading the tissues in the neighborhood of the artery was also intense.

When 0.1 mg of histamine phosphate was injected into the temporal artery, the first sensation was unilateral diffuse burning in the temporal bone (21 sec after injection). The pain became more severe and was soon of a dull aching nature and more widespread than that due to the puncture of the artery. This sensation was followed by the usual taste (after 26 sec) and then by a slight decline in the intensity of the headache (after 36 sec). A unilateral flush, heretofore barely perceptible, now (after 44 sec) became readily visible, persisting for 3 min. The headache then returned in greater intensity (after 50 sec), to remain unilateral and in the general area mentioned, namely, the temporal and parietal regions. It became a deeper, poorly localized headache, but remained unilateral; it was dull and throbbing, but still not severe. It covered the right temporoparietal region, extending upward about two-thirds of the way to the vertex, posteriorly to the anterior border of the occipital area and anteriorly to the lateral margin of the frontal area. After 2 min the deeper component increased in intensity and was felt also in the frontal region. Most of the pain remained unilateral, but later (2½ min) there was slight headache on the other side. The deep, aching, throbbing pain was still present in the temporoparietal and frontal regions on the side of the injection. The scalp in the region of the injection was "sore" to pressure, and compression of the temporal artery here increased the pain, but reduced it in the remainder of the involved area. The headache was gone 3½ min after the injection.

These experiments suggest that the temporal artery, possibly also the frontal, supraorbital, and occipital arteries, may participate in the headache produced by histamine.

It seems probable from the data presented that the contribution of the extracranial arteries does not determine the intensity of the histamine headache. Though local headache was produced by direct injection into the temporal artery, it must be remembered that a comparatively high concentration of histamine was permitted to act directly on the arterial wall, and that extreme stretching probably occurred. Under such circumstances, an artery known to be sensitive to pain might well give rise to local headache. But during generalized headache following injection of histamine into the antecubital vein, in the absence of such extreme local dilatation of extracranial arteries, it is doubtful whether the contribution made by these arteries predominates.

Middle Meningeal Arteries

Inferences concerning the contribution to histamine headache by pain impulses from the middle meningeal artery were drawn from experiments on seven subjects who had incomplete rhizotomy of the trigeminal nerve for tic douloureux.

In all seven New York Hospital patients the approach to the gasserian ganglion and its root included ligation and section of the middle meningeal artery and destruction, over 1 to 2 cm, of the periarterial nerve fibers. (The fact that "bleeding back" occurred demonstrated that the ligated arteries were subsequently filled with blood). If, therefore, in these subjects there was no difference in an induced histamine headache on the two sides, the inference could be drawn that the middle meningeal artery did not make a perceptible contribution to the pain of the histamine headache. The interval between ligation and injection of histamine varied in the seven cases, but in no instance was it great enough to afford regeneration of the sensory fibers.

Experiment 1. Histamine was administered intravenously. The headache that resulted was equal on the two sides of the head. Moreover, for four of the seven patients the operative approach involved ligation of the ipsilateral temporal artery. As indicated in experiment 3, above, these four subjects did not differ in their reactions to histamine in any way from the others, who had the temporal artery intact.

Though the pain contributed by the middle meningeal arteries is not as great as was first suggested by Pickering and Hess (1933) one may not infer that they are not involved. It is evident, however, that the absence of a pain-sensitive middle meningeal artery on one side does not appreciably decrease the intensity of the headache. Also, the contribution of pain from the temporal artery can similarly be considered imperceptible.

The evidence just presented suggests that the dural arteries are not the major contributors to the pain of histamine headache. It also adds further weight to the opinion previously expressed regarding the minor role of the extracranial arteries. Observations of Northfield (1938) support these views. After injection of histamine into the internal carotid artery in six cases, that investigator obtained homolateral headache in five cases and no headache in one. After injection of histamine into the external carotid artery in six cases, headache was absent in five and was faint and generalized in one.

Effect of Increasing the Intracranial Pressure

The following experiments are based on the assumption that certain of the cranial arteries, by virtue of their location, can be supported extramurally by increasing the cerebrospinal fluid pressure, thereby diminishing their amplitude of pulsation and thus reducing headache.

The large cerebral arteries at the base of the brain, notably those forming the circle of Willis and its branches, are obviously susceptible to extramural compression by increase in cerebrospinal fluid pressure. Extracranial (scalp) arteries, of course, are outside the direct influence of changes in intracranial pressure. The effect on dural arteries will be considered subsequently.

A method has therefore been devised to increase cerebrospinal fluid pressure rapidly by connecting the subarachnoid space with a high column of fluid (sterile physiologic solution of sodium chloride) in order to observe the effect of such increase in pressure on the intensity of the headache. As has been stated, the experiments rest on the premise that reduction in headache by this means is due to increased support of stretched cranial arteries. In headache due to dilatation of cranial arteries reduction in pain would indicate that intracranial arteries are responsible, whereas no change in intensity would bespeak an extracranial origin.

On 13 patients in whom spinal puncture was necessary for diagnosis, the effect of increasing intracranial pressure on headache induced by histamine was investigated.

Severe headache was induced within 60 sec by the intravenous administration of 0.10 to 0.15 mg of histamine phosphate. Such a headache reached its maximum intensity quickly, remaining there for 5 to 8 min in most instances, after which it gradually subsided and was gone within 10 to 12 min.

Method. In the experiments on subjects with histamine headache, the level of the column of fluid was elevated 800 to 1000 mm above the spinal canal. A

HISTAMINE HEADACHE

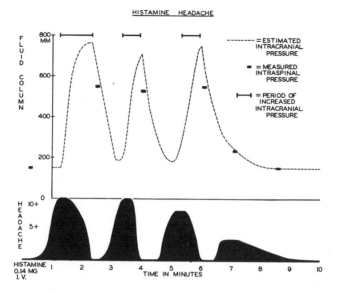

FIG. 9-3. Abolishing effect of repeated experimental increases in the intracranial pressure on a headache induced by the intravenous injection of 0.14 mg of histamine phosphate.

clamp was removed from the connecting tube when it was desired to increase the cerebrospinal fluid pressure rapidly and was replaced when further increase in pressure was no longer desired. To reduce pressure rapidly the clamped tube was disconnected and the fluid allowed to flow freely from the subarachnoid space. Pressure readings by means of the usual glass water manometer were taken at intervals.

Shortly after the onset of headache, and approximately at the time when it reached its maximum intensity, the pressure was suddenly raised as described to 800 to 1000 mm of physiologic solution of sodium chloride. If headache subsequently was abolished the fluid was then allowed to flow from the subarachnoid space until the pressure was greatly reduced. If headache recurred the pressure was again raised until the headache was eliminated. This sequence of events was repeated as often as the duration of a given histamine headache permitted.

Results. Of the 13 subjects, there were two from whom adequate information could not be obtained, owing to apprehension or difficulty in understanding. In 11 the headache was eliminated or grew less when the intracranial pressure was increased. In seven of the latter there was a constant relationship between increase in cerebrospinal fluid pressure and abolition of the headache. In these subjects there was always a recurrence of severe headache following

rapid reduction in pressure. In the other four patients, because of distracting paresthesias or insufficient severity of the headache, the relation of increase in pressure to decrease in intensity of headache was not clearly defined, but in three of the four subjects headache recurred when the pressure was diminished.

In seven headaches induced by histamine the pain was abolished 14 times, each time by increasing the cerebrospinal fluid pressure, and was brought back in every instance by an immediately ensuing reduction in the pressure. In two of the seven subjects headache was abolished once and recurred once on decreasing pressure. In three it was abolished and allowed to recur twice. In two headaches, pain was abolished and reinduced by this procedure three times (Fig. 9.3). Furthermore, in none of these seven induced headaches was there an instance in which increase in pressure failed to eliminate the pain.

The average initial pressure, measured before the headache was induced, was 145 mm of solution of sodium chloride. The average manometric pressure at which headache was eliminated was 480 mm of solution of sodium chloride (with a range of 350 to 550 mm). The average pressure on return of headache was 190 mm (with a range of 185 to 240 mm). Cerebrospinal fluid pressure after each increase in pressure was rapidly reduced until the headache returned to its former severity. The average amount of fluid removed to reach this state was 12 cc (with a range of 8 to 15 cc).

The average time from the moment of increasing the cerebrospinal fluid pressure to the first definite awareness of reduction in the headache was 35 sec (with a range of 15 to 90 sec). The average time from the moment of increase in pressure to elimination of the headache was 70 sec (with a range of 25 to 120 sec). The average length of time required for headache to recur (from the moment that pressure began to fall) was 45 sec (with a range of 15 to 90 sec).

Cerebral Arteries

By a process of elimination it is possible to infer that the cerebral arteries are the chief sources of histamine headache. This view is based, in summary, on the following data which have been presented: (1) demonstration of afferent nerves on the larger cerebral vessels, especially those near the base of the brain (Levine and Wolff, 1932); (2) observed cerebral vasodilatation following injections of histamine (Wolff, 1936); (3) abolition of histamine headache following elevation of intracranial pressure (Pickering and Hess, 1933; Clark *et al.*, 1936); (4) ineffectiveness of blocking afferent impulses from the superficial tissues of the scalp in diminishing histamine headache; (5) ineffectiveness of anesthetizing the extracranial arteries themselves; (6) lack of proof that compressing the arteries of the scalp reduces the intensity of histamine headache; (7) lack of appreciable decrease in histamine headache on one side following ligation of the middle meningeal or the temporal artery, or both arteries, on that side; and (8) development of homolateral histamine headache following the injection of the internal carotid artery.

The evidence thus far adduced indicates that many cranial arteries participate in headache, but that the cerebral arteries are the chief contributors to the pain of histamine headache and determine its intensity. The question as to which cerebral arteries are implicated may now be considered further.

That the circle of Willis at the base of the brain and the proximal portions of its main branches are pain sensitive has been demonstrated on patients during cerebral exposure under local anesthesia. Furthermore, the pain is intense, definite, and constantly localized. The branches of these vessels become insensitive as they spread over the convexity or become intracerebral arteries and arterioles.

Stimulation of the internal carotid and of the anterior, middle, and posterior cerebral arteries causes pain within, behind, or over the eye as far medial as the midline and as far lateral as the temporal region. Stimulation of pontile and internal auditory branches from the basilar artery causes pain behind the ear. Faradic stimulation of the vertebral and the basilar artery and the posterior inferior cerebellar branches near their origin causes pain in the occipital and the suboccipital regions.

The headache due to histamine is distributed to a variable degree in different persons over the areas just described. It is usually worse in the frontal and the temporal region, but sometimes begins in the occipital and the suboccipital area and moves forward. It is to be expected, therefore, that histamine headache arises from branches of several main arteries to the intracranial cavity: namely, the vertebral arterial branches of the subclavian artery; the basilar artery, which is derived from a confluence of the two vertebral arteries; the posterior cerebral arteries, resulting from a bifurcation of the basilar artery; and, finally, the middle and anterior branches of the internal carotid artery.

In short, it has been demonstrated that the arteries of the scalp are capable of contributing to headache experimentally induced by histamine, and that there may be variation in the contribution made by them in different persons, the implication of these arteries possibly adding to the distribution of the headache. Furthermore, evidence has been presented to show that the cerebral arteries are important sources of headache experimentally induced by histamine and that in the absence of pain contributions from the extracranial and dural arteries the intensity of the histamine headache is not diminished. It seems probable that the large arteries at the base of the brain, which include the internal carotid, the vertebral, the basilar artery, and the proximal portions of their branches, are the primary sites of origin of pain in the headache resulting from histamine.

SERIES II

PAIN PATHWAYS INVOLVED IN DISTENTION OF CEREBRAL AND PIAL ARTERIES

In the following experiments designed to demonstrate these pain pathways, headaches were induced by intravenous administration of histamine in subjects who had previously had section of various cranial and cervical nerves. Most of the patients had had partial or complete section of the sensory root of the fifth cranial nerve for trigeminal neuralgia. Others had had section of the seventh, eight, ninth, or tenth cranial nerve. Also studied were patients who had had section of cervical dorsal roots, patients who had disease of the bulb and of the cervical region of the cord, and those who had had section of the sympathetic trunk.

Based on common knowledge concerning the distribution of pain fibers to the skin over the head and neck, the assumption was made that the face and head as high as the vertex are supplied chiefly by the fifth cranial nerve and that the back of the head and neck are supplied chiefly by the second and third cervical nerves. Analgesia in these regions was assumed to be due to destruction of the aforementioned respective pathways or their nuclei. Though other afferent pathways are believed to carry pain fibers from the head, such as the first cervical and the eleventh and twelfth cranial nerves from the occiput, and the seventh, ninth, and tenth cranial nerves from the region

in and just behind the ear, interruption of these pathways did not result in demonstrable analgesia. In these experiments, therefore, anatomic inferences as to which pathways were interrupted were based whenever possible on surgical visualization rather than on the area of analgesia (Ray, 1954).

Pickering and Hess (1933) reported that in normal subjects headache induced by histamine affects both sides of the head equally; this we have confirmed. It usually begins in the forehead just above the orbits, occasionally in the temples, and while remaining maximal there, sometimes spreads over the vertex and frequently into the occipital region as it increases in severity. It may, however, begin in the occiput and move forward (Fig. 9-4).

In this study, subjects with unilateral analgesia were chiefly employed. Thus the normal side served as a suitable control for the abnormal side in each case. Because in the normal person headache induced by histamine was symmetric and equal on the two sides, the following assumption was made: If headache failed regularly to be induced in an analgesic area on one side of the head but occurred regularly in the corresponding area on the opposite intact side, the absence of headache on the analgesic side was due to the interruption of the afferent pathway conducting impulses interpreted as headache in that region of the head (Schumacher et al, 1949).

Method. Areas of anesthesia over the face, scalp, and neck of the subject were carefully mapped out and recorded. Perception of pin prick and of cotton wool was routinely tested, as was also sensation of the cornea. The subject then lay on a stretcher in prepa-

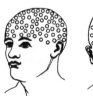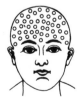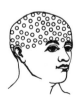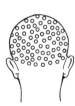

FIG. 9-4. Site of headache, indicated by circles, following the injection of histamine in a normal person.

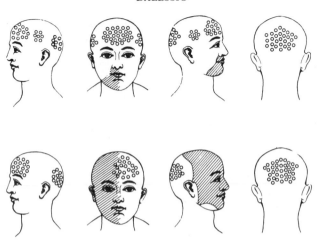

FIG. 9-5. Areas of headache following the injection of histamine, and of analgesia to pin prick in a person who first had partial section and then complete section of the sensory root of the fifth cranial nerve.

ration for an intravenous injection of 0.1 mg of histamine phosphate.

In order to be sure that the cranial arteries were stretched adequately during the experiments, photographic records of the pulsations of these arteries were made during each induced headache (Clark *et al.*, 1936).

Several control records of pulsations of the normal temporal artery with control readings of the pulse and blood pressure were made. After administration of the histamine while the arterial pulsations were being recorded and frequent readings of the pulse and blood pressure were being made, the subject was interrogated repeatedly as to the site and intensity of the headache. After subsidence of the headache, the experience was again carefully reviewed with the subject. In all cases of induced histamine headache, the photographic record indicated substantial increase in the amplitude of pulsations of the temporal artery.

This series of experiments was performed on 20 subjects, who were separated into several groups according to the afferent pathways interrupted. The location of the histamine headache in each of these groups was as follows:

Partial Section of the Sensory Root of the Fifth Cranial Nerve with No Analgesia. In one subject an incomplete

rhizotomy of the fifth cranial nerve had been performed, with resultant abolition of tic douloureux. Subsequently, no analgesia could be demonstrated. After injection of histamine the man had severe bifrontal headache.

Partial Section of the Sensory Root of the Fifth Cranial Nerve with Unilateral Analgesia of the Lower Part of the Face. Six subjects had unilateral loss of cutaneous sensation in the lower portion of the face due to partial section of the sensory root of the fifth cranial nerve on one side, the outermost fibers of the root having been cut. After intravenous injection of histamine all these persons had bilateral headache. In three it occurred only in the frontal region, but in two it involved the entire head (frontal, temporal, parietal, and occipital areas; Fig. 9-5). The sixth patient had headache which was confined to the center of the front of the head, extending somewhat to both sides.

Complete Section of the Sensory Root of the Fifth Cranial Nerve with Unilateral Analgesia of the Whole Face and Anterior Half of the Scalp. In eight subjects as a result of complete section of the sensory root of the fifth cranial nerve, hemianalgesia of the face and of the anterior half of the scalp (including corneal anesthesia) was found. In seven of these subjects, headache was not induced in the frontotemporoparietal region of the head on the side on which the nerve had been cut, but was present elsewhere in the head (Fig. 9-5). In three of the seven it was induced only in the frontotemporoparietal region of the opposite side; in the remaining four it occurred both in the frontotemporoparietal region of the opposite side and in the back of the head on both sides. The eighth subject had headache in the frontoparietal region on both sides, being more severe on the side on which the nerve had been cut.

Pickering and Hess (1933) induced headache with histamine in three patients in whom by surgical intervention cutaneous sensation over the area of distribution of the trigeminal nerve was completely abolished on one side. In all three headache was confined to the side of the head on which normal innervation was preserved.

Northfield (1938) likewise injected histamine into seven subjects who had had complete section of the sensory root of the trigeminal nerve on one side. In three persons the resulting headache was restricted to the forehead and temple of the opposite side and the back of the head on both sides. In two subjects headache was distributed over both sides of the front of the head, and in one of these it was worse on the side of the operation. In the remaining two persons no headache occurred, but in one of these injection of 10 cc of air into the lumbar theca produced bilateral headache in the back of the head, later involving only the front and side of the head on the normal side.

A comparison of the results described by Pickering and Hess (1933) and by Northfield (1938) with those obtained by us in cases of complete section of the sensory root of the trigeminal nerve shows incomplete agreement. In seven of eight subjects in the series reported here headache could not be induced in the analgesic region on the denervated side. Pickering and Hess found this to be true of all their three subjects. Northfield, however, obtained similar results for only three of seven subjects. Of the remaining four subjects, two had headache on the denervated side and two had none at all. The results for the latter may be omitted from consideration on the basis of an insufficient histamine effect; unless a headache is actually induced by an adequate intravenous amount of histamine, it is not possible to draw inferences as to the effect of interruption of a given afferent pathway on the site of headache. Northfield found, nevertheless, that in one of these two subjects headache produced by another means, namely, the injection of air into the spinal subarachnoid space, resulted in pain on only the normally innervated side of the front of the head and on both sides of the back of the head. Thus, in Northfield's series, four of six subjects had no pain in the denervated area but had it elsewhere in the head whereas two had headache also on the denervated side.

In combining the results of our investigations with those of the other workers, it is seen that of a total of 17 subjects with complete section of the sensory root of the trigeminal nerve, 14 experienced no headache in the frontoparietal region on the side of the root section after injection of histamine, though all experienced it in other parts of the head.

Lesion of the Brainstem and Upper Part of the Cervical Region of the Cord, with Hemianalgesia of the Head. One subject had hemianalgesia of the face, forehead, and scalp, including the occipital region, as a result of an injury to the head. The lesion involved, among other structures, the descending sensory nucleus of the trigeminal nerve, including the upper cervical sensory levels of the cord. On injection of histamine this subject had severe headache in the frontal and occipital areas on the normal side but none on the analgesic side (Fig. 9-6).

Multiple Section of the Roots of the Cervical and Cranial Nerve with Hemianalgesia of the Head. Two subjects with extensive infiltration of carcinoma (into the orbit and jaw, respectively) had had several nerves sectioned because of intractable pain. Both had had complete unilateral section of the sensory root of the fifth cranial nerve, the ninth cranial nerve, and the sensory roots of the second and third cervical nerves. In addition, one had section also of the tenth cranial nerve and of the sensory root of the first cervical nerve. In neither was the pain induced by the carcinoma completely abolished. In each pain was present on the denervated side of the head before the experiment was begun. The pain seemed to become worse after the administration of histamine, though the induced headache was felt also on the other side of the head. Cooperation was poor, and the reports were difficult to evaluate.

Syringomyelia with Unilateral Occipital Analgesia. In one patient occipital hemianalgesia had resulted from syringomyelia. After injection of histamine, headache occurred "in the center of the back of the head" and slightly in the front of the head, but was most intense in the back on the normal side. On the analgesic side of the back of the head pain was absent.

Headache following the injection of histamine was absent on one side of the back of the head in two subjects with lesions of the cervical portion of the cord and occipital analgesia (including the subject with complete hemianalgesia of the head mentioned above). This evidence suggests that the cervical nerves are afferent pathways for impulses giving rise to occipital headache.

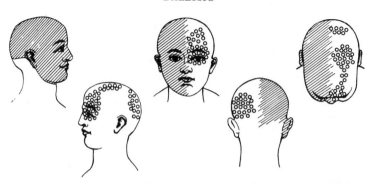

Fig. 9-6. Sites of headache in a person in whom a lesion of the brainstem has produced complete hemianalgesia.

It is relevant to consider further the afferent pathway for some of the painful impulses from the occiput and the posterior fossa. Stimulation of the dural arteries of the posterior fossa, with faradic current, causes pain to be experienced in the occiput. Similarly, stimulation of the vertibral artery and the proximal segment of the posterior inferior cerebellar artery gives rise to pain in the occiput and subocciput. The proximal segments of the pontile and the internal auditory artery are supplied by fibers, stimulation of which causes pain behind the ear. Section of cranial and cervical nerves followed by stimulation of pain-sensitive structures in the posterior fossa indicated further that these structures are supplied chiefly by branches of the ninth and tenth cranial nerves and the first three cervical nerves.

Section of the Seventh Cranial Nerve. In one patient extirpation of an acoustic neurinoma on the left side involved section of the left seventh and eight cranial nerves close to the brainstem. The operation required a transverse incision across the back of the head at the level of the external occipital protuberance. At the time of this experiment the patient had complete anesthesia of the occipital region from the external occipital protuberance to the vertex, left nerve deafness, and complete palsy of the left side of the face. The headache following intravenous injection of histamine was severe, bilateral, and equal on the two sides and was limited to the frontotemporal region.

This observation demonstrated that the seventh cranial nerve does not play a major part in conduction of the pain impulses resulting from effects of histamine on cranial arteries, since severe frontal and temporal headache was experienced by the subject when the nerve was sectioned close to the brainstem. This fact is of interest, since it has been shown that afferent nerves from the pial arteries enter the brainstem through the seventh cranial nerve. Apparently, this nerve is not an important afferent path for pain.

The effect of section of the eighth cranial nerve can be waived in a discussion of histamine headache, since it has been repeatedly demonstrated that no pain results from stimulation of the central end of this nerve.

Section of the Glossopharyngeal Nerve. In one subject the glossopharyngeal nerve had been sectioned as a therapeutic measure for anomalous tic douloureux. After section the patient was relieved of the symptoms and had poorly defined analgesia in the back of the throat and over the tonsil. Intravenous injection of histamine phosphate was associated with the usual generalized headache, which did not differ on the two sides of the head.

It may be inferred, therefore, that the glossopharyngeal nerve does not play a major role in conveying impulses essential to the headache experimentally induced by histamine.

It is, however, impossible to exclude both the seventh and the ninth cranial nerves, as taking no part in conduction of pain, for, according to the hypothesis stated previously, the absence of minor contributions to the headache could not be appreciated if the most intense contribution, conveyed along other pathways, was still present.

Section of the Sympathetic Trunk. One subject, who had had bilateral section of the cervical portion of the sympathetic trunk at the stellate ganglion for Raynaud's disease, experienced severe and generalized headache after injection of histamine. A second patient, who had had bilateral section of the second and third thoracic white rami communicantes, in addition to transection of the thoracic portion of the sympathetic trunk beneath the third ganglion, also had generalized headache after injection of histamine.

Although Dandy (1931) produced termination of severe hemicrania in two patients by resecting the inferior cervical and the first thoracic ganglion on the side of the pain, both Northfield (1932) and Pickering and Hess (1933), on injecting histamine into patients after this operation, found that resection of the ganglia did not modify the usual distribution of the headache experimentally induced by histamine.

The fact that the patients with unilateral analgesia in the occipital and suboccipital regions have less or no pain in these regions after administration of histamine, suggests that the sensory roots of the upper cervical nerves (first, second, and third) and the ninth and tenth cranial nerves are afferent pathways for these sensations. However, section of the fifth, seventh, ninth, and tenth cranial nerves and the sensory roots of the first, second, and third cervical nerves did not eliminate the headache due to histamine or that due to invasion of the skull and dura by carcinoma. Also, section of the seventh or the ninth cranial nerve alone failed to diminish perceptibly the headache experimentally induced by histamine. It is therefore evident that the afferent pathways are numerous, and that to ascribe the entire function of the sensation of headache to one or another nerve is an unjustified simplification.

OTHER HEADACHES RESULTING PRIMARILY FROM DISTENTION OF CEREBRAL AND PIAL ARTERIES

Headache Associated with Infection and Fever

Septicemia, bacteremia, and fever are commonly associated with headache. It is unlikely, however, that the agent responsible for the fever is identical to that resulting in the headache. The most intense, prolonged headaches associated with infections occurring in this part of the world, are those that accompany typhoid fever, typhus fever, and influenza. The headache is dull, deep, aching, generalized, but is often worse, especially at the beginning, in the back of the head. It is increased in intensity by bodily effort. It is often worse in the latter part of the day, especially if the patient is ambulatory, or when the patient is most exhausted or prostrated. The intensity of pain is decreased by manual compression of the common carotid artery. It is not modified appreciably by ergotamine tartrate, except possibly toward the end of the period of the headache.

A 19-year-old laboratory technician, who daily manipulated both murine and scrub typhus virus at her work, entered the hospital complaining of severe headache with occasional fever. Six days before admission she developed a moderately severe occipital headache. During the intervening five days this headache was of increasing intensity, recurred daily, was worse in the late afternoon and evening, and persisted through the night. It was usually absent the following morning. At the time of the headache her face was flushed. The headache was of a throbbing, aching quality, made worse by turning the head, by bending over, or by bodily effort. It became generalized, and was often most intense in the frontal region, especially during the three days before admission. The headache was not affected by acetylsalicylic acid, 0.6 gm but was appreciably diminished by codeine phosphate, 60 mg. The patient had no stiff neck, nausea, or vomiting. She was able to work until the day of hospitalization, and the fierce headache was out of all proportion to the general constitutional symptoms and signs. She had a moderate leukopenia and a temperature of 38.5°C. Two rose-colored macules were found under each breast.

Seven months before this illness the patient had been inoculated with both murine and scrub typhus vaccine. Three days after her hospital admission, or nine days after onset, the headache spontaneously ended, and she became symptom free. Tests of antibody titer established the diagnosis of murine typhus fever.

It was possible to observe in experimental animals, so prepared that the pial vessels could be visualized through a skull window, that the intravenous injection of foreign protein (typhoid vaccine) was followed by cerebral vasodilatation. Such vasodilatation was sometimes, but not always, associated with fever. Because of the use of barbiturates in inducing anesthesia which was necessary to the experiment, fever was inconstantly obtained. No change in the pressure of the cerebrospinal fluid was observed, though sometimes the pressure became slightly higher. The vasodilatation was usually extreme, and it was suggested that headache would probably follow such a state.

Since it has been observed that the fever induced by the intravenous administration of typhoid vaccine is frequently associated with headache or with sensations of fullness in the head, the relation of the cranial arteries to the headache was experimentally investigated in observations on patients who were undergoing fever therapy for chorea or rheumatoid arthritis.

Method. A tambour was placed on the temporal artery, a needle introduced into the lumbar sac, and the pulsations simultaneously recorded as heretofore described. After a suitable control period, during which records were made, an appropriate amount (25,000,000 to 1,000,000,000 bacteria per cubic centimeter) of typhoid vaccine was administered intravenously. If no chill or rise in temperature took place within 60 or 90 min, a second and smaller amount was given. Estimates of the state of the headache, determinations of the blood pressure, and records of the pulsations of the cerebrospinal fluid and the temporal artery were made at frequent intervals throughout the procedure.

Results. Twelve such experiments were performed. Because of the many hours of immobilization necessary for a complete record of the beginning and the end of the cycle of fever and the consequent discomfort to patients with arthritis, ex-

periments completely satisfactory from a technical point of view were not obtained. However, the observations were adequate and consistent and permitted inferences (Fig. 9-7).

Onset of a headache or a sensation of fullness in the head was found in all instances to follow increased amplitude of pulsations of the cerebrospinal fluid and of the temporal artery. Spontaneous lessening of the headache closely paralleled the decrease in amplitude of these pulsations, and as the amplitude of the pulsations again increased, the headache became more severe. With the ultimate decline in amplitude of these pulsations the headache ended. The pressure of the cerebrospinal fluid was at all times within the usual physiologic limits.

Observations of the temporal artery and the cerebrospinal fluid showed that here, too, the spontaneous increase and decrease of the headache paralleled the amplitude of pulsations.

The similarity between the pyrexial headache and those induced by histamine was previously noted. The amplitude of pulsations of the cerebrospinal fluid in headache induced by fever and by histamine was greatly increased, in contrast to that in migraine headache, in which there was no increase in amplitude. Pickering (1933) added the observation that increasing the cerebrospinal fluid pressure by means of a manometer attached to a needle in the lumbar subarachnoid space reduced fever headache.

The fact that increasing the intracranial pressure decreased the intensity of the headache indicates that the mechanism of the headache in fever and that of the headache following injection of histamine are similar, and that in both the intracranial arteries are the chief contributors to the pain. It is likely that the headache associated with acute infections, fever, sepsis, and bacteremia has such an explanation.

Although any fever or infection may be associated with headache, some of the common fevers and infectious diseases that have been linked with severe headache as initiating or accompanying symptom, but that in themselves have no special identifying characteristics are as follows:

Those of bacterial origin include: pneumonia, sep-

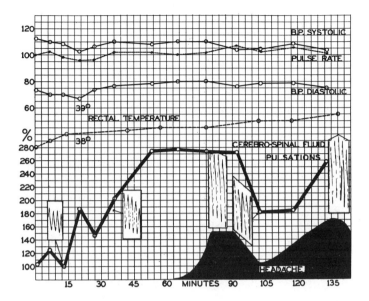

FIG. 9-7. Relation of the headache associated with intravenous injection of typhoid vaccine to the amplitude of pulsations of the cerebrospinal fluid. The onset, increase, and decrease in intensity of the headache paralleled the amplitude of pulsations of the cerebrospinal fluid. A spontaneous remission in the severity of the headache paralleled the decrease in the amplitude of pulsations of the cerebrospinal fluid.

ticemia, tonsillitis and adenoiditis, scarlet fever, chorea, typhoid fever, paratyphoid fever, undulant fever (brucellosis), tularemia, bubonic plague, Haverhill fever.

Those of probable viral origin include: acute coryza, influenza, herpes simplex, measles, mumps, smallpox, poliomyelitis, yellow fever, dengue, rabies, rubella, infectious mononucleosis.

Those of rickettsial origin include: typhus fever, trench fever, oroya fever.

Headache with the attack of malarial fever may be intense.

Accessory evidence that dilatation of intracranial vessels accompanies some acute systemic infections is provided by observations of changes in the force required to produce headache by rapid head movement during the illness. It has been noted, for example, that during a three-week period of recurrent chills and fever induced by therapeutic tertian malaria, the threshold to jolt headache (expressed in g units) fell from a control level of 6.9 to values as low as 1.6 g. This depression of threshold was not entirely dependent upon the presence of high body temperature, for it varied independently of the height of the fever.

Similarly, in another patient, a lowered threshold

to jolt headache could be demonstrated during the first stage of an acute nasopharyngitis accompanied by malaise and lethargy, and during an attack of acute gastroenteritis, also with systemic symptoms, and presumably of the winter viral type.

"Hangover" Headache

It is uncertain whether hangover headache belongs in the category under discussion. The mechanism of the headache that follows, usually the morning after the drinking of alcoholic beverages, is complicated. So-called impurities in alcoholic beverages may have significant pharmacodynamic effects, but their relevance to hangover headache is not established. Although ethyl alcohol causes cerebral vessels to dilate, the period of maximum alcohol concentration in the blood is not the period of headache. The latter usually occurs several hours later when the concentration is lower or minimal. Also, repeated trials with the experimental administration of 60 to 90 cc of 95% ethyl alcohol in our laboratory has not been followed by headache, even in those who often have headache. However, the taking of alcohol under laboratory conditions is quite different from social drinking. The discipline imposed by experimental situations precludes the excitement that accompanies its use in a party setting. Therefore it appears as though the action of the alcohol in inducing headache is indirect. although it is likely that the headache results from cranial vasodilatation. The throbbing quality, the increase in intensity with elevation of blood pressure or sudden head movement, the decline in intensity on carotid artery compression, which sometimes follows the administration of vasoconstrictor agents, i.e., of caffeine by mouth or of ergotamine tartrate by intravenous injection, support this view. It is unlikely that edema of the brain is relevant to the headache.

The common observation that hangover headache is readily aggravated by head movement offers suggestive evidence for dilatation of intracranial vessels as a factor in this type of headache. Accelerometer measurements in one patient revealed that jolts of 4.0 to 4.2 would intensify his usual right temporal hangover headache, whereas on symptom-free days jolts of 5.5 g or much higher would be required to induce headache.

It is suggested that the vasodilator type of headache results not only from the pharmacodynamic action of alcohol and impurities on cranial vessels, but also results from the effects on the subject of late hours, loss of sleep, excitement of social intercourse (talking, singing, and laughing), sustained effort and exhaustion, loss of restraint, and perhaps some remorse. In short, it is associated with psychobiologic factors akin to those operating in certain other types of vascular headaches.

However, since hangover headache is by no means a rare phenomenon and can be produced for experimental purposes so readily, it presents an inviting problem for further study.

It has been demonstrated that oral fructose increases the rate of alcohol metabolism in the healthy human (Pawan, 1968). Mean blood alcohol levels are lower after the ingestion of fructose, using the subject as his own control. Thirty grams of fructose will increase the rate of metabolism of alcohol by 15–30%. No other

sugars have this effect on alcohol metabolism, including glucose, galactose, and sucrose. Large amounts of vitamins including the B-complex vitamins, ascorbic acid, Vitamin E, and the like do not effect the rate of alcohol metabolism in the healthy human. This being the case, it is possible to reduce the intensity and frequency of hangover headache by employing fructose, either therapeutically or prophylactically.

The mechanism of action of fructose is uncertain. However, alcohol dehydrogenase is the rate-limiting enzyme in the degradation of alcohol and this is dependent to a considerable extent on the availability of the hydrogen acceptor, NAD (nicotinamide-adenine-dinucleotide). It is suggested that fructose stimulates the conversion of NADH to NAD which allows the rate of alcohol metabolism to be partially accelerated.

Post-seizure Headache

The headache that follows an epileptic attack with loss of consciousness, with or without convulsive movements, is a generalized, moderately intense, throbbing pain, usually of several hours' duration. It is noted when the patient regains consciousness, is often associated with a desire to sleep, and may be absent when the patient awakes.

The human brain has been repeatedly observed during the convulsive seizure. There may be noted an initial pallor just preceding and during the first part of the fit. However, whether or not initial pallor is noted, the latter part of the fit and the post-fit stage are always accompanied by widespread vasodilatation of cerebral vessels. The dilated vessels are first cyanotic, and then bright red. This bright red dilated phase persists for several hours, and it is therefore suggested that this cerebral artery dilatation is the basis of the post-epileptic headache.

Headache Associated with Hypoxia

Experimentally induced cerebral hypoxemia (Wolff and Lennox, 1930) especially when coupled with an increase in carbon dioxide tension in the blood, results in extreme dilatation of cerebral vessels, notably of the arteries and arterioles. This observation is probably relevant to the fact that some persons at high altitudes (Monge, 1942; Barcroft *et al.*, 1922) complain of headache that persists for hours or days until physiologic adjustments have been achieved, or until the individual returns to a lower altitude. Associated with the intense throbbing headache is a sensation of fullness of the head, hot flushes of the face, photophobia, injection of the ocular mucosa, and deep cyanosis. It is likely that such headaches are due to cerebral vascular distention.

An intense, throbbing headache of hours' or days' duration is a striking feature in persons exposed for a shorter or longer period to carbon monoxide. That the headache is due to distention of pial and cerebral vessels is extremely likely. Thus, hypoxemia resulting from inhalation of carbon monoxide has a dilator effect on the cerebral vessels. When, for experimental purposes, dilute mixtures of carbon monoxide and air were given to animals, and the cerebral blood vessels observed through cranial windows, cerebral vasodilatation and increased cerebrospinal fluid pressure were noted. An increased cerebrospinal fluid pressure in man as well as in animals has also been demonstrated, the result, probably, of vasodilation and a change in permeability of the blood vessel walls.

It has been demonstrated in animals that when after sudden local or generalized cerebral anemia, collateral or generalized circulation was reestablished, there followed an extreme cerebral vasodilatation comparable to the so-called reactive hyperemia of the skin. Indeed, a drop of blood pressure to a critical level, no matter what the cause, resulted in dilatation of cerebral vessels. From these observations it is possible to understand the headache associated with acute cerebral hypoxemia from various causes, such as fall in blood pressure associated with strong emotion or hemorrhage.

In a more recent paper, Appenzeller (1972) pointed out that headache may be associated with acute mountain sickness, acute pulmonary edema of altitude, and chronic mountain sickness in well acclimatized subjects. Altitude headache is uncommon below 8,000 feet, appears with increasing frequency at higher elevations, and above 12,000 feet is more or less universal in persons not acclimatized to altitude.

Altitude headache often appears hours after exposure to low oxygen tension and is not relieved by administration of oxygen. The headache is assumed to be related to vasodilatation and/or brain edema and is aggravated by maneuvers that increase intracranial pressure such as coughing, straining at stool, head jolting, and particularly exertion. Persons with altitude headache are uncomfortable when lying down. Papilledema and retinal hemorrhages have been observed in some patients with acute mountain sickness. Lumbar punctures in 34 subjects exposed to high altitude demonstrated a significant increase in cerebrospinal fluid pressure, and in one patient a biopsy of the brain revealed brain edema (Singh *et al.*, 1969).

Headache Associated with Anemia

Anemia associated with hypoxemia induces headache by causing dilatation of the intracranial vessels. According to J. R. Graham (1959), anemia from sudden loss of blood is more likely to be followed by headache than that due to slow loss; but even in chronic states of anemia when the hemoglobin falls below 7.0 gm, headache may follow. Nevertheless, except in the case of acute blood loss or hemolysis, anemia, with levels of hemoglobin above 11 gm, is rarely in itself the cause of headache.

Hemolytic crises, whether due to congenital or acquired hemolytic anemia, tranfusion reactions, sickle cell disease, Mediterranean anemia, paroxysmal hemoglobinemia, and favus bean poisoning; also, polycythemia vera and polycythemia secondary to hypoxia experienced with chronic pulmonary disease, congenital heart lesions, high altitude, and chronic exposure to carbon monoxide, may, because of the vasodilatation they induce, result in headache.

In addition to the cerebral oxygen deficit caused by the various anemias, similar deprivation occurs in the course of circulatory collapse, impaired pulmonary ventilation, pulmonary infiltration, pulmonary artery obstruction, and shunting cardiovascular anomalies.

Nitrite Headache

The headache experimentally induced by amyl nitrite was studied in five subjects (Wolff, 1929). The inhalation of amyl nitrite produced a prompt fall both in systolic and in diastolic blood pressure. Headache was experienced when there had been a return of the blood pressure toward the previous level, with increase in the amplitude of pulsations of the cranial arteries. The headache subsequently disappeared, with return of the pulsations to the initial level.

Some individuals exposed to nitrites, either as medicament, food or in industry, complain of headache (Evans, 1912; Laws, 1910). Such headaches are of a dull aching quality and are usually acompanied by a flushed face (Henderson and Raskin, 1972). The gradually increasing tolerance to the nitrites of those exposed to them usually results after a time in the spontaneous reduction or elimination of headache. A too-sudden increase in the amount of nitrites absorbed, beyond the tolerance of the subject, is commonly followed by a recrudescence of the headache. Reduction in amount, or withdrawal of the agent, is then followed by recession of the headache. It is reported that the use of vasoconstrictors such as ephedrine and benzedrine has been followed by reduction in the intensity or elimination of nitrite headaches. This statement is difficult to accept without suitable evidence, since, as shown above, even the powerful constrictor effect of ergotamine tartrate is nullified by the nitrite dilator action. Moreover, no control series of subjects with such headaches who received only placebos has been studied.

Headache Caused by Chemical Agents, with and without Anemia Vasodilatation

Chief among these headaches are those caused by carbon monoxide. Acetanilid when used in excess may cause headache by converting hemoglobin to methemoglobin, with resultant hypoxemia. In addition to the methemoglobinemia and sulfhemoglobinemia such as follows the ingestion of nitrates, sulfonamides, aniline compounds, acetanilid, and phenacetin, are those headaches that occur in the acute stage of poisoning from ethyl alcohol, carbon tetrachloride, benzene, arsenic, lead, anticholinesterase, insecticides, and the nitrates including nitroglycerin. Apresoline and thorazine, by virtue of their vasodilatating action, may produce headache in some patients. Withdrawal of agents such as ergotamin, amphetamine, and methysergide from those who have been using them in excess for long periods, may precipitate severe headache.

Headache with Electrolyte Disturbance due to Ill-Defined Factors

Headache may also be associated with states of dehydration and disturbed electrolyte balance, i.e., excess loss of fluid and electrolytes in the course of diarrhea, vomiting, post-operative fistulas, heat exhaustión, diuresis, and removal of ascitic fluid.

Caffeine-Withdrawal Headache

In studies of two subjects, caffeine-withdrawal headache has been shown to have many features suggesting that the pain arises from distention of intracranial, and possibly of extracranial, arteries. Like the headache induced by histamine given intravenously, caffeine-withdrawal headache is reduced in intensity by sustained straining or jugular compression, is readily accentuated by 'jolt' movements of the head, and is eliminated during exposure to centrifugal force of 2.0 g in the head-to-seat direction.

"Hunger" Headache

When a meal is missed or postponed the subsequent hypoglycemia in persons who are subject to vascular headache may induce headache. Headache may also occur as a symptom of impending insulin shock in diabetics and patients with islet cell tumor of the pancreas. Headache as a manifestation of hypoglycemia may be a feature in patients suffering from hypopituitarism, adrenocortical insufficiency, hypothyroidism, and liver disease. Von Brauch (1951) called attention to the fact that headache may occur with hypoglycemic states. An important implication from this and other papers on the subject, is that a serious change in the internal environment of the organism such as occurs with low oxygen, high carbon dioxide, low sugar, or acidosis that threatens survival of the neuron, evokes extreme cerebral vasodilatation. This then becomes the essential element in inducing the headache.

In a small series of subjects, Kunkle and Barker of the New York Hospital demonstrated that there is a relation between headache, food deprivation, the blood-sugar level, and threshold of jolt headache. Food deprivation, either with or without a fall of blood-sugar level, may be associated with lowering of the threshold. Thus, in one subject after eight hours of fasting, the jolt headache threshold dropped from 7.0 to 5.1 g. In another subject, after insulin injected intravenously, when the blood-sugar level fell from 85 to 24 mg/100 cc, the threshold of jolt headache fell from 5.9 to 3.3 g. And inversely, after ingestion of 50 gm of glucose, when the blood-sugar rose to normal (95 mg/100 cc) the threshold of jolt headache also rose to 6.3 g. These data further support the view that hunger headaches stem from pain-sensitive intracranial vessels.

Salzer (1960) who has examined and treated many patients with functional hyperinsulinism, describes a patient who had had resection of the right temporal artery for what was assumed to be a temporal arteritis of two years' duration. She also had had a laminectomy for removal of bony spurs impinging on the second cervical root—all without beneficial effect. A 6-hr glucose tolerance test revealed a blood-sugar fall to levels of 25 mg/100 ml at the fourth hour. The author, unfortunately, does not state if headache was precipitated during these periods of low glucose level! The patient was free of headache after a few weeks on a modified diet.

It is freely conceded that vascular headache may result during some episodes of hyperinsulinism and during the hunger that results from missing a meal. Sometimes under these circumstances there is fatigue, tension, irritability, and mood changes. It is in such a setting that headache of the vascular type or of the muscle-contraction variety may develop. On the other hand, low blood sugar, so-called functional hyperinsulinism, may be but one aspect of a patient's reaction to the difficult situation in which he finds himself and not of necessity the direct mediator of the headache.

Thus, granting that some persons with headache probably do develop a headache with low blood-sugar levels, functional hyperinsulinism still cannot be considered a common primary cause of headache.

Clinical Application. The headaches associated with fever, sepsis, bacteremia, anoxia, nitrites, and convulsions are modified by acetylsalicylic acid in 0.3- to 0.6-gm amounts, and by codeine phosphate in 60-mg amounts, the agent to be used depending upon the intensity of the pain. However, it is obvious that the eradication of the underlying infection is most pertinent.

An increase in the oxygen content of the blood is followed by narrowing of cerebral and pial arteries (Wolff and Lennox, 1930). Hence, the breathing of high concentrations of oxygen may sufficiently oxygenate the blood so that headache due to dilated intracranial arteries may be diminished in intensity or eliminated. The headaches associated with carbon monoxide poisoning and other anoxemias, and the postseizure headache, may be modified by the inhalation of high concentrations of oxygen.

"Ice Cream" Headache

Raskin and Knittle (1976) have noted the tendency for "ice-cream headache" and orthostatic symptoms to occur in patients with migraine. This occurs provided the stimulus is cold enough, prolonged, and applied to the pharynx. Application of similar cold materials in the esophagus or stomach does not cause headache. The pain may be situated at the vertex, is often felt behind the eyes, or is felt in the frontal areas; it is almost always associated with the ingestion of ice cream, hence the name. Raskin and Knittle suggest that patients with migraine are particularly susceptible to ice-cream headache; they imply that this phenomenon is a biological marker for migraine.

Post-Endarterectomy Hemicrania

Leviton *et al.* (1975) have described postendarterectomy hemicranial headache, a benign and self-limited condition occurring in patients three to four days after the operative procedure has been performed. The pain is hemicranial, throbbing, and indistinguishable from the usual migraine episode. It occurs primarily in those who have had migraine attacks prior to the carotid surgery. This disorder is perhaps due to a sudden increase in blood flow through a vascular system conditioned to low flow because of atherosclerosis.

Effort (Exertional) Migraine

Exertional headache is an uncommon disorder in which head pain appears to be related to exertion or straining (Rooke, 1968). It commonly affects men in a broad age range from 10 to 70 years. Almost always, exertional headache is a benign, though disconcerting, symptom. Approximately 30% of patients are improved or free of this symptom within five years, and over 70% are free of headache within ten years. Diamond (1977) has suggested that indomethacin 75 mg per day may be helpful in patients with this disorder.

Jokl (1965) was perhaps the first to note migraine occurring after exercise. His own description of this problem is graphic:

During my freshman year in medical school I ran as an anchor man in the mile relay team of my university and the German track championships of Jena, Thuringia. We won by the smallest possible margin. I was then 17 years old and this was the first time I had been clocked in under fifty seconds. A few minutes after the race my happiness over the victory was interrupted by an attack of nausea, headache, prolonged weakness and vomiting. It lasted fifteen minutes whereupon it quickly subsided. None of my professors were able to explain this episode, nor could I find appropriate reference in any textbooks of physiology or medicine.

Jokl and Jokl (1977) noted several profound cases of effort migraine during the recent Olympic games in Mexico City and described these to the author (Dalessio, 1974). The high altitude was an obvious predisposing factor as was heat, humidity, and perhaps lack of training. Migraine after effort tended to occur with prolonged running rather than sprints. These highly conditioned athletes developed scotomata, unilateral retro-orbital pain, nausea, vomiting, and in some cases a striking prostration.

Summary

The intravenous injection of histamine results in dilatation of the intracranial arteries, which, with normal systemic arterial pressure, causes increased cerebral blood flow, cerebral vasodilatation, and increased amplitude of intracranial pulsations. The intense headache associated with these changes has been studied as a means of analyzing other, nonexperimental headaches. The following conclusions were drawn.

1. The intensity of the headache experimentally induced by histamine is proportional to the degree of dilatation and stretch of the pial and dural vessels and the perivascular tissue.

2. Headache does not result from vascular dilatation unless the intracranial vessels are sufficiently distorted. Carbon dioxide, when used as a vasodilator, is less effective than histamine in increasing the amplitude of intracranial pulsations, and does not commonly produce headache.

3. Headache experimentally induced by histamine does not depend on the integrity of sensation from the superficial tissues.

4. The extracranial arteries play a minor role in contributing to the pain of headache experimentally induced by histamine.

5. Cerebral arteries, principally the large arteries at the base of the brain, including the internal carotid, the vertebral, and the basilar artery and the proximal segments of their main branches, are chiefly responsible for the quality and intensity of headache experimentally induced by histamine.

6. Although there may be other less important afferent pathways for the conduction of impulses interpreted as headache following injection of histamine, (a) the fifth cranial nerve on each side is the principal afferent pathway for headache resulting from dilatation of the supratentorial cerebral arteries and felt in the frontotemporoparietal region of the head, and (b) the ninth and tenth cranial nerves and the upper cervical nerves are the most important afferent pathways for headache resulting from dilatation of arteries of the posterior fossa and felt in the occipital region of the head.

7. The headaches associated with fever, bacteremia, and sepsis; the headaches resulting from carbon-monoxide poisoning; the headaches that follow the industrial and therapeutic use of nitrites; the headaches associated with polycythemia vera, chronic mountain sickness, and other hypoxemias; and probably the so-called "hangover headache"; the "post-seizure headache"; result primarily from distention of cerebral and pial arteries and resemble in mechanism the headache that follows the intravenous injection of histamine.

References

Appenzeller, O. (1972). Altitude headache. *Headache 12*, 126–130.

Barcroft, J. C., C. A. Binger, A. V. Bock, J. H.

Doggart, H. S. Forbes, G. Harrop, J. C. Meakins, and A. C. Redfield (1922). Observations upon the effect of high altitude on the physiological process of the human body, carried out in the Peruvian Andes, chiefly at Cerro de Pasco. *Phil. Trans. Roy. Soc. (London) Ser. B. 211*, 351.

Bronk, D. W. (1935). The nervous mechanism of cardiac-vascular control. *Harvey Lect., p. 245.*

Clark, D., H. B. Hough, and H. G. Wolff (1936).Experimental studies on headache: observations on histamine headache. *Assoc. Res. Nerv. Dis. Proc. 15*, 417.

Clark, D., H. B. Hough, and H. G. Wolff (1936). Experimental studies on headache: observations on headache produced by histamine. *Arch. Neurol. Psychiat. 35*, 1054.

Dalessio, D. J. (1974). Effort migraine. *Headache 14*, 53.

Dandy, W. E. (1931). Treatment of hemicrania (migraine) by removal of the inferior cervical and first thoracic sympathetic ganglion. *Bull. Johns Hopkins Hosp. 48*, 357.

Diamond, S. (1977). Recurrent exertional headache. *JAMA 237*, 580.

Evans, E. S. (1912). A case of nitroglycerine poisoning. *JAMA 58*, 550.

Forbes, H. S., S. Cobb, and F. Fremont-Smith (1924). Cerebral edema and headache following carbon monoxide asphyxia. *Arch. Neurol. Psychiat. 11*, 264.

Graham, J. R. (1959). Headache in systemic disease. *Headache: Diagnosis and Treatment* (A. P. Friedman, and H. H. Merritt, eds.), Chap. 7. F. A. Davis, Philadelphia.

Hardy, J. D., H. G. Wolff, and H. Goodell (1940). Studies on pain. A new method for measuring pain threshold: observations on spatial summation of pain. *J. Clin. Invest. 19*, 649.

Henderson, W. R., and N. Raskin (1972). Hot dog headache: individual susceptibility to nitrite. *Lancet 2*, 1162-1163.

Jokl, E. (1965). Indisposition after running. *Medicina Dello Sport 5*, 363.

Jokl, E., and P. Jokl (1977). Der Beltrag der Sportmedizin zur Klinischen Kardiologie—das Sportherz. In *Altern Leistungsfahigkeit Rehabilitation*, pp. 47-56. F. K. Schattauer Verlag.

Laws, C. E. (1910). The nitroglycerine head. *JAMA 54*, 793.

Levine, M., and H. G. Wolff (1932). Afferent impulses from the blood vessels of the pia. *Arch. Neurol. Psychiat. 28*, 140.

Leviton, A., L. Caplan, and E. Salznan (1975). Severe headache after carotid endarterectomy. *Headache 15*, 207-210.

Monge, C. (1942). Life in the Andes and chronic mountain sickness. *Science 95*, 79.

Northfield, D. W. C. (1938). Some observations on headache. *Brain 61*, 133.

Pawan, G. L. S. (1968). Vitamins, sugars, and ethanol metabolism in man. *Nature 220*, 374.

Pickering, G. W. (1939). Experimental observations on headache. *Brit. Med. J. 1*, 4087.

Pickering, G. W., and W. Hess (1933). Observations on the mechanism of headache produced by histamine. *Clin. Sci. 1*, 77.

Raskin, N. H., and S. C. Knittle (1976). Ice cream headache and orthostatic symptoms in patients with migraine. *Headache 16*, 222-225.

Ray, B. S. (1954). The surgical treatment of headache and atypical neuralgia. *J. Neurosurg. 2*, 596.

Rooke, E. D. (1968). Benign exertional headache. *Med. Clin. North Am. 52*, 801-808.

Salzer, H. M. (1960). Cephalgia; questions and answers. *JAMA 173*, 146.

Singh, I., P. Khanna, and M. G. Srivastava, (1969). Acute mountain sickness. *New Eng J. Med. 280*, 175-184.

Schumacher, G. A., B. S. Ray, and H. G. Wolff (1940). Experimental studies on headache. Further analysis of histamine headache and its pain pathways. *Arch. Neurol. Psychiat. 44*, 701.

von Brauch, F. (1957). Hypoglycemic headache. *Dtsch. Med. Wochenschr. 76*, 828.

Weiss, S., G. P. Robb, and L. B. Ellis (1932). The systemic effects of histamine in man, with special reference to the responses of the cardiovascular system. *Arch. Intern. Med. 49*, 360.

Wolff, H. G. (1929). The cerebral circulation: 11a. The action of acetylcholine. 11b. The action of the extract of the posterior lobe of the pituitary gland. 11c. The action of amyl nitrite. *Arch. Neurol. Psychiat. 22*, 686.

Wolff, H. G. (1936). The cerebral circulation. *Physiol. Rev. 16*, 545.

Wolff, H. G. (1938). Headache and cranial arteries. *Trans. Assoc. Am. Physicians 53*, 193.

Wolff, H. G., and W. G. Lennox (1930). Cerebral circulation: 12. The effect on pial vessels of variations in the oxygen and carbon dioxide content of the blood. *Arch. Neurol. Psychiat. 23*, 1097.

10

CRANIAL ARTERITIS

REVISED BY DONALD J. DALESSIO

Inflammation of cranial arteries occurs in two varieties of syndromes: (1) that in which the cranial arteritis is but part of a widespread vascular disease; (2) that in which the cranial arteritis is the only arterial disease. The headache phenomena are identical in both, and distinction between them rests on the concomitant presence or absence of systemic arterial disease of inflammatory nature.

Polyarteritis nodosa is the prototype of widespread vascular disease which also involves cranial arteries. So-called *temporal arteritis,* or *cranial arteritis,* or *giant cell arteritis* is usually but not always limited to the head and neck.

Of the three terms used to describe this syndrome, the most descriptive is giant cell arteritis, which is probably employed least. Temporal arteritis is in fact misleading, since it implies localization of the inflammatory process to the superficial temporal arteries, whereas in the usual case the disease is widespread. We will employ the term *cranial arteritis* in this chapter. See also Chapter 12, p. 278.

In polyarteritis nodosa, there are multiple areas of arterial necrosis and inflammation affecting many organs. The arterial lesion appears to be identical to that found in serum sickness. Gamma globulin may be identified in areas of fibrinoid necrosis. The role of gamma globulin in the production of the arterial lesion is the subject of intensive investigation. Gocke *et al.* (1970) describe four of eleven patients with biopsy proven polyarteritis who were found to have Australian antigenemia, suggesting that an immunological reaction to a

virus or virus-like partical produced the systemic vasculitis. Circulating immune complexes composed of Australian antigen and immunoglobulin were found in three of these patients. Studies of tissue from one patient showed deposition of Australian antigen, IgM, and β_1C in blood vessel walls.

Much of headache pain relates to anatomical changes in blood vessels. In particular, arterial inflammation is sometimes painful, and angiitis occurs as a frequent complication of immunological disorders (Table 10-1).

Headache is especially associated with polyarteritis nodosa and cranial arteritis. Headache is not characteristic of systemic

TABLE 10-1 Immunological Diseases Frequently Complicated by Angiitis

Polyarteritis nodosa (periarteritis nodosa)
Cranial arteritis (temporal arteritis)
Connective tissue disease (collagen disease)
    associated with:
  rheumatoid arthritis
  scleroderma
  poly- and dermatomyositis
  rheumatic fever
  erythema nodosum
  Sjogren's syndrome
Hypersensitivity angiitis
  drug reaction
  Henoch-Schonlein purpura
  systemic lupus erythematosus (SLE)
  mixed cryoglobulinemia
  Goodpasture's syndrome
  hypergammaglobulinemic purpura
  C2 deficiency with vasculitis
  Australian antigenemia with vasculitis

lupus erythematosus (SLE) unless diffuse involvement of the nervous system is present (Atkinson and Appenzeller, 1975).

THE EXTRACRANIAL BLOOD VESSELS AS PAIN-SENSITIVE STRUCTURES

It has long been observed that persons with certain headaches have distended, tender scalp arteries. Furthermore, from the earliest days such arteries have been more or less successfully resected for the relief of intractable pain. Headache from vascular structure on the outside of the cranium may be of high intensity and, even more important, such headache is exceedingly common. The focus of the ensuing discussion will, therefore, be upon these pain-sensitive extracranial structures.

The effects of traction on and dilatation of the intracranial blood vessels in producing pain have been demonstrated by Ray and Wolff in the series of experiments reported in Chapter 3. That the extracranial vessels are also sensitive to pain has been shown by the same investigators in a further series of experiments associated with operative procedures (Ray and Wolff, 1945). Their observations are as follows:

Scalp, Galea, Fascia, and Muscle. One-hundred fifty observations were made on 30 subjects.

The skin of the scalp was sensitive to all the usual forms of thermal, chemical, mechanical, and electrical stimulation. The galea was sensitive to pain but otherwise insensitive. Where the blood vessels were in close contact with the galea there was usually greater sensitivity to pain than at other places. The fascia covering the temporal and occipital muscles and also the muscles themselves were everywhere sensitive to pain. The pain arising in all these structures was usually experienced somewhere near the region of the stimulus.

Extracranial Arteries and Veins. All the arteries of the scalp were found to be sensitive to pain, whereas the veins were much less so or not at all (Fig. 10-1). The principal extracranial artery is the superficial temporal, which is a branch of the external carotid artery and supplies the larger portion of the parietal region. The sup-

raorbital and the frontal arteries are branches of the ophthalmic artery (itself a branch of the internal carotid artery) and supply the frontal region. The occipital arteries and the post-auricular arteries are branches of the external carotid artery and supply the occipital and suboccipital regions. There are veins corresponding to each of these main arteries. By various methods it was demonstrated that the main trunks of all of these arteries were sensitive to pain. The stimuli employed included faradic current, burning, distending, stretching, and crushing (temporal artery, 6 subjects, 24 observations; occipital artery, 5 subjects, 20 observations; frontal and supraorbital arteries, 2 subjects, 8 observations).

Stimulation of two different points 3 cm or more apart caused pain that was localized at slightly different sites. Charts of the observations showed that in each instance the pain was felt in the general region of the point of stimulation and that stimulation of both points at once produced pain over a larger area than a combination of the two painful areas produced previously (Fig. 10-2).

Distention of an artery by stretching its walls with the spread of a clamp inside its lumen elicited pain, and an intermittent pain followed alternate spreading and closing of the clamp. Distention was effected in still another way, by means of three fine silk threads attached to the wall of the temporal artery and so spaced in relation to each other that when they were pulled simultaneously the temporal artery was distended without interference with the blood flow. Passing the fine curved needles through the outer layers of the arterial wall produced no sensation. Gentle pressure likewise was not perceived, although pinching was associated with pain. It was observed that distention induced by pulling the three threads simultaneously, produced a well-localized pain in the temporal region, in an area about 5 cm in diameter. The pain was aching, persisted as long as distention was maintained, and promptly ceased when it was discontinued. Repeatedly and rhythmically distending and collapsing the artery gave a throbbing quality to the headache. When the threads were applied in the aforementioned manner in two places, one

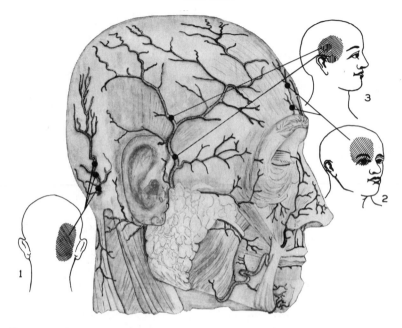

FIG. 10-1. The arteries of the scalp; indicates the point of stimulation causing pain. The diagrams show the area of pain following stimulation of (1) the occipital arteries; (2) the supraorbital and frontal arteries; and (3) the superficial temporal artery.

nearer the ear and one about 1.5 cm farther toward the temporal region, distention by pulling on either group of threads produced pain similar to that just described, but the areas of discomfort were separately located, the one nearer the ear and the other over the temple. When the two groups were pulled simultaneously, so that distention occurred at two separate sites, the ache seemed to be more widespread than the sum of the two painful areas produced previously, and the headache then seemed to reach from the front of the ear to the middle of the supraorbital ridge. The headache resulting from this distention was associated with a feeling of nausea or sickness. Longitudinal stretch of an artery was painful in the same manner as the lateral stretch of distention.

Constriction of the lumen was not painful. The repeated application of epinephrine to exposed and otherwise pain-sensitive arteries caused vigorous constriction of the vessels but no pain. Crushing and stroking of the arterial wall always resulted in pain.

In all such experiments no procaine hy-

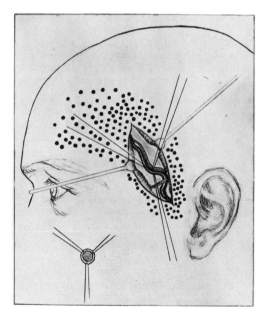

FIG. 10-2. Traction sutures symmetrically placed in the wall of the superficial temporal artery. The mechanical distention of the artery resulting from simultaneous traction on all three sutures caused pain in the dotted area.

drochloride was employed in the region about the artery. The introduction of procaine hydrochloride into the adventitia of the temporal artery immediately produced anesthesia to all stimuli a few centimeters distal to the point of injection. The implication is that the sensory nerve supply originates near, and travels along with, the arteries. It should be pointed out that sometimes a number of small visible nerves were seen passing along the course of these arteries, and this was particularly true of the supraorbital and occipital arteries. To be sure, direct stimulation of these nerves was painful, but the tests referred to were all on the artery itself after it had been separated from any visible adjacent nerve trunk. Since the temporal artery has a rich anastomosis with the supraorbital and frontal arteries anteriorly and the occipital arteries posteriorly, there is reason to assume that there is also a free overlapping of the nerves supplying these vessels. Hence, even when the nerve supply of the temporal artery was blocked in the temporal region, if one of the main branches of this artery was traced far enough anteriorly or posteriorly it was again found to be sensitive, presumably because of an additional nerve supply from these areas.

The anterior and posterior arteries of the scalp, that is, the frontal, supraorbital, postauricular, and occipital arteries, were found to be sensitive to crushing, burning, and stretching, just as were the temporal arteries.

To summarize, all of the arteries of the scalp have been found to be sensitive to pain. Distention of a scalp artery by stretching its walls will elicit pain, but constriction of the lumen of the artery has not been found to be painful. The introduction of procaine into the adventitia of the temporal artery has produced anesthesia to all stimuli distal to the point of injection. This implies that the sensory nervous supply of the artery originates near and travels along with the arterial trunk.

PATHOGENESIS OF CRANIAL ARTERITIS

Cranial arteritis is a rare, febrile, usually self-limited disease of variable duration and unknown etiology. It afflicts the aged of both sexes and is characterized by painful inflammation of the cranial arteries and the general systemic signs and symptoms of malaise, weight loss, anorexia, fever, sweating, and weakness.

Symptomatology

The symptomatology of the disease may be divided into the nonspecific complaints of a generalized systemic nature, and specific complaints directly attributable to inflammation and distention of the temporal and other arteries.

Not all patients with cranial arteritis have headache, but when present, the headache is of high intensity, of a deep aching quality, throbbing in nature, and persistent. In addition to the aching and throbbing, there is often a burning component, unlike most other vascular headaches. The headache is slightly worse when the patient lies flat in bed, and is diminished in intensity by the upright or half upright position. It is somewhat reduced in intensity by digital pressure on the common carotid artery on the affected side and is made worse by stooping over. There is hyperalgesia of the scalp, and the distended arteries are extremely tender, so that any pressure greatly increases the pain.

Some patients may suffer pain on mastication, and in some it may be the initial symptom. Facial swelling and redness of the skin overlying the temporal arteries, with the addition of the burning component of pain, are usually noted after the onset of headache. Immediate relief from burning pain and headache may follow biopsy of the inflamed temporal artery, and it is assumed that this follows the interruption of the afferents for pain about the vessel.

Prior to the onset of the full-blown picture of cranial arteritis, there is often pain in the teeth, ear, jaw, zygoma and nuchal region, and occiput. The distribution of these symptoms suggests primary involvement of other branches of the external carotid artery, notably the external and internal maxillary arteries.

Other arteries may also be involved, including the major vessels of the aorta, the coronaries, and the arteries of the limbs. Large- and medium-sized arteries are the principal sites of the inflammatory process.

Aneurysm formation may occur in association with the arteritis.

OCULAR SYMPTOMS

The presenting complaint may be of ocular symptoms (Russell, 1959). It has become evident that more than a third of patients with cranial arteritis are threatened with partial or even complete loss of vision. Diplopia and photophobia have been noted, ophthalmoscopic evidence of occlusion of the central retinal artery has been apparent in some cases, and many cases with complete loss of vision have been reported (Crompton, 1909).

CEREBRAL SYMPTOMS

Some patients have presented signs suggestive of cerebral damage and encephalitis (1940) during the acute stage of the illness, and Sprague (Heptinstall *et al.*, 1954) and MacKenzie (1940) report that their patient was considered by his intimates never to have recovered fully from his symptoms of lethargy and mental retardation. Mental sluggishness, dizziness, vomiting, dysarthria, stroke, delirium, and even coma have been described.

Enzmann and Scott (1977) describe two cases of giant cell arteritis with involvement of intracranial arteries. In addition to the usual constitutional symptoms of weight loss, anorexia, low-grade fever, and headache, their patients also demonstrated lethargy, depression, and cranial nerve palsies. One developed a left hemiparesis and the second became stuporous and died, presumably of the disease. Angiograms demonstrated marked irregularity of the arteries, presumably associated with the inflammatory changes, with localized narrowing and dilatation of the arterial lumens. These changes are nonspecific but the authors suggest that if intracranial giant cell arteritis is suspected, angiography may be a worthwhile diagnostic procedure.

OTHER SYMPTOMS

In every case there have been signs and symptoms that cannot be plausibly related to sterile inflammation of the temporal arteries alone, and are more suggestive of systemic arteritis.

Prevalent symptoms and signs are: weight loss, anorexia, general malaise, fever, sweating, and weakness. The weight loss may be profound (30 lb.), and the patient emaciated. This is probably secondary to anorexia, which, while in certain cases a concomitant of the excrutiating pain and headache, may antedate the onset of pain. Sweating is a common symptom.

Inconstant low-grade fever unassociated with shaking chills is recorded in 70% of the cases. The average temperature is 37.8°C, although recordings as high as 39.5° have been made.

Other complaints of a nonspecific nature are weakness, lassitude, malaise and "grippy feelings," and fatigue (occasionally to the point of prostration).

Laboratory Findings

A constant finding is a moderate leukocytosis ranging from 7500 to 14,500 and averaging 12,000 to 13,000. Eosinophilia is rarely seen.

In addition to elevated sedimentation rates, characteristically patients with cranial arteritis have a mild to severe anemia, elevation in the fibrinogen levels in the serum, a slight decrease in albumin on protein electrophoresis, and elevations of the alpha$_2$ globulins, Serum iron and iron saturation are characteristically low, though normal to increased iron stores are present in the bone marrow. Muscle enzyme determinations and tests for rheumatoid factors are usually negative.

Serum haptoglobin values are over 200 mg/100 ml in almost all cases, and beta globulins are frequently elevated (Wadman and Werner, 1972). Liver function studies show significant elevation of serum alkaline phosphatase in more than half of personally observed cases. Elevations are common in serum transaminase values, both SGOT and SGPT. The bromsulphalein test is consistently elevated.

In several cases percutaneous liver biopsies have been performed. Not infrequently there is stasis in the fine bile ducts with intracellular deposition of bile pigment, characteristic of cholestasis. In one personally observed case, in addition to cholestasis, a granuloma was present in the biopsy specimen.

Biopsy Findings

In cranial arteritis the involved arteries are grossly seen as tortuous, swollen, nodular vessels with or without pulsation, with cellulitis of contiguous tissue. Biopsies of temporal arteries have been performed in more than half of the cases reported, and some patients have come to autopsy. Microscopic examination reveals a panarteritis. The typical section reveals hypertrophy of the intima, medial necrosis associated with the formation of granulomatous tissue and the presence of foreign body giant cells, periarterial cellular infiltration, and thrombus formation (Figs. 10-3, 10-4). Eosinophilic invasion of the artery in cranial arteritis is rare. The presence of giant cells has suggested a tuberculous etiology, but no tubercules have been seen and no acid-fast bacilli have been demonstrated.

Consecutive biopsies on three cranial arteritis patients were studied by electron microscopy by Kuwabara and Reinecke (1970). All biopsies showed a combination of pathologic changes of various stages of the disease with confirmation of the smooth muscle cell involvement. Biopsies obtained in the clinically acute periods showed predominantly inflammatory elements. Later biopsies from the same patients showed granulomatous reactions and muscular regeneration.

Klein *et al.* (1976) called attention to the intermittency of pathological changes (skip lesions) which may occur in cranial arteritis. They identified skip lesions in 17 of 60 patients with temporal arteritis, based on a retrospective and prospective examination of temporal artery biopsy speciments. Examining more than 6,000 serial sections of arteries from patients with skip lesions, they found foci of arteritis as short as 330 mm in length in an otherwise normal biopsy specimen. Their study suggests the need to biopsy long segments of the artery, to examine multiple his-

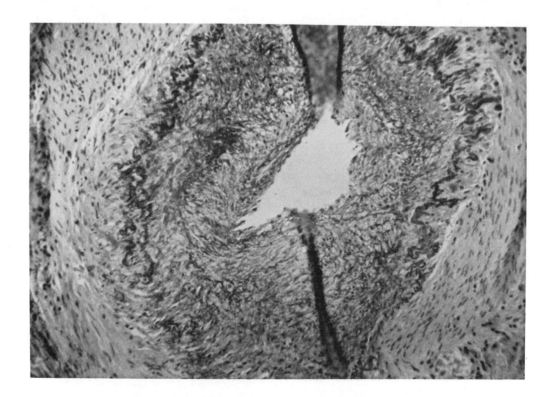

FIG. 10-3. Temporal arteritis. Section of a biopsy of temporal artery showing acute inflammatory cells and giant cells. H & E stain.

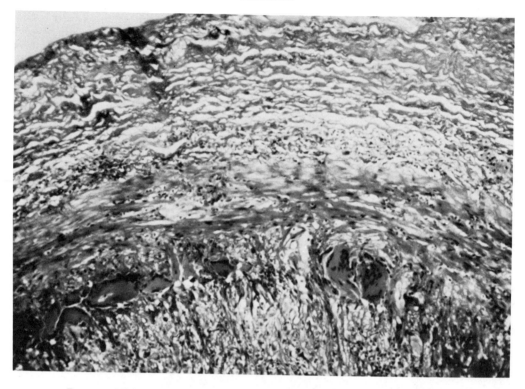

FIG. 10-4. Higher power view of Fig. 10-3, graphically demonstrating the giant cells.

tologic sections, and perhaps to consider performing a contralateral temporal artery biopsy
when frozen section examination of the first
side is normal.

Lie, Brown, and Carter (1970) made a study
of 150 temporal arteries from cadavers and
described senile changes in these arteries occurring with advancing age. There was progressive intimal thickening and alteration of
the internal elastic lamina from infancy to senil-
ity without development of atheroma.

Senile changes in temporal arteries are not
associated with giant cell reaction and should
not be confused with the active phase of cranial
arteritis. The residual changes of cranial arteritis which may persist for many years are
sufficiently different from the ordinary
changes of senescence to enable one to distinguish between the senescent arteries and the
arteries previously involved with the inflam-

matory reaction characteristic of temporal
arteritis.

Postmortem examination carried out by Cooke *et
al.* (1946) on two cases disclosed the characteristic
histologic picture occurring not only in temporal
arteries, but also in the aorta, radial, subclavian,
femoral, coronary, renal, retinal, celiac, and mesenteric arteries, indicating the more generalized
character of the disease, at least in some of those who
die. Andersen described a patient who had glaucoma
as an early manifestation of the disturbance in cranial circulation.

Hollenhorst *et al.* (1960), have reported on 175
patients with cranial arteritis who were seen at the
Mayo Clinic between 1931 and 1959. There were 95
women and 80 men. Seven patients were age 50 to 59
and the rest were 60 years or older. Some form of
ocular involvement resulted from temporal arteritis
in 102 patients; 73 patients (42%) had lost part or all
of their vision permanently at the time of their
discharge from the clinic, and 22 (12%) had diplopia.

Eighty-eight patients were seen in consultation by a neurologist because of headaches, blindness, and other symptoms that often suggested the presence of an intracranial lesion. The results of neurological examination were normal in 69 of the 88 patients, and abnormal in 19. If one excludes paresis of the ocular muscles, the incidence of objective neurological or electroencephalographic findings was exceedingly low; the abnormalities that were present probably resulted from involvement of the intracranial arteries and the arteries coming off the aortic arch.

ETIOLOGY AND PROGNOSIS

The majority of patients suffering from cranial arteritis present evidence, by sign and symptom, of a generalized, debilitating, subacute disease. And to this extent the condition superficially resembles generalized, inflammatory diseases of blood vessels such as polyarteritis and disseminated lupus. With rare exception, however, those diseases are progressive and unremitting processes that terminate fatally. It can be said with reasonable certainty that most cases of cranial arteritis have shown recovery despite the advanced ages of the persons affected, and that any residual damage is secondary to thrombosis of the branches of the carotid, and not the result of continued, active inflammation of a polyarteritic nature. Furthermore, in patients with cranial arteritis there is no impairment in visceral circulatory function such as has been noted in polyarteritis nodosa.

Cranial arteritis is usually a self-limiting disease of from several to many months' duration which may be attended by relapse, but which is apparently nonfatal. With the exception of visual defects secondary to arterial occlusion, recovery is often complete. The course of the illness is affected by treatment, and relief has followed arterial biopsy in a few cases (Scott and Maxwell, 1941).

In patients who suffer visual loss, recovery of this function did not always occur, and, as noted above, patients may incur permanent cerebral damage during the acute illness.

In 11 of the 21 cases studied by Wolff and colleagues there were signs, symptoms, or other evidence of preceding or concomitant infection in the head. Seven cases presented evidence of periapical tooth or other mouth infection. One patient recovered soon after tooth extraction (Horton, 1937), whereas another showed a recrudescence of symptoms following removal of three diseased teeth. In two patients large tender cervical lymph nodes were noted during the period of arteritis.

IMMUNOLOGIC STUDIES

Liang *et al.* (1974) performed immunofluorescent studies on 15 consecutive temporal artery biopsy specimens and on control specimens obtained from 10 patients with unrelated diseases. They found four different patterns of immunoglobulin deposition. Immunoglobulins were prominent in nuclei outlined by cytoplasmic staining, and were also at the disrupted internal elastic membrane, in 7 of 15 patients. These patterns were not present in the 10 control temporal artery specimens obtained at autopsy. The authors suggest that the cytoplasmic staining for IgG, IgM, IgA, and the third component of complement resulted from phagocytosis of antibodies, complexed with antigen and complement within the vessel wall. They suggest further that the elastic pattern is consistent with two mechanisms: (1) elastic tissues may bind antibody specific to the tissue or, (2) immune complexes may penetrate the endothelium and then lodge passively against the internal elastic membrane. These findings parallel those for other forms of vasculitis and suggest that antibodies participate in the pathogenesis of cranial arteritis. The immunoglobulins in these vessels may be antibodies to a component of the arterial wall, presumably elastin, or they may result from the deposition of circulating immune complexes.

Reyes *et al.* (1976) described a 67-year-old woman with a five-month history of progressive, multiple neurological deficits; an autopsy revealed virus-like particles associated with granulomatous angiitis of the central nervous system. The small parenchymal and leptomeningeal blood vessels of the brain and spinal cord were particularly affected. Electron microscopic studies of formalin-fixed brain disclosed intranuclear particles resembling herpes virus. Although definitive proof cannot be established, Reyes and his collaborators suggest that some cases of granulomatous angiitis of the central nervous system may result from virus infection.

Malmvall and associates (1976) studied immunoglobulin levels in the serum of 36 patients (25 women and 11 men) having a mean age of 70 years. Twenty-four (15 women and 9 men) had histologic findings of cranial arteritis in temporal biopsy specimens. Complement levels were determined in 30 of the patients. A control group consisted of 39 hospitalized patients with a mean age of 74 years, none of whom had fever or elevated sedimentation rate, and in whom there was no evidence of immunologic, malignant, or infectious diseases. In the group with giant cell arteritis the mean values of IgE, total complement, and

complement factors C_3 and C_4 were statistically significantly higher than in the control group. There was no increase of IgM concentration. The concentration of IgA was higher in men with giant cell arteritis as compared to men in the control group, but no difference was seen in women.

We have surveyed 36 temporal artery biopsies obtained from 1975 through 1978. All were examined with standard pathologic techniques, hematoxylin and eosin staining (H&E), and with immunofluorescent methods (IF). Of the 36 patients, 21 were women and 15 were men. In some selected cases, elastic stains were done. IF included IgG, IgA, IgM, C_{1_q}, C_3, and fibrinogen (Fig. 10-5). Results from nine representative patients with giant cell arteritis are presented in Table 10-2.

In addition, only H&E and IF studies were done in eight other cases. Of these, one-half

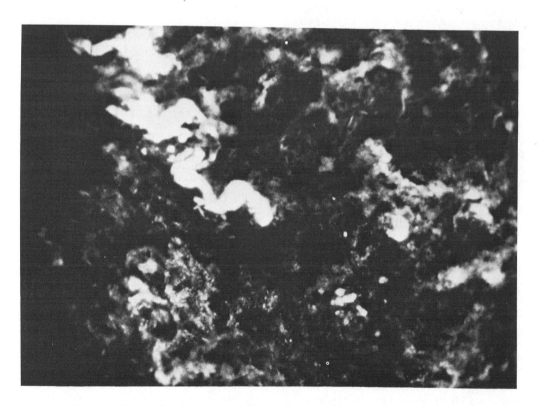

Fig. 10-5. Temporal arteritis. Immunofluorescence showing deposits of IgG in the vessel wall.

TABLE 10-2 Hematoxylin/Eosin and Immunofluorescence Findings in Nine Patients with Cranial Arteritis

AGE	H/E STAIN Diagnosis (Dx)	IgG	IgA	IF IgM	C1q	C3	Fib
74	temporal arteritis	luminal	—	luminal	—	—	luminal
68	giant cell arteritis	internal elastic membrane	—	—	—	—	diffuse
71	consist. with temp. arteritis	linear in smooth muscle	min. amt. in smooth muscle	min. amt. in smooth muscle	linear in smooth muscle	—	linear in smooth muscle
74	giant cell arteritis	—	—	—	—	—	—
68	giant cell arteritis	—	—	—	—	—	luminal
69	giant cell arteritis	—	—	—	—	—	—
62	giant cell arteritis	—	—	—	—	—	—
78	arteritis with intact elastica "not temporal"	scattered in intima/media	—	fine granular deposits at elastica	—	—	deposits in all parts
76	temporal arteritis	in media and intmia	—	—	in media	in media	in media

H/E = hematoxylin and eosin.
IgA, IgG, IgM = immunoglobulins A, G, M.
C1q, C3 = complement components.
Fib = fibrinogen.

showed fibrinogen within the lumen, and IgG on the internal elastic membrane.

These data suggest that giant cell arteritis probably represents a disorder of immunologic vasculitis associated with the deposition of immune complexes within the walls of affected blood vessels. This would lead to localized vascular injury and inflammation, producing the systemic signs of the disease.

POLYMYALGIA RHEUMATICA AND CRANIAL ARTERITIS

A rather common form of rheumatism which afflicts the elderly with pains in the head, neck, back, and proximal limbs may be associated with systemic signs of disease, an elevated erythrocyte sedimentation rate, and a very prompt therapeutic response to corticosteroids. This condition is best known as polymyalgia rheumatica. A significant number of patients with polymyalgia rheumatica will eventually develop cranial arteritis in the course of their illness, suggesting that the two diseases are in fact one, and that the myalgias of polymyalgia rheumatica may represent an early stage of cranial arteritis.

PAINFUL OPHTHALMOPLEGIA (TOLOSA-HUNT SYNDROME)

Six cases of retro-orbital pain and involvement of the structures lying within the cavernous sinus and its wall were studied by Hunt, Meagher, LeFever, and Zeman (1961). Pain may precede the ophthalmoplegia by several days, or may not occur until some time later. It is not a throbbing hemicrania occurring in paroxysms, but a steady pain behind the eye that is often described as "gnawing" or "boring." The defects are not confined to the third cranial nerve; the fourth, sixth, and first division of the fifth cranial nerves are also implicated. Periarterial sympathetic fibers and the optic nerve may be involved. The symptoms last for days or weeks. Spontaneous remissions occur, sometimes with residual motor or sensory deficit. Attacks recur at intervals of months or years. Exhaustive studies, including angiography and surgical exploration, have produced no evidence of involvement of structures outside the cavernous sinus. There is no systemic reaction. The syndrome is presumably caused by an inflammatory lesion of the cavernous sinus. Eduardo Tolosa (1954)

of the Neurological Institute of Barcelona published the report of a single case that met the above criteria. His patient expired after an exploratory operation, and autopsy showed an inflammatory lesion of the cavernous sinus. The syndrome, also called "pseudotumor of the orbit," has been carefully considered, reviewed, and discussed by Ingalls (1953) and as "syndrome of the superior orbital fissure," it has been studied by Lakke (1962) who supplies an additional bibliography.

Occasional cases of Tolosa-Hunt syndrome still appear in the medical literature. Smith and Taxdal (1966) have emphasized the dramatic response of the syndrome to systemic corticosteroid therapy. Recently Takeoka et al. (1978) have described angiographic findings in a patient with the Tolosa-Hunt syndrome. During the acute episode, at a time when a right third nerve paresis was present, there was evidence of irregular narrowing in the carotid siphon and incomplete opacification of the anterior cerebral artery when angiography was repeated. Ten days later, after treatment with corticosteroids, there was a remarkable improvement in the prior stenosis.

A few observations on the Tolosa-Hunt syndrome deserve emphasis. There is a close relationship between the oculomotor paresis which occurs and the angiographic abnormalities. In most patients pupillary function remains normal, with only 20% showing some pupillary involvement. The onset of the third-nerve paresis is rather rapid but recovery is almost always complete when appropriate therapy is provided.

TREATMENT OF CRANIAL ARTERITIS

Corticosteroids should be used promptly in the therapy of cranial arteritis, and should be begun as soon as the diagnosis is made, if necessary, prior to the temporal artery biopsy. The corticosteroids control the progress of the arteritis, reducing symptoms, and preventing the development of ocular complications. Blindness or defects in vision do not always correlate with the severity of the cranial arteritis, so that all patients should be treated promptly. Usually treatment is initiated with 40–60 mg of Prednisone daily. Therafter, this dose may be rapidly tapered to a maintenance level, depending upon the relief of symptoms, and the decline in the sedimentation rate toward normal. The duration of therapy is uncertain. It may be necessary to continue corticosteroids for months or even years, although eventually it is possible to discontinue treatment in almost all patients.

SUMMARY

1. Inflammation of cranial arteries occurs in two varieties of syndromes: (a) a generalized type in which the cranial arteritis is but part of a widespread vascular disease; (b) a focal type in which the cranial arteritis is the only arterial disease. The headache phenomena are identical in both, and distinction between them rests on the concomitant presence or absence of systemic arterial disease of inflammatory nature.

2. The head pain of cranial arteritis is of high intensity, and is throbbing in nature. In quality the pain is both aching and burning. There is an associated hyperalgesia of the scalp, and the distended temporal arteries are found on light palpation to be extremely tender. The headache may persist for one week to several weeks or months.

3. Most of the patients studied presented signs and symptoms generally associated with inflammation, namely, anorexia, prostration, fever, sweats, weight loss, and leukocytosis; and locally, over the artery, there was heat, swelling, tenderness, redness, and pain.

4. The association of polymyalgia rheumatica and cranial arteritis seems likely.

5. Cranial arteritis probably represents an example of immunologic vasculitis associated with the deposition of immune complexes within the walls of the affected blood vessels, thereafter producing localized vascular injury and inflammation.

6. Prompt therapy with corticosteroids is indicated in all patients with cranial arteritis.

REFERENCES

Atkinson, R., and O. Appenziller (1975). Headache in small vessel disease of the brain: a study of patients with SLE. *Headache 15*, 198.

Cooke, W. T., P. C. P. Cloake, A. D. T. Govan, and J. C. Colbeck (1946). Temporal arteritis: a generalized vascular disease. *Quart. J. Med. 15*, 47.

Crompton, M. R. (1959). The visual changes in temporal (giant-celled) arteritis. *Braine 82*, 377-390.

Enzmann, D., and W. R. Scott (1977). Intracranial involvement of giant cell arteritis. *Neurol. 27*, 794-797.

Gocke, D. J., C. Morgan, M. Lockshin, K. Hsu, S. Bombardier, and C. L. Christian (1970). Association between polyarteritis and Australia antigen. *Lancet 2*, 1149-1153.

Heptinstall, R. H., K. A. Porter, and H. Barkley (1954). Giant cell (temporal) arteritis. *J. Pathol. Bact. 67*, 507-519.

Hollenhorst, R. W., J. R. Brown, H. P. Wagener, and R. M. Shick (1960). Neurologic aspects of temporal arteritis. *Neurol. 10*, 490.

Horton, B. T., and T. B. Magath (1937). Arteritis of temporal vessels; report of seven cases. *Proc. Mayo Clin. 12*, 548.

Hunt, W. E., J. N. Meagher, H. E. LeFever, and W. Zeman (1961). Painful ophthalmoplegia. Its relation to indolent inflammation of the cavernous sinus. *Neurol. 11*, 56.

Ingalls, R. G. (1953). *Tumors of the Orbit*. C. C. Thomas, Springfield, Ill.

Klein, R. G., R. J. Campbell, G. Hunder, and J. Carney (1976). Skip lesions in temporal arteritis. *Proc. Mayo Clin. 51*, 504-510.

Kuwabara, T., and R. Reinecke (1970). Temporal arteritis. *Arch. Ophthalmol. 83*, 692-697.

Lakke, J. P. W. F. (1962). The superior orbital fissure syndrome caused by local pachymeningitis, with a case report. *Arch. Neurol. 7*, 289.

Liang, G. C., P. Simkin, and M. Mannik (1974). Immunoglobulins in temporal arteritis. *Ann. Intern. Med. 81*, 19-23.

Lie, J. T., A. L. Brown, Jr., and E. T. Carter (1970). Spectrum of aging changes in temporal arteries. *Arch. Pathol. 90*, 278-285.

Malmvall, B., B. Bengtsson, B. Kaijser, L. Nilsson, and K. Alestig (1976). Serum levels of immunoglobulin and complement in giant cell arteritis. *JAMA 236*, 1876-1878.

Ray, B. S., and H. G. Wolff (1945). Studies on pain. "Spread of pain"; evidence on site of spread within the neuraxis of effects of painful stimulation. *Arch. Neurol. Psychiat. 53*, 257.

Reyes, M. G., R. Fresco, S. Chokroverty, and E. Salud (1976). Virus-like particles in granulomatous angiitis of the central nervous system. *Neurol. 26*, 797-799.

Russell, R. W. (1959). Giant cell arteritis; a review of thirty-five cases. *Quart. J. Med. 28*, 471-489.

Scott, T., and E. S. Maxwell (1941). Temporal arteritis; a case report. *Intern. Clin. 2*, 220-222.

Smith, J. L., and D. J. R. Taydal (1966). Painful ophthalmoplegia: the Tolosa-Hunt syndrome. *Am. J. Ophthalmol. 61*, 1466-1472.

Sprague, P. H., and W. C. MacKenzie (1940). Case of

temporal arteritis (Horton-Magath syndrome). *Can. Med. Assoc. J. 43,* 562–564.

Takeoka T., F. Gotoh, Y. Fukuuchi, and Y. Inagaki (1978). Tolosa, Hunt syndrome. *Arch. Neurol. 35,* 219–223.

Tolosa, E. (1954). Periarteritic lesions of carotid siphon with clinical features of carotid infraclinoidal aneurysm. *J. Neurol. Neurosurg. Psychiat. 17,* 300.

Wadman, B., and I. Werner (1972). Observations in temporal arteritis. *Acta Med. Scand. 192,* 377–383.

11

THE MAJOR NEURALGIAS, POSTINFECTIOUS NEURITIS, INTRACTABLE PAIN, AND ATYPICAL FACIAL PAIN

REVISED BY DONALD J. DALESSIO

Perhaps no subject in medicine is as confusing to patient and physician alike as that of recurrent chronic facial pain. Often unilateral, frequently unresponsive to therapy, long-lasting, and discomforting, some chronic facial pains have resisted even simple nosologic classification. Some patients with severe protracted facial pain will develop complications related to attempts at pain relief as significant as the original cause of their problem. Drug addiction or dependence, serious (even suicidal) depression, disability, and invalidism are among the most frequently encountered complications of long-term intense facial pain. This knowledge notwithstanding, a physician who understands how to deal with patients with chronic facial pain and who understands the mechanisms behind their pain-centered behavior, may be able to affect a significant improvement in the lifestyle of many of these patients by using a judicious combination of drug therapy, surgery, and other modalities.

In evaluating facial pains, a working classification is a necessity, and is provided in Table 11-1. Rather than listing one long series of facial pain syndromes, we have grouped them into six categories: vascular, muscular, neuritic, rheumatic, traction and inflammatory, and psychogenic.

TRIGEMINAL NEURALGIA (TIC DOULOUREUX)

Trigeminal neuralgia (tic douloureux), an episodic, recurrent, unilateral pain syndrome, occurs for the most part in persons over 50

years of age. Tic douloureux is a disorder of adult life. It seldom begins before 30 or after 60 years of age. It occurs more commonly in women than in men, in a ratio of 2:1, and more often on the right side. It is a disorder characterized by high-intensity pain with peculiar temporal features. The pain is experienced chiefly in the tissues supplied by the second, and to a lesser extent in those supplied by the third and first divisions of the fifth cranial nerve. It may, however, be felt in any part of the face, but never below the ramus or in back of the ear, and rarely in the entire distribution of the fifth nerve at one time. The pain, of an aching and burning quality, may occur spontaneously, but is often initiated by cold air or a light touch on the skin of the cheek (powderpuff, veil, kiss, towel), by biting, chewing, swallowing, laughing, talking, yawning, sneezing, blowing the nose, or drinking cold water. Such sites from which an attack may be initiated (trigger zones) may occur in any part of the face, the most common being in the structures supplied by the second division of the fifth cranial nerve, and commonly near the lateral border of the nose.

The pain is usually a high-intensity jab of 20 to 30 seconds' duration followed by a period of relative freedom from pain of a few seconds to a minute, to be followed again by another jab of high-intensity pain. The attack, or series of such brief, fierce pains, usually lasts one or more hours. Sometimes after hours of such severe short-lived pains, there may be a steady, low-intensity aching pain. It occurs in periods

TABLE 11-1 Classification of Chronic Facial Pain

Vascular

A. Paroxysmal Recurrent
   a. Migraine
      1. classic
      2. common
      3. complicated
   b. Cluster
   c. Lower Half
B. Toxic/Metabolic
C. Hypertensive
D. Arterial, Degenerative
   a. Atheromatous
   b. Embolic
   c. Aneurysmal
   d. AVM
   e. TIA
E. Arteritis, Cranial
   a. Giant Cell
   b. Granulomatous/Infectious
   c. Immune Complex
   d. Tolosa-Hunt
F. Thrombophlebitis
G. Carotidynia
H. Obscure

Muscular

A. Myositis
B. Fibromyalgias
C. Neoplastic

Neuritic

A. Paroxysmal
   a. Trigeminal Neuralgia
   b. Glossopharyngeal
   c. VII, X nerve neuralgias
B. Chronic
   a. Post-traumatic
   b. Postherpetic
   c. Toxic
   d. 2°collagen disease

Rheumatic

A. TMJ disease
B. Infections
C. Neoplastic

Psychogenic

A. Burning Tongue and Mouth
B. Atypical Facial Pains
C. Conversion Reactions
D. Depressive Equivalents

Traction and Inflammatory

Mass lesions
Disease of eye, ear, nose, throat, and teeth
   Infections
   Degenerative
   Edematous
   Neoplastic

of two to three months or longer and may diminish or be absent for a year or more. Some patients have seasonal recurrences. Once begun, such attacks commonly recur for the remainder of life or until terminated by therapeutic precedures. Spontaneous total recovery is rare, but remissions are common.

Although attacks may occur any time in the 24 hr, and do occur predictably at night, they seldom begin during sleep unless the face is inadvertently rubbed. Examination reveals no defect in motility or sensory function except very slight hyperalgesia during an attack, and rarely a minimal hypalgesia between attacks. During a period of frequent attacks the cheek may become reddened, the tongue furred, and the eyes watery. The face takes on a cramped, painful expression. Between repeatedly recurring attacks the patient holds his face immobile and talks cautiously, often through closed jaws and lips. Although trigeminal neuralgia is a unilateral disorder involving always the same side, in rare instances the other side may also become involved in later life.

Pathophysiology

Kugelberg and Lindblom (1959) have studied the neuropathophysiology of trigeminal neuralgia. Their results indicate that the excitatory state necessary to fire an attack may be built up over a considerable time by temporal summation of afferent impulses. Antiepileptic drugs, when effective, raise an attack threshold and shorten the duration of attacks by diminishing the self-maintenance of the excitation. They postulate that periodic discharges in the brainstem, in structures related to the spinal nucleus of the fifth cranial nerve, may explain the suddenness, intensity, and brevity of the attack.

Tic douloureux is a unique disease in several respects. Patients with this disease give a consistent history, are often clustered in the older age groups, may have seasonal exacerbations of pain, and may be relieved of their pain by disparate drugs which are not commonly considered analgesic. Their tendency to manifest trigger zones is another characteristic. Such zones are quite precise areas of skin or mucous membrane which, when excited by the most trivial of stimuli, are capable of producing pain in one or another of the divisions of the trigeminal nerve. Patients learn to avoid these zones and may construct elaborate behavioral patterns to protect them, such as speaking or chewing from one side of the mouth only, to the wearing of face masks to protect the trigger zone from tactile stimuli or breezes. One patient in the author's experience, for example, learned to wash the area of his face containing the trigger zone with a soft shaving brush, and in this manner was able to avoid evoking typical tic pain when performing his morning rituals. In this condition, the patient practices avoidance behavior. Stated another way, he goes to great lengths to avoid stimulation of the face. Whereas patients with atypical facial pain and other pain syndromes will rub the face, or heat it, or ice it, or abrade it, or whatever, the patient with trigeminal neuralgia avoids any and all sensory stimuli. He will not touch the trigger zones, and he would prefer that others not touch them either.

Tic douloureux thus presents a singular opportunity to study pain in humans, both clinically and in the laboratory. Ordinarily, the laboratory study of pain is difficult, and results of studies, particularly pharmacologic studies comparing analgesics, have been disappointing. Too often in conscious man it requires a high-intensity stimulation, sometimes causing tissue damage, to produce pain. Given the standard conditions of most laboratories, the effects of fear and anxiety, conditioning, and previous experience, there is little wonder that studies in experimental pain have been difficult to reproduce consistently.

Patients with tic douloureux, however, have a reasonably consistent pain response from one day to the next during an exacerbation of their disease. Furthermore, their pain may often be elicited by recurrent and precise stimulation of a minute area, when such stimulation is little more than a slight tug or pull on the skin. Stimulation of even a single hair has been reported to produce pain in the trigger zone of a susceptible individual.

The trigger zones of ten patients with tic douloureux are illustrated in Fig 11-1. These zones are small, usually 2 to 4 mm in size, and cluster about the nares and mouth. Attacks of

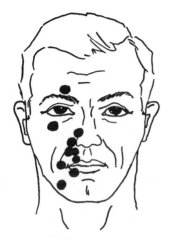

FIG. 11-1. Trigger zones in tic douloureux.

pain may be produced by some form of stimulation of the trigger zone, as when washing the face or brushing the teeth, or by simple movements of the mouth and jaw in talking or mastication. Differing forms of stimuli affect the trigger zones in strange ways. Painful stimulation of the trigger zone may not be an effective stimulus. Thermal stimuli are usually not effective. The application or relief of pressure on a trigger zone almost always evokes an attack in susceptible individuals. The vibratory stimulus is also effective.

We have made a study of the trigger zones of patients with a mechanical stimulator which delivers a light and tapping stimulus of variable dimensions at variable frequencies. It was possible to show that temporal summation of impulses occurred, and a specific curve could be developed by varying the number of impulses delivered to a trigger zone which would produce pain. Thus, for example, when one delivered a great number of impulses per second, pain was produced rapidly. When a few impulses were delivered, pain was produced only after a latent period, and sometimes not at all. These results suggest that the excitatory state necessary to provoke pain may be evoked by the summation of afferent impulses, and confirms previous, similar observations by Kugelberg and Lindblom (1959). These stimulus-response curves were repeated in three patients after the ingestion of carbamazapine, and a significant reduction in sensitivity of the trigger zone was noted in 24 (Fig. 11-2). After 48 hr, the trigger zone had effectively been abolished, at least as tested using this instrument. These data suggest that carbamazapine acts to reduce the sensitivity of the afferent projection system, without affecting cutaneous sensation. In other words, the trigger area in question is altered in terms of abnormal sensitivity, but is not anesthetized. Sensation remains normal, but the hyperexcitable state, which produces the trigger zone, is alleviated.

As an aside, it should be noted that there is a

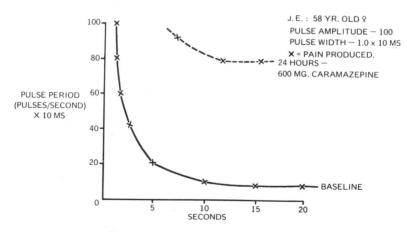

FIG. 11-2. Temporal summation of impulses

refractory period which is produced after these repetitive stimuli are applied, varying with the individual, sometimes lasting up to several minutes. If one attempts to evoke a painful attack by stimulating the skin during the refractory phase, one obtains either a diminished episode of pain, or no pain at all. The duration of the refractory phase seems to be a function of the duration, as well as the intensity, of the preceding painful attack. Attacks of a few seconds' duration show hardly any refractoriness, as tested with the stimulator. With a severe attack, the refractory phase is longer.

Drug Therapy

Three drugs were found to be effective in this situation at the Scripps Clinic (Fig. 11-3). All have similar pharmocologic effects, though their chemical structures are different. Carbamazepine (Tegretol) is a tricyclic compound related to imipramine. It finds its primary

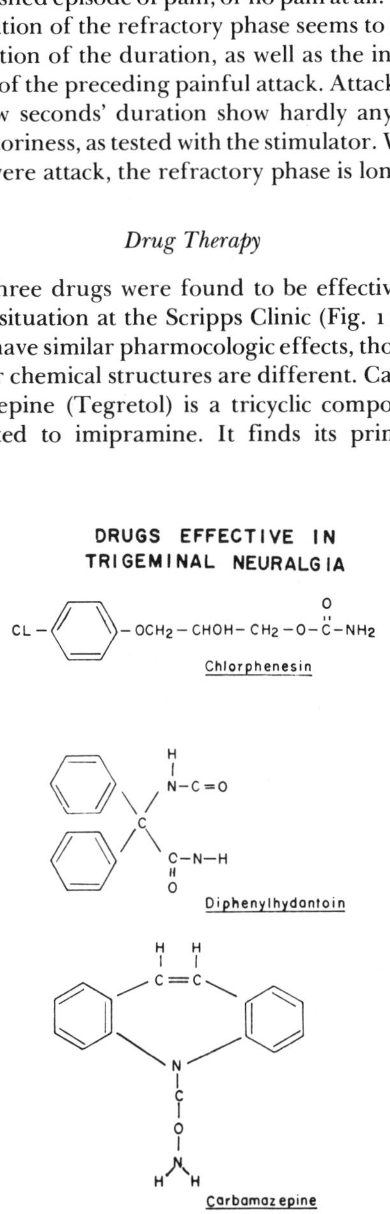

FIG. 11-3. Drugs effective in trigeminal neuralgia

use in this country in the treatment of trigeminal neuralgia, but is becoming increasingly important in the therapy of complex seizures of the temporal-lobe type. Diphenylhydantoin (Dilantin) a hydantoin derivative, is the most useful drug for major epilepsies. Acting to stabilize biological membranes, it is also useful in cardiac arrhythmias as well as trigeminal neuralgia. Chlorphenesin is a mephenesin-like compound, a series of drugs introduced primarily to alter skeletal muscle spasm of local origin.

The methods of action of the three drugs are similar. Diphenylhydantoin reduces post-tetanic potentiation of synaptic transmission within the spinal cord as well as the stellate ganglion of animals. Post-tetanic potentiation may be considered as an enhancement of synaptic transmission following rapid, repetitive, presynaptic stimulation. Carbamazepine also depresses post-tetanic potentiation at the spinal cord level in animals, and significantly inhibits polysynaptic reflex activity in the spinal cord. It depresses synaptic transmission in the spinal trigeminal nucleus (Fromm, 1969). Laboratory studies have shown that these anticonvulsants depress synaptic transmission in the trigeminal system, as evidenced by decreasing amplitude and increasing latency of evoked potentials (Fromm and Landgren, 1963). Depressant effects on polysynaptic potentials in spinal cords are also reported.

Chlorphenesin depresses transmission to a number of spinal and supraspinal polysynaptic pathways. It also depresses polysynaptic potentials in spinal cords of animals and inhibits convulsions induced by strychnine (Matthews et al., 1963). Our laboratory studies have demonstrated depression of synaptic transmission in the trigeminal system (Goodlett and Dalessio, 1973).

We have studied the effects of chlorphenesin on the trigeminal system of cats at Scripps. Recording were made from the spinal trigeminal nucleus, after stimulation of the ipsilateral infraorbital nerve. Reduction in postsynaptic component of the evoked stimulus curve was in the range of 40%, after chlorphenesin was given intravenously. Carefully controlled experimental observations have demonstrated that this reduction in the reactivity of the spinal trigeminal nucleus is a specific effect of chlorphenesin, similar to that demonstrated elsewhere for diphenylhydantoin and carbamazepine.

Chlorphenesin, as well as carbanazepine, strongly inhibits strychnine convulsions in animals. It may therefore be stated that all of these medications tend to depress polysynaptic activity and to stabilize transmission, either in the gasserian ganglion, or the spinal trigeminal nucleus, or both. If the neuropathophysiology of trigeminal neuralgia is best understood as a problem in the temporal summation of afferent impulses, with the excitatory state necessary to set off an attack presumably built up over a considerable period of time, related to lack of inhibition in the sensory pathways of the fifth cranial nerve, then medical therapies effective in this disease should raise the attack threshold and shorten the duration of attacks by diminishing the self-maintenance of the excitation.

How may one use these data in the clinical situation of trigeminal neuralgia? Our experience with this condition is outlined in Table 11-2. We have treated 19 patients. Three who eventually required triple drug therapy, were referred for surgery. Nine of our patients were managed on either carbamazipine or chlorphenesin alone. The dose of chlorphenesin ranged from 800 to 2400 mg per day, and in general the medication was well tolerated. Side-effects are few and not dangerous.

Carbamazepine, 200 mg three times daily, is the drug of choice. This should be given until the pain syndrome is suppressed. Thereafter, the medication should be gradually reduced to

TABLE 11-2   Summary of Patient Therapy Trigeminal Neuralgia 1973–78

	MEDICAL	SURGICAL
Carbamazepine	5	
Chlorphenesin	4	
Diphenylhydantoin	2	
Carbamazepine and chlorphenesin	4	
Diphenylhydantoin and chlorphenesin	1	
All three	3	7
Totals	19	7

the point that the pains are kept under control with the least possible dose. The medication should then be continued for several months before stopping it completely, presuming the patient entered a period of remission.

If carbamazepine is not entirely effective, diphenylhydantoin, 100 mg times daily, may be added as a third drug if the pain persists. If pain continues in spite of multiple medical therapies, then surgical procedures are probably indicated (Table 11-3).

The specific role of chlorphenesin in the therapy of trigeminal neuralgia remains conjectural. Certainly, based upon clinical experience, the medication is effective, at least as a secondary drug. Since it tends to cause less in the way of side effects than either carbamazepine or diphenylhydantoin, particularly when the latter is used in high doses, it may in some cases be the drug of choice in the treatment of this condition. Or, conversely, we would suggest that until further clinical experience is obtained, it be used as a secondary

TABLE 11-3   Medical Therapy of Trigeminal Neuralgia

NAME				
Generic	Brand	DOSAGE	PRECAUTIONS	PREPARATIONS
Carbamazepine	Tegretol	200–600 mg/day	monitor for blood disorders weekly ———→ monthly	oral
Diphenylhydantoin	Dilantin	200–400 mg/day	CNS, hemopoietic, oral	oral
Chlorphenesin	Maolate	800–2400 mg/day	drowsiness	oral

TABLE 11-4   Pharmacologic Activity of Chlorphenesin, Diphenylhydantoin, and
Carbamazepine

	CHLORPHENESIN	DIPHENYL.	CARBAMAZEPINE
1. Anticonvulsant	+	+ + +	+ +
2. Muscle relaxant	+ + +	+	+ +
3. Sedative	+ +	+	+ +
4. Anesthetic	0	0	0
5. Analgesic	±	0	±

or complimentary agent, given concomitantly with either carbamazepine or diphenylhydantoin (Table 11-4).

In summary, trigeminal neuralgia may be considered a disorder of excitation, wherein facial pain occurs after a temporal summation of afferent impulses. Medications such as carbamazepine, diphenylhydantoin, and chlorphenesin raise the attack threshold and shorten the duration of attacks by diminishing self-maintenance of excitation. They seem to reduce the sensitivity of the afferent projection system without altering normal facial sensation. The trigger zones are alleviated, and as they disappear, the symptoms of trigeminal neuralgia are alleviated.

Trigeminal Neuralgia and Multiple Sclerosis

Sensory disturbances in the distribution of the trigeminal nerve are relatively common in multiple sclerosis and may even involve the inside of the mouth. The usual descriptions of facial hypesthesia are nonspecific. Often patients speak of numbness of deadness of the face, or of a feeling that part of the face has been anesthetized by novocaine. Pain may or may not be associated with these sensations, which may be quite transient, last for a day or two or more, or sometimes become permanent. Objective signs of sensory loss are difficult to elicit but there may be associated impairment of pain and temperature sensitivity, and loss of touch in the region involved. The corneal reflex may be diminished or absent when the loss of sensation affects the first division of the trigeminal nerve.

Intermittent trigeminal neuralgia as opposed to the condition described above (which might be termed trigeminal neuritis) is uncommon in multiple sclerosis, and varies between a 1 and 2% incidence (Harris, 1950; Garcin et al., 1960). Conversely, the incidence of multiple sclerosis among patients with trigeminal neuralgia is approximagely 3%. Typically, the classical history of trigeminal neuralgia (Parker, 1978) will be obtained in patients with multiple sclerosis except that it may appear in those of younger age than is usual when the disease occurs in its idiopathic form. Some patients with multiple sclerosis manifest recurrent episodes of face pain, generally long-lasting and not stabbing or lancinating without associated trigger zones. These patients are assumed to have a form of atypical facial pain and not true trigeminal neuralgia.

In our experience trigeminal neuralgia almost never occurs as the first manifestation of the disease, and all of the patients seen with trigeminal neuralgia in association with multiple sclerosis have had very significant physical signs of multiple sclerosis before the facial pain began. Most, for example, have paraparesis or paraplegia, disorders of sensory function including posterior column signs, and the like, Single cases of trigeminal neuralgia appearing as the first manifestation of multiple sclerosis are rare.

The treatment of trigeminal neuralgia occurring in association with multiple sclerosis is the same as that given previously for the idiopathic variety.

With regard to the pathogenesis of trigeminal pain in multiple sclerosis, it can be stated that in this situation demyelinating plaques may be found at the point of entry of the fifth root, or involving the main sensory nucleus or the descending root of the trigeminal nerve.

Demyelinating plaques may also be found in the gasserian ganglion. If this is the case, plaques are often found in adjacent structures also involving the facial nucleus, sometimes producing facial weakness and continuous rhythmic fascicular contractions, termed facial myokymia. Presumably the plaques occurring either in the ganglion or in the main sensory nucleus alter the electrophysiology of facial sensation, allowing hyperactive sensory circuits to appear, producing trigger zones and the characteristic manifestations of trigeminal neuralgia, as we have come to know them.

PATHOLOGICAL ANATOMY OF THE TRIGEMINAL (GASSERIAN) GANGLION IN TIC DOULOUREUX

Alterations in the anatomy of the gasserian ganglion and sensory root have been reported for years. In 1934 Dandy found aberrant arteries and other vascular anomalies in 40% of patients with tic douloureux as he exposed the fifth nerve root through the posterior fossa. More recently, Jannetta (1967) has demonstrated small arterial loops impinging upon nerve fibers during subtentorial microdissection of the trigeminal root in patients with tic douloureux. Separation of these vessels from the root, combined with partial rhizotomy, relieved the neuralgia without producing a major sensory abnormality. Following an elegant anatomical study, Kerr (1963) has proposed that contact between the internal carotid artery and the under surface of the gasserian ganglion may be a significant factor in the development of tic douloureux. He based this proposal on sections of the petrous tip which demonstrated that a lacuna in the bony root of the carotid canal may be frequently present in normal patients. He found considerable variability in the fascial reinforcements of this lacuna, with a tendency for it to become reduced in thickness with age. Kerr felt that this structural variant was compatible with features peculiar to tic douloureux. In addition, electron-microscopic abnormalities in the gasserian ganglion itself have been described.

From the evidence presented above we may conclude that the primary cranial neuralgias, exemplified by trigeminal neuralgia, have in fact a pathologic anatomical basis, albeit a subtle one. These subtle anatomic factors may be responsible for the production of a focus of irritability within the trigeminal or other systems. This would produce pathological reflex activity in the area of the brain stem, central to the site of noxious irritation evoked by the pathological lesion. This would explain the appearance of pain evoked by a normal sensory stimulus produced peripherally, and the obvious and rapid response to anticonvulsant agents which act primarily centrally.

SURGICAL PROCEDURES FOR THE ELIMINATION OF MAJOR TRIGEMINAL NEURALGIA (SEE ALSO CHAPTER 15)

Alcohol injection into the gasserian ganglion or one or more branches of the trigeminal nerve root for the elimination of tic pain, a method long and widely used, has been abandoned at many institutions. Alcohol injection is in itself a painful procedure, not always successful, and is almost always impermanent.

There are two operative approaches for section of the sensory root behind the ganglion:* the transtemporal through the middle fossa, cutting the root immediately posterior to the ganglion; and the suboccipital, popularized by Dandy (1925), sectioning the root where it enters the pons. Dandy, in 1945, had performed over 500 such operations with a morality rate of less than 1%.

Although able neurosurgeons find that the suboccipital approach affords better visualization of the operative field and that accurate graduated section of the fifth cranial nerve root is easier to perform, such suboccipital root section requires more time and usually depletes the patient more than the transtemporal approach. A distance a little over a cm separates these two points of section. Also it is the intradural rather than extradural approach which carries with it the danger of meningitis.

A serious complication of complete sensory

---

*Because complete or partial section of sensory roots may be followed by numbness or paresthesias, such procedures should not be undertaken until the patient is convinced that no other means affords relief.

root section, keratitis in the ipsilateral eye, can be avoided by appropriate subtotal section of the root. Facial paralysis occurs in about 5% of patients, comes on four to five days postoperatively, is never permanent, and disappears in from three to six months. Another complication following root section is the anesthesia of the face necessary to eliminate pain and which is permanent. Approximately 25% of patients complain of stiffness, numbness, swollen feeling, apparent lack of mobility in the affected side of the face, fullness in the ear, and stiffness of the tongue which follow nerve section. In 5% a persistent hot, burning sensation develops in this anesthetic area. This paresthesia is continuous and may be almost as disturbing to some patients as the former intermittent neuralgia. Furthermore, if preoperative history reveals that the cheek or lip burns between the paroxysms of pain, this sensation may persist after root section has relieved the major pain.

Saunders and Sachs (1971) suggest that in patients undergoing surgery for trigeminal neuralgia, a significantly higher recurrence rate is seen if the motor root is surgically preserved. They suggest that the motor root is a mixed nerve and is a possible avenue for the pain of trigeminal neuralgia. It may also have a role in the pathogenesis of that diease.

A minimal and graded root section by the transtemporal or suboccipital approach creates an area of anesthesia just large enough to eliminate pain. But the absence of anesthesia or anaglesia always exposes the patient to the possibility of a recurrence of the pain and the necessity of a second operation.

Dandy (1934) in his initial drawings of the anatomy of the posterior root, described a number of accessory fibers entering the pons between the major sensory portion of the root and the more cephalad motor root.

The use of the binocular dissecting microscope and its modifications in surgical procedures has added a significant refinement to the field of surgery in general and to neurosurgery, ophthalmological surgery, and otolaryngology in particular. The anatomical and clinical studies of Jannetta and Rand (1967) have confirmed Dandy's often contested opinion that these accessory fibers exist and might be concerned with the perception of light touch on the face.

Jannetta and Rand have reported a number of successful procedures in which the major sensory root of the trigeminal nerve was sectioned and the accessory fibers preserved. In these patients complete relief of trigeminal pain has been afforded with preservation of light touch and corneal sensation in all instances. The length of follow-up, of course, is yet too short to be certain that recurrences of pain will not be seen; however, one cannot help but conclude that these reports constitute a major breakthrough in the surgery of trigeminal neuralgia.

Controversial Aspects of Neurosurgical Treatment

The neurosurgical management of trigeminal neuralgia remains a surprisingly controversial topic. Surgical approaches to neuralgic face pain range from simple ablative procedures of peripheral nerves to extensive craniotomies of the posterior fossa using microscopic neursurgical techniques. Three of the opposing points of view will be presented below (see also Chapter 15).

Peter Jannetta (1977) has presented his clinical observations on the treatment of trigeminal neuralgia by suboccipital and transtentorial cranial operations. Before surgery 15 of 46 patients had mild sensory abnormalities in the region of the tic pain, and abnormal sensory evoked potentials could be elicited in many of the patients. In 100 operated patients he noted evidence of compression of the trigeminal nerve, in 88 by aberrant arteries, and in six by tumors, two of whom had arterial venous malformations. The other six patients had multiple sclerosis. Jannetta's operative procedure is extensive, requiring an open craniotomy and the use of an operating microscope. His results seem to be excellent.

Thomas Morley (1977) takes the opposite operative approach, which is to do the minimum needed to stop the pain, and to repeat the simplest of procedures if the pain returns. He advocates initial evulsion of the peripheral nerve to the trigger zone, or alcohol injections, and if these are not successful, percutaneous radio frequency lesions. Denervation under direct approach of the trigeminal branch and/or ganglion involved is a last resort. Morley states that 50% of the patients who require operative procedures need only peripheral evulsions, but that multiple evulsions may be necessary.

J. M. Tew reported on 400 ptaients with trigeminal neuralgia, all of whom were first treated medically, and many of whom had had spot treatment, or "spot welding," as he termed it (Tew and Keller, 1977). Despite these therapies, the patients continued to complain of facial pain. He reviewed the requirements for stereotaxic surgery, which include a controlled current, a patient who is awake or easily rousable, careful sensory testing, the preservation of touch, and the ability to relieve pain at the time the patient is on the operating table. That surgical technique permitted precise localization of the various divisions of the trigeminal nerve as demonstrated by electrical stimulation. When the needle was in the proper position physiologically and radiographically, a radio frequency generator was turned on to a low voltage setting. The process was then repeated until the correct degree of sensory deficit had been created. Careful incremental lesions were necessary in order to prevent the creation of too much sensory deficit. Appropriate anesthesia was provided while the procedure was being done. Dr. Tew reported excellent results in pain control, but noted significant side effects in that 23% had masseter weakness, 11% had numbness of the face on the same side, and 10% lost the corneal reflex. These problems lasted variable lengths of time. Sometimes reoperation was necessary as well.

Tic-Like Neuritides of the Fifth Cranial Nerve Associated with Brain Tumors and Other Pathologic Processes

These relatively uncommon painful states resemble tic douloureux, but can usually be differentiated, because each painful paroxysm is commonly a sustained high-intensity ache of several minutes' duration, whereas the true tic is characterized by recurrent, brief, painful jabs of approximately 30 seconds' duration. Cushing (1920), in describing these neuralgias resulting from tumor involvement of the sensory root, the trigeminal ganglion, or the fifth nerve, has divided them into four groups, on the basis of the site of the precipitating cause.

1. Tumors of the cerebellopontile recess upon the trigeminal root may rarely be accompanied by paroxysms of pain which resemble tic douloureux. The pain is not eliminated by trigeminal ganglion operation. Sometimes there is a low-intensity, steady, dull ache, but usually little or no pain is produced by such tumors, and there is a gradual hypesthesia in the distribution of the fifth cranial nerve.

2. Tumors of the middle fossa that involve the trigeminal ganglion by direct pressure from above, mainly upon the dura overlying the ganglion, are growths with a meningeal attachment, such as endothelial tumors, granulomas, and occasional gliomas. The pain, again, rarely resembles tic douloureux as to its temporal features. Furthermore, it is an inconspicuous symptom of the underlying disorder. Usually when pain occurs it is of a sustained aching and burning character, and is associated with hypesthesia of an appropriate area of the skin. Paroxysms of high-intensity pain of 10 to 15 minutes' duration may occur.

3. Tumors that arise in the cranium or in the extracranial tissues beneath the ganglion, often metastatic, are almost certain to involve the ganglion in the course of time. Occasionally the nerve may be completely destroyed, resulting in total anesthesia in its territory, without production of pain; but more often the process is accompanied by aching and burning pain of high intensity occurring in paroxysms of 10 to 15 minutes' duration.

4. Endothelial tumors originating from the envelopes of the trigeminal ganglion give rise to pain in the region supplied by one or more branches of the fifth nerve. The character of the pain, a more or less sustained, steady ache, readily distinguishes it from true trigeminal neuralgia. It is also inevitably accompanied by a hypesthesia, if not anesthesia, and motor paralysis. Also, the third, sixth, and eighth

nerves may be involved by the tumor. Avulsion of the sensory root on the side affected, resulting in total anesthesia, eliminates the pain.

When true tic douloureux is found to occur in a young person, particularly a young woman, the patient should be carefully examined for evidence of a demyelinating disease or multiple sclerosis. Pain usually persists between paroxysms, but the symptoms may be indistinguishable from those of true tic. Every opportunity for remission should be exploited, but should the pain become intractable, the patient should be treated in much the same way as are patients with true tic douloureux. The symptom is sometimes associated with a plaque in the pontine and adjacent regions of the brainstem.

Thus, a specific gross pathological lesion is only rarely associated with true trigeminal neuralgia. Some patients with persistent burning sensations involving one of the three divisions of the trigeminal nerve may be said to have a form of trigeminal neuritis related to such a lesion. For example, advanced multiple sclerosis can produce a syndrome indistinguishable from idiopathic tic douloureux. Occasionally posterior fossa lesions, extracerebral in type such as arteriovenous malformations, epidermoids, acoustic neuromas, meningiomas, arachnoiditis, and basilar artery aneurysm will produce similar complaints, but almost always in the context of other neurological findings. Even more rarely, osteomas of the foramen ovale may evoke facial pain. In general it may be said that such lesions are rare and usually, if the history is carefully obtained, the character of the pain will be seen to be somewhat different from that of idiopathic tic douloureux.

GENICULATE NEURALGIA OF HERPETIC ORIGIN

Generally, geniculate neuralgia is related to herpes zoster infection of the geniculate ganglion and is characterized by severe pain in the tympanic membrane, the walls of the auditory canal, the external auditory meatus, and the external structures of the ear. The pain is typically deep, may be associated with a herpetic rash in the auricle, or the rash may be present in the external auditory canal. The disease may be associated with facial palsy, difficulty with hearing, vertigo, and tinnitus. Treatment is symptomatic.

HEMIFACIAL SPASM

J. C. Maroon (1978), a member of Jannetta's group, has reviewed the literature on hemifacial spasm and described his therapy of this syndrome. Recent surgical observations indicate that hemifacial spasm is most likely caused by normal or pathological vascular structures that cross-compress the facial nerve. The critical area of compression is found at the brainstem exit zone of the seventh nerve. In this area the central glial investment of the facial nerve changes to peripheral or Schwannian myelin. It is suspected that this anatomic junction zone may be of pathophysiologic significance when directly compressed or irritated. Maroon recommends a retromastoid craniectomy and vascular decompression operation to relieve hemifacial spasm, while at the same time preserving facial nerve function. This is in contrast to commonly used destructive operations for hemifacial spasm. He emphasizes, however, that microsurgical techniques must be employed or high morbidity and mortality may occur, using the retromastoid approach. Interestingly, in Maroon's series of cases, facial pain or headache associated with clonic facial spasm was extremely rare. He emphasizes that the problem is primarily a muscular one related to predominant contraction of the orbicularis and zygomatic muscles.

Hemifacial spasm should be differentiated from blepharospasm and the synkinesis that may occur following a Bell's palsy. In our experience, blepharospasm is always bilateral, affects primarily the periorbital muscles, but may spread to the upper facial muscles as well. In a small number of patients with Bell's palsy, hemifacial synkinetic movements may develop as the patient recovers from the episode but is left with persisting weakness. This history is clearly different from that of hemifacial spasm. Also, facial myokymia may appear as a form of fascicular twitching of the facial muscles, especially the orbicularis oculi. This is often a transitory occurrence in normal persons related to fatigue. Occasionally it is also found in hemifacial spasm. In none of these conditions is pain a prominent feature of the muscular movements.

PAINFUL TIC CONVULSIF

Painful tic convulsif is characterized by periodic contractions of one side of the face, accompanied by great pain. It may be confused with the facial contortions and masticatory movements on the involved side which sometimes accompany the paroxysms of true trigeminal neuralgia. Cushing (1920) has reported five cases of the disorder, which is extremely rare.

The following is a protocol of one of his patients:

J. L., aged 52, was first seen at the Johns Hopkins Hospital in May 1909. He complained of paroxysms of motor spasms of the right side of the face, accompanied by very high-intensity burning, twisting pain, of 12 years' duration. In the interims between attacks there was a distressing "hypesthesia dolorosa" over the lower part of the right face.

When the attacks began, in 1897, pain was confined to the ophthalmic division of the trigeminal, and was mainly localized in the eyeball. His right eye was therefore removed. A year later a supraorbital neurectomy was performed; in 1904 all his teeth were extracted, and in 1905 and 1907 unsuccessful attempts were made to remove the ganglion. In 1909 the ganglion and its sensory root were removed, resulting in total anesthesia of the trigeminal area, but the spasms and pain continued unabated. A few months later an attempt was made to destroy the geniculate ganglion, and on the right an anastomosis was made between the spinal accessory and the facial nerves. Destruction of the ganglion resulted in a temporary disappearance of the tic and some of the pain, the jaw still continuing to be painful. Six months later the spasm returned, accompanied by an increasingly high-intensity pain which extended into the ear.

The patient was desperate and contemplated suicide. He died during a further attempt to relieve the spasm and the pain by aural operation in October 1913.

Postmortem examination was unrevealing as to the cause of these complaints.

Painful tic convulsif is reported to be more severe in women than in men. It may begin in or about the orbicularis oculi as a fine intermittent myokymia, with some spread thereafter into the muscles of the lower part of the face. Occasionally strong spasms may involve all of the facial muscles on one side almost continuously. Rarely, the face may become weak and some of the facial muscles may atrophy. If the chorda tympani is involved, taste will be lost over the anterior two-thirds of the tongue.

The experience at Scripps Clinic with use of anticonvulsants in this situation is limited. Three patients have been treated without success. If the facial movements become disabling, then certainly operation can be considered as an alternative form of treatment.

GLOSSOPHARYNGEAL NEURALGIA

Glossopharyngeal neuralgia (tic) is characterized by severe pain in the region of the tonsil and ear. It has timing features like those of trigeminal neuralgia, and may be initiated by yawning and swallowing or contact of food with the tonsillar region. Rarely the patient may become unconscious during a paroxysm of pain (probably due to asystole). Examination reveals no evidence of reduction in perception of pinprick or touch, or of motility function in the nasopharynx.

Often the pain of glossopharyngeal neuralgia can be relieved by temporarily cocainization of the involved side of the throat. Extracranial block of the glossopharyngeal nerve with alcohol is not recommended since the injection of alcohol in the region of the jugular foramen might well cause paralysis of the tenth, eleventh, and twelfth cranial nerves and could conceivably also involve the sympathetic trunk.

If the patient does not respond to carbamazepine, the treatment of choice for glossopharyngeal neuralgia is intracranial section of the nerve. Usually the exposure is through a unilateral suboccipital craniectomy. The nerve can be identified as it passes along the floor of the posterior fossa to emerge through the jugular foramen.

Some authors use the term glossopharyngeal

and vagal neuralgia or vagoglossopharyngeal neuralgia instead of glossopharyngeal neuralgia, implying that the pain can radiate into the distribution of the vagus nerve as well as that of the glossopharyngeal nerve. The original term, glossopharyngeal neuralgia, is recognized by most neurologists and is more commonly used.

Since the ear and its adjacent structures are supplied by pain fibers from the fifth, seventh, ninth, and tenth cranial nerves, neuralgias of these structures often closely resemble each other and sometimes become inseparable. It is therefore not surprising that there has been controversy concerning the existence of separate neuralgias of these nerves, and conflict as to the best surgical procedures. It is likely that the mechanism of the pain in all is the same.

HEADACHE AND DIABETIC NEUROPATHY

Isolated cranial nerve palsies, especially of the third and sixth nerves, are known to occur in diabetics. Neuralgia of the fifth nerve with diabetic ocular paresis may occur.

No suitable explanation for the pain is available. It appears likely that the third, fourth, and sixth cranial nerve defects stem from vascular occlusive disease of the vasa nervorum, and that the fifth cranial nerve may rarely become similarly involved.

HERPETIC AND POSTHERPETIC NEURITIS (See also pp. 251–253)

Posterior Poliomyelitis (Herpes Zoster) with Involvement of the Gasserian Ganglion and Trigeminal Nucleus

The pain of herpes zoster, in contrast to tic as regards timing features, is steady and sustained. Although the pain often spontaneously regresses within two or three weeks, it may persist for several months, and when it occurs in persons past 70, as it frequently does, its duration may be a year or more. Rarely, it may persist indefinitely. The pain is unilateral and the quality and the quality of the pain is both burning and aching. It may be experienced in any part of the distribution of the fifth cranial nerve, although involvement of the forehead is most common. The pain is nonthrobbing, relatively uniform, and it usually diminishes gradually in intensity. Examination soon after onset reveals erythema and the typical herpetiform lesion of the skin associated with hyperalgesia and paresthesia. Examination later reveals hypesthesia and paresthesia of the involved areas, and sometimes scarring and pigmentation of the skin. There may be weakness of the masseter muscle and pterygoid muscle on the homolateral side. The judicious use of codeine and salicylates with reassurance of better days to come makes the period of spontaneous regression tolerable. Sensory root section does not usually give complete relief. Often it may have no effect.

Posterior Poliomyelitis (Herpes) and Involvement of Other Dorsal Root Ganglions and Nerve Tissues

Steady pain in the face and ear, back of the head, and neck, associated with vertigo and palsy of the homolateral side of the face, results from widespread inflammation involving the gasserian and glossopharyngeal and the first two or three dorsal root ganglions, and dorsal horns of the cervical portion of the cord. The pain has the qualities and duration described above. As with all herpes, there may be a slight or moderate palsy. There may or may not be herpetiform lesions.

OCCIPITAL NEURITIS DUE TO HERPES, OTHER INFECTIONS, AND CERVICAL CORD TUMORS

Occipital headache due to inflammation, injury, or pressure on the occipital nerves, upper cervical spinal roots, dorsal horn or root ganglions is a long-lasting, sustained, nonthrobbing ache of moderate intensity. It is difficult to separate from muscle contraction headache, since it is also always associated with muscle contraction and tenderness. The characteristic feature is paresthesia or algesia of the tissues of the scalp and the skin of the neck. Discoloration or scarring of the skin, such as follows herpes, may also occur. When the headache is postherpetic, section of nerves or roots will probably not eliminate the pain, although it may be somewhat reduced, Procaine injections about the sensory roots have a similar slight effect in reducing the intensity of pain.

Occipital headache due to tumors of the upper cervical cord, especially to those masses attached or adjacent to the first two or three roots, closely resembles that first described. In most such instances, in addition to the pain there is disturbance in sensory perception within the dermatomes involved. Spinal fluid protein is increased above the average in about one-half the patients. Also in many instances, a partial or complete block is demonstrable during manometric studies. Rarely, X-ray pictures show bony defects. Removal of the tumor or rhizotomy, when removal is impossible, eliminates or reduces the intensity of headache.

Sustained contraction of the neck with the X-ray picture of a straight cervical spine may also be associated with a variety of cervical defects, including displaced cervical intervertebral disc nuclei. Unilateral neck-ache extending to the occiput and sometimes also including the temple and forehead may appear in patients with mid- and upper-cervical joint disorders.

Cautious extension of the neck by manual or other traction may have therapeutic effect.

Patients who survive after rupture of the odontoid ligament have severe headache in the neck and the suboccipital region.

Headache and Diseases of the Cervical Spine (see also Chapter 19)

Russell Brain *et al.* in 1952 called attention to the headache and other clinical manifestations of cervical spondylosis. Commonly, pain is referred to the deep structures about the neck and back of the head, as well as into the arms and digits, which is likely to be worsened by moving of the neck and pulling on the arms. Hyperalgesia, wasting, and fasciculations may be present. In addition there may be symptoms arising from the impairment of function of the cervical spinal cord. Brain and his colleagues defined cervical spondylosis as a degenerative disorder of the cervical spine, leading to narrowing of the intravertebral spaces and protrusion of the intravertebral discs. These changes can cause pressure on the spinal nerves in their foramina as well as pressure on the spinal cord. Since the disorder is degenerative rather than inflammatory, he selected the term spondylosis rather than spondylitis. He considers trauma and the degeneration of the intravertebral discs with age as the main precipitating factors. It is commoner in men than in women and produces symptoms chiefly in the fifth and sixth decades. As a result of the morbid process the nerve roots are compressed in the formina, now the site of a secondary formation of fibrous tissue. Thus nerve fibers undergo degeneration. The cord is directly compressed and tethered by the adhesions around the nerve root, and normal neck movement causes continual mild injury. Blood supply may be affected by compression of the spinal veins and the anterior spinal artery. Spinal fluid may show a slight rise in protein, and when the neck is extended there may be a demonstrable obstruction on manometric tests. Brain finds that rest by immobilization with a plastic collar for three months usually eliminates the pain, rendering operative intervention unnecessary. However, when the spinal cord is compressed, surgical procedures are sometimes helpful if the operation takes place early in the course of the disorder.

A number of other workers have called attention to the occurrence of headache with pathological changes of the cervical spine and especially to the possibility of painful implication of the frontal part of the head.

Headache is said to be a common accompaniment of cervical disc lesions. High cervical bony defects or root damage do indeed become linked with headache which may become frontal. Conspicuous in this category is the headache that accompanies the development of Paget's disease involving the bones of the base of the skull and the upper cervical spine. The distortions and the displacements that occur under these circumstances may also be linked with occipital headache. But it is striking that large numbers of patients with discogenic root diseases involving the fifth, sixth, or seventh cervical roots who have great discomfort in shoulders and arms, do not have pain in the head.

Further critical analysis is necessary for a proper appraisal of the significance of low cervical discogenic disease to headache.

A number of transient disturbances resulting from interference in the blood supply of the brainstem, such as vertigo, nausea, light-headedness, and even visual disturbances could stem from vertebral artery obstruction. It is difficult, however, to see how recurrent attacks of headache over many years with complete freedom of headache in the interval between attacks which are preceded by vertigo, nausea, and visual disturbances and which last many hours, could stem from gross mechanical interference of the vertebral artery by bony changes in the cervical spine. Such changes being constant, it is not immediately apparent how they could give rise at intervals to such severe, long-lasting discomfort, and be followed again by periods of complete freedom from pain. Other explanations for the pain would seem more suitable.

ATYPICAL FACIAL PAIN

THE head and face pains included for consideration in this section differ from the typical or major facial neuralgias chiefly as follows.

1. In the atypical neuralgias the pain is seldom limited to the distribution of the fifth or ninth cranial nerves, but usually spreads over the area supplied by the cervical roots.

2. The pain is not significantly reduced or eliminated by division of the fifth or ninth cranial nerves.

3. The pain is of a steady, diffuse, aching quality of hours' or days' duration: it does not occur in paroxysms of short duration (1 to 30 sec) followed by freedom from pain, as in tic douloureux.

4. The atypical facial neuralgia syndromes do not present trigger zones.

5. These disorders occur in a younger age group than the major neuralgias, and far more commonly in women.

6. Attacks are not precipitated by cold, drafts, cold water in the mouth, swallowing, talking, chewing, shaving, or washing the face, as in typical trifacial neuralgias considered in the previous sections.

Sphenopalatine Ganglion Neuralgia—Lower-Half Headache

The syndrome of sphenopalatine ganglion neuralgia was first described by Sluder (1908) and further defined by Eagle (1942). The following features are described as characteristic.

The pain is unilateral; it involves the lower half of the face and never extends above the level of the ear. It is episodic, recurrent, and lasts from a few minutes to several days. It occurs predominantly in whites; about 60% of the patients are between the ages of 30 and 50. There are twice as many women as men with the syndrome, and it may be associated with menopause. There are two sites of maximum pain: one in the region of the orbit and the base of the nose, and the other just posterior to the mastoid process in the temporal bone. Only one of these pain sites may be present, the more common one being that in the orbit and nose. The pain may be of high intensity and is continuous. It originates in the nose, extends to the orbit, and is associated with tenderness of the eyeball. It may further, extend back through the eye to the region of the ear, sometimes causing earache and a sensation of fullness in the ear with tinnitus and vertigo. From the ear the pain extends to a point about 5 cm behind the auditory canal. Occasionally the pain spreads to the neck, sometimes involves the shoulder blade, but more often the top of the shoulder. Rarely, the pain extends from the top of the shoulder to the elbow and to the finger tips, involving usually the middle and index fingers. Occasionally there is itching of the skin of the upper extremity, taste disturbances, feelings of stiffness and muscle weakness in the upper extremity, and fortification scotomata.

During the attacks there is swelling of the nasal mucous membrane on the involved and painful side with outpouring of mucoid and serous nasal secretions, and nasal obstruction. Pain may emanate from the teeth of the upper and lower jaws on the affected side. In addition, burning, stinging, and tingling sensations have been noted to emanate from the skin over the lower part of the jaw. Eagle (1942) emphasized that "the diagnosis is conclusive if the symptoms are relieved within one to three minutes by cocainization of the sphenopalatine ganglion on the affected side." Also, he alleges that the attacks of pain may be alleviated permanently by a single application of 10% procaine in the area of the ganglion. Eagle further states that since there may be a recurrence from a few hours to weeks later, additional therapeutic aid may be necessary. When a "septal deviation or a spur or ledge of the nasal septum is involved and is thought to be the cause of the irritation of the sphenopalatine ganglion, it is necessary to perform a submucous resection of nasal septum," In Eagle's group of 159 patients, 80% were found to require intranasal operative procedures; and according to his records, therefore, "a submucous resection of the nasal septum was found to be the most efficient method of treating sphenopalatine ganglion neuralgia in the largest number of cases." However, the doubtful basis for such a procedure will be considered below in the discussion of the closely related syndrome of vidian neuralgia.

Vidian Neuralgia

Vidian neuralgia, according to Vail (1932), is a pain in the nose, face, eye, ear, head, neck, and shoulder, occurring in severe attacks and similar to that described by Sluder as "sphenopalatine ganglion neuralgia." These attacks cannot be induced by external stimulation, and are not associated with loss of perception of surface sensation. The attacks are typically unilateral, are often nocturnal, and may or may not be associated with the symptoms of nasal sinusitis. The condition is one of adult life and is most frequently found in women.

Vail is of the opinion that this syndrome is due to an irritation or inflammation of the vidian nerve in the vidian canal, and is always secondary to a latent or frank infection of the sphenoid sinus. It is Vail's conclusion that the syndrome that has been described as sphenopalatine ganglion neuralgia is actually a vidian neuralgia, and is due to an irritation of

inflammation of the vidian nerve. For this reason it seemed proper to Vail that the term *vidian neuralgia* be applied to this syndrome rather than the term *sphenopalatine ganglion neuralgia.* The treatment, according to Vail, should be directed toward the disease in the sphenoid sinus.

Comment. It was suggested by Sluder (1908) that vasoconstriction of the vascular bed supplying the nasal mucous membrane was the basis of the pain experienced by patients with lower-half headache. Such a view is not readily acceptable, since there is no evidence that vasoconstriction within the nasal mucous membrane or adjacent structures is accompanied by pain. Extreme vasoconstriction within the intact nasal mucous membrane has been noted during fear and panic without an accompanying pain. Experimentally induced vasoconstriction of arteries elsewhere except perhaps in the case of "cold pain" has not in itself resulted in pain, although if muscles so deprived are caused to contract, pain usually follows. Furthermore, pallor of the mucous membrane during the attack of so-called sphenopalatine ganglion neuralgia has not been noted. In fact, the opposite occurs. Hence the inference of Sluder regarding the cause of pain is unsupported. The relief of lower-half headache after cocaine was applied to the region of the sphenopalatine ganglion could result from the block of afferent pain fibers.

Vidian neuralgia, like sphenopalatine neuralgia, is a periodic, recurrent, unilateral, painful disorder with associated smooth muscle and gland disturbances. It is conceivable, as suggested by Vail, that "irritation or inflammation of the vidian nerve" would cause severe pain, but it is not likely that recurrent attacks of pain over many years with complete freedom from discomfort between attacks, and without disturbances in sensation of the parts supplied by this nerve, would result from inflammation of the peripheral nerve.

It is conceivable that some patients with primary mucous membrane disease could have one or possibly two attacks of pain in the face with spread to adjacent structures, but sphenoid sinus disease or inflammation in the region of the sphenopalatine ganglion could not explain the peculiar timing features demonstrated by this group of patients.

Since major portions of the turbinates and adjacent mucous membrane and vascular structures receive their sensory nerve supply from afferent nerves that pass through this so-called nerve ganglion and adjacent branches of the internal maxillary nerve, it is to be expected that the application of cocaine, phenol, or alcohol to this region would dramatically stop pain having its source in noxious stimulation of the vascular structures or the mucuous membranes in this region. It does not stop pain from afferent nerves that do not pass via this relatively small pathway.

Since lower-half headache may be abolished in a high percentage of persons by correction of a septal defect, according to Eagle, and by drainage of the sphenoidal sinus, according to Vail, or by the application of cocaine and phenol to the sphenopalatine ganglion and artery, according to Sluder, it is apparent that a variety of operative procedures may have a similar therapeutic effect. It therefore raises a doubt as to whether there is any specific etiologic relationship of the structures of the nose to the syndrome. Indeed, there is no good basis for accepting the thesis that the sphenopalatine ganglion plays any significant role.

The evidence indicates that quite different structures are involved and, because of the similarity to the group of neuralgias about to be considered, it seems likely that the so-called sphenopalatine or vidian neuralgia is actually a vascular syndrome involving the internal maxillary artery and especially the third portion that supplies the sphenopalatine region and adjacent structures. This point of view will be discussed further in the following section.

Atypical Facial Neuralgia (Episodic)

A group of patients with so-called "atypical facial neuralgia" with complaints that closely resemble those described by Sluder, Vail, and Eagle, has been carefully studied. There is unilateral spread of pain from the nose, eye, cheek, and ear, ultimately involving the neck and shoulder. Such patients have recurrent attacks of variable duration. There may be associated redness of the nasal mucous membrane, swelling of the turbinates, and increased secretion and obstruction in the nose. Serious disturbances in mood, attitude, and behavior were conspicuous.

The pain had an aching quality and seemed to arise deep in the bones or the eyeball, in contrast to that of trigeminal neuralgia, which has both an aching and a burning component. The pain emanated from the region of the nose, the upper and lower jaws, the eyeball and above it, the ear and behind it, and from the occipital region, the suboccipital region, and the neck and shoulder. There was considerable variation in the distribution. The pain was not eliminated by any of the following procedures. Section or alcohol injection of any branch of the trigeminal nerve; operations on structures in the painful areas, as teeth, nasal structures, and sinuses; cocainization of the sphenopalatine ganglion; resection of the superior cervical sympathetic ganglion; supraorbital and infraorbital nerve evulsion; stripping of the periarterial (carotid) plexus; subtotal section of the sensory root of the trigeminal nerve; mastoid operations; pelvic operations.

A series of patients with painful disorders in this distribution and of the nature described in the preceding paragraphs has been studied at the Scripps Clinic and Research Foundation. The investigators have determined that it is not possible to further define this bewildering group of facial pains and syndromes on the basis of any consistent history, and since the diagnosis rests entirely on the history, we choose to consider all unfortunate patients with these syndromes as having, simply, atypical facial neuralgia. We recognize that multiple factors may be responsible for the production of this syndrome, and when this diagnosis is made, we suggested a careful search be made for local pathology of the nose, eyes, teeth, sinuses, and pharynx. Atypical facial neuralgia may be associated with autonomic symptoms including cutaneous pallor, sweating, flushing, lacrimation, pupillary changes, rhinitis, and the like. If vasodilator phenomena are obvious, suggesting a lower-half headache, a trial on a vasoconstrictor agent of the ergot type may be worthwhile. But the physician should not be surprised if the patient does not respond to this or other forms of therapy.

CAROTIDYNIA

Fay (1932) introduced the word *carotidynia* to describe a variety of pain that arises in the neck. He suggested that the pain originated in the common carotid and external carotid arteries and its maxillary branches, and that the course of afferent impulses to the central nervous system was indirect, involving in part the vagus nerve. Carotidynia is a syndrome which is featured by tenderness, swelling, and sometimes conspicuous pulsation of the common carotid artery on the affected side. If the thumbs are placed on the common carotid arteries just below the bifurcation and the structures pressed back against the transverse cervical processes with a rolling movement, a severe pain is produced. Patients who already have a dull aching pain referred to the eye, deep in the malar region, spreading back to the ear, behind the ear, and down the neck, have the pain accentuated. The attacks are usually periodic, more likely to occur on the same side, and are not associated with visual disturbances.

Roseman (1967) has reviewed the literature on carotidynia and reported his observations in young and middle-aged adults. He describes a unilateral or bilateral neck pain of high intensity but of relatively short duration lasting 11 days on the average. In 90% of cases the disease was self-limited. Systemic signs of illness were absent. (see also Laskin and Ausiner, 1977). Treatment of carotidynia is usually supportive. Simple analgesics such as aspirin may be helpful. Corticosteroids are rarely necessary.

Lovshin (1977) has reported on a series of 100 cases of carotidynia from the Cleveland Clinic. All of the patients were examined, treated, and followed by the author. There were 82 females and 18 males, and 67 patients had a history of vascular headache. Forty-five patients volunteered the information that the glands in the neck had been swollen. Lovshin finds that the most common form of carotidynia is related to over distention, relaxa-

tion, and increased pulsation in the carotid artery. This syndrome of vascular neck pain is closely associated with various forms of extra-cranial vascular headache. It is more common in women than in men, the ratio being about 4 to 1. The syndrome occurs at almost any age but is more prevalent during the fourth and fifth decades, and there is often a history of vascular headache. The only significant abnormality on physical examination is the presence of a tender, throbbing, often dilated carotid artery. The condition is frequently misdiagnosed and therefore not properly treated. Lovshin states that preferred treatment is similar that of migraine and other painful vasodilating conditions of the head. In particular, he suggests various oral preparations of ergotamine tartrate, or methysergide 2 mg three or four times daily in a short course. Apparently carotidynia is not characterized by an inflammatory arteritis. The condition is not related to cranial arteritis.

Raeder's Syndrome and the Pericarotid Syndrome

Raeder's paratrigeminal syndrome (1924) is a rare illness characterized by oculosympathetic paralysis, the sudden onset of severe frontotemporal burning, aching pain of rapid onset, with associated ptosis and meiosis, often in a periorbital distribution, no previous history of headache, and normal sweating in the supraorbital area of the ipsilateral forehead. Raeder based his conclusions on five cases in which there were cranial nerve dysfunctions, usually involving the optic, oculomotor, trochlear, trigeminal, and abducens nerves. Raeder's first patient had a tumor arising from the region of the trigeminal ganglion infiltrating all of these cranial nerves. Two of his cases had multiple cranial nerve lesions and sympathetic paralysis related to head injury. In two cases, no particular cause could be identified. In essence then, Raeder's patients had multiple cranial nerve involvements, primarily parasellar, associated with oculosympathetic paralysis and intact facial sweating. Others have since described almost any lesion in which there is oculosympathetic paralysis associated with head pain as Raeder's syndrome. Given this confusion, it would probably be best to abandon the eponym and more precisely classify patients with oculosympathetic paralysis and headache, who may or may not have disturbances of sweating as well.

Many patients with cluster headaches have an associated oculosympathetic paralysis, but in this situation the tempo of the cluster headache establishes the diagnosis, rather than the autonomic dysfunction.

Vijayan and Watson (1978) have described a pericarotid syndrome characterized by oculosympathetic paralysis, ipsilateral head pain, and anhidrosis over the forehead with otherwise intact facial sweating. They suggest that the site of the lesion involving the oculosympathetic fibers in their patients is pericarotid. Their patients had no previous history of headache. They were able to establish a pathogenesis in only one of their six patients in whom a left internal carotid artery occlusion had occurred. In the other five patients, the etiology was unknown.

Long-Sustained or Chronic Atypical Facial Neuralgia (Psychogenic)

In contrast to the probable vascular origin of pain in the episodic variety of atypical facial neuralgia, the pathophysiology of long-sustained or continuous atypical facial neuralgia is ill defined. The failure of ergotamine tartrate to eliminate or reduce the pain, the inconstancy of the edema and the persistence of the pain for months or years invalidates the vascular hypothesis as regards patients with this chronic syndrome. Long-lasting alterations in mood, attitude, and behavior in this latter group of patients are conspicuous. The depressive, hypochondriacal, or hysterical features support the view that the pain is of a delusional nature, or at least that the delusion of pain is the outstanding feature of the patient's illness and far outweighs in significance any peripheral changes that might give rise to pain. The prognosis in this latter group of patients is grave regardless of therapy.

In a psychiatric study of atypical facial pain, Smith et al. (1969) from the Mayo Clinic found evidence of significant psychopathology. They studied 32 patients with atypical facial pain seen in the sections of Neurology and Dentistry of the Mayo Clinic during an eight-month period. Psychiatric diagnoses grouped the majority of the patients into three categories: depressive reaction, conversion reaction, and hysterical personality with a conversion reaction or a depressive equivalent. In general, the patients were found to be perfectionistic, striving, success-oriented, hypochondriacal, and depressed. Smith and his associates postulate that the patients demonstrate a considerable resentment and anger which was repressed and internalized, resulting in depression as well as in the painful condition of atypical facial pain. The writers concur with the literature indicating that the condition is psychiatric and conclude that patients with this syndrome seem to be in need of an understanding, reassuring medical regimen with psychotherapy made available for those who would benefit from this approach.

CENTRAL PAIN, POSTHERPETIC NEURITIS, AND TRANSCUTANEOUS NEUROSTIMULATION

Recent reports of the analgesic effects of transcutaneous electrical neurostimulation (TNS) have emphasized peripheral mechanisms (Ignelzi and Nyquist, 1976; Loeser et al, 1975). Although the possibility of a central effect has remained open, these reports have noted an apparent "fatigue" of peripheral nerve fibers, which could account for the analgesia obtained.

We have recently had some success with TNS in reducing the severity of central pain states in a small series of patients. It is of interest to review these cases because they demonstrate a central inhibitory effect of TNS.

Method and Results The eight patients whose experience is charted in Table 11-5 have had either thalmamic pain following a cerebrovascular accident (CVA) or postherpetic neuralgia. Three of four patients who had thalamic pain have obtained some relief with TNS (cases 1–3), and 5 of 14 patients with postherpetic neuralgia have likewise obtained significant relief (cases 4–8). We have no clear explanation for the failures except that several of these patients reported that TNS made them "nervous," or expressed displeasure at wearing the device.

The thalamic pain patients required electrode placement in the distribution of their pain, and one (case 3) obtained additional ben-

TABLE 11-5   Patients with Central Pain Partially Relieved by TNS

CASE	AGE	SEX	DIAGNOSIS	PAIN DISTRIBUTION	PAIN DURATION PRE-TNS	PAIN SEVERITY PRE-TNS (0-100)
1.	73	male	post-CVA	right foot	1½ yrs	75
2.	40	female	post-CVA	left arm, left leg, left side of head	6 mo.	95
3.	61	male	post-CVA	entire left side except abdomen	4 yrs	60 (if inactive) 90 (if active)
4.	79	female	post-herpetic	T4–5, left	3½ yrs	?
5.	65	male	post-herpetic	T8–10, left	5 yrs	50
6.	76	male	post-herpetic	C1–2, right	5 yrs	50
7.	16	male	post-herpetic	C2–3, right	1 yr	60
8.	68	male	post-herpetic	L4–5, left	14 mo.	80

efit from adding electrodes to the contralateral side as well. However, none of the patients with postherpetic neuralgia could tolerate such a "peripheral" placement, as it exacerbated their pain; electrodes at either side of the spinal vertebrae at the dermatomal level of their pain were better tolerated.

All patients wore the stimulating device throughout the day, except case 7, who did not wear it to school, but applied it on arriving home each day. Case 3 has tried on several occasions to determine how long he could do without TNS, and has found that after three or four days his pain is unbearable.

Discussion In herpes zoster, a varicella virus causes an inflammatory reaction in peripheral nerve and dorsal root ganglion (Adams, 1976). Most cases appear to recover uneventfully, but a variety of complications may arise, including myelitis and encephalitis (Gardner-Thorpe *et al*, 1976). Lesions include inflammatory necrosis in the dorsal root ganglion and associated destruction of the nerve cells and fibers in the cord, particularly in the anterior horns, sub-

stantia gelatinosa, and Clarke's column (Denny-Brown *et al.*, 1944). If, in the acute stage, there has been such severe inflammation and necrosis, then the subsequent loss of neurons and fibrosis may be associated with postherpetic neuralgia (Gordon and Tucker, 1945). The vascular dilatation and hemorrhage, which are frequent findings at the spinal level of the neuraxis in herpes zoster, suggest that the pathologic lesions may be comparable to the thrombotic CVA's associated with thalamic pain (Mumenthaler, 1976).

The fact that lesions at various levels of the neuraxis may give rise to pain has stimulated a number of theories to account for the phenomenon: irritable foci, disinhibition of thalamic functions, and/or alteration of functional balance in sensory systems. Irritability, resulting in epileptiform activity in partially damaged cells surrounding the area of destruction (sensory epilepsy) may occur in some cases; the condition sometimes responds to anticonvulsants, such as carbamazepine. How-

ANALGESICS PRE-TNS	TNS ELECTRODE PLACEMENTS (PAIR)	DURATION TNS FOLLOW-UP	PAIN SEVERITY POST-TNS (0–100)	ANALGESICS POST-TNS
meperidine 100 mg prn	right ankle	7 months (deceased)	0–10	none
oxycodone q4h	1. left wrist 2. high cervical	6 weeks (lost to followup)	0–45	none
Valium	1. both legs 2. both shoulders	1 yr 9 mo.	0 (if inactive) 60 (if active)	none
acetaminophen 650 mg q4h	thoracic paraspinals	5 mo.	?	none
none	thoracic paraspinals	1 yr	0–50 (intermittent use)	none
none	high cervical	8 mo.	20	none
ASA 650 mg q4h	high cervical	18 mo.	25	ASA occasionally
Fiorinal 2/day	lumbar spine	2 mo.	50	occasional propoxyphene

ever, the quality of pain and failure of the drug in many cases, suggests this is not an adequate explanation. In recent years, a model emphasizing the loss of normal inhibitory input from the periphery has gained favor (Melzack and Wall, 1965).

Previous reports on the effectiveness of TNS in a variety of pain states have incidentally noted some success in central pain (Davis and Lentini, 1975; Ebersold et al., 1975), but the implications of this finding appear to have been overlooked. What the earlier reports and the present series demonstrate is precisely what the gate-control theory would predict, namely, that peripheral stimulation can produce a central pain-inhibiting effect (see Chapter 2). Although peripheral nerve fiber "fatigue" may also occur with TNS, the partial analgesia produced in these cases of central pain is consistent with an inhibition at spinal or higher levels. Furthermore, it is unlikely that the results reported here are due to a placebo effect, inasmuch as our experience suggests that pain relief which is maintained for two to four weeks is likely to persist indefinitely (Sternbach et al., 1976).

SUMMARY

1. Tic douloureux may be associated with a state of abnormal reactivity of the spinal trigeminal nuclei. A subtle anatomic lesion of the gasserian ganglion itself commonly accompanies this syndrome.

2. Medications which reduce polysynaptic reflex activity in the spinal trigeminal nuclei are effective in the therapy of tic douloureux.

3. Anticonvulsant therapy, beginning with carbamazepine, is the treatment of choice of the major neuralgias.

4. Surgical procedures should be reserved for those patients who respond poorly to medical therapy.

5. Anticonvulsants are not helpful in postherpetic pain syndromes.

6. Atypical facial neuralgia is a general term used to cover a variety of head and face pains which are poorly defined and which may not

deserve separate clinical status. These include sphenopalatine neuralgia, vidian neuralgia, carotidynia, and autonomic facioplegia, amongst others.

7. The pathogenesis of the atypical facial neuralgias is uncertain and multiple causation seems likely. Search for local inflammatory pathology, vasomotor phenomena, and depressive symptoms is indicated, with treatment guided by the findings.

8. Three cases of thalamic pain and five cases of postherpetic neuralgia have shown a significant decrease in pain levels with transcutaneous electrical neurostimulation (TNS). Such a favorable response in central pain states suggests that, in addition to any peripheral nerve fiber "fatigue" which TNS may cause, it has central inhibitory effects as well.

REFERENCES

Adams, J. H. (1976). Virus diseases of the nervous system. In *Greenfield's Neuropathology* (W. Blackwood and J. A. N. Corsellis, eds.), pp. 301–302. Arnold, London.

Brain, W. R., D. W. C. Northfield, and M. Wilkinson (1952). The neurological manifestations of cervical spondylosis. *Brain 75*, 187.

Cassinari, V., and C. A. Pagni (1969). *Central pain: A Neurosurgical Survey,* pp. 93–108, 139–158. Harvard Univ. Press, Cambridge.

Cushing, H. (1920). The major trigeminal neuralgias and their surgical treatment, based on experiences with 332 Gasserian operations. The varieties of facial neuralgia. *Am. J. Med. Sci. 160*, 157.

Dandy, W. E. (1925). Section of the sensory root of the trigeminal nerve at the pons. *Bull. Johns Hopkins Hosp. 36*, 105

Dandy, W. E. (1934). Concerning the cause of trigeminal neuralgia. *Am. J. Surg. 24*, 447.

Dandy, W. E. (1945). *Surgery of the Brain.* W. F. Prior, Hagerstown, Md.

Davis, R., and R. Lentini (1975). Transcutaneous nerve stimulation for treatment of pain in patients with spinal cord injury. *Surg. Neurol. 4 (Suppl.)* 100–101.

Denny-Brown, D., R. D. Adams, and P. J. Fitzgerald (1944). Pathologic features of herpes zoster. *Arch. Neurol. Psychiat. 51*, 216–231.

Eagle, W. W. (1942). Sphenopalatine ganglion neuralgia. *Arch. Otolaryngol. 35*, 66.

Ebersold, M. J., E. R. Laws, Jr., H. H. Stonnington, and G. K. Stillwell (1975). Transcutaneous electrical stimulation for treatment of chronic pain: a preliminary report. *Surg. Neurol. 4 (Suppl.)* 96–99.

Fay, T. (1932). Atypical facial neuralgia, a syndrome of vascular pain. *Ann. Otol. 41*, 1030.

Fromm, G. H. (1969). Pharmacological consideration of anticonvulsants. *Headache 9*, 35.

Fromm, G. H., and S. Landgren (1963). Effect of diphenylhydantoin on single cells in the spinal trigeminal nucleus. *Neurol. 13*, 34.

Garcin, R., S. Godlewski, and J. leLapresle, (1960). Nevralgie du Trijumeau et Sclerose en Plaques. *Rev. Neurol. 102*, 441.

Gardner-Thorpe, C., J. B. Foster, and D. D. Barwick (1976). Unusual manifestations of herpes zoster: a clinical and electrophysiological study. *J. Neurol. Sci. 28*, 427–447.

Goodlett, R., and D. J. Dalessio (1973). *Unpublished Observations.*

Gordon, I. R. S., and J. F. Tucker (1945). Lesions of the central nervous system in herpes zoster. *J. Neurol. Neurosurg. Psychiat. 8*, 40–46.

Harris, W. (1950). Rare forms of paroxysmal trigeminal neuralgia and the relation to disseminated sclerosis. *Brit. Med. J. 1*, 831.

Ignelzi, R. J., and J. K. Nyquist (1976). Direct effect of electrical stimulation on peripheral nerve evoked activity: implications in pain relief. *J. Neurosurg. 45*, 159–165.

Jannetta, P. J. (1967). Structural mechanisms of trigeminal neuralgia. *J. Neurosurg. 26*, 159.

Jannetta, P. J. (1977). Treatment of trigeminal neuralgia by suboccipital and transtentorial cranial operations. *Clin. Neurosurg. 24*, 538–549.

Jannetta, P. J., and R. W. Rand (1967). Gross (mesoscopic) description of the human trigeminal nerve and ganglion. *J. Neurosurg. 26*, 109.

Kerr, F. W. L. (1963). The etiology of trigeminal neuralgia. *Arch Neurol. 8*, 15.

Kugelberg, E., and U. Lindblom (1959). The mechanism of the pain in trigeminal neuralgia. *J. Neurol. Neurosurg. Psychiat. 22*, 36.

Loeser, J. D., R. G. Black, and A. Christman (1975). Electrical stimulation in the nervous system: the current status of electrical stimulation of the nervous system for relief of pain. *Pain 1*, 109–123.

Lovshin, L. (1977). Carotidynia. *Headache 17*, 192–195.

Maroon, J. C. (1978). Hemifacial spasm. *Arch. Neurol. 35*, 481–483.

Matthews, R. J., J. P. DaVanzo, and R. J. Collins (1963). The pharmacology of chlorphenesin carbamate. *Arch. Intern. Pharmacodyn. 143*, 574.

Melzack, R., and P. D. Wall (1965). Pain mechanisms: a new theory. *Science 150*, 971–979.

Morley, T. P. (1977). The place of peripheral and subtemporal ablative operations in the treatment of trigeminal neuralgia. *Clin. Neurosurg. 24*, 550–556.

Mumenthaler, M. (1976). The pathophysiology of pain. In *Epileptic Seizures—Behavior—Pain* (W. Birkmayer, ed.), pp. 303–305. University Park Press, Baltimore.

Parker, H. L. (1978). Trigeminal Neuralgia Associated With Multiple Sclerosis. *Brain* 51:46.

Raeder, J. G. (1924). Paratrigeminal paralysis of oculopupillary sympathetic. *Brain 47*, 149–158.

Raskin, N. H., and S. P. Prusiner (1977). Carotidynia. *Neurology 27*, 43–46.

Roseman, D. M. (1967). Carotidynia. A distinct syndrome. *Arch. Otolaryngol. 85*, 81.

Saunders, R., and E. Sachs (1971). The role of the motor root in trigeminal neuralgia. *Headache 10*, 144.

Sluder, G. (1908). The role of the sphenopalatine (or Meckle's) ganglion in nasal headaches. *N.Y. Med. J. 87*, 989.

Smith, D. P., L. F. Pilling, J. S. Pearson, J. G. Rushton, N. P. Goldstein, and J. A. Gibilisco (1969). A psychiatric study of atypical facial pain. *Can. Med. Assoc. J. 100*, 26.

Sternbach, R. A., R. J. Ignelzi, L. M. Deems, and G. Timmermens (1976). Transcutaneous electrical analgesia: a follow-up analysis. *Pain 2*, 35–41.

Tew, J. M., and J. T. Keller (1977). The treatment of trigeminal neuralgia by percutaneous radiofrequency technique. *Clin. Neurosurg. 24*, 557–575.

Vail, H. H. (1932). Vidian neuralgia. *Ann. Otol. 41*, 837.

Vijayan, N., and C. Watson (1978). The Pericarotid Syndrome. *Headache 18*, 244.

12

ALLERGY, ATOPY, NASAL DISEASE, AND HEADACHE

REVISED BY DONALD D. STEVENSON

The term *allergy* was derived by von Pirquet (1906), from the greek words ALLOS (other) and ERGON (action). He used *allergy* to describe the "changed reactivity" which occurred in a minority of animals after immunization with antigens (allergens). The most striking example of "changed reactivity" is anaphylaxis. A susceptible animal, which has had prior immunization by specific antigens, undergoes a clearly defined, predictable systemic reaction when antigen is reintroduced. This reaction is the consequence of union between specific antigens; specific cell-fixed IgE antibodies; release of chemical mediators; and their rapid effects upon smooth muscles, vascular beds, and mucuous membranes.

Although an antigen-induced anaphylactic reaction is universally accepted as an allergic event, physicians agree less frequently when the term *allergy* is used to describe other immunologic inflammatory reactions and agreement disappears when nonimmunologic

	TYPE I	TYPE II	TYPE III	TYPE IV
Immuno-chemical reaction	IgE-mediated chemical mediator release	cytotoxic or cytolytic Ab. (IgM or IgG)	circulating complexes of Ab. Ag and complement	sensitized lymphocytes
Time of reaction	Immediate (15 min)	Immediate to delayed (minutes to hours)	Intermediate (4–24 hr)	Delayed (24–72 hr)
Clinical state	Anaphylaxis Allergic rhinitis	Hemolytic anemia	Vasculitis	Contact dermatitis

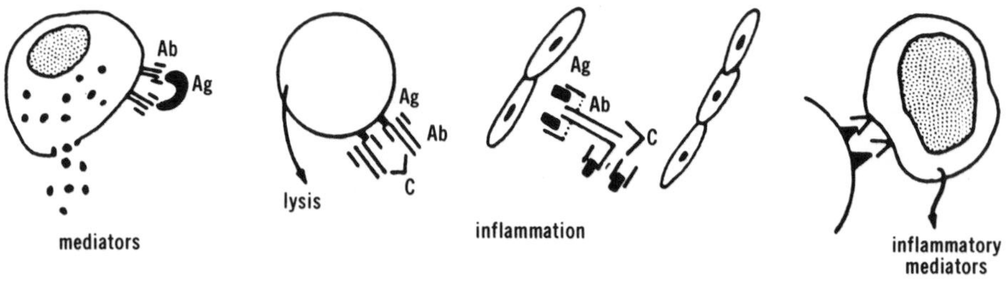

FIG. 12-1. Types of allergic reactions.

untoward reactions are included in a classification of "allergic" reactions. Since the 1960's, the classification of Gell and Coombs (1968) has gained widespread acceptance as a reasonable description of directions by which the immune system can respond to the introduction of specific antigens (Fig. 12-1).

The atopic state refers to allergic reactions (such as asthma and hay fever) which are familial, and in which intracutaneous injection of the offending allergen leads to immediate wheal and erythema of the skin.

Type I Reactions

When IgE antibodies, which are fixed to tissue mast cells or circulating basophils, combine with specific antigens, a cascade of intracellular biochemical events is initiated which culminates in the release of chemical mediators from their intracellular storage granules into surrounding tissue or fluid (Kaliner and Austen, 1973). A number of mediators have been identified.

Histamine can combine with receptors in certain tissue cells to produce a variety of special events depending upon the response of the tissue where the receptors reside. For pharmacologic convenience, these receptors are called H_1, which are blocked by standard antihistamines (chlorpheniramine, diphenhydramine, etc.) or H_2 which are blocked by the newer antihistamines (cimetidine). Table 12-1 summarizes the tissues which contain H_1 or H_2 receptors and the consequences of their stimulation by histamine molecules (Goth, 1978). Important counter mechanisms exist for degrading histamine rapidly. Radiolabelled histamine, injected intravenously, disappears from the circulation in about 1 min (Beall and Van Arsdel, 1960).

Slow Reacting Substance of Anaphylaxis (SRS-A) is more powerful and has a more prolonged effect upon smooth muscle constriction than does histamine (Brocklehurst, 1960). SRS-A is a complicated acidic lipid with a molecular weight of 400 (Stechschulte *et al.*, 1973). It has not been satisfactorily purified and study of its isolated effects upon the peripheral or cerebral vascular systems are therefore unknown.

Eosinophilic Chemotactic Factor of Anaphylaxis (ECF-A) is a glycopeptide with a molecular weight between 500 and 1000. When released from tissue storage cells, eosinophiles are attracted to this site of anaphylactic activity by ECF-A through counter gradient mechanisms (Kay and Austen, 1971). Although the precise role of eosinophiles in anaphylaxis is not set-

TABLE 12-1   Locations and Actions of Histamine Receptors (H_1 and H_2) in Humans

H_1 RECEPTORS	ORGANS	ACTIONS
Blocked by		
Diphenhydramine	Lacrimal glands	Increased secretions
Chlorpheniramine	Salivary glands	Increased secretions
Cyclizine	Capillary	Vasodilatation and increased permeability
Promethazine	Heart	Tachycardia
Cyproheptadine	Vascular	Vasodilatation (hypotension)
	CNS	Stimulation
	Mast cells	Inhibition of histamine release
	Cutaneous	Pruritus
	Bronchial tree	Bronchoconstriction
H_2 RECEPTORS		
Blocked by	Cutaneous vasculature	Cutaneous vasodilatation
Cimetidine	Larger arteries	Vascular dilatation
Metiamide	Heart	Excitation
	Leukocytes	Inhibit functions
	Gastrointestinal	Secretion HCl and pepsin

tled, the presence of eosinophiles can serve as a marker for type I IgE-medicated reactions.

Neutrophil Chemotactix Factor (NCF-A) was identified by Wasserman *et al.* (1977) in the sera of patients with cold urticaria. Partial purification of this material indicates it has a high molecular weight (> 750,000) and shows a preferential chemotactic activity toward neutrophilic polymorphonuclear leukocytes. Its release into the venous effluent follows a time course which is identical with that of histamine and low-molecular weight eosinophil chemotactic factor, suggesting that these mediators are released together, during anaphylactic cellular discharge.

Kinin Activating Factor is released from IgE-sensitized basophiles after antigen challenge, with a time course similar to histamine release (Newball *et al.*, 1975). Leukocyte kallikrein behaves similarly to plasma kallikrein by cleaving kininogen into the potent plasma mediator, bradykinin.

Platelet Activating Factor (P.A.F.) is released from basophilic leukocytes after antigen challenge. It combines with platelet receptors, stimulating release of serotonin and histamine from rabbit platelets (Benveniste, 1974). However, human platelets contain only serotonin and a role for P.A.F. in man awaits clarification.

Although Type 1 reactions can produce rapid and profound changes in the caliber of circular smooth muscles, vasodilatation, increased vascular permeability, infiltration of eosinophiles and neutrophiles, aggregation of platelets, and activation of the kinin and coagulation systems; the compensatory and counter-regulatory systems which either destroy the circulating mediators or block their effects by activating the sympathomimetic autonomic responses are also well developed. These balances serve to either localize IgE-mediated (Type 1) reactions to the site of antigen–antibody interaction or to shorten the time of their systemic effects.

Type II Reactions

Cytolytic or cytotoxic reactions occur when the antigens are constituents of cell walls, as in autoimmune hemolytic anemia or transfusion reactions, or when the antigens are adherent to the cell walls. When penicillin or quinidine adheres to red blood cells, they can initiate Type II reactions if circulating antibodies of the IgG or IgM classes, which have been synthesized in response to the antigens above, combine with these antigens. This union, by itself, does not damage the cells. However, antibodies from both IgG and IgM classes have the capability of activating the complement system through the classical pathway, beginning with the C_1 trimolecular complex, through C_4, C_2, C_3, and $C_{5,6\&7}$, C_8, and C_9. With the addition of the terminal complement components spaces are formed in the lipid membrane of the cell wall, the contents extrude into the extracellular space, and cytolysis with cell death occurs (Ruddy *et al.*, 1972). Type II hypersensitivity reactions are not involved in the pathogenesis of headache.

Type III Reactions

Immune complex reactions occur within the vascular spaces when circulating soluble antigens (drugs, nuclear antigens, virus particles) combine with IgG or IgM antibodies, and then fix complement components. This active immune complex of antigen, antibody, and complement adheres to the endothelial surface of blood vessels, greatly aided by certain properties of activated complement. These include: release of C_{3a} and C_{5a} anaphylatoxins which stimulate nonimmunologic release of stored mediators from circulating basophils, activation of the kinin system through C_2, and release of chemotactic complexes of complement cleavage proteins which attract neutrophils to the site of complement activation (Kohler, 1978).

In Type III reactions, inflammation occurs in the walls of blood vessels where immune complexes are deposited. The renal endothelial surfaces are frequent sites of immune complex deposition, presumably because immune complexes leave the plasma when the rate of blood flow diminishes. Biopsy and immunofluorescent staining for antibody or complement shows a lumpy bumpy arrangement of complexes in the subendothelial cell walls with infiltration of inflammatory cells, particularly PMNS. Type III reactions can produce headache if immune complexes are deposited in those arteries which carry blood to both intra/and extracranial structures.

Type IV Reactions

Cellular immune reactions occur when thymus-derived or T lymphocytes, previously sensitized to specific antigens, arrive at the site of antigen introduction. When the original antigen is either introduced through the skin or arrives when certain lipids (as in *Mycobacterium tuberculosis*), lymphocytes are preferentially sensitized or stimulated by such antigen-adjuvant combinations. Reintroduction of specific antigens stimulate sensitized lymphocytes to migrate toward the site of antigen entry or concentration. Activated lymphocytes secrete bioactive chemicals or factors (David and David, 1972) which produce inflammation in the area of their release. The tuberculin cutaneous reaction, occurring 24 to 72 hr after introduction of killed *M. tuberculosis* antigens is the classic example of a delayed cellular reaction. With the possible exception of tuberculous and fungal meningitis, cellular immune reactions probably do not produce headaches.

Other Mediator Systems

The prostaglandins are a group of closely related chemicals with a common basic structure. They are not stored in intracellular granules, but are derived from a common essential fatty acid, arachidonic acid, contained in the wall of many mammalian cells and, released by the enzyme phospholipase A_2. Prostaglandin synthetase converts arachidonic acid to hydroperoxide, then into nedoperoxide PGH_2 and eventually into PGF_2 and PGE series. For the most part, these mediators appear as a consequence of any inflammation and tend to modulate or amplify other systems. For instance, PGF_2 will directly stimulate bronchoconstriction and decrease cyclic AMP levels in mast cells and basophiles. PGE_1, on the other hand, stimulates bronchodilatation and

increases intracellular cyclic AMP levels in mast cells, diminishing or interrupting mediator release from storage cells (Vane, 1976).

The role of prostaglandins in neurovascular biology is incompletely defined. Some prostaglandins, particular thromboxanes, can aggregate platelets with disruption and release of stored serotinin, a potent vasodilator. Bergstrom *et al.* (1959) showed that intravenous injections of prostaglandin E_1 in susceptible individuals was associated with the onset of vascular headaches, whereas all patients experienced burning pain along the vein where PGE_1 was infused.

Kinins

A circulating globulin, kininogen is the precursor protein for bradykinin. Kininogen is cleaved by the enzyme kallikrein to produce the active peptide bradykinin (Lewis, 1961). Kallikrein is generated from prekallikrein after interaction with activated Hageman factor (from the coagulation cascade), or can be released from basophiles or mast cells during Type I reactions. The generation of the nonapeptide, bradykinin, produces a potent mediator which: increases vascular permeability, contracts smooth muscles, and interacts with sensory nerve endings to produce a painful stimulus (Kaplan and Austen, 1975).

For the most part, kinin activation appears to be a secondary system, resulting from release of mediators from basophiles, activation of the complement system, or intravascular coagulation. Bradykinin is a potent vasodilator, but is rapidly cleaved in normal plasma to an inactive octapeptide, limiting its systemic effects in normal humans and animals. Because of the lability of bradykinin in normal mammalian circulations, it has been extremely difficult to study its *in vivo* effects and to assign a clear role for the kinin system in disorders such as vascular shock, asthma, pain syndromes, or vascular dilatation of the cerebral circulation.

PARANASAL HEAD PAIN AND ALLERGIC RHINITIS

Paranasal head pain develops in some patients when IgE-mediated reactions occur in nasal mucous membranes. Thus, allergic rhinitis can be responsible for paranasal headache, with or without associated inflammation in the paranasal sinuses. The percentage of patients with allergic rhinitis who also report paranasal head pain is unknown. Many individuals with allergic rhinitis experience mild "pressure" in the paranasal structures but their individualized definition of pain plays a substantial part in whether or not they report paranasal pain during allergic rhinitis episodes. In our allergy clinic, only 20% of patients with proven IgE-mediated rhinitis report paranasal discomfort when directly questioned about this issue. These patients rarely seek medical attention because of their head pain, but instead describe rhinorrhea, nasal congestion, or sneezing as their chief complaints.

Other Types of Rhinitis

The term rhinitis is nonspecific. A number of inflammatory mechanisms can induce swelling and congestion of the nasal membranes, and all can lead to paranasal pain. Important variables in the production of paranasal pain include: (1) the anatomical arrangements between the nasal septum, turbinates, and sinus ostia; (2) the relative size of the nasal passages; and (3) the presence or absence of nasal polyps.

The characteristics of all forms of rhinitis are compared to allergic rhinitis in Table 12-2. *Allergic rhinitis* is the only type which is initiated by antigen–antibody interaction. *Infectious rhinitis* is usually the consequence of a viral agent infecting the nasal membranes and inciting an inflammatory response. A viral infection frequently extends to the paranasal sinuses, pharynx, larynx, and trachea. Primary or secondary bacterial infections, usually *Staphylococcus aureus, Hemophyllis influenza, Pneumococcus pneumonia,* or *Streptococcus hemolyticus,* also occur in the nasal and sinus membrane. Paranasal head pain is more prominent during infectious rhinitis than in any other forms of rhinitis (Solomon, 1967).

Vasomotor Rhinitis mimics allergic rhinitis, but antigens and antibodies do not initiate this type of nasal congestion. Instead, a variety of stimuli, including temperature changes, exercise, change in position, change in barometric pressure or humidity, anger, and certain odors, precede the onset of nasal congestion. How these nonallergic stimuli induce nasal congestion is not entirely clear, but most evidence favors dysfunctional control of nasal

TABLE 12-2 Characteristics of the Major Forms of Rhinitis

	ALLERGIC RHINITIS	INFECTIOUS RHINITIS	VASOMOTOR RHINITIS	IRRITANT RHINITIS
Seasonal incidence	frequent	increased in winter	none	smog
Itching & sneezing	usual	rare	unusual	unusual
Collateral allergy	common	occasional	occasional	occasional
Family history allergy	common	occasional	occasional	occasional
Sore throat	rare	common	rare	rare
Fever	rare	common	rare	rare
Conjunctivitis	itching common	occasional	rare	burning common
Nasal pallor	usual	rare	common	occasional
Nasal polyps	occasional	occasional	occasional	occasional
Injection of pharynx	rare	common	rare	rare
Eosinophil nasal secretions	usual	absent	absent	absent
Purulent nasal secretions	rare	usual	occasional	occasional
Positive allergy skin tests	usual	rare (coincidental)	rare	rare (coincidental)
Paranasal pain	occasional	common	occasional	occasional

vascular beds by the autonomic nervous system. Interruption of the cervical sympathetic nerves is followed by unilateral nasal obstruction and hypersecretion. Disruption of the parasympathetic fibers produces dry, crusted atrophic nasal membranes (Millonig *et al.,* 1950). If a cold stimulus is applied to the nasal membranes or to skin of the extremity, there is prompt engorgement of the nasal turbinates in patients suffering from vasomotor rhinitis (Ralston and Kerr, 1945).

Irritant Rhinitis is sometimes classified as a form of vasomotor rhinitis. As implied by its name, irritant chemicals activate congestion and inflammation of the nasal membranes through direct contact with these structures. The precise role of the vasomotor autonomic reflexes in the resulting nasal congestion is unclear. Normal individuals who inhale volatile acidic fumes, smoke, or smog invariably develop mild to moderate tearing and nasal congestion. At the other end of the spectrum, selected "sensitive" individuals experience severe conjunctival or nasal congestion upon contact with minimal atmospheric concentrations of smog, cigarette smoke, perfumes, or cocaine. Although many of these patients also have vasomotor rhinitis, others experience nasal congestion only when their nasal membranes are in contact with irritant fumes.

Rhinitis Medicametosa is the rebound response of the nasal vascular beds to topical application or sympathomimetic drops or sprays. Neosynephrine and oxymetazoline HCl are the preparations usually applied to the nasal membranes. Rhinitis medicametosa almost never occurs by itself and attention to the underlying rhinitis mechanism is necessary, both to wean the patient away from sympathomimetic nasal sprays and also to initiate a treatment plan which will prevent the need for using topical sympathomimetic drugs in the future. By the time these individuals seek medical attention, the syndrome of underlying rhinitis with superimposed rhinitis medicametosa is frequently associated with paranasal head pain. However, despite their discomfort and desire to receive medical assistance, these patients are usually reluctant to disclose their use of sympathomimetic sprays. Close questioning

and even observation may be necessary to obtain this essential information.

Finally, although the features of rhinitis are presented in Table 12-2 as separate entities, few individuals experience only one type of rhinitis during their lifetime. An individual with IgE-mediated rhinitis to grass pollen in the spring, may experience irritant rhinitis in the fall, vasomotor rhinitis while skiing in the winter, and a viral upper respiratory infection with rhinitis in March. This relatively simplistic chronology can be further complicated by the simultaneous appearance of two or more rhinitis mechanisms. Diagnostic and treatment ingenuity can be severely strained when several types of rhinitis occur simultaneously (Tennenbaum, 1972). Many unfortunate patients with vasomotor rhinitis, who coincidentally have positive allergy skin tests, are inappropriately treated with allergy desensitization injections.

Clinical Features of Paranasal Head Pain

The headache associated with frontal sinus disease is localized diffusely over the frontal region. Antral disease produces headache over the maxillary region. The headache associated with sphenoid and ethmoid sinus disease is experienced between and behind the eyes and over the vertex of the skull. Commonly, when sinus disease is of sufficient duration, there is pain in the back of the head, neck, and shoulders, in addition to the headache experienced in the front and top of the head.

Headaches are less frequent when the patient has been in the supine position and are less prominent at night then during the day. Moreover, the pain associated with maxillary sinus disease gradually diminishes over about 30 min when the patient lies down with the diseased sinus uppermost.

The headache associated with frontal sinus disease commonly begins about 9 a.m., gradually becomes worse, and terminates toward evening, or upon retiring. The pain associated with maxillary sinus disease usually has its onset in the early afternoon.

In all instances, the pain is of a deep, dull, aching, nonpulsatile quality. It is seldom, if ever, associated with nausea. Chronic sinus disease produces headache pain of lower intensity than that associated with acute sinus disease. In both instances, the intensity of pain if increased by shaking the head or assuming the head-down position. The headache is intensified by procedures that increase the venous pressure, such as "straining," coughing, or wearing a tight collar.

The headache associated with disease of the nasal and paranasal structures is commonly reduced in intensity or abolished by nasal decongestant sprays or pills. Aspirin may reduce the intensity of the pain, but usually does not abolish it. Patients frequently report the simultaneous disappearance of nasal congestion and paranasal head pain after appropriate decongestant therapy is initiated.

Experimental Study of Pain From the Nasal and Paranasal Structures

In a number of studies carried out by Harold Wolff and his associates, the intensity and distribution of pain originating from the nasal and paranasal structures was elucidated. The cartilaginous and bony portions of the external auditory canal, the drumhead, the pharynx and nasopharynx, and the nasal structures were examined and touched and pressed with a probe, and stimulated with faradic current. Cotton tampons, soaked with epinephrine solution (1:1000) and inserted along the turbinates for the purpose of shrinking tissues to give access to the sinuses, were also used because of the irritant nature of epinephrine solution which induces local and referred pain from the structures with which they were in contact. Sensation in the rim of the soft palate and the fossa of Rosenmuller was elicited by contact of a catheter, and in the eustachian tube by blowing air through it.

The faradic current stimulator was a wire insulated to the tip with flexible varnish, which could be bent to probe and stimulate the ostium and the maxillary sinus, the nasofrontal duct, and the frontal sinus.

Sphenoid and ethmoid sinuses were stimulated by pressure against their outer walls by a probe. The mucosal lining of the sphenoid sinus in one patient was stimulated directly through an eroded sella turcica.

Subjects covered the tip of their index finger with soft red wax and were instructed to press the pigment-covered finger against the skin at the site where pain was experienced during these explorations. This left an easily discernible record of the site of pain. Pain was described as 1 plus, 2 plus, 3 plus, etc., on the basis of 10 plus being the worst or intolerable pain. The intensity of the faradic current used for stimulation was that which would elicit a 1 plus pain when applied to the tip of the tongue.

The normal subjects were two investigators, a medical student, a physician especially interested in the problem of headache, and a young woman volunteer. Also investigated were ten subjects who had had a complete extirpation of a left acoustic neuroma with section of the left facial nerve; five subjects with chronic, and four with acute, sinus disease. Also studied was one subject with a fistulous opening into the maxillary sinus following extraction of the left upper second molar. Through the kindness of Dr. Bronson Ray it is possible to report upon the sensitivity of certain paranasal cavities during surgical operations on the head.

SENSATION FROM STIMULATION OF THE PHARYNX, THE NASOPHARYNX, AND THE EUSTACHIAN TUBE

A 1 to 2 plus aching pain was elicited by pressing against the mucous membrane of the pharynx and posterior nasopharynx. The pain was described as being felt deep in the throat, and was marked on the skin as being approximately along the thyroid cartilage of the larynx and at the edge of the hyoid bone, extending to the border of the tragus. Stimulation of the tonsils with faradic current was felt as an uncomfortable tickle at the site of stimulation, but pain was occasionally referred to an area in back of the ear.

Contact of a nasal catheter with the rim of the soft palate and the fossa of Rosenmüller was felt as touch which was described as unpleasant but not painful. Inflation of the eustachian tube was felt as "air blowing through and striking the ear drum." Section of the fifth or seventh cranial nerve did not disturb sensation in these structures. One patient, who had both the fifth and seventh cranial nerves cut on the right side stated that he did not feel the catheter engage the rim of the soft palate, nor impinge upon the fossa of Rosenmüller, but that he felt air blowing through the right eustachian tube. In another patient with both the fifth and ninth nerves cut, the pharynx and fossa of Rosenmüller were reported to be insensitive, but blowing air through the eustachain tube produced the usual sensations.

SENSATION FROM STIMULATION OF THE NASAL FLOOR AND THE SEPTUM

In all subjects with intact cranial nerve supply, touch and pressure stimuli were recognized as such on the nasal floor, and local unpleasant sensations were elicited by passage of a nasal catheter. In subjects with complete section of the fifth cranial nerve root, the septum on that side was insensitive and the passage of a catheter through the nose was not felt until it impinged upon the soft palate and the fossa of Rosenmüller. Such patients, however, stated that they felt "a pressure from the posterior portion of the nasal floor."

The nasal septum in normal subjects was sensitive throughout to light touch, and both faradic current stimulation and pressure with a probe elicited moderate pain (1 to 2 plus) which was felt locally and was sometimes referred as follows: Stimulation of the middle part of the septum caused pain to be felt along the zygoma and toward the ear. On stimulation

of the ethmoid portion, pain was felt in both the outer and the inner canthus of the eye on the homolateral side (see Fig. 12-2).

The lower, middle, and upper turbinates, whether stimulated mechanically with a probe, or by faradic current, were considerably more sensitive than the nasal floor or the septum. A sharp, burning pain was felt at the site of stimulation and along the lateral wall of the inside of the nose. A duller, aching pain was referred into the upper teeth when faradic current or pressure was applied to the anterior portion of the lower turbinate. When the middle and posterior portions of the lower turbinate were stimulated, pain was also felt under the eye, along the zygoma, and toward the ear. On stimulation of the middle turbinate, pain was felt along the zygoma, extending back toward the ear and into the temple, and occasionally deep in the ear. On stimulation of the anterior tip of the superior turbinate, pain was felt in the inner canthus of the eye and spread to the forehead and along the lateral wall of the nose (see Fig. 12-3).

Pain elicited by inserting a cotton tampon soaked with epinephrine (1:1000 solution) along the turbinates usually reached an intensity of 4 to 5 plus. The intensity of pain elicited

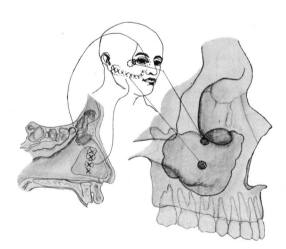

FIG. 12-2. The points stimulated on the septum are shown by crosses and on the lateral wall of the maxillary sinus by cross-hatched circles. The areas in which pain of 1 to 2 plus intensity was felt are indicated by crosses within an outline on the small head above. Note that widely separated stimuli cause pain to be felt in the same areas.

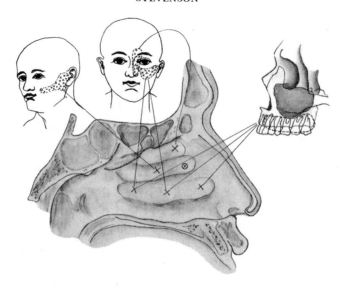

Fig. 12-3. The points stimulated on the turbinates are indicated by crosses, from which lines lead to the indicated areas in which pain of 4 to 6 plus intensity was felt.

by stimulation of these structures, and its extent of spread, varied from subject to subject. It was observed in subjects with engorged mucous membranes of the nose, especially of the turbinates, that experimentally induced pain was more intense, was referred to a larger area, and was longer lasting than when mucous membranes showed no injection or purulent secretion.

The following experiment was typical of subjects who had deep red, swollen nasal mucous membranes. When a cotton tampon soaked with epinephrine (1:1000 solution) was inserted in the right naris along the inferior turbinate, pain was felt as follows: within 1 min there was a bright, burning pain along the medial and lateral walls of the inside of the nose. In the second minute after insertion of the epinephrine pack, pain has spread to the floor of the posterior nasopharynx, and soon involved the entire nasopharyngeal wall. This was of a dull, aching quality. During the next 2 min, profuse lacrimination and dilatation of the pupils was observed, and there was photophobia. Within 5 min a dull, aching pain was felt in the right frontal region, along the supraorbital ridge, in both temples, and there was a feeling of fullness in the head.

At the end of 11.5 min, the sense of fullness and of dull, aching pain of a 2 to 3 plus intensity had extended up to the hair line and deep into the right ear. The intensity of the pain was increased by swallowing and by deep inhalation. It quickly subsided after the removal of the irritant tampon.

The mucous membrane of the opposite or left naris showed a greater degree of injection than did that of the right, and there was purulent secretion over the anterior tip of the inferior turbinate. Another cotton tampon soaked with epinephrine was then inserted into the left naris along the inferior turbinate. The experience of pain was similar to that on the right, and quickly spread to include the entire upper portion of the head on the left, and the supraorbital region on the right as well. At the end of 10 min there was a dull, throbbing, aching pain of 4 or 5 plus intensity. After the tampon was removed the intensity diminished, but pain persisted for approximately 8 hr. During this time the skin of the left side of the face was slightly hyperalgesic, and the intensity of the pain in the head could be increased by quick, forced inhalations, shaking the head, or by breathing cold air.

In patients with complete section of the fifth cranial nerve root, stimulation of the turbinates by pressure, faradic current, or epinephrine tampons elicited no sensation at the site of stimulation, except for a feeling of pressure "deep in." Two such patients also said they felt a pain deep in the ear when the middle turbinate was pressed upon with a probe, but they could feel nothing at the site of stimulation, and there was no referred pain.

SENSATION FROM STIMULATION OF THE OSTIUM OF THE MAXILLARY SINUS

The normal ostium in three subjects was stimulated by a probe or faradic electrode. As soon as the probe touched the walls of the ostium there was a sharp, burning pain of 6 plus intensity at the site of stimulation, accompanied by profuse lacrimation and injection of the eye on the side stimulated. When attempts were made to push the probe or electrode through the ostium into the antrum, a 5 to 8 plus sharp, burning pain was felt at the site of stimulation, and an intense 4 plus aching pain was felt in the posterior nasopharynx, in the

back teeth, along the zygoma, and back into and well above the temple on the side stimulated. There was a deep aching pain in the pharynx. The skin over the zygoma was flushed and hyperalgesic (see Fig. 12-4). The skin over the zygoma and the temple remained hyperalgesic, and the upper teeth were "sore" for approximately 24 hr following this procedure.

SENSATION FROM STIMULATION OF THE NASOFRONTAL DUCT

The nasofrontal duct and the lower part of the channel leading to the frontal sinus were likewise found to be exceedingly pain sensitive. Figure 12-5 illustrates the areas in which pain was felt when the duct of the frontal sinus was stimulated with faradic current, or merely with the passing of the electrode or a metal probe into the frontal sinus. Pain was felt at the inner canthus of the eye, and in a wide band under the eye along the zygoma and into the temple,

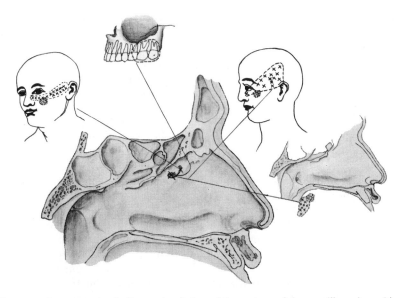

FIG. 12-4. Large crosses indicate stimulation of the ostium of the maxillary sinus. Lines lead to the areas indicated by small crosses in which pain of 6 to 9 plus intensity was felt. A dotted circle over the zygoma indicates the area of erythema and hyperalgesia that long outlasted stimulation of the ostium.

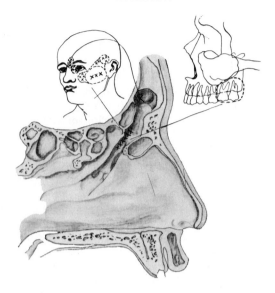

FIG. 12-5. Lines lead from the points stimulated in the nasofrontal duct to the areas in which pain of 5 to 7 plus intensity was felt. On stimulation of the inner wall of the frontal sinus minimal pain of no more than ½ plus intensity was felt only in the area indicated directly over the sinus.

on the side stimulated. Pain was also felt at the angle of the jaw and in the last two or three upper teeth. There was profuse lacrimation and injection in the eye, and there was photophobia.

SENSATION FROM STIMULATION OF THE SINUSES

(a) The Frontal Sinus. When the walls and roof of the frontal sinus were stimulated by pressure with a probe, or by faradic current, minimal pain of no more than a ½ plus intensity was felt directly over the site of stimulation. More intense faradic current stimuli were felt as a vibrating sensation in the frontal bones and along the bridge of the nose, but these sensations did not outlast the stimulus. Faradic current was never applied for longer than 10 sec.

It was concluded, therefore, that the nasofrontal duct and lower part of the channel leading to the frontal sinus is exceedingly pain sensitive, but that the walls lining the frontal sinus itself are relatively insensitive.

(b) The Superior Nasal Cavity. In two of the normal subjects it was possible to investigate the pain sensitivity and sites of pain reference from stimulation in the vicinity of the ethmoid sinuses. The sinuses themselves were not explored. By pressing a probe against the wall of the superior nasal cavity in the general region of the anterior cells of the ethmoid sinus, pain of 6 plus intensity was felt directly over the eye and deep in the eye at its inner canthus. Pain was also felt in the upper jaw just above the superior nasal cavity over the posterior cells of the ethmoid, the conjunctiva adjacent to the nose became injected, and there were profuse lacrimation and photophobia.

When this region of the superior nasal cavity over the posterior ethmoid cells was pressed upon by a probe, there were an intense aching pain of 5 to 6 plus intensity in the upper teeth including the canine, the cuspids, and the first molar, profuse lacrimation in both eyes, and photophobia. The pupils were observed to be dilated. There was moderate aching pain just under and over the outer canthus of the homolateral eye. Also, pain extended from the teeth up the side of the nose (see Fig. 12-6).

(c) The Sphenoid Sinus. When the wall of the

superior nasal cavity in the region of the sphenoid sinus was pressed upon by a probe, pain of 5 to 6 plus intensity was felt immediately, and most intensely deep in the pharynx, which was described by the subject as seeming to be deep in the head. Pain of lesser intensity was referred over the eye and into the upper teeth on the side stimulated (see Fig. 12-6).

During an operation on the head for removal of a pituitary tumor, Dr. Bronson Ray stimulated the mucosal lining of the interior of the sphenoid sinus. In this patient pain of slight degree (1 to 2 plus) was felt at the vertex of the skull (see Fig. 12-7).

(d) The Maxillary Sinus. The maxillary sinuses in the normal subjects investigated could not be entered through the ostia. However, in three patients who had had operative procedures performed on the nose and paranasal sinuses, the ostia were accessible and so large that a faradic stimulator could be introduced into the antrum with ease, and the walls of the latter could be stimulated by faradic current and by pressure. It was doubtful if the mucous membrane linings of these antrums were free of

inflammation, since all of these patients had had sinus disease. Stimulation of the upper wall was felt up through the eye. Stimulation of the lower lateral wall was felt in the jaw and the back teeth. The sensation elicited from the walls of the sinus was of the same intensity and quaity as that elicited by this same amount of faradic current from the tip of the tongue and from the mucous membrane of the septum (see Fig. 12-2), whereas, when it was applied to the lower and middle turbinates in the same patient, a pain of 3 to 4 plus intensity was elicited. Pressure with a probe against the walls of the maxillary sinus was felt as pressure, but was not reported as painful in these three patients.

In two of the patients with complete fifth cranial nerve root section, pressure on the posterior wall of the maxillary sinus was felt as "pressure deep in." Faradic stimuli were not felt on the walls of the sinus, nor was any sensation experienced in the teeth in three of these patients when faradic current was applied to the lateral wall. The ostia on the side of the fifth cranial nerve root section in these patients were also insensitive.

It was possible, however, to explore a normal

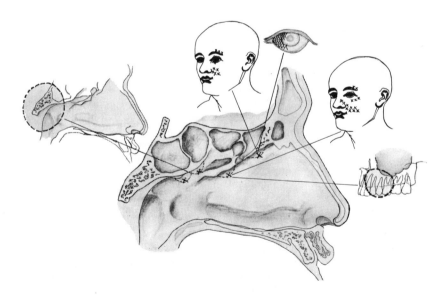

FIG. 12-6. Crosses indicate the points of pressure against the walls of the superior nasal cavity in the region of the sphenoid and ethmoid sinuses, with the indicated areas in which pain of 5 to 6 plus intensity was felt.

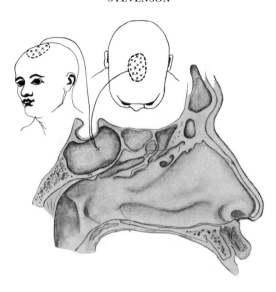

FIG. 12-7. The area is indicated in which pain of 1 to 2 plus intensity was felt on faradic stimulation of the mucosal lining of a sphenoid sinus by Dr. Bronson Ray.

maxillary sinus in a unique way. A 28-year-old woman was studied, who had a sinus tract into the left maxillary sinus following extraction of the first left molar in the upper jaw. This opening was large enough to allow the entrance of a Holmes laryngoscope for visualization of the mucous membrane lining the sinus cavity.

Experiment 1. The mucous membrane of the sinus was seen to be smooth and glistening throughout and was free of inflammation or of atrophy. The normal ostium could also be observed as open, and without surrounding inflammatory reaction or scar tissue.

When the wall of the maxillary sinus in this subject was stimulated with faradic current just under the orbital plate, there was a vibrating sensation felt at the site of stimulation, and a ½ plus pain up through the eye and over the eye along the supraorbital ridge. On the lateral wall and the posterior wall, faradic stimulation was felt as an electric shock along the upper jaw and in the teeth, but the subject stated that the sensation was not painful. When faradic current was applied to the mucous membrane close to the ostium, however, 2 plus pain was experienced, and pain was felt in the upper teeth, in and over the eye, and alone the zygoma toward the left temple.

Experiment 2. The effect of prolonged positive pressure within the maxillary sinus: A thin rubber balloon was attached with adhesive tape binding over the end of a small perforated rubber catheter. This was inserted into the maxillary sinus through the fistulous opening after injection of procaine into the gum around the opening. The catheter was attached to a manometer so that pressure applied inside the sinus could be measured in millimeters of mercury (see Fig. 12-8).

A positive pressure of 15 to 25 mm Hg elicited a sensation of pressure and fullness in the side of the face, but was maintained for 3½ hr without eliciting pain. The pressure in the sinus could be gradually raised to 200 mm Hg before pain was immediately experienced.

Pressure was maintained between 50 and 80 mm Hg for a period of two and a quarter hours before the subject experienced a 1 plus pain in and just below the area of the zygoma, and in the upper teeth, radiating back toward the ear. However, quick, forced inhalations of air through the left naris increased the intensity of the pain from 1 to 3 and 4 plus and enlarged the area in which it was felt. Reducing the pressure to 0 mm Hg did not immediately abolish pain, but its intensity gradually diminished during a ten-minute period.

The state of the turbinates was noted at fixed intervals throughout a 6-hr period of inflation. The left turbinate gradually became swollen during this

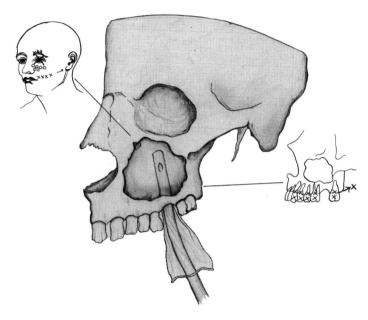

FIG. 12-8. The thin rubber balloon is shown in the maxillary sinus. The areas are indicated in which pain was felt when positive pressure was applied to the walls of the sinus for prolonged periods.

time, but it was not until this engorgement had occluded the left naris that pain was experienced with a pressure of 50 mm Hg. Moreover, at the beginning of this period, pressure could be raised to 200 mm Hg before pain was experienced, whereas when the turbinates had become swollen and engorged, pressures over 50 mm Hg caused pain.

This pain associated with pressure in the maxillary sinus and swollen, engorged turbinates could be materially reduced in intensity, or almost entirely abolished, by procainization of the engorged turbinates, in spite of continued pressure and a feeling of fullness in the side of the face.

Comment. It may be inferred from the above that sustained increased intramural pressure within the antrum may be associated with pain. However, such sustained stimulation of the walls of the sinus evokes engorgement of the turbinates. It is the reflex engorgement of these nasal structures that is responsible for most of the pain, since procainization of the inferior and middle turbinates markedly reduces its intensity, although pressure within

the sinus be still maintained and be still felt as pressure in the side of the face.

Experiment 3. The effect of negative pressure within the maxillary sinus: The nasal side of the ostium was occluded by inserting a cotton and petroleum jelly tampon under the middle turbinate well over the ostium. Negative air pressure was then applied to the sinus by inserting a tube through the fistulous opening. There was immediately felt a drawing sensation in the face, which the subject described as the feeling that "my face will collapse." This sensation was elicited with a negative pressure of 100 to 150 mm Hg. The experience was accompanied by considerable apprehension on the part of the subject, but in spite of this she maintained that she felt no immediate pain. However, if subsequently the negative pressure were increased to 250 mm Hg, there was an immediate 4 plus pain felt in the side of the nose and in the teeth.

Comment. When the cotton tampon occluding the ostium was removed at the termination of the experiment, a portion of its surface presented the appearance of having been drawn into the ostium. It is quite likely that the pain that was experienced with high negative pressures resulted from such stimulation of the ostium. Thus, although the effects of negative pressures were not as intensively explored as were those of positive pressure, the available evidence made it seem likely that most of the pain that resulted was secondary to stimulation of nasal structures.

Experiment 4. A thin rubber balloon was inserted into the sinus, and was filled with hot (45° C) and cold 19° C) water. Of these stimuli, the cold was not distinguished immediately, and the hot not at all. After 10 min the cold water was recognized as "a slight feeling of coolness." While the balloon was in the antrum, filled, under pressure with a syringe, with either hot or cold water, the teeth in the upper jaw felt sore when pressed upon, but these procedures did not elicit any aching pain anywhere in the side of the face.

When the maxillary sinus was irrigated through the fistulous opening with saline, no pain was elicited other than irritation of the fistulous opening itself. When the sinus was irrigated with saline through the nose and the ostium, however, a 4 to 5 plus pain was felt in the nasal wall, along the zygoma into the temple, over the eye, and all through the upper teeth. Similar pain was induced by inserting a cotton tampon soaked with epinephrine under the middle turbinate and over the ostium.

Comment. The feeling of cold after 10 min of exposure to cold within the sinus could have resulted from cooling of neighboring structures. The soreness of the teeth probably resulted from direct stimulation of the dental nerves.

"Sinusitis," Headache, and Anesthetization of the Turbinates

The following experiments are from a series of investigations that illustrate the effects of surface anesthetization of nasal mucous membranes in patients with headache associated with disease of the nasal and paranasal structures.

Experiment 1. This patient had pain in the jaws and teeth and on both sides of the face along the zygomas and into the temples. There was also pain in the frontal region, increased lacrimation, and photophobia. The pain was described as a steady ache of a 3 plus intensity except in the forehead, where is was 4 plus.

With transillumination and in roentgenograms both maxillary and both frontal sinuses were shown to be opaque. The nasal mucous membrane was bright red, and the turbinates were swollen. The inferior turbinate was in contact with the septum. There was purulent secretion beneath both middle turbinates, in the region of the ostia.

Cotton tampons soaked with procaine hydrochloride (1% solution) were inserted along the inferior turbinates. At the end of ten minutes the tampons were removed. The subject stated that the pain in the teeth and jaws was nearly gone. Similar tampons were inserted under the middle turbinates approximately 5 mm beneath the ostia for 10 min. Within 8 min all the pain in the jaws, teeth, and face was gone, but a 1 plus pain remained in the frontal region. In another 10 min the subject stated that all of the pain in the head was gone, and shaking the head vigorously produced no pain.

Experiment 2. On the eighth day of an upper respiratory infection the patient had pain over the right side of the face, from the side of the nose, under the eye along the zygoma, into the temple and ear, and in the upper teeth and jaw. The pain was of 1 plus intensity, an of a dull, aching quality. The nasal mucous membranes were injected throughout. The turbinates were swollen and in contact with the septum. The middle turbinate was bright red in color, redder than the inferior turbinate, and was extremely pain sensitive. When touched with a probe, pain in the right side of the face was intensified to 3 plus. There was purulent secretion beneath the middle turbinate in the region of the ostium. A procaine-soaked cotton tampon was inserted along the inferior turbinate and left in place for 10 min. There was a slight decrease in pain, especially along the side of the nose. Another tampon was inserted under the middle turbinate, approximately 5 mm below the ostium, for 10 min, and when it was removed all pain in the side of the face, temple, ear, and teeth was gone, with only a sense of fullness and stiffness remaining. Within an hour all discomfort was gone, and did not return.

Comment. The effect of placing procaine under the middle turbinate and about 5 mm beneath the ostium cannot be explained as a direct procaine effect on nerves entering the ostium to innervate the walls of the sinus. Such nerves as enter the ostium through the nose enter for the most part posteriorly and along the upper margin.

Experiment 3. Pressure symptoms associated with a cyst in the left antrum. This patient, with a history of pain for three days in the left side of the face and head, was observed to have engorged turbinates which were in septal contact, with complete occlusion of the nares. A local anesthetic was placed on the mucous membranes of the inferior and middle turbinates. Within 15 min the patient was left with a sense of fullness in the left side of the face and beneath the eye, with almost complete alleviation of the pain. The left antrum was entered with a trochar, and straw-colored fluid escaped from the needle under a pressure sufficient to send a stream in a straight line for 10 to 12 inches. Thereafter the subject had no sensation of head fullness or pain.

Comment. This experiment is further evidence that increased pressure in the maxillary sinus per se produces sensations of head fullness, and that such pain as the subject experienced had its origin in the inflammation of the turbinates. This experiment further illustrates that increased pressure in the antrum may exist for a long period without symptoms. It was only with the onset of an upper respiratory infection and the associated inflammation of the turbinates that pain was experienced.

Variations in Venous Pressure and the Size and Appearance of the Turbinates

Experiment 1. This subject had no gross infection of the nose. The jugular outflow on the left side of the neck was occluded for three minutes, which caused a gradually increasing engorgement of the turbinates. Ultimately the inferior turbinate was in contact with an anterior deviation of the septum, so that the air passage was occluded. Toward the end of the 3 min period there was an increase of watery secretion.

Experiment 2. When the appearance of the nose was again normal, the experiment was repeated so that venous occlusion was produced on the opposite side. The same engorgement effect resulted except that occlusion was not complete because there was no septal deviation on this side.

Experiment 3. The head was tilted to the horizontal in such a way as to avoid pressure on the neck and to minimize venous stasis. No change in the appearance of the turbinates was noted within three minutes.

although over a 45-min period some swelling on the dependent side gradually occurred.

Experiment 4. In addition to tilting the head as in Experiment 3, the face and neck were firmly pressed against by a pillow or the supporting hand. The turbinates on the dependent side were noted to become swollen to the point of occluding the air passage within 1 to 3 min.

The Effect of Vigorously Shaking the Head on Subjects with Engorged Turbinates

The intensity of headache associated with disease of the nasal and paranasal sinuses was increased by shaking the head. That this increased pain results from the sudden displacement of swollen, inflamed structures is shown by the following experiments.

The subject, about 12 days after the onset of an upper respiratory infection, and during a headache-free period when the turbinates in the right naris were moderately engorged, induced further engorgement by occluding venous return in the right jugular vein with pressure with the hand, and by lying on the right side for 5 min. The air passage in the right side of the nose was completely occluded, and there was a sense of fullness in the right side of the head, but no pain. The turbinates were observed to be swollen, the middle turbinate being especially engorged and in septal contact. At this time, shaking the head vigorously induced pain over the right side of the face from the side of the nose, along the zygoma, into the temple, and in the right upper teeth and jaw. The pain was of a dull, aching quality, of a 1 plus intensity, and persisted through two hours. A cotton tampon soaked with a vasoconstrictor (neosynephrine hydrochloride) was then inserted along the inferior turbinate and in contact with the middle turbinate, and left in place for 10 min. When the pack was removed the turbinates were observed to be pale and shrunken, and all pain in the side of the face was gone. Vigorously shaking the head now elicited no pain.

The Site of Origin of Headache from Disease of the Nasal and Paranasal Structures

It is evident from these studies that the linings of the sinuses are relatively insensitive as compared with their extremely sensitive ducts and ostia, and the turbinates. Even though with inflammation the threshold for pain in the sinuses is lowered so that they become more pain sensitive, the situation is altered relatively little, since with inflammation the ostia, ducts, and turbinates become even more pain sensitive.

Although the term *sinus headache* is commonly assigned to those headaches associated with sinus disease, proof that the major portion of the pain has its source in the paranasal structures is lacking. The issue has been confused by the fact that sinus inflammation rarely occurs without concomitant inflammation of the nasal structures. The rare exception is sinus infection secondary to periapical abscess, but this type of sinus disease causes but minor discomfort until the nasal structures are directly or indirectly inflamed as well. The vast majority of instances of sinus disease pain have associated inflammation and engorgement of the nasal structures.

It is inferred, therefore, that the site of the headache is related chiefly to the region of the nose that is most diseased. Disease of the superior nasal structures causes headaches primarily in the front and top of the head, and in and between the eyes. Disease of the middle and inferior nasal structures causes headaches primarily over the zygomas and temples and in the teeth and jaws. It has not been proven that disease of the paranasal sinuses underlying these areas of headache makes important contributions to the intensity of the pain.

THE PATHOPHYSIOLOGY OF HEADACHE FROM DISEASE OF NASAL AND PARANASAL STRUCTURES

Variations in Venous Pressure

Variations in venous pressure modify the intensity of the headache. Unilateral pressure on the jugular veins, both internal and external, increases turgescence of the turbinates on the homolateral side. When the turbinates are inflamed and engorged, the effect is more striking than when they are normal. When the turbinates are already moderately painful, the pain is augmented by further turgescence, and is still further augmented by shaking the head and by lowering the head between the knees. When a subject with turgescent turbinates rests

in a lying-down position on his side, there is a momentary slight increase in pain as the swollen, reddened turbinates are displaced. Gradually the uppermost turbinates shrink slightly, whereas the dependent turbinates become more turgescent, and occlude the air passages.

On the other hand, venous pressure is not a factor of first importance in sinus headache, since intensity is usually greatest when the subject is in the erect position, and the cranial venous pressure is lower.

Exudate in the Sinuses

The presence of purulent secretion in the sinuses is not in itself a basis for headache. In the lying-down position when the opportunity for drainage is least and for filling maximal, the pain experienced is least.

Negative and Positive Air Pressure

The fact that the headache is usually worse in the upright position and better when the patient is lying down has been used in evidence that pain is due to negative or positive air pressure in the sinuses, resulting from the draining out, or filling up with purulent secretion. However, since changes in pressure have been demonstrated to be inadequate stimuli for producing serious discomfort from these cavities, other factors must be more important as causes of pain.

Irritants on the Nasal Mucosa

Toxic or noxious chemicals, either in the liquid or gaseous phase, can produce inflammation in the nasal mucosa by direct interaction with the mucous membranes. This is not immunologically mediated, although variations in the degree of sensitivity of dose–effect relationship in certain patients have been observed by careful clinicians. Some individuals with exquisite sensitivity to inhaled cigarette smoke, smog, and chemical fumes are already suffering from other forms of nasal mucosal inflammation (allergic or vasomotor rhinitis). The superimposition of chemical molecules upon already inflamed surfaces, increases the inflammation and swelling and this may be enough to exceed pain thresholds, producing a paranasal pain syndrome. In the absence of underlying rhinitis, chemical fumes would not be an adequate stimulus to produce paranasal pain in this subgroup of patients.

Vasomotor Changes in the Nasal Linings

Local vasomotor changes in the erectile tissues of the nose as accompaniments of stress, exhaustion, anxiety, sexual excitement, and various emotional states have been observed. Ordinarily such variations are not associated with nasal symptoms, but sometimes, the effects of these changes produce enough congestion of the turbinates to induce obstruction of the nasal passages with or without associated paranasal head pain.

NASAL DYSFUNCTION AND HEADACHE IN PATIENTS HAVING ADAPTIVE DIFFICULTIES

Functional alterations in the structures in the nose of man have been studied and correlated with a wide variety of circumstances including noxious stimulation inside the nose by chemical agents, noxious stimulation of other portions of the head, variations in environmental temperature, interruption of afferent nerve pathways, weeping, and numerous threatening life situations with their accompanying affective states.

In general two patterns of disturbance of nasal function were recognized. The first involved vasoconstriction in the nose with shrinkage of the membrane and increase in the size of the air passages. Such changes in reaction to threats accompanied feelings of fear, sadness, and other emotions which, although strong, involved minimal conflict (Fig. 12-9).

The second type of disturbance in the nose appeared to have greater significance with relation to disease. It was characterized by the initial hyperemia associated with turgescence of the erectile tissues in the turbinates and nasal septum, engorgement of the nasal mucosa, and increased secretion. These changes were accompanied by obstruction to breathing and often by pain. Often, after the subsidence of hyperemia, secondary pallor ensued with

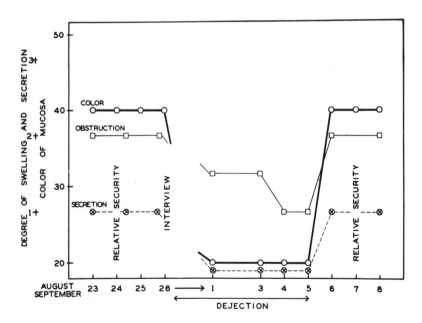

FIG. 12-9. Pallor and shrinkage of nasal membranes associated with feelings of sadness, fear, and dejection.

the mucous membranes of the nose remaining boggy and edematous. This second type of nasal disturbance characterized by hyperfunction occurred in reaction to a variety of environmental threats against the individual and appeared to constitute part of a defense mechanism for shutting out and washing away a noxious environment at the head of the organism. Such a pattern was found to occur in response to local stimulation by the noxious fumes of ammonium carbonate (Fig. 12-10) or by pollens from grasses to which the subject was sensitive (Fig. 12-11). It also occurred following noxious stimulation, not directed specifically at the nose or respiratory passages as, for example, the painful tightening of a metal headband. In fact this defensive pattern of shutting out occurred even in response to noxious environmental stimuli which did not involve physical contact with the organism, such as situational threats from difficulties of interpersonal adjustment. Weeping which followed frustrating or humiliating experiences was accompanied by swelling, hyperemia, hypersecretion, and obstruction in the nose (Fig. 12-

12). Such changes also accompanied anger and feelings of frustration without weeping.

One subject, a 25-year-old physician, was studied in detail and continuously over 8 months. He exhibited alterations in nasal function which were observed during naturally occurring day-to-day life stresses. Pallor of nasal membranes with increase in size of the air channels occurred in a setting of abject fear and dejection following his wife's hemoptysis. In situations of conflict, however, when decisions were required regarding threats to his career or to his position as head of his household, nasal hyperemia with swelling, hypersecretion, and obstruction to breathing occurred. At such times he had frequent colds with sneezing and coughing, postnasal discharge, and sinus headache.

He approached his problems in an energetic, aggressive, outgoing and self-confident fashion. Situations within his realm of responsibility were rarely out of his control. His system of security rested on three props: (1) the approval of his superiors; (2) his ability to be assertively independent in the economic and social spheres; (3) his achievement of a recognized position in a competitive society—i.e., 'success in his career.'

At the time when the subject's wife was five months

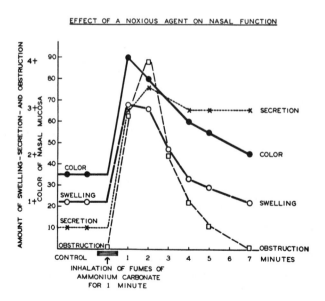

FIG. 12-10. Nasal hyperfunction following inhalation of the noxious fumes of ammonium carbonate.

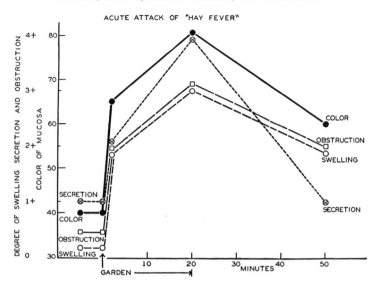

FIG. 12-11. Nasal hyperfunction after exposure to pollens.

pregnant a decision had to be made to relinquish their own apartment and go to live with the wife's aunt in a suburb of the city.

During this period, in which the subject was exposed to serious threats to his independence, he was also subjected to threats to his 'career' and to danger of losing the approval of his superiors. Working with him under his supervision was an intern about four years his senior, who found it difficult to perform the menial but essential chores which were customarily assigned to an intern, and who was unwilling to accept the responsibility for his patients. The subject

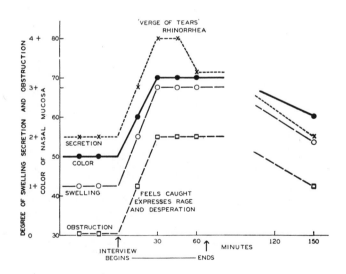

FIG. 12-12. Nasal hyperfunction during an interview in which the subject experienced rage and desperation.

hesitated, because of his subordinate's experience and age, to reprimand him openly and frankly. He first tried to cope with the situation by suggesting a plan to maintain the ward's efficiency. When this failed the subject began, in addition to his own work, to perform the neglected duties himself. He finally frankly confronted the intern with the issue, but the latter refused to accept criticism from a younger, less-experienced man.

In this setting of threat to his career, with feelings of anger and resentment, and the fear of loss of the approval of his senior colleagues, as well as the conflict arising from his being forced to sacrifice those symbols of independence which his own home represented, the subject was aware of an increase in postnasal accumulations of secretions and 'cleared his throat' frequently. His nose felt occluded, and there was burning pain in both nostrils. Figure 12-13 demonstrates the increase in redness of the nasal mucosa associated with a significant increase in the amount of secretion, swelling, and obstruction sustained throughout this 12-day period.

During weeping, not only the eyes but also the nose were found to participate in this reaction, and in two individuals in this study, deep-

er structures including the bronchae constricted during threatening situations, thus participating in the bodily reaction of exclusion. Against local intrusion by dust, for example, or noxious fumes, the reaction of shutting out and washing away proved highly effective. Against situational threats involving interpersonal relations, however, the nasal changes afforded incomplete relief and were often productive of discomfort.

When the nasal changes in the bodily pattern of shutting out and washing away were unduly sustained, they gave rise to troublesome symptoms including burning pain of low intensity. This was increased by forced inspiration; and a dull, aching pain spread from the bridge of the nose into the orbit and along the zygoma to the ear on each side of the swollen nasal structure. When the swelling shifted to the opposite nostril, the pain correspondingly changes position. The pain, which also involved the teeth, especially those of the upper jaw, alternated with a feeling of fullness, which was worse during the working hours of the day, especially

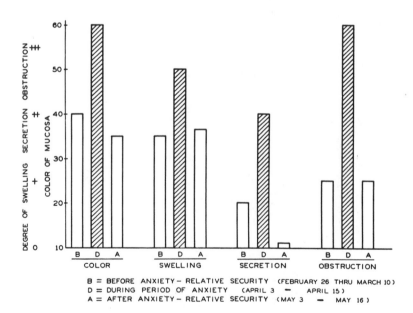

FIG. 12-13. Sustained nasal hyperfunction during 12 days of anxiety and resentment compared with control periods before and after.

during periods of stress, and was minimal in the early morning and late evening. When pain was relatively intense, local deep tenderness was also noted. Photophobia occurred, especially on the painful side, with injection of the sclerae and the skin of the cheek. Distribution of headache is shown schematically in Fig. 12-14.

The data presented indicate that during sustained conflict there may occur prolonged nasal hyperfunction accompanied by obstruction, facial pain, and tenderness. Such symptoms are often attributed to acute sinusitis. In this case no infection of the sinuses was demonstrated, however, and the disturbance with accompanying symptoms subsided completely when the subject's conflicts were resolved.

ANGIOEDEMA AND HEAD PAIN

Soft tissue swelling after release of vasodilating mediators can occur in tissues of the face, tongue, pharynx, or larynx. Antigens such as penicillin, sulfa, horse serum, or insulin can combine with specific IgE antibodies to initiate a Type I hypersensitivity reaction, manifested by either urtication, angioedema, or both.

In urticaria, crops of wheals, frequently surrounded by erythema and associated with pruritus, occur in either specific locations or over most of the body's surface. Angioedema, by contrast, is a condition characterized by nonpitting localized edema without associated pruritus (Mathews, 1974). These two forms of abnormal cutaneous or subcutaneous vasodilatation can appear separately or at the same time.

Both urticaria and angioedema are associated with vasodilatation and increased permeability of small venules and capillaries; vascular congestion occurring in the upper corium vessels in urticaria and in the subcutaneous vessels in angioedema (Lever, 1961).

Intradermal injection of histamine produces local wheal and flare urticarial lesions which are indistinguishable from spontaneous urticaria (Lewis, 1927). However, many patients who have urticaria do not respond to antihistamines (H_1 blockers) and the pathogenetic mechanisms which produce urticaria and angioedema are now recognized to be heterogeneous with immunologic, nonimmunologic, emotional, neural, and physical inciting events triggering a complicated chain of mechanisms culminating in vasodilatation and increased permeability of cutaneous vessels (Fink, 1972; Kaplan, 1978).

Although most angioedema is painless, in certain forms and/or locations it causes head pain. For the most part, these instances are obvious. Pain will be directly related to the area of soft tissue swelling on the scalp or face. Angioedema of the tongue, pharynx, and larynx is almost always manifested by other symptoms, such as obstruction, sensation of a mass, or difficulty with swallowing or speaking. Pain is rarely a manifestation of these latter angioedema locations and referred pain is even more unusual. Generalized, severe angioedema has been reported in at least one patient with associated headaches, epilepsy, hemiplegia, and coma (Fowler, 1962). We have observed a patient who reacted to parabens (stabilizer chemicals in injectable medications) by developing generalized erythrodermia with tissue edema, including cerebral edema, headache, and semicoma. She was treated with

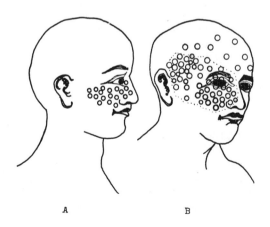

A   B

FIG. 12-14. Distribution of pain and hyperalgesia during nasal hyperfunction associated with emotional conflict.

corticosteroids (without parabens) and recovered.

CEREBRAL ARTERITIS SYNDROMES

Systemic Lupus Erythematosis (SLE) is a disease manifested by deposition of toxic complexes of DNA, antibody, and complement in arterial walls (Type III reactions). The resulting inflammation or arteritis can produce systemic symptoms, such as fever, malaise, myalgias and arthralgias, or localized symptoms which are the consequences of occlusion and perinflammation of specific arteries. When cerebral arteries or the choroid plexus are involved by SLE, the patient can develop head pain adjacent to inflamed superficial arteries, as a consequence of arterial obstruction with ischemic pain or as a generalized cerebritis with a dull, pressure-type pain (Atkins, Kondon, and Quismorio, 1972).

Giant Cell Arteritis may occur in the cranial arteries. Because the superficial temporal arteries are accessible and can be sacrificed for biopsy, the term *temporal arteritis* has gained popular acceptance. Actually, in this syndrome, giant cell arteritis is present in arteries which supply the skeletal muscles (polymyalgia rheumatica syndrome) (Healey and Wilske, 1977) and viscera (O'Neill *et al,* 1976); axillary brachial, femoral, and heart arteries (Stanson, et al, 1976).

Evolving evidence supports the hypothesis that giant cell arteritis (temporal arteritis, cranial arteritis, and polymyalgia rheumatica) are diverse manifestations of Type III, toxic complex arteritis appearing in a number of large and medium-sized vessels. Immunofluorescent studies of biopsied arteries (superficial temporal) show deposits of IgG, IgA, sometimes IgM, fibrin, and complement components (Waaler *et al,* 1976) in a number of biopsy specimens, depending upon the stage of disease and the biopsy site with respect to skip lesions (Klein *et al,* 1976). Hazelman *et al.* (1975) reported lymphocyte stimulation by arterial wall antigen extracts in polymyalgia rheumatica, suggesting that cellular immune hypersensitivity or Type IV reactions may be occuring in this syndrome. If these observa-

tions are supported by further studies, the possibility of combined hypersensitivity (Type III and Type IV) responses will have been identified. However, the main deterrent in categorizing giant cell arteritis as an immune disease has been our failure to identify the inciting antigen(s). In SLE, on the other hand, a variety of nuclear antigens have been separated and studied by Nutmon *et al.* (1975).

The relationship between the arteritis syndromes and headaches is described in greater detail in Chapter 10.

HEADACHE REACTIONS TO DRUGS USED TO TREAT ALLERGIC DISEASES

Common and frequently overlooked causes of head pain in patients with allergic disease are reactions to the drugs used to treat these patients. Individuals with allergic rhinitis receive antihistamine and sympathomimetic decongestants; asthmatics received theophylline, sympathomimetic bronchodilators, and corticosteroids; and patients suffering from systemic arteritis syndromes frequently receive high dosages of corticosteroids. Therefore, when evaluating a patient who has one or more of the above diseases and also complains of head pain, it can be very productive to examine the consequences of those drugs to treat the disease, rather than assuming that the disease is responsible for the head pain syndrome.

In Table 12-3, the major drugs used to treat allergic diseases, along with their side effects, are listed.

RELATIONSHIP BETWEEN ALLERGY AND MIGRAINE HEADACHE

Migraine is a common disorder which occurs in 15% of the adult population, twice as frequently in women as in men (Dalsgaard-Nielsen, 1974). Because migraine headaches tend to occur intermittently, some clinical investigators have attempted to identify provoking factors responsible for each migraine attack. Infrequent exposure to allergens or antigens constitutes a hypothetical provoking event for each or even occasional migraine headaches. Unfortunately, some physicians

TABLE 12-3   Side Effects of Drugs Used to Treat Allergic Diseases

| | | CONSEQUENCES OF DRUGS | |
Drugs	Head-Pain Type	Other Side Effects and Manifestations
Decongestants Antihistamines and sympathomimetics	Vascular, pounding headaches	Somnolence, or excitation
Sympathomimetics Epinephrine Ephedrine Isoproterenol Metaproterenol	Vascular, pounding headaches	Tremor, palpitations, tachyarrythmias
Aminophylline or Theophylline	Toxic, sick headache, generalized	Nausea, emesis, tremor, excitation, convulsions, tachyarrhythmias
Corticosteroids Prednisone Methyl prednisolone	Cervico-occipital headaches Vascular headaches	Hypertension, Cushing's features, Osteoporosis

have assumed that this hypothesis has been proven, even as accumulated data have shown no relationship between immune reactions to inhaled or ingested antigens and the pathogenesis of spontaneous migraine headaches.

History of Allergy and Migraine Headaches

Pagniez, Vallery-Radot, and Nast (1919) were among the first to hypothesize an allergic mechanism in migraine. The reports of De Gowin (1932), Rinkel (1933), Balyeat and Brittain (1930), Hahn (1930), Hamburger (1935), Gonzales (1953), Ogden (1951), and others followed. Vaughan's works (1927, 1934) are representative of these publications. On the basis of a clinical history of migraine attacks after ingesting certain foods and the presence of positive skin tests to these foods, he concluded that hypersensitivity was a causative factor in 70% of patients with vascular headache of the migraine type. In half his patients, there was a reduction in migraine headaches after diet modification. The chief food offenders have varied in different studies: wheat, milk, chocolate, and eggs in the opinion of Balyeat and Brittain (1930); and celery, peas, and onions in the report of De-Gowin (1932).

Other physicians have attempted to link migraine headache to allergy by identifying common associations. For example, Neusser (1892) reported eosinophilia during a migraine attack. Van Leeuwen and Zeydner (1922) described an activity in the blood of patients with asthma, urticaria, epilepsy, and migraine which induced smooth muscle contraction in vitro, but was absent from the blood of normal control subjects.

One of the strongest and earliest relationships discovered between migraine and allergy was from the outset based upon definitions. In 1873, Trousseau stated that migraine was one of the allergic manifestations of the atopic state. He declared, without evidence, that periodic headache, along with hay fever, urticaria, and eczema were all features of an "asthmatic state." This position was championed in the United States by Vaughan and others (Rowe, 1932) (Unger and Unger, 1952). By defining migraine as an allergy, Rinkel in 1933 was able to show that migraine patients had a family history of "allergy." Although a small number of migraine patients came from families where atopic diseases, such as allergic rhinitis, asthma, urticaria, and eczema existed, in the majority of family members the "allergy" was migraine headache. Another interpretation of the same data would be that the majority of migraine patients came from families where other members also had migraine headaches. Despite the evolution of time, the controversy continues. Recent publications by Unger and colleagues (1970, 1974) and Speer (1975) continue to reveal a strong belief that allergy causes spontaneous migraine headaches.

Dietary Migraine

The major arena of controversy with respect to a cause-and-effect relationship between allergic reactions and migraine has been the area of food allergy. From the outset, those who favored the allergic migraine hypothesis observed migraine headache attacks after food ingestion in many of their patients. Wolf and Unger recorded migraine headache attacks in one patient after he consumed food extracts which had given positive skin tests. They then failed to produce headache in the patient after administering harmless extracts presented as the known offending allergen.

Hyslop (1934) reported a patient who suffered migraine after ingesting pork when the patient was wired or under emotional stress.

However, in most of the studies, a critical experimental control had been omitted. If the allegedly offending foodstuff had been administered without the patient's being aware that it had been given, and headache then predictably occurred, a direct cause-and-effect relationship between food and headache would be more convincing. When this step was carried out at the New York Hospital, with the administration of chocolate, disguised in capsules for those allegedly sensitive to chocolate, or milk given through a stomach tube to those who were said to be sensitive to milk, the results did not confirm the earlier work. No headache ensued. Moreover, in 1950 Mary Loveless gave, in disguised form, milk, corn, arrowroot, and tapioca, as well as placebo preparations, to persons alleged to have had headache attacks precipitated by the ingestion of these foods. She noted, in her well-controlled study, no predictable relationship between the administration of these substances and the occurrence of headache.

In another well-controlled, double-blind food challenge and elimination study, Walker (1960) showed that there was no predictable relationship between disguised offending foods and the occurrence of migraine headache attacks. Many of us have concluded that the effect of the doctor-and-patient *belief* that the allergen offered would produce a migraine headache could have triggered migraine attacks through fear and psychic anticipation of stress in the earlier, uncontrolled feeding experiments.

The reduction in frequency and intensity of migraine attacks by the ingestion of so-called elimination diets cannot be relied upon as supporting the relevance of ingested allergens to migraine. The list of allegedly therapeutic regimens in migraine is long. Wolff (1955) has put forth the thesis that the interest and good will of the physician and the expectation of improvement on the part of the patient may effect relief in many patients through neural rather than antiallergic mechanisms.

The presence of positive wheal-and-flare skin test responses to certain foods has been used as evidence for "food allergy" in migraine patients (Vaughan, 1927). Unfortunately, positive skin tests occur in up to 25% of asymptomatic, nonallergic control populations (Smith, 1978). Not only are positive food skin tests found in asymptomatic individuals, but a cause-and-effect relationship between food addition and elimination in known atopic conditions has been difficult to prove. These difficulties of establishing a diagnosis of food hypersensitivity have been outlined by May and Bock (1978). In migraine, the problem is further compounded by a psychic factor such that a positive skin test to a food can induce fear or stress in the susceptible patient, which, in turn, can precipitate a migraine headache when that forbidden food is reintroduced.

The many problems in the interpretation of skin tests make it difficult to establish their relevance to migraine. It is noteworthy that although the gastrointestinal tract is more permeable to food allergens in the very young, Vahlquist (1955) has shown that the incidence of migraine in children is at most one-third to one-half that found in adults. If food allergy, which has a high incidence in children compared to adults, were important in the pathogenesis of migraine, the opposite relationship should exist with migraine headaches being 2 to 3 times as common in children as they are in adults.

The term "dietary migraine" has been used by Dalessio (1972) to describe the relationship between eating certain foods and the onset of migraine headaches. Despite the lack of evidence to support food-induced allergic reactions, the observation that certain patients develop headaches after ingesting selected foods remains valid. It is now clear that those foods which produced migraine have one thing in common. In addition to their food antigens, they contain vasoactive chemicals or substrates for enzyme systems which synthesize vasoconstrictors. These chemicals and substrates have direct or indirect effects upon cerebral blood vessel receptors, stimulating vasoconstriction of the susceptible migraine arteries. From a practical standpoint, since the presence or absence of a positive food extract skin test is irrelevant, migraine patients should not undergo allergy skin testing for evaluation of migraine, but should avoid those foods containing vasoactive chemicals. See Chapter 5.

Epidemiologic Investigations of Migraine and Atopic Populations

Lance and Anthony (1966), in their headache clinic, studied 500 patients with migraine headaches and 100 patients with tension headaches. Seventeen percent of the migraine patients were found to have allergic disorders, including asthma, hay fever, hives, and eczema. Thirteen percent of the patients with tension headaches had similar allergies. There were no statistical differences between 17 and 13%, strongly implying that migraine sufferers had no greater propensity toward allergies than did a control group of patients with muscle contraction headaches. Furthermore, an epidemiologic study of an entire Michigan community (pop. 11,305) showed that the incidence of asthma and allergic rhinitis was 21.8% for males and 25.3% for females (Broder et al., 1974). Urticaria is extremely common, occurring at least once in 20% of the population

(Smith, 1978). Atopic dermatitis or eczema is common in children, frequently associated with the above conditions in 63% of cases and tends to disappear in adulthood. Our best available information leads to the conclusion that 20% of the adult population suffers from one or more manifestations of allergy or atopy, an incidence exceeding that found in Lance and Anthony's headache populations.

In a neurology clinic in Chicago, Bassoe (1933) found that only 3% of his 270 migraine patients had any manifestations of allergy. Ziegler and colleagues (1972) studied 289 migraine patients and also found a very low incidence of associated allergic rhinitis and asthma.

In looking at the allergic population for the incidence of migraine, Schwartz (1952) examined 241 asthmatics and 200 nonallergic controls as well as their 3,815 relatives. He found an incidence of approximately 5% for migraine headache in the asthmatics, the normal controls and their relatives. This figure is actually lower than the 15% incidence of migraine in the general population reported by Dalsgaard-Nielsen (1974). In another study by Kallow and Kallow-Deffner (1955), the incidence of migraine in their allergic population was 15%.

Therefore, since migraine and allergy are frequently found in the total population, it is not surprising that nonrandom studies will show some degree of association. It would appear that approximately 20% of migraine patients will have allergy and 15% of allergy patients will have migraine headaches. Figure 12-15 illustrates this point.

Because of the difficulty in identifying some patients with allergic disease even by allergy specialists, a potential criticism of studies which attempted to identify allergies in a migraine population has been that the nonallergist investigators failed to accurately identify allergic patients. Medina and Diamond (1976) measured total serum lgE levels in 89 unselected patients with migraine headaches and 27 control patients with muscle contraction headaches. Elevated levels of serum lgE were found in 5.7% of patients with migraine and 3.7% of patients with muscle contraction

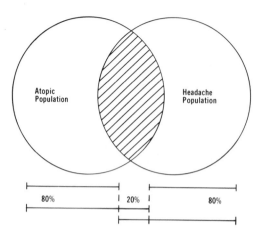

FIG. 12-15. Schematic representation of the overlap between the atopic and migraine populations. The hash-marked area between the circles represents those atopic patients who also have migraine headaches.

headaches, incidences not significantly different from each other or the rate in the general population. By contrast, elevated levels of serum IgE were found in 41% of patients with both eczema and respiratory allergy and in 79% of patients with severe atopic dermatitis and respiratory allergy (Smith, 1978).

Although there is no universal test to identify atopy and one must rely upon the history to identify migraine patients, there are no data which link these two conditions into a mono- or even polygenetic defect. There is no evidence that classical or common migraine or other forms of vascular headache, such as cluster headache, are truly allergic in origin. However, since both allergy and migraine are common conditions, the presence of one does not appear to protect against the other. Some patients will have both. In these individuals, it is important to deal realistically with both disorders.

Migraine Headaches in the Allergic Patients

Allergic patients may develop paranasal sinus headaches, muscle contraction headaches from tension and worry over their diseases, and (in susceptible individuals) typical or classical migraine headaches. Is there any evidence that Type I IgE-mediated reactions precipitate migraine headaches in the allergic subgroup of migraine patients?

The experiments by Kallos and Kallos-Deffner (1955) are particularly interesting. They carefully selected a small group of 28 patients who had both migraine headaches and urticaria, rhinitis, or asthma which was provoked by specific allergens. They then injected extracts of specific allergens into these patients, using concentrations great enough to produce typical IgE-mediated reactions of rhinitis, asthma, or urticaria. In most patients, the parenteral injections of large dosages of allergenic extracts were also followed by a vascular headache. However, two important clarifying observations were made. Headache always appeared in association with rhinitis, asthma, or urticaria and never as the only manifestation of allergen-induced reaction. Second, the migraine aura (phase 1 or the vasconstrictive component) was universally absent. The nasopulmonary reaction could then be prevented by pretreating the patient with antihistamine (H_1 blockers) but the vascular headache continued to occur unless the patient was pretreated with ergotamine, which blocked the headache, but had no effect upon the respiratory tract reactions. These very interesting observations suggest on the surface that mediators released during IgE-mediated anaphylaxis can produce vascular headaches, possibly by stimulating the second (or vasodilator) phase of a vascular-type headache. If this mediator is histamine, it would require H_2 cerebral arterial receptors, since H_1 antihistamines do not block vascular headache.

The role of histamine in vascular headaches was first reported by Pickering (1933) who injected 0.1 mg of histamine intravenously, producing a vascular headache in everyone. Keeney in 1946 systematically reviewed this subject and studied 37 patients with periodic vascular headache. Twenty-four developed typical vascular headaches after s.q. injections of 0.1 mg histamine. In 7 of 10 patients 0.6 mg of nitroglycerine s.l. also produced vascular headache, suggesting that vasodilatation, rather than a specific susceptibility to histamine, represented the pathogenic event in vascular head pain.

Although it is clear that s.q. or intravenous injections of large dosages of histamine or other vasodilators will produce cerebral vascular dilatation and headaches in susceptible individuals, it is not at all clear whether these observations have any relevance to migraine occurring as a consequence of spontaneous IgE-mediated rhinitis, asthma, or urticaria. In a study which measured venous plasma histamine during spontaneous asthma, Simon et al. (1977) were able to demonstrate only 1–5 ng/ml of plasma histamine during active and moderately severe asthmatic attacks. When asthma was induced during antigen bronchial inhalation challenge, Bhat et al. (1976) were able to show a rise of 1–6 ng/ml in venous plasma histamine. In both instances, the concentrations of plasma histamine/ml were on the order of 1000 times more dilute than the 0.1 mg of histamine given by Pickering (1933) to provoke vascular headaches. Therefore, in spontaneous rhinitis, asthma, or urticaria, it seems unlikely that enough histamine molecules spill into the vascular space, escape active degradation enzymes, and become available to vascular receptors in the cerebral arteries to effect significant vasodilatation.

However, there are several artificial systems whereby a large intravascular discharge of mediators can occur. In systemic anaphylaxis, antigen is circulating in the vascular space with IgE fixed to circulating basophils, and this leads to the release of mediators from these storage cells as well as most cells in the lung and other organs. Under such circumstances, 100 ng/ml of histamine may be measured in the plasma and patients frequently develop generalized peripheral vasodilatation and hypotensive shock. Selected patients also develop vascular headache. These have been recorded in the absence of treatment with epinephrine, another pharmacologic cause of head pain. Systemic anaphylaxis occurs in the following instances: after bee sting, injection of drugs (penicillin) or proteins (horse serum), food anaphylaxis, and as a side effect of desensitization for hay fever treatment.

Mary Loveless in 1950 studied the occurrence of headache, as well as other effects of overdoasage of allergens, in 177 pollen-sensitive persons. Headache, when it occurred in these subjects after allergen overdosage,

was generalized and not hemicranial. It occurred both in those with and in those without histories of frequent headache attacks. Of the 177 subjects, there were 925 overdosage reactions. Twelve of the 177 subjects experienced headaches as part of such overdosage reactions on one or more occasions. Indeed, these 12 persons experienced 26 headaches during 121 overdosage reactions, or 21% of the time. For the entire group, the incidence of headache as an aspect of allergen overdosage effects was 2.8%, and then always as part of a widespread allergen overdosage syndrome, including urticaria, rhinitis, asthma, and hypotension. In the Loveless study, headache never occurred as an isolated phenomenon during induced antigen IgE reactions.

Since most allergy practices have an incidence of overdosage or systemic reactions to injected allergy extracts in the order of 1 in 500 treatments, this artificial or iatrogenic event cannot begin to account for spontaneous vascular or migraine headaches, even in the atopic population receiving immunotherapy.

Walker (1960) emphasized again the insignificance of the effects of food allergens in the migraine headache attack. She was not able to demonstrate a significant therapeutic effect from elimination diets, but was convinced that for some patients the occurrence of allergic phenomena is in itself so disturbing and exhausting as to constitute a sufficient basis for the precipitation of migraine attack by entirely independent mechanisms.

SUMMARY

1. Allergic reactions can be categorized into four types, which depend on the immunochemical reaction involved, and its time span.

2. Some forms of rhinitis are associated with paranasal head pain. The headache is dull, deep, aching, and nonpulsatile. It is associated with nasal congestion.

3. The mucosa covering the approaches to the paranasal sinuses was found to be the most pain sensitive of the nasal and paranasal structures and cavities, whereas the mucosa lining of the sinuses was of relatively low sensitivity. When a given faradic stimulus to the tongue

was experienced as a 1 plus pain; when applied to the turbinates, it elicited a 4 to 5 plus pain; when applied to the nasofrontal duct, a 5 to 7 plus pain; when applied to the ostium, a 6 to 9 plus pain; and when applied to the lining of the frontal or maxillary sinuses, a 1 to 2 plus pain.

4. Most of the pain arising from faradic, mechanical, and chemical stimulation of the mucosa of the nasal and paranasal cavities was referred pain, i.e., it was felt at a site other than that stimulated. It was referred chiefly to those areas supplied by the first division of the fifth cranial nerve. When severe enough, or of sufficient duration, the pain spread over most of the region supplied by the division of the fifth cranial nerve to which it was initially referred, and sometimes spread from the region of the second to that of the first division.

5. The stimulation of several different sites resulted in pain referred to the same region. Thus, stimulation of the nasal structures near the midline resulted in the same area of referred pain as did stimulation of the ostium and the more lateral wall of the maxillary sinus.

6. Section of the fifth cranial sensory nerve root in most instances caused the nasal mucosa on the same side to be insensitive, whereas the pharynx, tonsils, fossa of Rosenmüller, eustachian tubes, external auditory canals, and the eardrum continued to be sensitive to faradic stimulation.

7. Painful sensations were described as diffuse, sustained, nonpulsatile, and of a deep, aching nature. Pain was associated with lacrimation, photophobia, erythema, and hyperalgesia. The pain and associated effects outlasted the period of stimulation.

8. Inflammation and engorgement of the turbinates, ostia, nasofrontal ducts, and superior nasal spaces are responsible for most of the pain emanating from the nasal and paranasal structures.

9. Sustained positive pressure of 15 to 25 mm Hg applied within the antrum did not produce pain. A positive pressure of 200 mm was required to elicit immediate pain, although sustained pressure of 50 mm produced pain after 2½ hr. There was no perception of pain when a brief negative pressure of 100 to 150 mm Hg was produced within the antrum.

10. If a headache is not associated with turbinate engorgement and inflammation, it is in all probability not the result of disease of the nasal or paranasal structures. Headaches secondary to neoplastic invasion of paranasal structures and to antral infection through the dental roots are rare exceptions and are easily detected by sinus roentgenograms.

11. The phenomena of migraine and certain allergic responses are similar in many respects. In both, attacks are paroxysmal with associated edema and hyperemia, presumably mediated by protein breakdown products and terminated by vasoconstrictor agents. There is, however, no predictable relationship between most allergens and the occurrence of migraine headaches. Serum levels of IgE are approximately the same in patients with migraine as they are in the general population. The cellular infiltration prominent during allergic reactions is absent in migraine, and responses to antihistamines and to adrenal steroids are different in the two disorders. Hence, there is no conclusive evidence that histamine or ingested allergens are implicated in the etiology of migraine or that migraine results from ingestion of such allergens as a part of an antigen-antibody reaction.

REFERENCES

Atkins, C. J., J. J. Kondon, and F. P. Quismorio (1972). The choroid plexis in systemic lupus erythematosus. *Ann. Intern. Med.* 76, 65–72.

Balyeat, R. M., and F. L. Brittain (1930). Allergic migraine—based on a study of 55 cases. *Am. J. Med. Sci.* 180, 212–220.

Bassoe, P. (1933). Migraine. *JAMA* 101, 599–605.

Beall, G. N., and P. P. Van Arsdel (1960). Histamine metabolism in human disease. *J. Clin. Invest.* 39, 676–684.

Benveniste, J. (1974). Platelet-activating factor, a new mediator of anaphylaxis and immune complex deposition from rabbit and human basophils. *Nature* 249, 581–582.

Bergström, S. H. Duner, U. S. Von Euler, B. Pernow, and J. Sjovall (1959). Observations on the effects of infusions of prostaglandin E in man. *Acta Physiol. Scand.* 45, 145–153.

Bhat, K. N., C. M. Arroyave, S. R. Marney, D. D. Stevenson, and E. M. Tan (1976). Plasma histamine changes during provoked bronchospasm in asthmatic patients. *J. Allergy Clin. Immunol.* 58, 647–656.

Brocklehurst, W. E. (1960). The release of histamine and formation of a slow reacting substance (SRS-

A) during anaphylactic shock. *J. Physiol. (London)* *151*, 416–425.

Broder, E., M. W. Higgins, K. P. Mathews, and J. B. Keller (1974). The epidemiology of asthma and hay fever in a total community: Tecumseh, Michigan (32). *J. Allergy Clin. Immunol.* *54*, 100–112.

Dalessio, D. J. (1972). Dietary migraine. *Am. Fam. Physician 6*, 60–65.

Dalsgaard-Nielsen, T. (1974). The nature of migraine. *Headache 14*, 13–18.

David, J. R., and R. R. David (1972). Cellular hypersensitivity and immunity: inhibition of macrophage migration and lymphocyte mediators. *Prog. Allergy 16*, 300–332.

DeGowin, E. L. (1932). Allergic migraine: review of sixty cases. *J. Allergy 3*, 557–564.

Fink, J. N. (1972). Urticaria and physical allergy. In *Allergic Diseases* (R. Patterson, ed.), p. 341. Lippincott, Philadelphia.

Fowler, P. B. S. (1962). Epilepsy due to angioneurotic edema. *Proc. Roy. Soc. Med. 55*, 13–15.

Gell, P. G. H., and R. R. A. Coombs (1968). The allergic response and immunity. In *Clinical Aspects of Immunology*, pp. 423–456. F. A. Davis, Philadelphia.

Gonzales, S. (1953). Association of asthma and headache of allergic origin. *Med. Ibera 2*, 747–753.

Goth, A. (1978). Antihistamines. In *Allergy: Principles and Practice* (Middleton, Reed, and Ellis, eds.), pp. 454–463. C. V. Mosby, St. Louis.

Hahn, L. (1930). Relation between migraine and allergy. *Med. Klin. 26*, 1219–1226.

Hamburger, J. (1935). Migraine: role of food allergy. *Rev. Immunol. (Paris) 1*, 102–109.

Hazelman, B. L., I. C. M. MacLennan, and R. G. Earler (1975). Lymphocyte proliferation to artery antigen as a positive diagnostic test in polymyalgia rheumatica. *Ann. Rheum. Dis. 34*, 122–128.

Healey, L. A., and K. R. Wilske (1977). Manifestations of giant cell arteritis. *Med. Clin. North Am. 61*, 261–270.

Hyslop, G. H. (1934). Migraine: suggestions for its treatment. *Med. Clin. North Am. 17*, 827–842.

Kaliner, M., and K. F. Austen (1973). A sequence of biochemical events in the antigen-induced release of chemical mediators from sensitized human lung tissue. *J. Exp. Med. 138*, 1094–1102.

Kallos, P., and L. Kallos-Deffner (1955). Allergy and migraine. *Intern. Arch. Allergy Appl. Immunol. 7*, 367–392.

Kaplan, A. P., and K. F. Austen (1975). Activation and control mechanisms of Hageman factor—dependent pathways of coagulation, fibrinolysis and kinin generation and their contribution to the inflammatory process. *J. Allergy Clin. Immunol. 56*, 491–503.

Kaplan, A. (1978). Urticaria and angioedema. In *Allergy: Principles and Practice* (Middleton, Reed, and Ellis, eds.), pp. 1080–1099. C. V. Mosby, St. Louis.

Kay, A. B., and K. F. Austen (1971). The IgE-mediated release of an eosinophil leukocyte chemotactic factor from human lung. *J. Immunol. 107*, 899–906.

Keeney, E. L. (1946). Periodic vascular head pain. *Clinics 5*, 550–567.

Klein, R. G., R. J. Campbell, G. G. Hunder, and J. A. Carney (1976). Skip lesions in temporal arteritis. *Mayo Clin. Proc. 51*, 504–510.

Kohler, P. F. (1978). Immune complexes and allergic disease. In *Allergy: Principles and Practice* (Middleton, Reed, and Ellis, eds.), pp. 155–176. C. V. Mosby, St. Louis.

Lance, J. W., and M. Anthony (1966). Some clinical aspects of migraine. *Arch. Neurol. 15*, 356–361.

Lever, W. F. (1961). Urticaria and angioedema. In *Histopathology of the Skin*, pp. 114–120. Lippincott, Philadelphia.

Lewis, G. P. (1961). Bradykinin. *Nature 192*, 596–600.

Lewis, T. (1927). *The blood vessels of the human skin and their responses*, p. 90. Shaw and Sons, London.

Loveless, M. H. (1950). Milk allergy. A survey of its incidence: Experiments with a masked ingestion test. *J. Allergy 21*, 489–501.

Mathews, K. P. (1974). A current view of urticaria. *Med. Clin. North Am. 58*, 185–196.

May, C. D., and S. A. Bock (1978). Adverse reactions to food due to hypersensitivity. In *Allergy: Principles and Practice* (Middleton, Reed, and Ellis, eds.), pp. 1159–1171. C. V. Mosby, St. Louis.

Medina, J. L., and S. Diamond (1976). Migraine and atopy. *Headache 15*, 271–274.

Millonig, A. G., H. E. Harris, and W. J. Gardner (1950). Effect of autonomic denervation on the nasal mucosa. *Arch. Otolaryngol. 52*, 359–365.

Neusser, E. (1892). Klinisch-hamatologische Mittheilungen. *Wien. Klin. Wscher. 5*, 41–45.

Newball, H. H., R. C. Talamo, and L. M. Lichtenstein (1975). Release of leukocyte kallikrein mediated by IgE. *Nature 254*, 635–637.

Nutman, D. D., N. Kurata, and E. M. Tan (1975). Profiles of antinuclear antibodies in systemic rheumatic diseases. *Ann. Intern. Med. 83*, 464–469.

Ogden, H. D. (1951). The treatment of allergic headache. *Ann. Allergy 9*, 611–619.

O'Neil, W. N. Jr., S. P. Hammar, and H. A. Bloomer (1976). Giant cell arteritis with visceral angiitis. *Arch. Intern. Med. 136*, 1157–1160.

Pagniez, P., P. Vallery-Radot, and A. Nast (1919). Therapeutique preventive de certaines migraines. *Presse Med. 27*, 172–176.

Pickering, G. W. (1933). Histamine headache. *Clin. Sci. 1*, 77–101.

Ralston, H. J., and W. J. Kerr (1945). Vascular responses of the nasal mucosa to thermal stimuli with some observations on skin temperature. *Am. J. Physiol. 144*, 305–312.

Rinkel, H. J. (1933). Considerations of allergy as factor in familial recurrent headache. *J. Allergy 4*, 303–312.

Rowe, A. H. (1932). Allergic migraine. *JAMA 99*, 912–917.

Ruddy, S., I. Gigli, and K. F. Austen (1972). The

complement system in man. *New Engl. J. Med. 287*, 489–495.

Schwarz, M. (1952). Is migraine an allergic disease? *Acta Allerg. 5 Suppl. II*, 426–432.

Simon, R. A., D. D. Stevenson, C. M. Arroyave, and E. M. Tan (1977). The relationship of plasma histamine to the activity of bronchial asthma. *J. Allergy Clin. Immunol. 60*, 312–316.

Smith, J. M. (1978). Epidemiology and natural history of asthma, allergic rhinitis and atopic dermatitis (eczema). In *Allergy: Principles and Practice* (Middleton, Reed, and Ellis, eds.), p. 637. C. V. Mosby, St. Louis.

Solomon, W. R. (1967). Hay fever, allergic rhinitis and asthma. In *A Manual of Clinical Allergy* (J. M. Sheldon, ed.), pp. 78–88. W. B. Saunders, Philadelphia.

Speer, F. (1975). The many facets of migraine. *Ann. Allergy 34*, 273–285.

Stanson, A. W., R. G. Klein, and G. G. Hunder (1976). Extracranial angiographic findings in giant cell arteritis. *Am. J. Roentgenol. 137*, 957–963.

Stechschulte, D. J., R. P. Orange, and K. F. Austen (1973). Detection of slow-reacting substance of anaphylaxis (SRS-A). *J. Immunol. 111*, 1585–1592.

Tennenbaum, James I. (1972). Allergic rhinitis. In *Allergic Diseases* (R. Patterson, ed.), pg. 172. Lippincott, Philadelphia.

Trousseau, A. (1873). Clinique medicale de L'Hotel-Dieu de Paris. 4e. ed. Vol. 2. Baillieu, Paris, p. 460.

Unger, A. H. and L. Unger (1952). Migraine is an allergic disease. *J. Allergy 23*, 429–436.

Unger, L., and J. L. Cristol (1970). Allergic migraine. *Ann. Allergy 28*, 106–112.

Unger, L., and M. C. Harris (1974). Stepping-stones in allergy. *Ann. Allergy 33*, 353–363.

Vane, J. R. (1976). The mode of action of aspirin and similar compounds. *J. Allergy Clin. Immunol. 58*, 691–712.

Vaughan, W. T. (1927). Allergic migraine. *JAMA 88*, 1383–1394.

Vaughan, W. T. (1934). Analysis of allergic factor in recurrent paroxysmal headache. Trans. Assoc. Am. Physicians 49, 348–358.

Vahlquist, B. (1955). Migraine in children. *Intern. Arch. Allergy 7*, 348–360.

Von Leeuwen, W., and Z. Zeydner (1922). Occurrence of toxic substance in blood in cases of bronchial asthma, urticaria, epilepsy and migraine. *Brit. J. Exp. Path. 3*, 282–287.

von Pirquet, C. (1906). Allergie. *Munchen. Med. Wsch. 53*, 1457–1465.

Waaler, E., O. Tonder, and E. J. Milde (1976). Immunological and histological studies of temporal arteries from patients with temporal arteritis and/or polymyalgia rheumatica. *Acta Pathol. Microbiol. Scan. 84*, 55–63.

Walker, V. B. (1960). *Report to the Ciba Foundation Conference on Migraine*. London, England.

Wasserman, S. I., N. A. Soter, D. M. Center, and K. F. Austen (1977). Cold urticaria: Recognition and characteristics of a neutrophil chemotactic fac-characterization of a neutrophil chemotactic factor which appears in serum during experimental and cold challenge. *J. Clin. Invest. 60*, 189–196.

Wolf, A. A., and L. Unger (1944). Migraine due to milk: feeding tests. *Ann. Intern. Med. 20*, 831–843.

Wolff, H. G. (1955). Headache mechanisms. *Intern. Arch. Allergy 7*, 210–225.

Ziegler, D. K., R. Hassanein, and K. Hassanein (1972). Headache syndromes suggested by factor analysis of symptom variables in a headache prone population. *J. Chron. Dis. 25*, 353–362.

13

HEADACHE AND BRAIN TUMOR

REVISED BY JOHN F. ALKSNE

Although no single headache pattern is pathognomic of brain tumor, and brain tumors can occur without headache, some headache patterns are more often associated with brain tumor than others. Whatever the headache pattern, brain tumor must be suspected in all patients with chronic headache and appropriate measures taken to establish or rule out the diagnosis. For example, the patient whose head scan is shown in Fig. 13-1 complained of headache 1½ years before this large tumor was detected. She had no other symptoms and was thought to have "tension headaches".

On the basis of a careful study of 72 patients

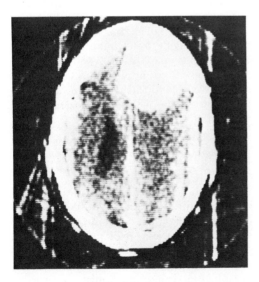

FIG. 13-1. Computerized brain scan showing large right-frontal tumor.

with primary brain tumor (Kunkle *et al.*, 1942), and a general review of the literature, we can attempt to:

1. define the quality and intensity of brain tumor headache,

2. outline the common mechanisms of brain tumor headache,

3. define when headache might be expected to have value in diagnosis and localization of brain tumor.

I. The Quality and Intensity of Brain Tumor Headache

The headache was of a deep, aching, steady, dull nature. It was not rhythmic and seldom throbbing. It was usually intermittent, but in one-tenth of the patients it was continuous. The headache was sometimes severe, but rarely was it as intense as that of migraine or the headache associated with ruptured cerebral aneurysm, meningitis, or certain febrile illnesses, or that induced by certain drugs. It was usually relieved by acetylsalicylic acid, or cold packs applied to the scalp, both indications of its moderate intensity. It rarely interfered with sleep. It was aggravated by coughing, or straining at stool, and sometimes it was worse in the erect than in the recumbent position. It was also commonly aggravated by the onset of a minor infection. If there were any variation in intensity during the 24 hr cycle, it was worse in the early morning.

Even when the tumor directly compressed or extensively stretched cranial nerves containing pain afferents, the pain was not equal in inten-

287

sity to that of tic douloureux, and indeed was often mild or absent (Cushing, 1917, Cohen, 1939, Dandy, 1945, Pollock, 1941).

Unless the pain were severe, nausea with tumor headache was slight. Vomiting occurred with displacement or compression of the medulla and was sometimes projectile, perhaps because it was unexpected when unaccompanied by nausea. The headache when occipital or suboccipital, was sometimes associated with stiffness or aching of the muscles of the neck and tilting of the head toward the side of the tumor.

II. The Pathophysiology of Brain Tumor Headache

Two sets of observations on headache directly introduce the present study. First of all, data obtained during the operative exposure of intracranial contents have identified those structures that are pain sensitive to mechanical stimulation, and the sites of the headache thus induced (Fay, 1936; Ray and Wolff, 1940) (see Chapter 3). These structures are, in brief, the great venous sinuses and their tributaries from the surface of the brain, the dural arteries, the internal carotid arteries, the cerebral arteries at the base, the basilar and vertebral arteries, the other arteries near their sites of origin from the basilar and vertebral trunks, parts of the dura at the base, and the intracranial portions of the trigeminal, glossopharyngeal, vagus, and upper cervical nerves. It was noted, furthermore, that stimulation of the pain-sensitive structures on or above the superior surface of the tentorium cerebelli resulted in pain transmitted by the fifth nerve and located in regions on the anterior half of the head.

Stimulation of the pain-sensitive intracranial structures on or below the inferior surface of the tentorium cerebelli resulted in pain over the posterior half of the head, the pain pathways being chiefly in the ninth and tenth cranial nerves and the upper three cervical nerves (Ray and Wolff, 1940).

Organization of the data available from these studies has indicated six basic mechanisms of headache, involving distortion or inflammation of intracranial pain-sensitive structures (Ray and Wolff, 1940).

1. Traction on the large venous sinuses or their tributaries from the surface of the brain.

2. Traction on the middle meningeal artery.

3. Traction on the large arteries at the base of the brain.

4. Direct pressure upon the cranial and upper cervical nerves which carry pain fibers.

5. Dilatation of intracranial arteries.

6. Inflammation in or about any of the intracranial pain-sensitive structures.

The first four of these six mechanisms play a part in the headache associated with brain tumor.

A fact important to an understanding of brain tumor headache is that increased intracranial pressure is not essential to its production (Kunkle et al, 1943). Thus, elevation of the intracranial pressure in normal human subjects to levels as high as 510 mm of saline by the intrathecal injection of normal saline consistently failed to cause headache (Chapter 14). Evidence even more compelling that increased intracranial pressure and tumor headache are not closely related was obtained in the study of a man with a left parietal oligodendroglioma in whom bifrontal headache had been present intermittently for two months but happened to be absent at the time the following experiment was performed. By drainage of cerebrospinal fluid with the patient horizontal, moderate headache, chiefly left frontal, was induced. The headache was then relieved at once by restoration of fluid and elevation of pressure to its initial level, and furthermore could not be produced by pressure elevation to a high level, 550 mm of saline.

1. Tumor Headache and Increased Intracranial Pressure not Essentially Related

In this series of 72 patients, headache occurred almost as commonly in those patients (19 of 23) without increased intracranial pressure as it did in those (46 of 49) with increased pressure. Moreover, of the seven patients (about 10% of all cases) who were headache-free, three had increased intracranial pressure.

These data demonstrate that increased pressure per se is neither an essential nor a major factor in tumor headache.

2. Tumor Headache in Patients with Normal Intracranial Pressure—The Mechanism of Local Traction

Of the 23 patients with normal intracranial pressure, 19 had headache as a symptom. In all but three patients with hypophysial adenoma, the existence and location of the headache could be explained by traction upon or distortion of directly neighboring pain-sensitive structures, and in some at operation the headache was thus reproduced. These adjacent structures were: (1) for the four supratentorial meningiomas—the superior sagittal sinus and its tributaries, the middle meningeal artery and the large arteries at the base: (2) for the one glioma—the superior sagittal sinus and its tributaries; (3) for the three craniopharyngiomas—the large arteries at the base; (4) for the four hypophysial adenomas—the large arteries at the base and in one patient the lining of the sphenoid sinus; and (5) for the four cerebellopontile angle tumors—the internal auditory artery, the pontile arteries, the dura about the internal auditory meatus, and the transverse sinus. In Fig. 13-2 are shown examples of this group.

Another example of the headache produced by local traction may be cited (Fig. 13-3). A 37-year-old male with a trigeminal "neuroma" in the right cerebellopontine angle and no evidence of increased intracranial pressure had had for four months three separate kinds of head discomfort. These with the sites of origin of the symptoms, were: (1) right temporal tightness—fifth cranial nerve; (2) soreness in the right eyeball, superior surface of the right transverse sinus, and fifth cranial nerve; (3) pain and tenderness in the right postauricular area, right internal auditory and pontile arteries, and inferior surface of the transverse sinus.

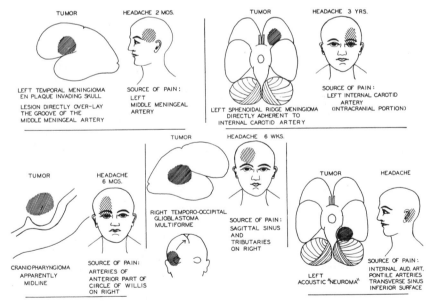

LOCAL TRACTION HEADACHE IN PATIENTS WITH NORMAL INTRACRANIAL PRESSURE

FIG. 13-2. Five examples of patients with tumor headache produced by local traction. Intracranial pressure was normal in all. The structures that were the probable sources of the pain are listed in each case.

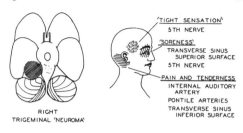

RIGHT
TRIGEMINAL 'NEUROMA'

'TIGHT SENSATION'
5TH NERVE

'SORENESS'
TRANSVERSE SINUS
SUPERIOR SURFACE
5TH NERVE

PAIN AND TENDERNESS
INTERNAL AUDITORY
ARTERY
PONTILE ARTERIES
TRANSVERSE SINUS
INFERIOR SURFACE

HEADACHE WITH AN ANGLE TUMOR

FIG. 13-3. Demonstration of headache from local traction in a man with three separate types of head discomfort, due to a trigeminal "neuroma" in the right cerebellopontile angle. The intracranial pressure was normal.

This mechanism of tumor headache may be termed local traction. While independent of increase in intracranial pressure, it may well be augmented by generalized displacement of the brain associated with cerebrospinal fluid pressure rise.

The three patients with hypophysial adenoma in whom local traction did not entirely account for the headache had pain in the occiput or subocciput in addition to frontotemporal headache. The pain in the back of the head in these three of the seven patients with hypophysial adenoma is unexplained.

3. Tumor Headache in Patients with Increased Intracranial Pressure—Consideration of Local and Distant Traction

In less than one-half (18) of those patients (46) with headache and increased intracranial pressure could the locations of the headache be explained or the pain induced by local traction. Most of the remaining half of the patients had posterior head pain in association with supratentorial tumors and frontal headache in association with infratentorial tumors. The following analysis of the group illuminates this seeming paradox.

(A) DISTANT TRACTION THROUGH EXTENSIVE DISPLACEMENT OF THE BRAIN

Slightly less than one-half (14 of 32) of the patients with supratentorial tumor with headache had pain in the posterior half of the head—occipital, suboccipital, or postauricular areas. In seven patients this pain was bilateral. In the seven in whom it was unilateral it was homolateral to the tumor in all but one. In each instance pain was also present in one or several other head regions.

Headache so located in these patients could not be explained by local traction, for there is no evidence that any supratentorial structure can be the direct source of posterior head pain. Pressure downward upon the tentorium cerebelli from above has been shown experimentally to cause only fronto-orbital pain, probably by traction upon the upper surfaces of the transverse sinuses. Such a mechanism, therefore cannot be relevant to posterior head pain. It has been recognized, however, that when supratentorial lesions are large enough to cause generalized increase in pressure, there is often a widespread shift in the brain causing distortion of supra- and infratentorial structures. Thus, traction or pressure upon the transverse and occipital sinuses, the basilar and vertebral arteries, the ninth and tenth cranial, and upper cervical nerves is probably a common occurrence. However, with supratentorial tumor the extent of such distortion in the posterior fossa is much less and the establishment of a "cerebellar pressure cone" is less likely than in patients with intratentorial tumor.

Herniation of the hippocampal gyri through the incisura tentorii may also be responsible for posterior head pain from supratentorial tumors. In a 1941 review of autopsied cases of supratentorial neoplasms such a complication was found in about 80% of the series (Schwarz and Rosner, 1941). The distortion produced by this "temporal pressure cone" has been shown to affect not only the hippocampal gyri but also the adjacent brainstem, and presumably the basilar artery and its branches. This mechanism must be considered to be of minor importance as regards the present problem, for in the autopsied series reported, posterior head pain was no more common in the patients with such herniation than in those without it.

In brief, posterior head pain in patients with supratentorial tumor appears to depend upon expansion of the mass to such an extent that coincident with generalized rise in intracranial pressure, traction is produced upon pain-sensitive structures in the distant posterior fossa by displacement of the whole brain. In contrast to local traction this may be conveniently termed distant traction and may be considered as a second mechanism of brain tumor headache. It is evident that in extensive shift of the brain, traction effected at a distance from the tumor may involve structures on the same side as the tumor or on both sides. The data indicate that both situations are common.

(B) DISTANT TRACTION THROUGH INTERNAL HYDROCEPHALUS

Frontal headache was a symptom in two-thirds (10 of 14) of the patients with infratentorial tumor and increased intracranial pressure, all of whom had headache. This fact likewise required explanation in terms other than local traction by the tumor. Analysis revealed that nine of the ten with frontal headache, comprising two patients with angle tumors and seven with cerebellar or fourth-ventricle tumors, had block to the cerebrospinal fluid outflow at the aqueduct or the fourth ventricle and had internal hydrocephalus with increase in intracranial pressure. The frontal headache was bilateral in all but one patient.

The association of internal hydrocephalus with frontal headache in patients with infraten-

torial tumor has been noted by others (Cushing, 1931, Dandy, 1945). Direct evidence that the hydrocephalus is causally related to the headache has been provided by the demonstration that distention of one lateral ventricle with a balloon at operation induces homolateral frontal headache by traction upon the veins over the convexity of the brain anchoring it to the superiorsagittal sinus. Experimental distention of the third ventricle has been found to cause diffuse headache arising from traction upon the many large vessels at the base (see Figs. 3-17 and 3-18). There is further evidence that significant distortion of adjacent structures at the base is produced by enlargement of the third ventricle in internal hydrocephalus, for in such patients a visual field defect indicative of chiasmal pressure has often been found (Wagener and Cusick, 1937). The usual bilaterality of the frontal headache in these patients may therefore be understood.

Hence, frontal headache of this kind is like the posterior head pain discussed in the previous section in that it is produced by traction at a distance from the tumor.

An example of a small tumor producing headache entirely by distant traction is outlined in Fig. 13-4. A 16-year-old male had had intermittent bifrontal and bioccipital headache for five years. On admission moderate papilledema was noted. The ventriculograms showed advanced dilatation of the third and

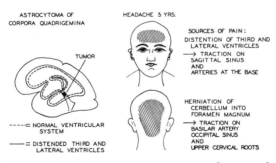

FIG. 13-4. Demonstration of distant traction headache produced by a small astrocytoma in the roof of the aqueduct. The frontal headache was due to internal hydrocephalus, the occipital headache to distortion of posterior fossa structures by wedging of the cerebellum into the foramen magnum.

lateral ventricles. Exploration confirmed the presence of internal hydrocephalus. The foramina of Monroe were widely stretched. The largest diameter of the left opening measured 2.5 cm. Moreover, as seen in a second exploration, the tonsils of the cerebellum were herniated in part into the foramen magnum. No tumor could be found, but autopsy revealed a small fibrillary astrocytoma of the corpora quadrigemina occluding the aqueduct of Sylvius. The frontal headache was due to distention of the lateral, and possibly the third, ventricles. The occipital headache was due to traction upon the basilar artery, the occipital sinus, the ninth and tenth cranial nerves, and upper cervical roots by the wedging of the cerebellum down into the foramen magnum. The site of origin and the location of both frontal and occipital headaches were remote from the tumor itself.

(C) TUMOR HEADACHE UNEXPLAINED BY LOCAL OR DISTANT TRACTION

In two patients with increased intracranial pressure the headache could not clearly be related to these mechanisms. One, a 24-year-old female, had had a left temporal headache for five months. She had a right acoustic "neuroma," increased intracranial pressure, and internal hydrocephalus.

The other, a 44-year-old female, had had right occipital headache for six months. She had a left cerebellar hemangioblastoma, increased intracranial pressure, and internal hydrocephalus.

Headache in this pattern, sparing the homolateral side but involving the contralateral side, appears bizarre. The direction and distribution of the stress and strain in these two cases are conjectural and the factors that make them atypical are not apparent. There is no evidence, however, that mechanisms other than traction upon pain-sensitive structures are involved.

Thus, in 44 of the 46 patients with headache and increased intracranial pressure the existence and location of the headache could be accounted for on the basis of the mechanisms thus far outlined. In many (18) local traction alone appeared to be responsible. In a few (four) traction at a distance alone was responsible either through displacement of posterior

fossa structures in patients with supratentorial tumors or through internal hydrocephalus in patients with intratentorial tumors, but, in the largest group (22) both local and distant traction were concerned. In two patients the headache could not be clearly explained by either mechanism.

It is to be emphasized that the association of increased intracranial pressure with headache due to distant traction does not justify the inference that increased intracranial pressure of itself causes headache. It indicates rather that the same factors that bring about distant traction, that is, extensive displacement of the brain directly by the tumor or indirectly by internal hydrocephalus, will also cause generalized elevation of intracranial pressure (see Fig. 13-5).

4. Continuous vs. Intermittent Headache with Brain

Tumor. As mentioned above, the headache of brain tumor is usually intermittent. In this series continuous headache was noted in only seven cases or about a tenth of the patients (all with supraentorial tumor). Four of these had increased intracranial pressure. Local traction appeared to be the mechanism in all seven cases. The persistence these cases is not surprising, for it is reasonable to expect local traction to be continuous, and in fact progressive, if the tumor growth is moderately rapid. There is no explanation of the inter-

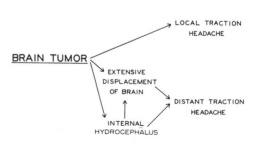

FIG. 13-5. Schematic outline summarizing common mechanisms of brain tumor headache.

mittency of the headache that will apply to all the remaining large group of patients. In some, intermittent block to cerebrospinal fluid outflow, either because of varying states of brain hydration or by movable tumors in the fourth or third ventricles, appears to have been responsible. In others the increase in intracranial venous pressure with straining and coughing might have been the basis for occasional headache.

5. Patients with Brain Tumor without Headache

Seven patients, or about a tenth of the entire series, had no headache in association with their lesions. The tumors represented were all supratentorial; in three of the seven increased intracranial pressure was present.

Associated with increased intracranial pressure and no headache were:

TUMOR TYPE	SITE
Meningioma	left parasagittal parietal
Glioblastoma multiforme	right frontocallosal
Glioblastoma multiforme	left frontal (subcortical)

Associated with normal intracranial pressure and no headache were:

TUMOR TYPE	SITE
Meningioma	right frontotemporal (invading the skull)
Oligodendroglioma	left frontotemporal
Oligodendroglioma	right temporoparietal
Craniopharyngioma	suprasellar (sella and dorsum destroyed)

Review of these patients disclosed that the only characteristic common to all was a supratentorial location of the tumor.

The absence of headache in patients with brain tumor may be related to the slow growth of the neoplasm. Thus five of the abovementioned seven patients had lesions that are notably slow in expanding, i.e., meningioma, craniopharyngioma, and oligodendroglioma. Moreover, in one of the two patients who were free of headache with glioblastoma mul-

tiforme, ordinarily a rapidly growing neoplasm, the clinical course indicated unusually slow growth of the tumor. When expansion of the tumor mass is slow, mechanical adaptation of adjacent structures may be sufficient to prevent pain production. This may represent the return of distorted pain endings to normal contour even though gross distortion of the tissues in which the pain endings are embedded persists. When the pace of growth is fast, such adaptation is inadequate (Cohen, 1939; Pollock, 1941).

It may be noted that in contrast to tumors above the tentorium, posterior fossa tumors, whatever their rate of growth, usually cause headache, undoubtedly because many of these lesions cause internal hydrocephalus (Cushing, 1931; Dandy, 1945). In consideration of headache, the speed of growth of the posterior fossa tumor is less significant, since it bears no direct relation to the completeness of occlusion of the iter or the fourth ventricle. A block once induced results in a relatively sudden displacement of the brain and stimulation of local and distant pain-sensitive structures.

Serious sensorial defects produced by the tumor, particularly with frontal lobe lesions, may be a second cause for absence of headache. For example, in the second of the two patients with glioblastoma multiforme without headache listed in the table above, the tumor was in the right frontocallosal region, and apathy and confusion were early and dramatic symptoms. Under such circumstances, gross defects in reaction to pain may veil or completely mask headache.

Invasion of the skull by meningiomas may be still a third factor in preventing or delaying headache. The bone of the skull is insensitive and extension in this direction may take the place of greater intracranial expansion toward pain-sensitive structures.

6. Brain Tumor and Headache Resulting from Sustained Contraction of Skeletal muscles of the Head and Neck

An additional and significant factor in the generalized headache associated with brain tumor is the pain that originates from the sustained contraction of skeletal muscle of the head and neck (discussed in detail in Chapter 19). As mentioned elsewhere, afferent impulses from any portion of the head may by spread of excitatory effects within the brainstem and upper cord cause skeletal muscle in the same and adjacent segments to contract. The sensations from such contraction are described as tight, cap-like, band-like, vise-like, but when sustained and sufficiently intense, cramping pain or ache may result. Thus, sometimes patients with posterior fossa tumors, involving one cerebellar lobe or the cerebellopontile angle, have in addition to the pain emanating from intracranial sources, the pain resulting from unilateral muscle contraction in the neck and occipital regions with characteristic tilting of the head. Also, afferent impulses arising in the occipital region may cause frontal and temporal headache. The reason for this is that apart from skeletal muscle effects, and because of spread in the brainstem of the central excitatory effects of noxious stimulation, pain may be experienced in sites other than those in which the afferent impulses originated.

III. Headache in the Localization of Brain Tumor

I. Limitations of Headache as a Localizing Sign

(A) HEADACHE IN ASSOCIATION WITH INCREASED INTRACRANIAL PRESSURE OF LIMITED LOCALIZING VALUE

In the preceding section it was noted that headache in patients with normal intracranial pressure could, with rare exceptions, be explained entirely in terms of local traction. Of patients with increased intracranial pressure, in only 18 of 46, or about 40% was local traction solely responsible; in the remaining 26, distant traction was an accessory or the chief mechanism.

When distant traction is involved, the problem of localization of the tumor is complicated, for with this mechanism distortion of bilateral pain-sensitive structures is common, and the site of the expanding mass is often concealed. It is evident, therefore, that in the presence of increased intracranial pressure, which in patients with brain tumor is presumptive evidence of extensive displacement of the brain, the localizing value of tumor headache becomes reduced.

(B) FRONTO-OCCIPITAL HEADACHE OF NO LOCALIZING VALUE

The combination of frontal and occipital headache was noted in one-fourth of all the patients with headache. The group with fronto-occipital headache included patients with meningioma, cerebral glioma, third-ventricle cyst, hypophysial adenoma, cerebellopontile angle and cerebellar and fourth-ventricle tumors. Except for the two instances of hypophysial adenomas, all were accompanied by increased intracranial pressure. Internal hydrocephalus was present with only one of the supratentorial tumors, the third-ventricle cyst, but was present with all five infratentorial tumors.

The data indicated that fronto-occipital headache occurred almost as frequently with supratentorial tumors as with those below the tentorium. Moreover, they showed conclusively that the fronto-occipital headache combination cannot be considered diagnostic of internal hydrocephalus in patients with brain tumor. It is of additional interest that except for the hypophysial adenomas, all the patients with headache of this pattern had increased intracranial pressure.

HEADACHE AND BRAIN TUMOR

(C) HEADACHE OVER THE VERTEX—INFREQUENT AND OF LITTLE LOCALIZING VALUE

Headache over the vertex was noted infrequently in this series. In only three patients was the headache in the vertex alone; these were a midline olfactory groove meningioma, a craniopharyngioma, and an eosinophilic hypophysial adenoma. In the first two the intracranial pressure was elevated. In two other patients headache was vertical in part but not predominantly; the tumors found were a parasagittal parietal meningioma and a midline cerebellar astrocytoma, both with increased pressure.

HEADACHE FROM MIDLINE TUMORS NOT ALWAYS BILATERAL

Twenty-three patients with midline tumors and headache were included in this series. In 17 patients the headache was symmetrically bilateral, 11 having increased intracranial pressure. In six the headache was entirely or predominantly unilateral; none of these had increased intracranial pressure.

Local traction apparently was the pain mechanism for the headache when it was unilateral. The inequality of the distortion produced may have been due to unrecognized asymmetrical expansion of the growing tumor. Whatever the explanation, it is clear that unilateral headache may occur with midline tumors.

2. Assets of Headache as a Localizing Sign

The limitations of headache having thus been considered, its value may now be appraised.

(A) HEADACHE NEAR OR OVERLYING THE TUMOR

Headache to be of service as a localizing sign of brain tumor must be interpreted in terms of the headache mechanisms and principles of pain reference just outlined. Only when tumor headache is caused solely by local traction is it of direct value in localization. Even then the headache may not overlie the tumor, for in about 40% of the patients with headache due only to local traction the pain was not immediately over the tumor. In the following analysis certain tumors located at the base and anteriorly were not included since obviously they could not produce headache near to or directly overlying the tumor, other than in the nasopharynx. These lesions were the cranio-

pharyngiomas, hypophysial adenomas, a suprasellar meningioma, and a third-ventricle cyst. The evidence in summary, based on the remaining 22 patients with local traction headache, was as follows:

	HEADACHE NEAR TO OR OVERLYING THE TUMOR
Supratentorial tumors	
Meningioma	3 of 6
Glioma	4 of 9
Infratentorial tumors	
Cerebellopontile angle tumors	4 of 4
Cerebellar and fourth ventricle tumors	2 of 3
	13 of 22

When the analysis was broadened to include all the patients (again excluding those with tumors at the base) headache was found to overlie the tumor in only 19 of 51, or about one-third.

(B) HEADACHE AS FIRST SYMPTOM OF BRAIN TUMOR

With the exception of the cerebellopontile angle tumors, the presence of most of the posterior fossa tumors first was made manifest by headache. The tumors above the tentorium, on the other hand, were more likely first to cause other symptoms, such as visual disturbances, paresthesias, convulsions, and sensorial and personality changes. Other authors have reported similar observations (Brain, 1925; Cohen, 1939). Northfield's figures (1938) based upon a series of 100 cases, are presented in brackets for comparison with the data of this New York Hospital series. Headache as first symptom of brain tumor.

		NORTHFIELD
In 54 cases of supratentorial tumor		
Meningioma	5 of 15	(36%)
Glioma	11 of 22	(36%)
Third ventricle tumors	1 of 2	
Hypophysial adenoma	1 of 8	
Craniopharyngioma	2 of 7	
	20 of 54 or about one-third	
In 18 cases of infratentorial tumor		
Cerebellopontile angle tumors	1 of 7	(0)
Cerebellar and fourth ventricle tumors ..	9 of 11	(83%)
	10 of 18	

The usual occurrence of headache as first symptom in patients with cerebellar or fourth-ventricle tumors is related to the fact that internal hydrocephalus can easily result from such lesions. Angle tumors, however, are less frequently associated with internal hydrocephalus in the early stages and are directly adjacent to the several cranial nerves which traverse the angle region, potential sources of such symptoms as facial paresthesias, deafness, tinnitus, or weakness of face or jaw. Whether or not supratentorial tumors cause focal symptoms or signs before the occurrence of headache depends upon the region of the brain involved.

(C) THE SIGNIFICANCE OF HEADACHE IN THE BACK OF THE HEAD AND NECK WITH BRAIN TUMOR

Pain in the back of the head—occipital, or postauricular or suboccipital areas—was present in one-half the patients. As described in a preceding section, such pain was present in 17 of the 47 patients with supratentorial tumor with headache. In each of these, headache was present also in one or several other areas on the anterior half of the head. Except for the patients with hypophysial adenoma, headache in all was accompanied by increased intracranial pressure.

In contrast, pain in the back of the head was present in almost all the patients with infratentorial tumor. Of the 18 patients, 16 had acoustic "neuroma" and a cerebellar astrocytoma, both accompanied by increased intracranial pressure.

It seems generally true, therefore, that occipital, suboccipital, or post-auricular pain did not of itself identify a tumor as being above or below the tentorium. On the other hand, the evidence did indicate that when posterior headache was absent the tumor was rarely infratentorial.

(D) THE SIGNIFICANCE OF HEADACHE IN THE FRONT OF THE HEAD WITH BRAIN TUMOR

Frontal headache with brain tumor in this series was even more common than was pain in the back of the head. In 60% of all patients with headache, frontal headache was present, alone or with headaches elsewhere. In contrast to pain in or near the occiput, frontal headache was noted somewhat more often in association with supratentorial tumors (32 of the 47 with headache) than with infratentorial tumors (10 of 18).

Pain solely frontal was noted in 11 of the 47 cases of supratentorial tumor with headache but in only two of the 18 cases with infratentorial tumor or headache.

The predominance of frontal headache is not surprising in view of the diverse ways, direct and indirect, in which brain tumor may produce pain referred to the frontal areas. But from the data it may be inferred that although frontal headache was common in all types and locations of tumor, the pain when solely frontal was usually due to supratentorial tumor.

(E) THE SIGNIFICANCE OF UNILATERAL HEADACHE

It has been shown above that midline tumors may cause unilateral headache, probably because of asymmetric expansion of the mass. Further data concerning the significance of unilateral headache were derived from an analysis of the 42 remaining patients with headache and tumor not in the midline. The headache patterns were as follows:

Headache homolateral to the tumor 24
Headache contralateral to the tumor 5
Headache symmetrically bilateral 13

All five patients with headache contralateral to the tumor had increased intracranial pressure. In three of these five the contralateral location of the headache was the result of distant traction.

It is evident that headache chiefly on one side of the head was common in these patients, and that in most cases the headache was on the same side as the tumor (see also Pickering 1938). Contralateral headache may have resulted from the presence of anatomic asymmetries in the brain or skull such as the size or position of the lateral or third ventricles, or the relative position of the cerebellum, brainstem, and anchoring structures in the posterior fossa. In none of the patients with normal intracranial pressure was contralateral headache noted. The important inference from these considerations is that headache solely or chiefly unilateral is probably on the same side as the tumor when the intracranial pressure is normal.

3. Various Types of Tumors in Relation to Headache

Among patients with craniopharyngiomas, headache as an initial symptom was rare and its location unpredictable. The hypophysial adenomas also rarely produced headache as an initial symptom, and the site of the headache presented nothing of specific or helpful value.

Among most of the patients with headache due to cerebellopontile angle tumors the headache was a leading clue in the localization of the lesion, although headache did not occur as an early symptom. Headache solely in the postauricular area was almost specific, especially before gross displacement of the brain occurred.

Among patients with meningiomas (all but one being supratentorial), headache was a first symptom in one-third. In about one-half of the 14 patients with headache the headache was predominantly unilateral and on the same side as the tumor, and in all but two of the 14 cases the headache was due to local traction. It might be expected, situated as the meningiomas are in contact with pain-sensitive structures at the base and over the convexities, that headache as an initial symptom might occur in a higher proportion than the one-third indicated. It is probable, however, that the slow growth and bone invasion offset the effects of proximity to pain-sensitive vascular structures.

Gliomas, despite their lack of direct contact with pain-sensitive structures, presented headache as a first symptom in one-half of the patients when they occurred above the tentorium and even more frequently when they occurred below. Such tumors produced headaches as an early manifestation, probably because of their speed of growth and the likelihood of their occluding the lateral, third, and fourth ventricles.

In the patient with an intracranial space-occupying lesion, the frontal and temporal headache induced by sudden head rotation may be of diagnostic value (Wolff et al, 1947). Headache may sometimes be induced by this technique with ease and in areas of the head that point to the side of the lesion (although not the nature of the mass).

HEADACHE FROM NON NEOPLASTIC INTRACRANIAL MASS LESIONS

Non neoplastic intracran;ial mass lesions suc as hematomas and abscesses also cause headache and follow the same general rules as already discussed. Because their clinical presentation is different, however, they will be discussed separately.

(A) The Headache Resulting from Parenchymal and Epidural Abscess

Since parenchymal abscess is often associated with disease of adjacent nasal and aural structures, it is common to have headache from the latter source long preceding the actual involvement of brain tissue. Moreover, the brain abscess does not become of adequate size to cause headache by traction and displacement until about two months after parenchymatous breakdown has begun. At this time the abscess is of maximal size and is usually walled off. It is in essence, then, a cystic tumor that has gradually increased in size through the accumulation of fluid. Therefore headache from the abscess manifests itself with the development of papilledema and other evidence of local traction and generalized displacement of the brain. The mechanisms and clinical features are thus like all other parenchymatous tumors. The headache of brain abscess is usually associated with leukocytosis, fever, and pleocytosis. It is noteworthy that brain abscess from infections of the ear may occur either above or below the tentorium. In the latter case the evidence of brainstem embarrassment—hiccoughing, vomiting, and occipital headache—occurs early in the course of the illness.

Ray and Parsons (1943) emphasized that if headache associated with sinus disease and osteomyelitis of the adjacent bony wall persists after drainage of the sinus, it is likely that epidural abscess is also present. Such epidural abscesses occur in the frontal region adjacent to the diseased frontal, ethmoid, and sphenoid sinuses and, following osteomyelitis of the mastoid bone, in the postauricular occipital region.

(B) The Headache Resulting from Intracranial Hematoma

The headache resulting from intracranial hematoma cannot be discussed adequately without subdividing hematomas into a number of groups. These will be presented separately although on some occasions it may not be possible to differentiate them clinically (Fisher, 1968; Appenzeller, 1978).

EPIDURAL HEMATOMA

If the patient is conscious, headache may be a prominent early symptom of epidural hematoma because the pain-sensitive vascular structures in the dura are being separated from their natural attachment to the bone. As the mass lesion increases in size, producing brain compression and deteriorating consciousness, the pain input may be manifest as restlessness and combativeness without a specific complaint of headache. The progression of a head-injured patient from headache to restlessness should therefore alert the physician to the possibility of an expanding intracranial mass.

SUBDURAL HEMATOMA

The hematomas that occur between the dura and the brain can be divided into five clinical entities:

1. Acute subdural hematomas become clinically significant within 48 hr of injury. They occur most commonly in patients who have experienced severe head injury and are unconscious. The complaint of headache therefore is not an important clinical sign.

2. Subacute subdural hematomas become clinically significant 2 to 14 days after injury.

They are usually found when a patient fails to recover as expected after a head injury. Headache may or may not be present but when it is, the manifestations are similar to those of chronic subdural hematoma described below. The major reason for making a distinction between these two groups is that the surgical therapy is different.

3. Chronic subdural hematomas become clinically significant more than 14 days after head injury. The antecedent injury is usually mild to moderate and in a significant number of cases, no history of injury can be elicited.

Headache is the commonest complaint in these patients and is usually more troublesome than the headache of brain tumor (Scheinberg and Scheinberg, 1964). If the headache is ignored, progressive signs of brain compression may ultimately ensue, but these may be nonspecific and nonlocalizing, e.g., apathy, inappropriate behavior, and confusion. Such symptoms may result in the patient's admission to a mental hospital.

The intracranial pressure may be normal in a patient with chronic subdural hematoma despite the fact that considerable shift of intracranial structures and papilledema is uncommon. The headache is presumed to be secondary to the stretching of tributary veins which pass from the cerebral hemispheres to the sagittal sinus. As the subdural collection gradually enlarges from recurrent bleeding or osmotic fluid shifts, the stretching of these veins becomes more marked and the headache more intense. It is not uncommon for these patients to note that sudden head movement or jolts accentuate the headache, and head tapping can be used as a clinical sign. One can visualize how a stretched vein could be easily stimulated by minor head movement.

4. Chronic subdural hematoma of the elderly should be recognized as a separate entity because it can be manifested as mental deterioration without headache. Brain atrophy may account for this as it permits a considerable subdural mass to be accommodated with only minimal shift or stretch of structure. In addition, these lesions are frequently bilateral so the potential for lateral displacement is counterbalanced.

5. Infantile subdural hematomas must be discussed separately because the expansivity of the infantile skull minimizes increases in intracranial pressure and the young child may not be able to complain of headache even if it occurs. (Till, 1968). Children with subdural hematomas are frequently restless and irritable, however, suggesting that head pain may be present.

INTRACEREBRAL HEMATOMA

Acute intracerebral hematoma may produce headache if blood leaks into the subarachnoid space or if sufficient brain distortion occurs before the patient loses consciousness to put traction on pain-sensitive structures. More commonly, headache is noted as the patient regains consciousness after an acute episode. This headache is usually dull and poorly localized but may become more severe due either to enlargement of the hematoma or localized brain edema.

SUMMARY

1. Brain tumor headache is produced by traction upon intracranial pain-sensitive structures, chiefly the large arteries, veins, venous sinuses, and certain cranial nerves. There are two types of traction which operate singly or in combination: local traction by the tumor mass upon adjacent structures; and distant traction by extensive displacement of the brain, either directly by the tumor or indirectly by ventricular obstruction (internal hydrocephalus).

2. The value of headache in the localization of brain tumor is limited by two facts: the headache may be remote from the site of its production, and the site of production of the headache may be remote from the tumor.

3. Despite these limitations, the headache of brain tumor may aid significantly in the localization of the lesion, especially when the headache is continuous. Thus, generally speaking, (a) in the absence of papilledema, when the headache is one-sided the side of the headache is usually the side of the tumor; (b) with tumor of the posterior fossa the headache is initially in the back of the head; (c) with tumor above the tentorium, in the absence of papilledema, the headache is usually in the front of the head; (d) when the headache is both frontal and occipital it is without localizing value.

4. Some patients with brain tumor have no headache whatsoever.

5. No headache pattern is absolutely characteristic of brain tumor.

6. Patients complaining of persistent headache after mild to moderate head injury should be evaluated for chronic subdural hematomas.

REFERENCES

Appenzeller, O. (1978). Headache and cerebrovascular disease. *Med. Clin. North Am.* 62, 467–479.

Brain, W. R. (1925). A clinical study of increased intracranial pressure in sixty cases of cerebral tumour. *Brain 48,* 105.

Cohen, H. (1939). Intracranial causes of headache. *Brit. Med. J.* 2, 713.

Cushing, H. (1931). Experiences with the cerebellar astrocytomas. *Surg. Gynec. Obstet.* 52, 129.

Cushing, H. (1917). *Tumors of the Nervous Acusticus,* p. 150. Saunders, Philadelphia.

Dandy, W. E. (1945). *Surgery of the Brain.* Prior, Hagerstown.

Fay, T. (1936). Mechanisms of headache. *Trans. Am. Neurol. Assoc.* 62, 74.

Fisher, C. M. (1968). Headache in cerebrovascular disease. In *Handbook of Clinical Neurology* (P. Vinken and G. Bruyn, eds.), Vol. 2, pp. 138–146. Amsterdam, North Holland.

Gibbs, F. A. (1932). Frequency with which tumors in various parts of the brain produce certain symptoms. *Arch. Neurol. Psychiat.* 28, 969.

Kunkle, E. C., B. S. Ray, and H. G. Wolff (1943). Experimental studies on headache: analysis of the headache associated with changes in intracranial pressure. *Arch. Neurol. Psychiat.* 49, 323.

Kunkle, E. C., B. S. Ray, and H. G. Wolff (1942). Studies on headache: the mechanisms and significance of headache associated with brain tumor. *Bull. New York Acad. Med. 18,* 400.

McNaughton, F. L. (1938). The innervation of the intracranial blood vessels and dural sinuses. *Assoc. Res. Nerv. Dis. Proc. (1937) 18,* 178.

Northfield, D. W. C. (1938). Some observations on headache. *Brain 61,* 133.

Penfield, W., and F. McNaughton (1940). Dural headache and innervation of the dura mater. *Arch. Neurol. Psychiat.* 44, 43.

Pickering, G. W. (1939). Experimental observations on headache. *Brit. Med. J.* 1, 4087.

Pollock, L. J. (1941). Head pains; differential diagnosis and treatment. *Med. Clin. North Am.* 25, 3.

Ray, B. S., and H. Parsons (1943). Subdural abscess

complicating frontal sinusitis. *Arch. Otolaryngol.*
37, 536.

Ray, B. S., and H. G. Wolff (1940). Experimental
studies on headache. Pain sensitive structures of
the head and their significance in headache. *Arch.
Surg. 41, 813.*

Scheinberg, S. C., and L. Scheinberg (1964). Early
description of chronic subdural hematoma: etiology, symptomatology, and treatment. *J.
Neurosurg. 21, 445.*

Schwarz, G. A., and A. A. ROSNER (1941). Displacement and herniation of the hippocampal tyrus

through the incisura temtorii. *Arch. Neurol. Psychiat.
46, 297.*

Till, K. (1968). Subdural hematoma and effusion in
infancy. *Brit. Med. J. 3, 400.*

Wagener, H. P., and P. L. Cusick (1937). Chiasmal
syndromes produced by lesions in the posterior
fossa. *Arch. Ophthal. 18, 887.*

Wolff, H. G., E. C. Kunkle, D. W. Lund, and P. J.
Maher (1947). Studies on headache: induced
mechanical stresses in the analysis of headache
mechanisms. *Trans. Am. Neurol. Assoc. 72, 93.*

14

HEADACHE ASSOCIATED WITH CHANGES IN INTRACRANIAL PRESSURE

REVISED BY JOHN F. ALKSNE

Although it is generally assumed that headache is a common sign of increased intracranial pressure, this is probably not the case unless the pressure is very high or is associated with shift of the intracranial contents. On the other hand, headache is one of the most troublesome symptoms of decreased intracranial pressure. This apparent paradox is best understood by recognizing that the cause of headache due to alterations in intracranial pressure is traction on pain-sensitive structures. These are primarily the vascular channels and meninges, which are only minimally distorted by elevated intracranial pressure without mass lesion or shift but are severely distorted when an individual with low intracranial pressure assumes the erect posture. A review of intracranial dynamics will assist the reader in appreciating this concept.

I. CEREBROSPINAL HYDRODYNAMICS

When the human subject is in a horizontal position the lumbar, cisternal, and presumably the intracranial (vertex) pressure are equal and approximately 50 to 180 mm of water. When the subject is erect these pressures diverge. Because the intraspinal dura is not a rigid tube, the lumbar dura distends and although the lumbar puncture pressure rises to between 375 and 550 mm, the top of the fluid in a recording manometer will be near or slightly below the level of the foramen magnum (Loman, *et al.,* 1935; Loman, 1934; Von Storch *et al.,* 1937).

The pressure above this level will be negative. The cisternal pressure of a person in the erect position may be as low as -85 mm water (Loman, 1934) and the intracranial pressure is -150 to -300 mm water (Fremont-Smith and Kubie, 1929). The depression noted over the open fontanel in infants who are placed in the erect position supports this contention.

Studies of venous pressure have shown that with postural shift, changes occur which parallel those in the cerebrospinal fluid. Weed and Hughson (1921) demonstrated that the intracranial cerebrospinal fluid pressure in animals is slightly greater than the venous pressure as measured in the sagittal sinus. In human beings, also, Myerson and Loman (1932) showed that with the subject in the horizontal position the lumbar pressure is slightly greater than the jugular pressure, and that with tilting of the body, head up, to an angle of 45 degrees the lumbar pressure rises to between 200 and 270 mm, whereas the jugular pressure falls to zero or lower; reverse changes occur when the patient is tilted head downward. Von Storch and co-workers (1937) correlated such changes in the venous and cerebrospinal fluid pressure, postulating that in the erect subject the rise in lumbar fluid pressure represents the transmission via distended intraspinal veins of the hydrostatic effect of the column of blood in the venous channels up to the level of the auricles. Since bilateral jugular compression led to as great an increment in lumbar pressure when the subject was erect as when he was horizontal, they asserted that the state of filling the intracranial veins is unaffected by the change in posture. Working with model systems and animals, Pollock and Boshes (1936) reached similar conclusions.

The essential relationship between the venous and the cerebrospinal fluid pressure within the cranium has been summarized by Weed and Flexner (1933) as follows.

The pressure equilibrium between cerebral veins and the cerebrospinal fluid [is] that of an elastic membrane separating two fluids which are normally under almost identical pressures but which can exist under very difficult pressures.

From these various data the following formulation seems tenable. In adjustments made to changes in posture, the cerebrospinal fluid pressure follows closely the venous pressure as measured at the same level in the intracraniospinal system. When the human subject is erect, both the venous and the cerebrospinal fluid pressure within the cranium fall to negative values, while the lumbar pressure rises. The height of the rise in lumbar pressure will depend on the height of the venous column above the lumbar sac; that is, on the height of the subject. The zero point lies usually a little above the auricles of the heart and below the cisterna magna. During postural changes the state of distention of intracranial veins is essentially unaltered, for the equilibrium between intravascular and extravascular pressure is maintained.

This balanced relation between the venous and the cerebrospinal fluid pressure in the cranium in spite of changes in position may be diagrammed, as in Fig. 14-1. For simplification, the slight excess of intracranial cerebrospinal fluid pressure over venous pressure is here waived.

A method by which intracranial pressure can be estimated is illustrated in simplified form by a model of the cerebrospinal fluid system (Fig. 14-2). Like its analogue in man, it represents a compromise between a completely closed and a completely open system. A rubber diaphragm, arbitrarily placed at the top, represents the distensible elements, venous and meningeal, in the human subject. In the typical

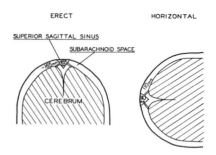

FIG. 14-1. Representative normal values for intracranial venous and cerebrospinal fluid pressures in man in the erect and in the horizontal position, illustrating that the balance between the intravascular and the extravascular pressure is probably little affected by change in position. The venous pressures are estimates derived from published measurements of sagittal sinus pressures in animals and jugular venous pressures in man.

situation shown in Fig. 14-2A, when the model was erect, the total height of the fluid column was 600 mm; yet the lumbar pressure was 440 mm. The point on the same horizontal level as the meniscus in the manometer, representing in man a point a little

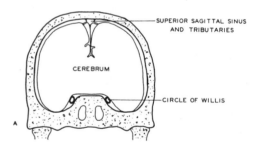

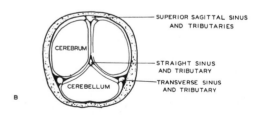

FIG. 14-2. Simplified model of the cerebrospinal fluid system, illustrating the method of calculation of intracranial pressure at the vertex in man. A, for the subject in the erect position; B, for the subject in the tilted position.

below the cisterna magna, must have a pressure of zero. This was confirmed in the model by opening the stopcock at S; there was then neither entrance of air nor escape of fluid. And, finally, the intracranial pressure at the vertex must be negative, and to a degree equal to its vertical height above the zero point, or—160 mm. The pressure at the vertex of the model by actual measurement was found to be identical with the calculated value. In short, in this model and in the human subject, the vertex pressure is equal to the lumbar pressure minus the distance from needle to vertex.

When the model was tilted, the vertical distance from needle to vertex was calculated in terms of the angle of tilt, which could readily be measured. It is clear from Fig. 14-2B that AB = AC × sin angle, and that therefore in the instance shown, with the lumbar pressure −AB, or 290 −600 sin 45 degrees, or −134mm. In the human subject similar deductions concerning vertex pressure should be possible provided the lumbar pressure, the angle of tilt, and the distance between the lumbar needle and the vertex are known.

Experiments have been performed in humans which indicate that lowering intracranial pressure to -200 to -300 mm water with the individual in the erect position invariably causes headache, whereas elevating intracranial pressure as high as 500 to 1000 mm H_2O does not produce headache (Schumacher and Wolff, 1941). The common realization that placing the head lower than the heart or coughing does not cause headache, although both maneuvers increase intracranial pressure, supports the conclusion that mild to moderate elevations of intracranial pressure are not symptomatic.

On the basis of the data thus far presented it is convenient to introduce at this point a hypothesis concerning the mechanism of the headache associated with removal of cerebrospinal fluid. The brain normally exerts traction on the structures that support it within the cranium, and this traction may under certain conditions be augmented enough to cause pain. The argument supporting this statement is as follows.

1.Within the dura mater the brain lies almost entirely surrounded by cerebrospinal fluid, being thus cushioned against sudden movement and protected from excessive sliding contact with the dura. It is not, however, supported entirely by the medium in which it is immersed, as comparison of the density of the solid and that of the liquid will indicate. Data concerning the density of the human brain are scanty, but Vierordt (1906) cited, from two separate sources, figures for the specific gravity as 1.039 and 1.040. In observations on a single specimen of material obtained 8 hr post mortem, with a modification of the Hammerschlag technique, the specific gravity of sections of cerebrum and cerebellum was 1.041 at room temperature. The specific gravity of cerebrospinal fluid, more readily obtained, is commonly given as 1.007 to 1.008 (Merritt and Fremont-Smith, 1938).

The weight of the normal adult brain varies within moderate limits, but averages 1300 gm (Appel and Appel, 1942). It may then be derived that a 1300-gm brain with a specific gravity of 1.040 immersed in fluid with specific gravity of 1.008 would have a net weight of 41 gm. The weight of the spinal cord, about 30 gm (Gray, 1930) with a specific gravity of 1.030 is relatively so small that it can be disregarded in these considerations. In the example cited here the extra 41 gm of brain weight must be supported within the cranium by something more than the buoyant effect of the cerebrospinal fluid. It is probable that this moderate weight is shared by suspension from the vault above and by support from structures at the base below. Suspension from above is probably largely through the cerebral veins tributary to the superior sagittal sinus, with a smaller contribution through the cerebellar veins tributary to the transverse and the straight sinuses. Supporting the brain from below, in addition to the floors of the anterior, middle, and posterior fossae, are the tentorium cerebelli and the large vascular structures at the base, chiefly the circle of Willis and its immediate branches. The relative contribution of each of these structures to the support of the brain is entirely conjectural. The relations of some of these structures and the direction of stress when the subject is seated in the erect position are outlined diagrammatically in Fig. 14-3.

2. These various anchoring vascular structures have been shown to be sensitive to pain

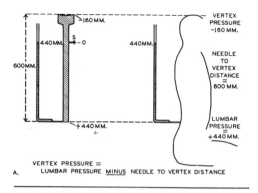

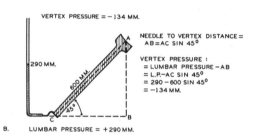

FIG. 14-3. Pain-sensitive structures sharing in the support of the brain within the cranium of the subject when in the erect position. A, coronal section through the head at the middle fossa, showing the venous tributaries to the superior sagittal sinus and the circle of Willis. The inferior sagittal sinus is omitted because its tributaries are so few. B, coronal section through the posterior third of the head, showing the veins tributary to the superior sagittal, straight, and transverse sinuses.

when, on operative exposure, they are stimulated by distortion or traction (Fay, 1937). Pain arising from structures on or above the superior surface of the tentorium cerebelli has been shown to be transmitted by the fifth cranial nerve and referred to the anterior half of the head. Pain arising from structures on or below the inferior surface of the tentorium cerebelli is transmitted chiefly by the ninth and tenth cranial nerves and the upper three cervical nerves and is referred to the posterior half of the head. Such observations indicate that the basic mechanisms of headache involve traction on these major intracranial vessels or on the cranial and upper cervical nerves which carry pain fibers as well as dilatation of intracranial

arteries or inflammation about any of these pain-sensitive structures of the head (see Chapter 3).

3. The mechanical adjustments that take place within the craniovertebral spaces of the erect human subject when cerebrospinal fluid is removed have never fully been analyzed. The problem indeed is not readily accessible to direct study. That some adjustments must occur can not be denied, and that they are complex is probable (Weed and Flexner, 1973).

One basic fact concerning the adjustment is that the lumbar and the intracranial cerebrospinal fluid pressure fall with removal of fluid. Since the intracraniospinal venous pressure is probably essentially unchanged by drainage of fluid, the intravascular and the extravascular pressures are then no longer in balance. Also, since veins are thin walled and, within moderate limits, passively adjust to the pressures within and about them, it may be inferred that dilatation of veins within the cranium and the spinal canal occurs. If the walls of the veins offered no resistance to distention, venous dilatation could completely compensate for a moderate loss of fluid and the intracranial pressure would remain unaltered, but because of their elasticity the compensation is incomplete. Accordingly, the intracranial cerebrospinal fluid pressure slowly falls when fluid is removed. Arterial size is much less dependent on extravascular support than is venous size, and whatever dilatation in the arteries may occur is largely active, rather than passive (Wolff, 1936).

Evidence that venous dilatation does occur after drainage of cerebrospinal fluid has been recorded by Forbes and Nason (1935).

Direct observations through cranial windows in cats revealed that after removal of fluid through the cisterna magna, the pial veins and venules dilated moderately, whereas the pial arteries did not. In addition, the bulk of the brain appeared to increase slightly, for its surface approached nearer the window. Confirmation of such venous dilatation and increased bulk came with the further observation by these authors that after the readjustment had occurred, the fluid removed could not be reinjected intrathecally without the pressure's being raised well above its initial level. The latter maneuver has been repeated on human subjects, with similar results (Masserman, 1934).

4. Another possible mechanical effect of the removal of cerebrospinal fluid from the subject in the erect position is that such a procedure may directly increase the degree of traction by the brain on the structures that suspend it from above and support it from beneath. There are no data or experimental methods to guide an exploration of this possibility. Yet it may be reasoned that the drainage of fluid from the lumbar sac and the consequent lowering of the intracranial pressure need have no direct effect on the support requirements of the brain. As fluid is removed and the venous bed dilates in partial compensation for the loss, the brain itself probably becomes slightly heavier. But since at the same time it increases in volume, the change in its density is minor, for the additional blood brought to the brain has a specific gravity of 1.060 (Hawk and Bergeim, 1935). Moreover, although the thickness of the layer of cerebrospinal fluid enveloping the brain may thus become less, the brain must still be virtually completely immersed in the fluid, for the brain case remains a closed box except for the distensible vascular bed. The increase in the "net" weight of the brain following drainage of fluid may thus be so slight as to be insignificant.

When air is introduced to replace lost cerebrospinal fluid, as in the pneumoencephalographic procedure, the situation pictured here is radically different. As fluid is progressively replaced by air, the buoyant support of the brain is diminished; its "net" weight increases from approximately 40 to 1300 gm, and traction on anchoring structures is augmented to such a degree that intense pain results. The severe headache that is induced during pneumoencephalographic examination may in part be explained on this basis (Brewer, 1937; Eisberg and Southerland, 1934). However, to repeat, no such series of circumstances follows simple drainage of cerebrospinal fluid.

This analysis indicates that the downward sag of the brain probably is not strikingly altered by drainage of moderate amounts of cerebrospinal fluid. Yet the presumptive increase in brain volume following drainage may itself effect increased traction on anchoring structures, and in a manner distinct from the downward sag of the brain due to gravity. Merely because of the expansion of the brain, the veins that course obliquely over the convexities to join the large sinuses may be subjected to an augmented "tug." Also, painful displacement of the vascular structures at the base may similarly result.

Hence, two potential factors in the production of drainage headache have become apparent in the preceding discussion (a) Granted that intracranial venous dilatation follows removal of cerebrospinal fluid, it may be inferred that such dilatation may cause pain, at least in those veins which in the erect subject are already under constant longitudinal traction by the brain mass. In other words, distention of an anchoring vein joined with lengthwise pull by the brain may distort the wall of the vein to such a degree that headache results. (b) The increase in brain volume secondary to extensive venous dilatation may conceivably produce such distortion of anchoring structures above and at the base that headache is produced.

Conclusion

It is suggested that a fall in intracranial pressure following the removal of cerebrospinal fluid in the erect human subject leads both to intracranial venous dilatation and to an increase in the usually mild and painless traction by the brain on its anchoring structures. With regard to the veins over the top of the cerebrum and cerebellum anchoring these to the superior sagittal, straight, and transverse sinuses, the two factors may act in combination. Drainage headache may thus be considered to be traction headache, with traction on dilated veins of primary importance.

An associated hypothesis must be that mild to moderate elevations of intracranial pressure do not cause distortion or traction of anchoring structures and therefore are not painful. In situations where these structures have increased sensitivity, however, such as meningitis or in which there are other causes of distortion such as mass lesion, headache does occur.

II. Headache Following Lumbar Puncture

The headache experimentally induced by drainage of cerebrospinal fluid has its clinical analogue in the headache that so frequently follows diagnostic lumbar puncture. The evidence for this linkage is of two types. First, the reports of many observers indicate that postpuncture headache is associated with loss of cerebrospinal fluid, and second, studies demonstrate the similarity of the responses of drainage and of postpuncture headache to certain experimental procedures.

Postpuncture headache may be defined as the headache, mild or severe, that may appear a few hours to several days after lumbar puncture, lasting a variable period of days or, rarely, weeks. It is a sequel to lumbar puncture in approximately one out of every four patients (Cooper, 1938; Perkel, 1925; Davenport, 1939; Kulchar and King, 1933). The pain is a dull, deep ache and may be throbbing. It is usually bifrontal and often also suboccipital. In the latter position it may be associated with moderate stiffness of the neck. Most characteristic are its occurrence when the subject is erect and its virtual elimination when he is horizontal. Shaking the head makes it more intense. Because of the frequency of its occurrence, the occasional severity of the discomfort, and the duration of the disability, headache of this type has been of clinical interest ever since the technique of lumbar puncture was introduced.

Although theories concerning postpuncture headache have been clearly contradictory, the weight of the evidence supports the view that it is usually related to a loss of cerebrospinal fluid secondary to leakage through the dural hole. The accumulated data may be summarized as follows.

1. Postpuncture headache is accompanied by lowered cerebrospinal fluid pressure. Without citing actual data, several observers (Targowla and Lamache, 1928; Merritt and Fremont-Smith, 1938; Solomon, 1929) have reported that in patients with postpuncture headache on whom a second puncture was done the lumbar pressure had fallen from its initial level. The studies of postpuncture headache by Nelson and Jacobeus and Frumerie present pressure data in detail (Nelson, 1930; Jacobeus and Frumerie, 1923). In each of several patients with postpuncture headache the pressure observed on a second tap was low. One of the group reported on by Jacobeus and Frumerie, a patient with severe headache, stiff neck, pallor, and bradycardia, had a lumber pressure of zero. Injection of 90 cc of physiologic solution of sodium chloride raised the lumbar pressure to 250 mm and caused immediate clinical improvement, which was maintained by elevation of the foot of the bed. Similar results were obtained with a second patient.

Manometric studies on a group of 16 patients with postpuncture headache were made by Pacifico (1934). The interpretation of the results is complicated by the fact that at least three of the patients had very high pressures on the initial tap, and eight of the remaining 13 patients had an unexplained elevation to 210 mm or above (in the horizontal position). In all but two of the group a second puncture 24 to 96 hr later, and after headache had begun, demonstrated that the pressure, measured in both the erect and the horizontal position, had fallen from the initial levels.

2. The dural hole at the site of lumbar puncture may persist for several days after the procedure. At laminectomy Mixter noted the presence of a dural hole six days after lumbar puncture, and Castro Silva confirmed this in observations made eight to 15 days after puncture (Mixter, 1932; Castro Silva, 1930).

3. Leakage of cerebrospinal fluid through the dural hole into the epidural space may occur. Such leakage, first suggested by Sicard as a factor in postpuncture headache, was observed by Pool (1942) in myeloscopic studies performed two to four days after lumbar puncture, as well as by Ingvar (1923) in the dissection of cadavers. The latter noted in one patient the presence of subcutaneous fluid following lumbar puncture. Moreover, in histologic studies of the repair reaction following

dural puncture, he observed that the plug which forms over the hole appears fragile and insecurely fixed.

4. Measures that diminish the likelihood of leakage have been claimed to be effective in reducing the frequency and severity of postpuncture headache. Cisternal rather than lumbar tap, the use of a small needle, the insertion of catgut in the dural hole, and the introduction of air into the epidural space to eliminate the hypothetical epidural negative pressure have all been said to be useful devices in the control of postpuncture headache (Nelson, 1930; Kulchar, 1940; Greene, 1926; Heldt and Mohoney, 1928). None of these techniques, however, is entirely effective. The value of the use of catgut has been shown to be slight (Heldt and Whitehead, 1936).

5. Temporary decrease in the intensity of postpuncture headache may result from procedures that increase the volume of cerebrospinal fluid. The intravenous administration of hypotonic solutions (of sodium chloride or distilled water) has been found by several observers to diminish postpuncture headache (Solomon, 1924; Alpers, 1925; Perkel, 1925). Conversely, it has been reported that a hypertonic solution of dextrose given intravenously augments the headache (Masserman, 1936).

Without exception, the various procedures adopted in the analysis of postpuncture headache have emphasized its similarity to the headache induced by drainage of cerebrospinal fluid. The two types of headache share the following features: (1) association with decreased intracranial pressure; (2) complete elimination by elevation of the intracranial pressure to normal when the subject is erect; (3) reduction in intensity by change in the subject's position from erect to horizontal or by tilting of the head; and (4) increase in intensity by bilateral jugular compression. Accordingly, the same headache mechanism may apply both to drainage and to postpuncture headache.

Unlike drainage headache, postpuncture headache may not have its onset until a few hours or days after the lumbar tap. The drainage of the small volume, 5 to 15 cc of fluid ordinarily removed for diagnostic tests is usu-ally insufficient to cause an immediate headache. The delayed headache presumably is due to the continued slow loss of cerebrospinal fluid after the initial removal of fluid. This type of headache may properly be termed "leakage" headache. Reflex inhibition of choroidal secretion following penetration of the dura has been suggested as the cause of the decreased volume and pressure of cerebrospinal fluid accompanying postpuncture headache (Targowla and Lamache, 1928), but this hypothesis lacks both experimental and clinical support.

It is relevant to note at this point that closure of the dural-arachnoid puncture hole may be aided by inflammatory changes in the meninges and an increase in the cell and the protein content of the spinal fluid such as may be associated with disease of the central nervous system. This may explain the fact noted by several authors, notably Perkel (1925), that in patients with a pathologic fluid, headache is less likely to develop after lumbar puncture than in those with a normal fluid. On the other hand, the difference between the two groups may reflect only that patients with normal fluids, as a group being less "ill," may attempt to resume activity sooner after the puncture.

Clinical Applications

It follows from the discussion above that, when and as long as the total spinal fluid is less than 90% of its usual amount, headache will occur when the subject is in the upright position. To prevent such losses, several methods exist. Taking spinal fluid from the cisterna magna by subarachnoid puncture avoids headache due to drainage because the pressure in the cisterna magna when the subject is in the upright position is negative or near zero. Therefore, no fluid runs out of the puncture hole. Unfortunately, most patients find this procedure distasteful and most physicians are not skilled in its performance.

Lumbar puncture must be considered the most practical procedure. The matter reduces itself to the following: (1) the hole should be as small as possible (i.e., small-bore needles produce smaller holes than large-bore needles; but manometric studies are difficult when the bore is too small; thus one evil must be balanced against the other); (2) the subject should remain completely immobile during the procedure so as not to enlarge the initially small hole (O'Connell, 1946); (3) there should be only one hole rather than several.

According to Noon (1949) the incidence of headache following spinal puncture has been reported variously as less than 1% and more than 56%. The author analyzed data from 1658 spinal punctures: 1158 for diagnostic purposes and 500 to induce spinal anesthesia. He found that previous administration of 180 mg of sodium 5-allyl-5(1-methylbutyl) barbiturate (seconal sodium) did not result in the lowering of the incidence of headache in those who were active soon after puncture or in those who were kept recumbent for 24 hrs. There was an overall incidence of postpuncture headache of 29% in 1658 patients. In only 7% of 500 cases of spinal puncture done for inducing spinal anesthesia did headache occur.

Sciarra and Carter (1952) studied the effects of lumbar puncture on 102 patients from whom cerebrospinal fluid was removed. Headache occurred in 46% of 62 patients who had cerebrospinal fluid removed. In the 40 patients in whom the dura was pierced but from whom no cerebrospinal fluid was collected in a test tube the incidence of headache was comparable (38%). It was concluded that 10 to 12 cc of fluid was the optimal amount to remove, since this did not increase the incidence of headache, as compared with the group who had no fluid removed. It is not clear how much cerebrospinal fluid was lost in the tissue.

It has been suggested by Brocker (1958) that the incidence of post-lumbar puncture headache can be appreciably reduced if in addition to the use of a smaller needle (No. 18) the patient then be placed on his abdomen for three hours. Headache under these circumstances occurred in 4 out of 894 patients tapped, an incidence of less than 0.5 per cent. In contrast were the results of 200 patients who, following lumbar puncture, were placed in the supine position. Under these circumstances, the incidence of headache was 36.5%. The difference, it was assumed, had to do with factors that reduced the loss of spinal fluid.

Gilland has made several suggestions regarding the headache associated with lumbar puncture (1969). He advises that, before the lumbar puncture needle be removed, a leather belt be tightened about the patient's waist until the cerebral spinal fluid pressure rises to approximately 200 mm of water. The patient is thereafter advised to rest prone for 30 min and supine for a further 30 min and then he is allowed to walk around, still wearing the belt. If the headache recurs, the patient is told to lie down again for 30 min, tightening the belt as much as possible. If no headache occurs, the belt is taken off on the morning following the lumbar puncture. Of 27 patients investigated with this procedure, only four had postpuncture headache. In three of these it was relieved by tightening the abdominal belt. In the fourth, a recumbent position had to be maintained until the second day when belt-tightening was effective in alleviating it. Gilland suggests that increased abdominal pressure, by raising the venous pressure, reverses the gradient for cerebral spinal flow and facilitates the repair of the meningeal puncture.

Aziz et al. have investigated the value of vasopressin in the prevention of lumbar puncture headache (1968). A series of 50 consecutive unselected patients who required lumbar puncture for diagnostic purposes was divided at random into two groups. Immediately after lumbar puncture, the patients received an intramuscular injection of either 20 units of aqueous vasopressin or isotonic saline. This injection was repeated at 12-hr intervals for 48 hr. The reaction to the lumbar puncture was assessed at 24 and 48 hr. No significant difference was found between the two groups in the number of patients unaffected by the lumbar puncture. Those treated with vasopressin tended to have less severe headaches, though statistically this did not reach significant levels. Side effects of varying severity occurred more often after vasopressin injection than after placebo.

Similar to drainage or postpuncture headache is that which follows the introduction of spinal anesthetics into the subarachnoid space. Although a number of procedures to prevent headache have been suggested, none seems to be entirely satisfactory. It is doubtful whether 24 hr of bed rest prevents headache (Levin, 1944) or allows for much healing or closure of the holes.

Treatment of Intractable Post-lumbar Puncture Headache

Despite all possible precautions some intractable postpuncture headaches do occur. These are most common after spinal puncture with a large needle or after inadvertent dural puncture during epidural catheter insertion. Craft *et al.* (1973) have suggested that in situations where a high incidence of postpuncture headache can be anticipated the prophylactic injection of 60 cc of saline into the epidural space should be considered. They report a reduction in postpuncture headache from 76 to 12% by this procedure in a series of 33 patients who had recognized inadvertent dural puncture during epidural anesthesia.

Severe, intractable postpuncture headaches have also been treated by a second puncture with saline injection (Rice and Dobbs, 1950), but recently the use of the "blood patch" has been more popular. The epidural injection of the patient's own blood at a site of previous spinal puncture was first advicated by Gormley (1960), and 45 cases have been reported by Di Giovanni and Dunbar (1970). In this procedure a spinal needle is reinserted at the same level as the previous lumbar puncture with care being taken to remain in the epidural space. Ten cc of the patient's nonheparinized venous blood is then injected slowly and the needle withdrawn. The authors report immediate relief of postural headache in 41 of their 45 cases. Walpole (1975) reported one case that required a second "blood patch" three days after the first, again with a good result. Although this procedure appears effective, it should probably be reserved for those patients who have failed to respond to more conventional methods.

OTHER CAUSES OF LOW CSF PRESSURE HEADACHE

Headache may accompany any condition that decreases intracranial pressure such as CSF rhinorrhea or inappropriately functioning ventricular shunt. In the former there is usually a history of head injury and in the latter, of course, a history of shunt insertion. In both instances, as one would expect, the headache is aggravated by standing upright or by rapid head movements and relieved by lying down. The appropriate therapy is correction of the offending lesion.

III. HEADACHE WITH CHRONIC OR MARKED ELEVATIONS OF INTRACRANIAL PRESSURE

Although it has been stated that headache does not occur with mild to moderate elevations of intracranial pressure because there is no associated traction or distortions of pain-sensitive structures, in at least two conditions this is not the case—acute hydrocephalus and benign intracranial hypertension. The mechanisms underlying the cause of head pain are not understood but we must assume that because of the severity or duration of the pressure change, shift of structures does occur which is sufficient to put traction on pain-sensitive areas.

Acute Hydrocephalus

The acute increase in intracranial pressure which occurs with ventricular obstruction or shunt malfunction in a treated hydrocephalic usually causes severe headache followed by visual disturbances. Because vascular perfusion of the brain is reduced as intracranial pressure approaches mean systemic arterial pressure, permanent neurologic deficit or death can result if emergency ventricular drainage is not instituted. Lumbar puncture is contraindicated if this situation is suspected, since papilledema may not always be present.

III. Benign Intracranial Hypertension

The term *benign intracranial hypertension* (B.I.H.) refers to a syndrome of increased intracranial pressure for which no specific cause can be determined. The diagnosis should not and cannot be made without excluding brain tumors or other intracranial mass lesions, infections, hypertensive encephalopathy, pulmonary encephalopathy (related to chronic CO_2 toxicity), and obstruction of the cerebral ventricles from whatever cause. The adjective "benign" is employed since spontaneous recovery usually occurs, though this is not invariable, and indeed, permanent visual loss may occur. Etiologic factors which may be associated with benign intracranial hypertension include, in addition to intracranial venous occlusion, menstrual dysfunction, deficiency of the adrenals, corticosteroid therapy, hypoparathyroidism, Vitamin A intoxication, and administration of tetracycline in infants.

Quincke (1893) was the first to describe cases of this syndrome and he supplied the name "serous meningitis." Nonne (1907) introduced the term "pseudotumor cerebri," at which time other writers were referring to the condition appropriately as "die Nonnesche Krankheit." The condition was designated by Symonds (1937) as "otitic hydrocephalus," by Dandy (1937) merely as "increased intracranial pressure without brain tumor," and by Foley (1955) by the reassuring term "benign intracranial hypertension."

Papilledema (sometimes with retinal hemorrhages) which reflects the increased intracranial pressure is the one finding common to all cases. Generalized headache, giddiness, and vomiting occur in the majority, but these symptoms are usually of mild degree. The headache is generalized, nonthrobbing, or low intensity, and is usually increased on suddenly jolting or rotating the head. Some degree of blurring of vision develops with persistence of papilledema, and occasionally visual acuity is significantly diminished; but blindness is rare.

Perimetry discloses only enlargement of blind spots and minimal restriction of peripheral vision. Diplopia as a result of abducens nerve palsy secondary to increased intracranial pressure sometimes occurs. Convulsions are rare. The patient's feeling and appearance of well-being are striking. They are out of keeping with the papilledema and increased intracranial pressure, and in contrast to what is so commonly observed in patients with papilledema due to brain neoplasm or subdural hematoma.

The term "otitic hydrocephalus" arose because of the frequent association of the syndrome with some infectious process of the ear, although "hydrocephalus" is a misnomer. Accumulated evidence has indicated that increased intracranial pressure in conjunction with ear infections results from thrombosis of the dural venous sinuses (transverse or superior sagittal sinus). Thrombosis or phlebitis of these sinuses has also been implicated in the presence of systemic infections, or in conjunction with phlebothrombosis or thrombophlebitis elsewhere in the body. Ray and Dunbar (1950, 1951) made a systematized attempt by sinusography to investigate the possibility that, in all cases having the syndrome of pseudotumor (Davidoff, 1956), there was a thrombosis of major venous sinuses. Later they reported (Ray *et al.*, 1955) that obstruction of venous channels could be demonstrated in less than half the patients studied. Thus, the cause of the increased intracranial pressure in half or more of such patients is still unknown. Among the latter, the incidence is greater in women than in men, in a ratio of 2 to 1, in the middle decades of life.

In the syndrome of pseudotumor (Davidoff, 1956), the resting spinal pressures-vary from 220 to 600 mm of water. The fluid is always clear, colorless, and without any abnormality of cellular or chemical constituents. Indeed, the protein content of the cerebrospinal fluid may be unusually low.

The electroencephalogram is usually normal. Occasionally diffuse slowing with high-amplitude waves has been reported. In pneumoencephalography the ventricles may appear narrowed, with little air in the cortical

subarachnoid spaces. Computerized axial tomography shows similar findings.

SUMMARY

1. Headache can be regularly induced in
normal, erect human subjects by the free
drainage of approximately 20 cc of cerebrospinal fluid, the estimated vertex pressure falling to between -220 and -290 mm from a
normal of approximately -150 mm. Moreover,
(1) drainage headache is reduced in intensity
by the intrathecal injection of physiologic solution of sodium chloride and the restoration of
the cerebrospinal fluid volume; (2) drainage
headache is reduced in intensity by tilting the
body toward the horizontal.

2. It is inferred that drainage headache is
caused primarily by traction by the brain on
various pain-sensitive structures which anchor
it to the cranium; dilatation of some of these
structures, particularly the intracranial veins,
and increase in brain volume are suggested as
joint factors in the augmented traction which
follows drainage of fluid and leads to
headache.

3. The headache that often follows lumbar
puncture has predictable and unique features,
all of which indicate its similarity to drainage
headache. Like drainage headache (1) postpuncture headache is associated with a decrease in cerebrospinal fluid volume, as evidenced by a fall in cerebrospinal fluid pressure; (2) it is completely eliminated by the
intrathecal injection of saline solution and by
the elevation of the intracranial pressure to
normal; (3) its intensity is reduced by change
from the erect to the horizontal position.

4. Elevation of intracranial pressure in
healthy human subjects to abnormally high
levels fails to cause headache.

5. For unexplained reasons, such marked or
chronic elevations of intracranial pressure as
may occur in acute hydrocephalus or essential
intracranial hypertension can cause headache.

REFERENCES

Alpers, B. J. (1925). Lumbar puncture headache.
   Arch. Neurol. Psychiat. 14, 806.

Appel, F. W., and E. M. Appel (1942). Intracranial
   variation in the weight of the human brain. *Hum.
   Biol. 14*, 48.

Aziz, H., J. Pearce, and E. Miller (1968). Vasopressin
   in the prevention of lumbar puncture headache.
   Brit. Med. J. 4, 677.

Brewer, E. D. (1937). Etiology of headache, occurrence and significance of headache during ventriculography. *Bull. Neurol. Inst. N. Y. 6*, 12.

Brocker, R. J. (1958). Technique to avoid spinal-tap
   headache. *JAMA 168*, 261.

Castro, Silva, cited by H. Koster and M. Weintrob
   (1930). Complications of spinal anesthesia. *Am. J.
   Surg. 8*, 1165.

Cooper, M. J. (1938). Clinical observations on effects
   of choline compounds in neurologic disorders,
   with special reference to Ménière's syndrome. *Am.
   J. Med. Sci. 95*, 83.

Craft, J. B., B. S. Epstein, and C. S. Coakley (1973).
   Prophylaxis of dural-puncture headache with
   epidural saline. *Anesth. Analg. 52*, 228-231.

Dandy, W. E. (1937). Intracranial pressure without
   brain tumor: diagnosis and treatment. *Ann. Surg.
   106*, 492.

Davenport, K. M. (1939). Post-puncture reactions.
   N. Y. State J. Med. 39, 1185.

Davidoff, L. M. (1956). Pseudotumor cerebri; benign intracranial hypertension. *Neurology 6*, 605.

Di Giovanni, A. J., and B. S. Dunbar (1970). Epidural
   injections of autologous blood for post-lumbar
   puncture headache. *Anesth. Analg. 49*, 268-271.

Elsberg, C. A., and R. W. Southerland (1934).
   Headache produced by injection of air for encephalography. *Bull. Neurol. Inst. N. Y. 3*, 519.

Fay, T. (1937). Mechanism of headache. *Arch.
   Neurol. Psychiat. 37*, 471.

Foley, J. (1955). Benign forms of intracranial hypertension: "toxic" and "otoxic". *Brain 78*, 1.

Forbes, H. S., and G. I. Nason (1935). The cerebral
   circulation: vascular responses to (A) hypertonic
   solutions and (B) withdrawal of cerebrospinal
   fluid. *Arch. Neurol. Psychiat. 34*, 533.

Fremont-Smith, F., and L. S. Kubie (1929). Relation
   of vascular hydrostatic pressure and osmotic pressure to the cerebrospinal fluid pressure. *Assoc. Res.
   Nerv. Dis. Proc. (1927) 8*, 104.

Gilland, O. (1969). How to take the headache out of
   spinal taps. *Headache 8*, 154.

Gormley, J. B. (1960). Treatment of post-spinal
   headache. *Anesthesiology 21*, 565–566.

Gray, H. (1930). *Anatomy of the Human Body*, 22nd
   ed., p. 749. Lea & Febiger, Philadelphia.

Greene, H. M. (1926). Lumbar puncture and prevention of post-puncture headache. *JAMA 86*,
   391.

Hawk, P. B., and O. Bergeim (1931). *Practical
   Physiological Chemistry*, 10th ed., p. 374. P. Blakis-
   ton's Son & Company, Philadelphia.

Heldt, T. J., and J. C. Mohoney (1928). Negative
   pressure in epidural space. *Am. J. Med. Sci. 175*,
   371.

Heldt, T. J., and L. S. Whitehead (1936). Clinical studies in postlumbar puncture headache. *Am. J. Psychiat.* 93, 639.

Ingvar, S. (1923). On the danger of leakage of cerebrospinal fluid after lumbar puncture. *Acta. Med. Scand.* 58, 67.

Jacobeus, H. C., and K. Frumerie (1923). About the leakage of spinal fluid after lumbar puncture and its treatment. *Acta Med. Scand.* 58, 102.

Kulchar, G. V. (1940). Cisternal puncture: a survey of reactions following one thousand two hundred and forty-six punctures. *Am. J. Syph.* 24, 643.

Kulchar, G. V., and A. D. King (1933). Use of sodium amytal in prevention of reactions associated with lumbar puncture. *Arch. Neurol. Psychiat.* 30, 170.

Levin, M. J. (1944). Lumbar puncture headache. *Bull. U. S. Army Med. Dep.* 82, 107.

Loman, J. (1934). Components of cerebrospinal fluid pressure as affected by changes in posture. *Arch. Neurol. Psychiat.* 31, 679.

Loman, J., A. Myerson, and D. Goldman (1935). Effects of alterations in posture on cerebrospinal fluid pressure. *Arch. Neurol. Psychiat.* 33, 1279.

McNaughton, F. L. Personal communication to the author.

Masserman, J. H. (1936). Cerebrospinal dynamics, effects of intravenous injection of hypertonic solutions of dextrose. *Arch. Neurol. Psychiat.* 35, 296.

Masserman, J. H. (1934). Cerebrospinal hydrodynamics: clinical experimental studies. *Arch. Neurol. Psychiat.* 32, 523.

Masserman, J. H., W. F. Schaller (1933). Intracranial hydrodynamics: influence of rapid decompression of ventriculosubarachnoid spaces on occurrence of edema of brain. *Arch. Neurol. Psychiat.* 30, 107.

Merritt, H. H., and F. Fremont-Smith (1938). *The Cerebrospinal Fluid*, pp. 224-226. Saunders, Philadelphia.

Mixter, W. J., in discussion on F. Fremont-Smith, H. H. Merritt, and W. G. Lennox (1932). Relationship between water balance, spinal fluid pressure and epileptic convulsions. *Arch. Neurol. Psychiat.* 28, 956.

Myerson, A., and J. Loman (1932). Internal jugular venous pressure in man. *Arch. Neurol. Psychiat.* 27, 836.

Nelson, M. O. (1930). Post-puncture headaches: clinical and experimental study of cause and prevention. *Arch. Derm. Syph.* 21, 615.

Nonne, M. (1907). Über Fälle von benignen Hirnhauttumoren; über atypisch verlaufene Fälle von Hirnabszess sowie weitere klinsche und anatomische Beiträge zur Frage vom "Pseudomotor cerebri." *Dtsch. Z. Nervenheilk 33*, 317.

Noon, Z. B. (1949). Postspinal puncture headache. *Ariz. Med.* 6, 19.

O'Connell, J. E. A. (1946). The clinical signs of meningeal irritation. *Brain* 69, 9.

Pacifico, A. (1934). Sui disturba da punctura lombare. *Riv. Pat. Nerv. Ment.* 43, 1215.

Perkel, J. D. (1925). Des accidents secondaires qui suivent la ponction lombaire. *Presse Med.* 33, 1320.

Pollock, L. J., and B. Boshes (1936). Cerebrospinal fluid pressure. *Arch. Neurol. Psychiat.* 36, 931.

Pool, J. L. (1942). Myeloscopy. *Surgery* 11, 169.

Quincke, H. (1893). Ueber Meningitis serosa. *Samml. Klin. Vortr. Leipzig 67*, 665.

Ray, B. S. *et al.* (1955). Unpublished observations.

Ray, B. S., and H. S. Dunbar (1951). Thrombosis of the dural venous sinuses as a cause of "pseudotumor cerebri." *Ann. Surg.* 134, 376.

Ray, B. S., and H. S. Dunbar (1950). Thrombosis of the superior sagittal sinus as a cause of pseudotumor cerebri: methods of diagnosis and treatment. *Trans. Am. Neurol. Assoc.* 75, 12.

Ray, B. S., and H. G. Wolff (1940). Experimental studies on headache. Pain sensitive structures of the head and their significance in headache. *Arch. Surg.* 41, 813.

Rice, G. G., and H. C. Dobbs (1950). The use of peridural and subarachnoid injection of saline solution in the treatment of severe post spinal headaches. *Anesthesiology* 11, 17–23.

Schumacher, G. A., and H. G. Wolff (1941). Experimental studies on headache: contrast of histamine headache with headache of migraine and that associated with hypertension. *Arch. Neurol. Psychiat.* 45, 199.

Sciarra, D., and S. Carter (1952). Lumbar puncture headache. *JAMA 148*, 841.

Solomon, H. C. (1929). Effect on human cerebrospinal fluid pressure of extraction and injection of fluid. *Assoc. Res. Nerv. Dis. Proc. (1927) 8*, 82.

Solomon, H. C. (1924). Raising cerebrospinal fluid pressure with especial regard to effect on lumbar puncture headache. *JAMA 82*, 1512.

Symonds, C. P. (1937). Hydrocephalic and focal cerebral symptoms in relation to thrombophlebitis of the dural sinuses and cerebral veins. *Brain 60*, 531.

Targowla, R., and A. Lamache (1928). Les accidents d'intolerance a la ponction lombaire. *Presse Med 36*, 1111.

Vierordt, H. (1906). *Anatomische Physiologische und Physikalische Daten und Tabellan*, pp. 59 and 449, Gustav Fischer, Jena.

Von Storch, T. J. C., E. A. Carmichael, and T. E. Banks (1937). Factors producing lumbar cerebrospinal fluid pressure in man in the erect posture. *Arch. Neurol. Psychiat.* 38, 1158.

Von Storch, T. J. C., L. Secunda, and C. M. Krinsky (1940). Production and localization of headache with subarachnoid and ventricular air. *Arch. Neurol. Psychiat.* 43, 326.

Walpole, J. B. (1975). Blood patch for spinal headache. *Anesthesia 30*, 783–785.

Weed, L. H., and L. B. Flexner (1933). Relations of the intracranial pressures. *Am. J. Physiol.* 105, 266.

Weed, L. H., and W. Hughson (1921). Intracranial venous pressure and cerebrospinal fluid pressure as affected by intravenous injection of solutions of various concentrations. *Am. J. Physiol. 58*, 101.

Wolff, H. G. (1936). The cerebral circulation. *Physiol. Rev. 16*, 545.

Wolff, H. G., E. C. Kunkle, D. W. Lund, and P. J. Maher (1947). Studies on headache: induced mechanical stresses in the analysis of headache mechanisms. *Trans. Am. Neurol. Assoc. 72*, 93.

15

THE SURGICAL TREATMENT OF HEAD AND NECK PAIN

RONALD J. IGNELZI

The surgical management of head and neck pain has changed appreciably in the last several years. Introduction of the radiofrequency thermocoagulation techniques to the treatment of trigeminal neuralgia as well as other cranial neuralgias, the even more recent development of the microsurgical approach to vascular compression of the trigeminal nerve at the pons, and finally techniques of central neurostimulation have revolutionized our concepts of the diseases as well as their surgical management. At the same time there has been an increasing awareness of the futility of surgical therapy for migraine, other vascular headaches, and atypical facial pains.

TRIGEMINAL NEURALGIA

Trigeminal neuralgia with its excruciating and incapacitating pain has led its sufferers and those treating them to attempt many manipulations of the trigeminal system in order to achieve relief. Early approaches such as injection of local anesthetics or alcohol into the peripheral divisions of the trigeminal nerve or ganglion (Stookey and Ransohoff, 1959) have given way to more refined methods of localization using specific roentgenographic guidance for localization (Perl and Ecker, 1959). The classic temporal approach with retrogasserian rhizotomy as developed by Spiller and Frazier (1901) provided the most successful and prolonged pain relief of the open ablative procedures, but carried with it the annoying numbness, paresthesias, and occasional anesthesia dolorosa produced by denervation. Other pro-cedures that have enjoyed short-lived prominence but still have their advocates are neurectomy and/or avulsion of peripheral branches of the trigeminal nerve (Horrax and Poppen, 1935; Henderson, 1965). The decompression and compression operations developed by Taarnhoj (1952, 1954) and Pudenz and Shelden (1952) had the attraction of simplicity and lack of postoperative anesthesia, but rather early and progressive rates of recurrence dampened the enthusiasm for these approaches (White and Sweet, 1969). Posterior fossa rhizotomy as pioneered by Dandy (1925, 1929, 1932, 1945), and quite successful in his hands, had the theoretical advantage of being able to selectively section the pain fibers of the trigeminal nerve at the brainstem where they are often separated from the main root carrying other modalities of sensation. However, the procedure did not prove applicable for technical reasons for most neurosurgeons after Dandy, and therefore the popularity was short-lived. Medullary tractotomy (Sjoqvist, 1938, 1948) again had the theoretical advantage of being able to produce a differential loss of pain perception. It carried a high complication rate and required rather sophisticated technical apparatus, so that it too never gained wide use.

Radiofrequency Thermocoagulation

In 1970 Sweet and Wepsic described their method for treatment of trigeminal neuralgia with radiofrequency lesions using the percutaneous approach to the gasserian ganglion.

European investigators had pioneered various electrocoagulation methods to the gasserian ganglion previously (Kirschner, 1942), but Sweet and Wepsic introduced the concept in this country and refined the technique using a radiofrequency generator to produce a controlled thermocoagulation allowing differential destruction of rootlets and pain fibers with relative preservation of touch sensation. The rationale behind the controlled thermocoagulation was based on experimental work that showed that the small c and A delta pain fibers were more sensitive to heat than the larger myelinated A beta fibers concerned with touch and proprioception (Bessou and Perl, 1969; Letcher and Goldring, 1968). In 1974 Wepsic and Sweet presented a series of 274 patients treated by this method for facial pain, 214 of whom had trigeminal neuralgia (Sweet and Wepsic, 1974). Of those patients with trigeminal neuralgia, 91% experienced pain relief initially. At 2½ to 6 years' follow-up, the recurrence rate was 22%, and the longer the patients were followed, the more likely a recurrence. The great advantage of the Sweet-Wepsic procedure from a surgical standpoint is that there was no mortality or neurological morbidity outside of the trigeminal nerve. Only six of their patients complained of postoperative paresthesias. However, in 28 patients, an anesthetic cornea was produced, leading to loss of eyesight in one patient due to corneal scarring. Later, Nugent (Nugent and Berry, 1974), refining the technique somewhat, reported on the ability to preserve touch but eliminate pain in eight of ten patients when the first division was involved in the tic. Today, surgeons experienced in the percutaneous radiofrequency coagulation techniques achieve good results with long-lasting relief in most patients (Thiry, 1962). And, in those patients whose symptoms recur, a repeat procedure can be performed with little increase in technical difficulty or operative morbidity.

Vascular Decompression

Jannetta's microsurgical approach to the trigeminal nerve has added new dimensions to our understanding of the pathogenesis of trigeminal neuralgia and has provided effective treatment for many sufferers. His introduction of the operating microscope for exploration of the root entry zone of the trigeminal nerve at the brainstem provided evidence that vascular compression-distortion of the nerve root entry zone could be the cause of trigeminal neuralgia. In a report of his operative findings in 100 consecutive patients with tic douloureux (Jannetta, 1976), he stated that 88% of the patients had some microvascular abnormality to explain the disorder in the trigeminal system. Another 6% had tumors or arteriovenous malformations to explain the cause of the pain, and another 6% had multiple sclerosis.

The concept that the etiology of trigeminal neuralgia might be related to vascular compression was synthesized by Jannetta but suggested by others earlier. The correlation of elongation of intracranial arteries with arterial sclerotic cerebral vascular disease was suggested by Lewy and Grant (1938), and they postulated that the development of the symptom in most patients paralleled the timing of the development of arteriosclerosis. However, they believed that the abnormality existed within the brain itself. Dandy noted several times that there was compression-distortion of the root entry zone of the trigeminal nerve in many patients with tic. He noted abnormalities in over 40% of his patients, and questionable abnormalities in another 18% (Dandy, 1934). Dandy reported finding an artery compressing the root in 30.7% of his cases and in another 14% found that a branch of the petrosal vein crossed the sensory root or passed directly through it. What is remarkable is that Dandy did this without the use of an operative microscope. With the development of the microsurgical approach to the root entry zone, Jannetta was able to appreciate an abnormality in virtually all patients operated upon. In a series of 60 consecutive patients (Jannetta, 1977a) he found that lower facial tic (V_2, V_3, $V_{2,3}$) was usually correlated with nerve root compression from an anterocephalad direction in 46 patients. Upper facial tic (V_1, $V_{1,2}$) was associated with compression from the caudal-lateral direction in eight patients. He found that the most frequent cause of trigeminal nerve root compression was a looping of the superior cerebellar artery (40 patients). The anterior-inferior cerebellar artery was the cause in four. A vein was incriminated in four patients. Seven patients had some vascular abnormality in combination with another anatomic variant such as a tight arachnoid. In the remaining series of five patients, tumors were found as a cause of the pain—three meningiomas and two acoustic neuromas.

Jannetta believes that the tendency to progression and frequency in the severity of the episodes may correlate with progressive elongation of the vascular loop. Waning of pain is the symptom to be explained by neural accommodation, and electron microscopy has shown simultaneous denervation and re-enervation such that short circuits may be obliterated only for others to reform (Beaver *et al.*, 1965). It appeared to Jannetta that the electron microscopy studies explained abnormal transmission of the trigeminal nerve in patients with tic douloureux. Treatment with some antiepileptic drugs does help some patients with tic douloureux. These are drugs which cut down neurotransmission—normal or abnormal. He believes that in occasional familial cases there must be some predisposition by direction of vessels into the area of the root entry zone of the trigeminal nerve (Jannetta, 1976). He noted this in his younger patients—especially those who had a family history of tic. In support of the vascular compression etiology for tic, Jannetta noted that in one patient with known trigeminal neuralgia who came to postmortem examination, vascular compression-distortion of the nerve root entry zone was demonstrated (Jannetta, 1976). He further points out that if careful sensory testing is done in these patients, subtle neurological deficits can be demonstrated and that if electromyograms are done, some denervation can also be found (Jannetta, 1977b; Saunders *et al.*, 1971). Jannetta goes on to state that microscopic inspection of the cranial nerve root entry or exit zones in patients operated upon for other problems (over 70 in number) revealed no abnormality. Studies of over 250 cadavers that did not have trigeminal neuralgia

in life did not reveal any vascular distortion of the root entry zone (Jannetta, 1977a).

Jannetta's (1976) surgical approach consists of a small posterior fossa craniotomy with superior medial retraction of the cerebellum and identification of the root entry-exit zone of the trigeminal nerve. After identification of the vascular abnormality compressing the nerve at this point, the vessel is freed and preserved and then strutted with a silastic sponge protecting the nerve from further compression. His results indicate that the operation has been a success in over 85% of 200 consecutive patients with trigeminal neuralgia who were operated on in a ten-year period (Jannetta, 1977b). In the same review of 200 patients, he reports one death, two cerebellar infarctions, one cerebellar hematoma, one bacterial meningitis, two patients with decreased hearing, ten aseptic meningitides, and nine recurrences. Six of the latter patients were actually not relieved of their pain at the first operation; and at reoperation a second vessel was thought to be the offender; and once it was dealt with, the patients were pain free. In the other three cases, reoperation revealed a slipped prosthesis, and when a larger one was inserted the patients were relieved of their pain.

Comparison of Radiofrequency Thermocoagulation and Vascular Decompression

Percutaneous radiofrequency coagulation of the gasserian ganglion and trigeminal rootlets and microvascular decompression of the trigeminal nerve are emerging as the two most productive surgical methods of treating trigeminal neuralgia. Which procedure should be undertaken for an individual patient will depend on the many factors involved. The percutaneous approach has earned its place as the safest and most effective procedure when it is determined that an ablative procedure is the treatment of choice. The complications of this technique can be serious but are rare. In approximately 15% of postoperative patients there is altered sensation in the form of a severe degree of numbness and/or dysesthetic sensations (Apfelbaum, 1977), as with any ablative procedure. Loss of corneal sensation can be serious, but if the ablation is carefully staged, this too can often be avoided (Nugent—comments on Apfelbaum article, 1977). In elderly patients or those debilitated for other reasons who might not be able to undergo a formal craniotomy, this procedure has its greatest benefit.

The microvascular decompressive technique has the distinct advantage of avoidance of most of the side effects of the percutaneous technique; however, it does involve a formal craniotomy under general anesthesia with its attendant risks and complications. Being a nonablative approach, its greatest advantage is that patients are not asked to exchange the symptom of pain for the symptom of numbness or dysesthesia, and corneal anesthesia is not a problem. It also offers the possibility of directly attacking the cause of the problem. Damage to nearby cranial nerves as well as the cerebellum can often be overcome with better microsurgical technique. However, in older and debilitated patients, the increased risk of surgery obviates against this technique. Operating in the lateral recumbent position offers the advantage of eliminating the potential of air embolus (Alksne, 1977).

Another advantage to the Jannetta procedure is that it allows a direct look at the cerebellar pontine angle, which might harbor an unsuspected tumor as the cause for the tic. In Jannetta's larger series there was a 4.5% incidence of tumors discovered at surgery that were otherwise unsuspected (Jannetta, 1977b). In Apfelbaum's comparison of the two techniques (Apfelbaum, 1977), he found that when patients were questioned about the procedures, 18% (7/39) of the series stated they would not repeat percutaneous neurolysis. Only 4% (2/55) would not repeat microvascular decompression. In Apfelbaum's series, success was achieved in 88% of the patients with percutaneous radiofrequency coagulation and 96% of patients with microvascular decompression. He found that severe recurrences of trigeminal neuralgic pain occurred in 13% of the patients who underwent the percutaneous technique and in only 5% of those who had microvascular decompression. However, his

follow-up was very short, and long-term follow-up will be necessary to make a final evaluation of the long-term results of either procedure.

GLOSSOPHARYNGEAL NEURALGIA

Glossopharyngeal neuralgia is fortunately a rare condition. Therefore, there are no large series of patients in which to systematically evaluate the possible etiologies and the mechanisms or the various treatments and results. In the experience of Spurling and Grantham (1942), glossopharyngeal neuralgia occurs only 1/70th as often as major trigeminal neuralgia. Weisenburg (1910) was the first to note this type of pain and describe it in a patient whose pain in life was found at postmortem to be the result of a tumor of the cerebello-pontine angle. Pain usually arises in the posterior third of the tongue; tonsillar pillars and fossa, nasal, oral, and laryngeal pharynx including the pyriform recess, larynx, eustachian tube, middle ear, external auditory canal, central parts of the pinna, and the small zone in front and back of the ear; it may also radiate to other areas of the face and neck. Often the pain is provoked by touching of the area (or swallowing in the case of the larynx), often beginning as a sudden, sharp pain in the abovementioned trigger areas. Generally, however, the pains go on to become paroxysms of very sharp pain very similar to the type found in trigeminal neuralgia. It is important in the differential diagnosis of this condition that one consider tumors as a more probable cause of the condition than is generally the case with trigeminal neuralgia. Nasal pharyngeal tumors—either by extension or direct involvement of the trigger areas—as well as metastases to the base of the skull, are frequent offenders. Cocainization of the trigger area is very useful in establishing the diagnosis and may in some instances be an effective form of therapy. Once the etiology is established, particularly in the case of tumor, local treatment may relieve the pain. However, often the cause is not found or the tumor cannot be resected, and therefore some other form of therapy must be considered. White and Sweet (1969) point out that because of the great overlap of sensory innervation of the ninth and tenth cranial nerves in the area of the throat as well as the ear, both nerves must be considered in the possible etiology of the condition which the authors prefer to call vagoglossopharyngeal neuralgia. In the same review they advocated section of the ninth nerve as well as the upper rootlets of ten in order to obtain permanent total relief of the pain because of the great sensory overlap. Furthermore, they feel that the upper cervical rootlets may be contributory to the innervation and should be stimulated during the procedure on the awake patient to see if they provoke the pain. Tew (1977) has used the percutaneous approach into the jugular foramen as a means of ablating the ninth and tenth nerves for pain in the appropriate areas secondary to malignancy. Interestingly, Jannetta (1977a) reported on two patients where vascular compression of the ninth and/or tenth nerve at their root entry zones at the brainstem appeared to be the cause of the glossopharyngeal neuralgia.

POSTHERPETIC PAIN

Although rare, postherpetic pain following an attack of herpes zoster occurs—particularly in older people—and is a constant burning ache with superimposed stabbing pains which may occur spontaneously or may be elicited even by very light sensory stimuli. In some cases a true anesthesia dolorosa exists, although most often there is some degree of sensation present. In a large series of all postherpetic neuralgias, 18% occurred in the distribution of the trigeminal nerve, making this site second in frequency to the thorax (Erokhina and Malkova, 1963). The ophthalmic division is most commonly affected and, in fact, in one series of 58 cases the only one so affected (Tatlow, 1952). However, other cranial facial sites have been reported as well as other cranial nerves (Engstrom and Wohlfart, 1949). During the acute bout there is often severe pain, however, in most cases it subsides with the illness. In a very small number of patients, the pain persists. If the pain is persistent, then electrical stimulation (Russell et al.,

1957) or massage (Russell, 1957) or intradermal injections of hydrocortisone (Lefkovits, 1961) may be of some help. Elevation of skin flaps was initially reported to bring short-term relief (De Vet, 1952); however, in another series with a longer follow-up, the pain often recurred (Tindall et al., 1962). Peripheral neurectomies (Taptas, 1953), as well as trigeminal denervation (Ray, 1954), thalamotomy (Mark and Ervin, 1969), and even frontal lobotomy (Falconer, 1948) have been attempted in intractable cases. Again, the results have been either disappointing, short-lived, or the accompanying deficits produced are often incapacitating. Central stimulation—to be discussed below—may be of some benefit, but to date only one patient has been reported, and he obtained significant relief (Adams et al., 1977).

CENTRAL PAIN STATES

The treatment of central pain is still one of the most difficult problems encountered. Such conditions as anesthesia dolorosa, postoperative facial dysesthesias, and post cerebral vascular accident pain in the face deserve special consideration in the context of this chapter. The classic ablative procedures of thalamotomy and frontal lobectomy have been used in the past for treatment of these difficult conditions —often with equivocal results or undesired side effects (White and Sweet, 1969e). Electrical stimulation of the brain has been successfully used recently to suppress these clinical pain states secondary to central nervous system lesions. The effective stimulation site has always been within the somatosensory system. Adams notes complete relief of pain in a patient with electrical stimulation prior to a Thalamotomy (Adams et al., 1977). Before making the therapeutic lesion, stimulation of the primary relay nucleus, ventralis posterior lateralis (VPL), was carried out for the purpose of anatomical localization. The stimulation resulted in immediate suppression of the patients spontaneous pain in association with the evoked sensory paresthesias. This suggested to Adams that stimulation of the third-order neuron in the sensory thalamus might be a means of clinically controlling pain. A similar observation was made by Mark and Ervin (1969). Adams then proceeded to stimulate the posterior ventralis medialis (PVM) of the thalamus by clinically implanting stimulating electrodes in five patients with severe facial anesthesia dolorosa after retrogasserian rhizotomy (Hosobuchi et al., 1973). Four of these patients obtained very satisfactory suppression of pain by these electrically induced paresthesias. Subsequently, Adams treated four patients with the thalamic syndrome by electrically stimulating the somatosensory system at the next highest level, namely the posterior limb of the internal capsule. In a 4–16-month follow-up, Adams reported the relief of anesthesia dolorosa and facial pain to be satisfactory in six of the seven patients so treated. In patients with the thalamic syndrome, he found that after 6–40 months, eight had obtained satisfactory relief (Adams et al., 1977). He suggested that the relief might be related to a direct inhibitory pathway passing through the posterior limb of the internal capsule to the parietal cortex and/or be related to the endogenous opiate system in the brain.

Richardson was the first to demonstrate that stimulation of the periventricular gray matter could produce analgesia in diverse peripheral pain syndromes in man (Richardson and Akil, 1977a). His work was based on experimental work by Liebeskind (Liebeskind et al., 1973) and Akil (Akil and Liebeskind, 1975), among others, who found they could obtain analgesia by stimulation of these areas in animals. At present, a great deal of experimental as well as clinical work suggests that the mechanism of analgesia obtained in central stimulation is probably related to a neural inhibitory system involving endogenous opiate neural transmitters and receptors (Mayer and Hayes, 1975). A large descending neural pathway has been found to be intimately related at the periventricular gray area which, when stimulated, leads to peripheral analgesia (Basbaum et al., 1976). In patients undergoing such stimulation, increased amounts of the endogenous opiates have been recovered from the spinal fluid (Richardson and Akil, 1977b). Endogenous opiates have been named enkephalins or endorphins, depending upon their origin in the central nervous system. These peptides presumably produce analgesia by directly binding with opiate receptors around the periventricular gray area, leading to increased firing in central inhibitory pathways involved in modulating more distal pain input centers. Stimulation of this centrifugal inhibitory system has provided a means of pain suppression without ablative procedures. An extremely interesting and, without doubt, clinically important observation about central stimulation-produced analgesia is that it can persist for long periods of time beyond the actual stimulation (Adams et al., 1977). This further suggests that poststimulation analgesia may be due to the release or activation of neurotransmitters which have long-lasting effects. Adams has reported that patients using this means of stimulation do develop tolerance to the stimulation if it is utilized constantly on a long-term basis, which is reminiscent of the use of opiate drugs (Mayer and Hayes, 1975). Regardless of the fact that the mechanisms of analgesia produced by central stimulation are yet to be completely elucidated, the significant contributions of these pioneers have revolutionized our concepts and treatment of central pain states.

HEAD AND NECK PAIN RELATED TO NEOPLASMS OF THE FACE, HEAD, AND UPPER NECK

Patients with pain from neoplasms of the head and neck represent difficult challenges, but if relief can be obtained they are among the most grateful patients encountered. Psychologically, these patients are often anxious and depressed about their obviously dismal future. As with cancer patients in general, treatment of their anxiety with mild tranquilizers and their depression with one of the tricyclic antidepressants will often allow a marked decrease in their analgesic intake. Often these patients are treated with large doses of narcotics and sent home to spend their remaining days in an obtunded state while the concomitant physical side effects of these drugs present difficulties for their families. The patients often linger in a subhuman state of existence for the remainder of their days. However, a rational combination of antianxiety and antidepressant agents with low-dose narcotics may be all that is necessary to control the pain—at least initially. If these measures fail, then a classic ablative procedure can often be utilized to produce the short-term pain relief needed in these patients. These patients are often willing to put up with the numbness and occasional dysesthesias that occur, in exchange for pain relief. The fact that they have a short life span means that the well-known recurrence of pain associated with ablative procedures in benign pain conditions is usually not a problem.

Since these tumors often lie deeply in the oropharyngeal, aural, or cervical zones supplied by overlapping cranial nerves V, intermedius, IX, and X, and by cervical nerves 1, 2, and 3, extensive rhizotomies must be performed in order to guarantee relief. Posterior fossa craniectomy and/or cervical laminectomy to reach these roots can be a formidable procedure in debilitated patients. If the pain is bilateral, staged thalamotomies or even bifrontal leucotomies may be more judicious than the rhizotomies. White and Sweet recommend a graduated radiofrequency inferior frontomedial leucotomy in the high-risk debilitative patients who have a few months to live. Summarizing the results in 20 cases with different forms of frontal leucotomy, they found that the radiofrequency coagulation gave good short-term relief with only mild psychological changes as opposed to unilateral or bilateral transections which brought good to satisfactory results, but often with marked apathy and other undesirable psychological changes (White and Sweet, 1969d). Vernon Mark summarized his experiences with thalamotomy in 24 cases of cancer pain of the head and neck and found that worthwhile improvement occurred in all but two of the cases (Mark and Ervin, 1969). Excellent relief of cancer pain in the head and neck with central neurostimulation of the medial thalamus has been reported by Adams *et al.* (1977). If the patients and their family are willing and cooperative enough to involve themselves in the care and use of the stimulating devices, this may prove to be the treatment of choice in the future. Again, the individual patient, his disease, life expectancy,

and technical availability of instrumentation will help determine the proper mode of treatment.

OCCIPITAL NEURALGIA

One should consider operation for occipital neuralgia only when medical therapy fails. One does not operate for pain alone and particularly not for posterior occipital headache. In general, operative section of the occipital nerves should be avoided. There may be an occasional case where an occipital compression neuropathy can be demonstrated, where the nerve can be blocked with the long-lasting relief of pain, and where a section of the nerve may be at least considered. In our experience, however, section of the occipital nerves is rarely curative, frequently leads to complications with denervation dysesthesias, and is certainly not the procedure of choice in treatment of posterior occipital headache. Extensive manipulation of the neck should also be done with extreme care when pain is the primary problem, especially in the elderly, if cervical spondylosis and early signs of cord compression are present. In general, cervical traction is not indicated in these cases.

We suggest the use of antiinflammatory and analgesic medications, particularly the newer antiinflammatory drugs such as ibuprofen and related compounds. The standard regimen is ibuprofen (400 mg three times daily) with some form of muscle relaxant taken at bedtime such as diazepam (20 mg) or chlorphenesin (800 mg). Gentle physical therapy with much laying on of hands and stimulation of the skin and subcutaneous tissues should be emphasized as the treatment of choice in this condition. Often, in addition, patients will respond to the use of the electrical neurostimulator. When muscle contraction is a persistent problem, biofeedback training is also helpful. We employ local injection of tender areas with anesthetic agents and/or corticosteroids, sometimes repeatedly, another modality of treatment which has been found to be helpful but not curative. We often suggest the use of a cervical orthopedic pillow, attempting to retain the cervical lordotic curve during rest and perhaps during sleep as well.

Our physical therapy group teaches body mechanics and a posture program to patients with chronic neck complaints. Generally, if an intensive conservative course such as that outlined above is followed, the patients complaints can be controlled at least to some extent, and more radical operative procedures can be avoided.

SUMMARY

1. In elderly patients or those debilitated by other illness, radiofrequency thermocoagulation is the procedure of choice in the surgical treatment of trigeminal neuralgia.

2. Microvascular decompression (Jannetta) of the trigeminal nerve should be offered to younger patients with trigeminal neuralgia who can withstand a formal craniotomy. This procedure has the advantage of reducing facial and corneal hypesthesia, and allowing direct visualization of the trigeminal nerve and the cerebellopontine angle.

3. Glosspharyngeal neuralgia, being rare, is not a common surgical problem. Nasopharyngeal tumors should be suspected if this disease occurs. The proper surgical procedure will depend on the expertise of the surgeon, but probably should include lesions of both the ninth and tenth cranial nerves.

4. Ablative surgical procedures are often ineffective in postherpetic neuralgia.

5. Treatment of central pain states often emphasizes stimulation of the nervous system rather than ablation.

REFERENCES

Adams, J. E., Y. Hosobuchi, and R. Linchitz (1977). The present status of implantable intracranial stimulators for pain. In *Clinical Neurosurgery* (E. B. Keener *et al.*, eds.), pp. 347–361. Williams & Wilkins, Baltimore.

Akil, H., and J. C. Liebeskind (1975). Monoaminergic mechanisms of stimulation produced analgesia. *Brain Res. 94*, 279–296.

Alksne, J. F. (1977). Prevention of air embolus by performing the Jannetta procedure in the lateral recumbent position. Presented at the Neurosurgical Society of America annual meeting, Colorado Springs.

Apfelbaum, R. I. (1977). A comparison of percutaneous radiofrequency trigeminal neurolysis and microvascular decompression of the trigeminal nerve for the treatment of tic douloureux. *Neurosurgery 1*, 16–21.

Basbaum, A. I., C. H. Clanton, and H. L. Fields (1976). Opiate and stimulus-produced analgesia: functional anatomy of a medullospinal pathway. *Proc. Natl. Acad. Sci. 73*, 4685–4688, 1976.

Beaver, D. L., H. L. Moses, and C. E. Ganote (1965). Electron microscopy of the trigeminal ganglion. III. Trigeminal neuralgia. *Arch. Pathol. 79*, 571–582.

Bessou, P., and E. R. Perl (1969). Response of cutaneous sensory units with unmyelinated fibers to noxious stimuli. *J. Neurophysiol. 32*, 1025–1043.

Dandy, W. E. (1925). Section of the sensory root of the trigeminal nerve at the pons. *Bull. Johns Hopkins Hosp. 36*, 105–106.

Dandy, W. E. (1929). Operation for cure of tic douloureux; partial section of the sensory root at the pons. *Arch. Surg. (Chicago) 18*, 687–734.

Dandy, W. E. (1932). Treatment of trigeminal neuralgia by the cerebellar route. *Ann. Surg. 96*, 787–795.

Dandy, W. E. (1934). Trigeminal neuralgia. *Am. J. Surg. 24*, 447–455.

Dandy, W. E. (1945). Surgery of the brain. A monogr. In *Practice of Surgery* (Lewis, ed.), Vol. 12, pp. 167–187. Prior, Hagerstown, Md.

De Vet, A. C. (1952). Cited by J. C. White and W. H. Sweet (1969). *Pain and the Neurosurgeon, A Forty-Year Experience*, pp. 382–383. C. C. Thomas, Springfield, Ill.

Engstrom, H., and G. Wohlfart (1949). Herpes zoster of the seventh, eighth, ninth and tenth cranial nerves. *Arch. Neurol. Psychiat. 62*, 638–652.

Erokhina, L. G., and E. V. Malkova (1963). Postgerpeticheskaia nevralgiia troinichnogo nerva. *Klin. Med. (Moskva) 41*, 45–49, 1963.

Falconer, M. A. (1948). Relief of intractable pain of organic origin by frontal lobotomy. *Res. Publ. Assoc. Res. Nerv. Ment. Dis. 27*, 706–714.

Henderson, W. R. (1965). The anatomy of the gasserian ganglion and the distribution of pain in relation to injections and operations for trigeminal neuralgia. *Ann. Rev. Coll. Surg. Engl. 37*, 346–373.

Horrax, G., and J. L. Poppen (1935). Trigeminal neuralgia. Experiences with and treatment employed in 468 patients during the past 10 years. *Surg. Gynecol. Obstet. 61*, 394–402.

Hosobuchi, Y., J. E. Adams, and B. Rutkin (1973). Chronic thalamic stimulation for the control of facial anesthesia dolorosa. *Arch. Neurol. 29*, 158–161.

Jannetta, P. J. (1976). Microsurgical approach to the trigeminal nerve for tic douloureux, *Prog. Neurol. Surg. 7*, 180–200.

Jannetta, P. J. (1977a). Observations on the etiology of trigeminal neuralgia, hemifacial spasm, acoustic nerve dysfunction and glossopharyngeal neuralgia. Definitive microsurgical treatment and results in 117 patients. *Neurochirurgia 20*, 145-154.

Jannetta, P. J. (1977b). Treatment of trigeminal neuralgia by suboccipital and transtentorial cranial operations. *Clin. Neurosurg. 24*, 538-549.

Kirschner, M. (1942). Die behandlumg der trigeminusneuralgia (Nach Erfahrungen an 1113 Kranken). *Munch. Med. Wochenschr. 89*, 263-269.

Lefkovits, A. M. (1961). Postherpetic neuralgia. A method of effective treatment. *Neurology (Minneap.) 11*, 170-171.

Letcher, F. S., and S. Goldring (1968). The effect of radiofrequency current and heat on peripheral nerve action potential in the cat. *J. Neurosurg. 29*, 42-47.

Lewy, F. H., and F. C. Grant (1938). Physiopathologic and pathoanatomic aspects of major trigeminal neuralgia. *Arch. Neurol. Psychiat. Chicago 40*, 1126-1134.

Liebeskind, J. C., G. Guilbrand, J. M. Besson, and J. L. Oliveras (1973). Analgesia from electrical stimulation of the periaqueductal gray matter in the cat: behavioral observations and inhibitory effects on spinal cord interneurons. *Brain Res. 50*, 441-446.

Mark, V. H., and F. R. Ervin (1969). Stereotactic surgery for relief of pain. In *Pain and the Neurosurgeon, A Forty-Year Experience* (J. C. White and W. H. Sweet, eds.), pp. 843-887. C. C. Thomas, Springfield, Ill.

Mayer, D. J., and R. L. Hayes (1975). Stimulation produced analgesia; development of tolerance and cross-tolerance to morphine. *Science 188*, 941-943.

Nugent, G. R., and B. Berry (1974). Trigeminal neuralgia treated by differential percutaneous radiofrequency coagulation of the gasserian ganglion. *J. Neurosurg. 40*, 517-523.

Nugent, G. R. (1977). Comments to article by R. I. Apfelbaum (1977). A comparison of percutaneous radiofrequency trigeminal neurolysis and microvascular decompression of the trigeminal nerve for the treatment of tic douloureux. *Neurosurgery 1*, 16-21.

Perl, T., and A. Ecker (1959). A roentgenologically controlled placement of the needle in the trigeminal root for the treatment of tic douloureux. *Am. J. Roentgenol. Radium Ther. Nucl. Med. 82*, 830-839.

Pudenz, R. H., and C. H. Shelden (1952). Experiences with foraminal decompression in the surgical treatment of tic douloureux. *Proceedings of Meeting of the American Academy of Neurological Surgery, New York.*

Ray, B. S. (1954). The surgical treatment of headache and atypical facial neuralgia. *J. Neurosurg. 11*, 596-606.

Richardson, D. E., and H. Akil (1977a). Pain reduction by electrical brain stimulation in man. Part I: Acute administration in periaqueductal and periventricular sites. *J. Neurosurg. 47*, 163-177.

Richardson, D. E., and H. Akil (1977b). Pain reduction by electrical brain stimulation in man. Part 2: Chronic self-administration in the periventricular gray matter. *J. Neurosurg. 47*, 184-194.

Russell, W. R. (1957). The facial neuralgias. *Trans. Ophthalmol. Soc. UK 77*, 331-336.

Russell, W. R., M. L. E. Espir, and F. S. Morganstern (1957). Treatment of post-herpetic neuralgia. *Lancet 1*, 242-245.

Saunders, R. L., R. Krout, and E. Sachs, Jr. (1971). Masticator electromyography in trigeminal neuralgia. *Neurology (Minneap.) 21*, 1221-1225.

Sjoqvist, O. (1938). Eine neue Operationsmethode bei Trigeminusneuralgie, Durchschneidung des tractus spinalis trigemini. *Zentralbl. Neurochir. 2*, 247-281.

Sjoqvist, O. (1948). Ten years experience with trigeminal tractotomy. *Brasil Med.-Cir. 10*, 259-274.

Spiller, W. G., and C. H. Frazier (1901). The division of the sensory root of the trigeminus for relief of tic douloureux; an experimental pathological and clinical study with a preliminary report of one surgically successful case. *Philadelphia Med. J. 8*, 1039-1049.

Spurling, R. G., and E. G. Grantham (1942). Glossopharyngeal neuralgia. *South. Med. J. 35*, 509-513.

Stookey, B., and J. Ransohoff (1959). *Trigeminal Neuralgia. Its History and Treatment.* C. C. Thomas, Springfield, Ill.

Sweet, W. H., and J. G. Wepsic (1974). Controlled thermocoagulation of trigeminal ganglion and rootlets for differential destruction of pain fibers. Part 1: Trigeminal neuralgia. *J. Neurosurg. 40*, 143-156.

Taarnhoj, P. (1952). Decompression of the trigeminal root and the posterior part of the ganglion as a treatment in trigeminal neuralgia; preliminary communication. *J. Neurosurg. 9*, 288-290.

Taarnhoj, P. (1954). Decompression of the trigeminal root. *J. Neurosurg. 11*, 299-305.

Taptas, J. N. (1953). *Maux de tête et névralgies. Douleurs cranio-faciales.* Masson & Cie, Paris, 230 pp.

Tatlow, W. F. T. (1952). Herpes zoster ophthalmicus and postherpetic neuralgia. *J. Neurol. Neurosurg. Psychiat. 15*, 45-49.

Tew, J. M., Jr. (1977). Percutaneous rhizotomy in the treatment of intractable facial pain (trigeminal, glossopharyngeal, and vagal nerves). In *Current Techniques in Operative Neurosurgery* (H. H. Schmidek and W. H. Sweet, eds.), pp. 409-426. Grune and Stratton, New York.

Thiry, S. (1962). Expérience personnelle basée sur 225 cas de névralgie essentielle du trijumeau traités par électrocoagulation stéréotaxique du ganglion de Gasser entre 1950 et 1960. *Neurochirurgie 8*, 86-92.

Tindall, G. T., G. L. Odom, and R. G. Vieth (1962).

Surgical treatment of postherpetic neuralgia. Results of skin undermining and excision in 14 patients. *Arch. Neurol.* 7, 423–426.

Weisenburg, T. H. (1910). Cerebello-pontile tumor diagnosed for six years as tic douloureux; the symptoms of irritation of the ninth and twelfth cranial nerves. *JAMA* 54, 1600–1604.

White, J. C., and W. H. Sweet (1969a). *Pain and the Neurosurgeon, a Forty-Year Experience*, p. 203 (Table XXX). C. C. Thomas, Springfield, Ill.

White, J. C., and W. H. Sweet (1969b). *Pain and the Neurosurgeon, a Forty-Year Experience,* p. 265. C. C. Thomas, Springfield, Ill.

White, J. C., and W. H. Sweet (1969c). *Pain and the Neurosurgeon, a Forty-Year Experience*, pp. 289–292. C. C. Thomas, Springfield, Ill.

White, J. C., and W. H. Sweet (1969d). *Pain and the Neurosurgeon, a Forty-Year Experience*, p. 321. C. C. Thomas, Springfield, Ill.

White, J. C., and W. H. Sweet (1969e). *Pain and the Neurosurgeon, a Forty-Year Experience*, pp. 386–406. C. C. Thomas, Springfield, Ill.

16

POST-TRAUMATIC HEADACHE

REVISED BY DONALD J. DALESSIO

Almost all persons who have had injury to their heads have local pain or tenderness at the site of impact for a few hours or even for a few days, after which many become symptom free.

Between one-third and one-half of all persons who injure their heads sufficiently to warrant hospitalization develop chronic post-traumatic headaches (Merritt *et al.*, 1944; Brenner *et al.*, 1944).

A small number of patients with headaches that persist after injury to the head have pain due to gross accumulations of blood in the epidural, subdural, or subarachnoid spaces. The headache of subdural hematoma begins at the time of the blow or the regaining of consciousness and persists often for months until the hematoma is removed, or until spontaneous resolution occurs. Large amounts of blood in the subarachnoid space about the base of the brain induce headache because of traction, displacement, distention, and rupture of pain-sensitive blood vessels and pia arachnoid (Kunkle *et al.*, 1942, 1943; Ray and Wolff, 1940). A still smaller group of patients have sustained headache after head injury due to adhesions involving pain-sensitive structures in the arachnoidea (Penfield, 1927; Penfield and Norcross, 1936).

The vast majority of patients with post-traumatic headaches that persist or recur for long periods of time after head injury have no such intracranial abnormalities to explain their headaches. It has been the purpose of the following study to ascertain the pathophysiology in this dominant group of post-traumatic headaches.

Sixty-three New York Hospital patients with the complaint of headache following injury to the head were studied. Most of the injuries were sustained in military situations, the remainder at home or in industry. All the patients were known to have no epidural, subdural, subarachnoid, or parenchymatous hemorrhage at the time of observation. Thirty-three of them were known to have had cerebral and meningeal damage as evidenced by operative visualization, electroencephalogram, or pneumoencephalogram. Some portion of the remainder may also have had cerebral or meningeal damage, but it was not demonstrable. Several patients had had more than one head injury with loss of consciousness with each accident. The headaches were of two months' to 14 years' duration. In no instance was headache the only complaint.

The headaches following injury to the head in this series were divided into three types. Headaches of types 1 and 2 are closely allied and often indistinguishable, yet for purposes of analysis they have been arbitrarily separated in this study. (1) a steady "pressure sensation" or aching pain in a cap- or band-like distribution, or, more commonly, in a circumscribed area elsewhere than at the site of injury and usually associated with deep tenderness on manual pressure; (2) in addition to type 1 headache, a circumscribed, relatively superficial tenderness at the site of impact or in a scar, often associated with aching pain of moderate intensity; (3) an aching pain, often throbbing, occurring in attacks, usually unilateral in onset, and chiefly in the temporal, frontal, postauricular, or occipital region, occasionally combined with type 1 headache.

Description and Pathophysiology-Muscle Contraction Headache (Headache, Type 1)

Headache, type 1, was the most frequent and troublesome variety of head sensation following head injury. All 63 patients suffered from this type, including 15 patients having type 2 headache and four patients with type 3. However, 44 patients had type 1 headache alone. The head sensations, when painful, were of a dull, aching quality. There was deep tenderness, and headache could often be reproduced by manual pressure upon these tender areas. The intensity of pain, when present, varied from mild to very severe (1 to 8 plus intensity on a scale of 1 plus to 10 plus, the latter being of maximal intensity). Head pains of this type often recurred for many years. The headache attacks were intermittent, varying from a few hours to ten days in duration.

It should be emphasized that for the greater part of the time and between the headache attacks, the head sensations that were the basis of complaint in this type of chronic post-traumatic headache syndrome were not actually pain. These sensations were experienced at the vertex, circumferentially over the eyes, or at the base. All patients were tense, anxious, resentful, fearful, and more or less dejected. The headache and other head sensations were commonly made worse by effort, stooping, coughing, or turning the head. Mental concentration and emotional tensions involved in making decisions or associated with conflicts from divergent drives also accentuated the pressure sensations. During periods of asthenia, exhaustion, and prostration, headaches and other head sensations were usually more frequent and more intense. The intensity of the head sensations or pain was reduced for shorter or longer periods by medication, by massage, or by any other device that induced relaxation.

Occasionally spinning sensations and frequently dizziness and photophobia were accompaniments of this type of headache. The giddiness was commonly a sensation of unsteadiness, swimming, uncertainty, or falling and was made worse by head movements, when the latter accentuated the pain. The giddiness was seldom accompanied by nystagmus, and the spinning sensation was rarely as severe as that of Ménière's, or labyrinthine, syndromes. It did not induce nausea or vomiting, but was sometimes associated with anorexia. The giddiness was increased by manual pressure upon tender regions about the base of the skull or behind the ear.

At or near sites of disagreeable head sensations the muscle potentials commonly increased with an increase in the intensity and decreased with a decrease in the intensity of pain.

Muscle potentials were registered and the records analyzed in the manner previously described.

The following protocol is illustrative of the relation between muscle potentials and the post-traumatic headache of type 1.

Patient F. S., a 23-year-old Marine, was rendered unconscious by a bomb burst. Because of persistent headache following this accident, his head was subsequently explored bilaterally for subdural hematomas. Xanthochromic fluid was found, but no hematomas. Following these surgical procedures he continued to complain of almost continuous headache of the type 1 variety, with 1 to 2 plus plain in the frontal and right temporal areas, and in the area to the right of the vertex, with 5 plus plain in the right frontal area (see Fig. 16-1). During one of the brief spontaneous remissions of this headache, on 9/3/43, the patient visited the laboratory, free of all complaints, and in good spirits. The electromyograms recorded on this headache-free day showed no increased muscle potential from the previously painful areas. On 9/8/43 he revisited the laboratory complaining of his usual headache, which on this day was of 5 plus intensity in the bifrontal and bitemporal areas. He was tense, dejected, and irascible. The electromyograms recorded at this time showed exaggerated muscle potential from all electrodes.

The electromyographic and other data on the 63 patients studied are presented briefly in the following paragraphs:

Sixty-two patients had definite headaches or other precisely definable and disagreeable head sensations; one had indefinite head sensations.

Of the 62 patients with definable sensations, all but one had headache for three months or more; 25 patients for three to nine months; 15 patients for 10

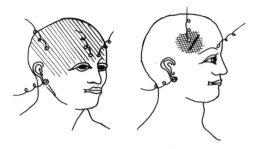

FIG. 16-1. The distribution of headache (single hatching) in patient F.S., the area of deep tenderness (cross hatching), the operative scar, and the location of electrodes.

to 18 months; and 19 patients for periods of a year and a half to ten years. One exceptional patient had had headaches for 13 years, and one other for 14 years.

Of the 62 patients with definable sensations who had headache at one time or another, 37 had headache at the time of the electromyographic study. In about three-quarters of the latter there was evidence of muscular activity in the head or neck muscles. In more than half, excessive muscle potentials indicated gross overactivity of the muscles of the head or neck. In the 12 remaining, there was minimal but abnormal activity.

In 28 of the 37, the muscle activity was greatest at the site of the head sensation, although such activity was noted elsewhere as well. In four, muscular activity was recorded in the neck, although the headache was frontal or temporal.

Records made during headache-free periods usually gave evidence of slight, sometimes no muscle contractions.

Comment. It was noteworthy that in about a third of patients with headache the amount of muscular disturbance was just above the physiologic limit at rest. It was probably the basis of complaint because it was sustained and because of an abnormal preoccupation with, and overreaction to, minimal head sensations.

Pressure, tightness, or other nonpainful experiences when persistent may be misinterpreted as pain if the patient is anxious, depressed, or alarmed as to the implications of the head sensations. Moreover, such contractions may become so intense as to give rise to a cramp-like aching pain that is intensified by

head movements, by arising from the lying-down position, or by mental concentration and conflict. There are then usually regions of tenderness when manual pressure is applied.

Thus, Elliott (1944) has shown in patients with painful muscle contraction in the leg that when the needle electrodes are placed directly into a small focus of tenderness, the so-called rheumatic nodule, violent action potentials can be recorded, whereas adjacent muscles may be relatively or even completely inactive. In other words, the muscle contraction may be in some instances extremely local, even though the pain is diffuse.

The injection of 1% procaine hydrochloride into zones of deep tenderness eliminated existing headache and made impossible the experimental reproduction of headache by deep manual pressure, indicating that headache and other head sensations were of extracranial origin.

The protocols on the following three patients who had pain in different areas and who received injections of 1% procaine hydrochloride were selected as representative of the 44 patients having type 1 headache alone.

Patient S. P. was a Coast Guardsman, aged 21. He complained of almost continuous headache, sometimes as intense as 7 plus, for three years following a fall on the ice when he had hit his head. On September 20 he visited the laboratory with a headache of 7 plus intensity in the left frontal, temporal, parietal, occipital, and cervical regions. He was pale, dejected, and tense. At this time electromyograms revealed a moderate amount of muscle potential abnormality in the temporal, occipital, and cervical areas. The occipital and upper cervical regions were found to be tender on manual pressure, which increased the intensity of the headache both locally and in the frontal and temporal regions. The injection of 10 cc of 1% procaine hydrochloride into the trapezius muscle on the left, fanwise from a point of 2 cm below the occipital attachment, was immediately followed by the complaint of intense (10 plus) pain in the area injected. The patient reacted with profuse perspiration, marked pallor, and nausea. During this period of intense pain, muscle potential was grossly exaggerated in the frontal, occipital, and cervical regions. Within a minute after the injection, the intensity of the pain diminished, and when deep analgesia about the area of injection was established, both the headache and muscle potential were minimal in all areas.

When Patient F. S., the 23-year-old Marine described in Series 1, visited the laboratory on September 8 with 5 plus headache in the bifrontal and bitemporal areas, he also had extreme tenderness on manual pressure in the right temporal area (Fig. 16-1). Furthermore, pressure upon this area increased the intensity showed exaggerated muscle potentials. Infiltration of 5 cc of 1% procaine hydrochloride into the right temporal muscle eliminated headache and exaggerated muscle potentials, and firm pressure upon the right temporal area no longer elected tenderness or pain.

The patient C. T., a 44-year-old automobile mechanic, had had similar complaints since he had fractured his skull two years before. This patient's accident had been followed by a three-week period of unconsciousness, a right-sided hemiplegia, and a subsequent aphasia, from which he recovered sufficiently to become ambulatory. He had, at the time of the observation, a slight mentation defect, as indicated by mental testing procedures, some residual motor and sensory disturbances, and records of abnormal electroencephalographic and pneumonencephalographic studies. However, when 8 cc of 0.5% procaine hydrochloride was injected deeply into the tender regions over the vertex and in the right lower occipital region, headache was eliminated, indicating again that despite the evidence of structural brain disease, headache was of extracranial origin.

In all the patients who were investigated with headaches of type 1 and who had headache at the time of the observation, it was possible to demonstrate in each patient that certain passive and active movements of the head and neck modified the intensity of the headache. The requisite movements varied from patient to patient. Electromyographic records from patients in whom pain was either increased or decreased by active or passive muscle movement showed corresponding increase or decrease in action potentials.

Simons, Day, Goodell, and Wolff (1943) have shown that contraction of the skeletal muscles in the head and neck may result reflexly and secondarily from noxious stimuli from any part of the head, either inside or outside. On the other hand, these skeletal muscle contractions may be part of a sustained postural contraction in a pattern of tension, anxiety, or fear. In both, the sustained contraction may result in paresthesia or pain. One may not infer from electrical overactivity in skeletal muscle which of the two varieties of circumstance is the precipitating factor. Furthermore, the elimination of pain by procaine injection of the muscle, by massage, or by other factors that lead to relaxation of the muscle may not be used as evidence concerning the basis of the sustained muscular contraction. All that may be inferred is that the major portion, if not all of the pain, arises in structures on the outside of the head and probably results from sustained contraction of skeletal muscle. That such a mechanism may operate to produce the type 1 variety of chronic post-traumatic headache follows from the evidence here presented.

Further, there may occur central spread of the effects of noxious stimulation from one part of a neural segment to ultimately include all structures supplied by the same segment and even adjacent segments. This phenomenon causes pain to be experienced remote from the original zone of noxious stimulation, in both superficial and deep structures.

Cyriax (1938) demonstrated that injections of 0.1 cc of 4% solution of sodium chloride into the posterior cervical muscles close to their occipital insertion, and into the occipitalis itself, gave rise to a pain that ran forward, forming a band half encircling the head and reaching its maximum intensity in the temple and forehead over the eye. Injections of salt solution in an area between 2 and 5 cm below the occiput induced pain in the back of the head up to the vertex. Similar injections below this area caused pain in the cervical muscles only. Injections into the upper end of the sterno cleidomastoid muscle caused pain to be experienced in the temporal region. Injections into the epicranial aponeurosis caused pain to be experienced behind the eyes.

Campbell and Parsons (1944) confirmed these observations, and patient S. P. offers further evidence of the spread of pain from the occipital region to the anterior portion of the head. With such spread of pain, action potentials from the muscles involved in the zone of spread may be present or absent, but procaine injected into such muscles will reduce the intensity of the headache only locally, whereas procaine injected into the primary site of noxious stimuli within the muscle will abolish the headache.

Description and Pathophysiology-Painful Site of Injury (Headache, Type 2)

Included in this group were 15 patients (about a quarter of the total) who in addition to type 1 headache had a clearly defined and relatively superficial tender zone at the site of the original injury, often but not always associated with a visible or palpable scar. This tender area sometimes became the basis of complaint only when some pressure such as that of a hat or a comb was applied to it. Such headaches were experienced for the most part about the site of noxious stimulation. But usually there was spontaneous aching pain in this region, either continuous or intermittent.

Palpation sometimes revealed adherence of the scalp to the scar. Sometimes the skin, without actually being ruptured, appeared atrophic. Such tender areas were irregularly ovoid in shape and were from 1 to 3 cm in their longest axis. The life span of the complaint was variable. Nine had had their symptom less than a year, although three patients had had aching pain in the region of tender sites or scars for two years or more.

Noxious stimulation, such as pressure, upon sites of local scalp tenderness or scars, reproduced the headache spontaneously experienced, or, if a headache was already present, increased its intensity. The injection of procaine into such sites eliminated headache and tenderness locally, but remote "cap" and "pressure" sensations and aches characteristic of the concomitant type 1 headache often persisted for some time or were not affected.

Patient F. D. complained of a constant ache and a tender spot on manual pressure in the right parieto-occipital region following a blow on the head in that region six months previously. Pressing upon and moving in a circular motion the skin and subcutaneous tissues of the tender area and injecting 2.5 cc of isotonic saline solution intra- and subcutaneously into the site of the injury increased the local pain from an intensity of 1 plus to an intensity of 3 plus. The subsequent injection of 0.5% procaine

hydrochloride subcutaneously and intracutaneously in the same area eliminated both local tenderness and pain.

Comment. Aching pain does not arise from the superficial layers of the skin, and yet aching pain and tenderness in this patient were first increased by distending these tissues with saline and then eliminated by intra- and subcutaneous injection of procaine. It is likely, therefore, that the distention resulting from the saline displaced deeper pain endings and that the procaine infiltrated perivascular and other deeper pain structures.

It is inferred that the tender zones and aching pain of type 2 headache result from stimulation of nerve endings involved in the locally damaged tissue, because of lowered threshold associated with local nerve defect and abnormal healing.

Jones and Brown (1944) have also noted that chronic post-traumatic headache may have its origin in injured soft tissues about the head and neck. Thus upon surgical exploration on several patients they found varying degrees of connective tissue reaction. Such scar formation about a "neurovascular bundle" they considered to be a cause of post-traumatic headache. They were able to eliminate tender points and headache in some of their patients by procaine infiltration of such areas.

It is therefore suggested that the type 2 headache results from traumatic myositis, fibrositis, or periostitis, which causes also the local tenderness at the sites of injury.

Pathophysiology (Headache, Type 3)

Four of 63 patients had type 3 headache as a primary complaint. It was characterized by its relatively short duration, recurrence, and periodicity, its throbbing, dull, aching quality, and associated anorexia, nausea and vomiting. It was usually temporal, but sometimes frontal, postauricular, or occipital, and sometimes it involved the eye. It was usually unilateral in onset, often becoming generalized, often began in the early hours of the morning, or was present when the patient awakened, and continued all day. Frequently, distended arteries could be seen or palpated at the site of the headache. The intensity of pain varied from 2 to 8 plus and was increased by effort, coughing, bending, or lying down. It was not modified by massage, heat, or sedation; but icebags, cold compresses, digital compression of the common carotid artery on the corresponding side of the neck of the region of the head involved, and codeine sulfate reduced the intensity of the pain. Ergotamine tartrate eliminated all but the type 1 components: sensations of head tightness, "bands," or "weights," and steady ache, which were intermittently present between the above-described headache attacks.

A profound depression and anxiety accompanied the headache, and prostration was usual, often persisting for hours after the headache attack was ended; and then gradually the individual recovered completely or he became aware once again of the tightness, band, or weight sensations in his head. Tension, exhaustion, and fatigue usually precipitated these attacks. Such patients had had infrequent headaches of a similar nature before the head injury, and it was inferred that they were vascular in origin, resulting from painful distention of cranial arteries.

The following protocol is representative. Patient J. M., a Puerto Rican merchant marine cook, aged 33, complained of headache since a head injury sustained three months before. He had fallen several feet to the floor from his bunk, striking the back of his head, and was unconscious for 2 hr. Though long a tense, anxious, rigid, perfectionistic person, since the accident he had grown increasingly irritable, and complained of poor memory and attention. He was especially anxious and disturbed because of the probability of induction into the Army within a short time. Electroencephalograms revealed evidence of brain damage.

He had two varieties of headache. The first was throbbing and of high intensity, and occurred in recurrent attacks in the frontal and temporal regions once or twice a week, lasting eight to ten hours. It was increased in intensity when lying flat, and reduced by sitting upright. Also, it was reduced in intensity or eliminated by digital pressure on the temporal artery. Associated with the headache were anorexia and nausea. This type of headache he had had at infrequent intervals for many years.

The second type of headache was also intermittent, but of less intensity. It was sometimes associated with, but occurred independently of, the throbbing headache attacks. It was chiefly occipital, and was of a steady cramp-like quality, alternating with a feeling of a "band" or tightness.

Electromyograms revealed exaggerated muscle potentials in the occipital and temporal regions. An intramuscular injection of 0.5 mg ergotamine tartrate eliminated the throbbing frontal and temporal headache in 17 min. The occipital sensations were not significantly modified by the ergotamine tartrate.

GENERAL DISCUSSION OF TYPES 1, 2, AND 3 HEADACHE AND THE SIGNIFICANCE OF BRAIN DAMAGE TO POST-TRAUMATIC HEADACHE

Small amounts of blood in the subarachnoid space and the injury of bone and meninges usually fail to induce pain for long periods, a statement supported by the fact that long-lasting headache as a sequel to head injury produced by neurosurgery is uncommon. Chronic headache is rare after craniotomy and complete removal of meningiomas, gliomas, neuromas, and hematomas. Actually, the characteristic sequence after operation is a few days to a week of headache, rarely, two weeks, and then a subsidence of all discomfort.

Sustained, chronic, or recurrent headache persisting longer than two months following spontaneous subarachnoid hemorrhage is rare in patients who have not had headaches before the accident (Wolff et al., 1945). Yet the opportunity for arachnoidal adhesions is as great as after subarachnoid hemorrhage from a head injury. Similarly, after meningococcus meningitis, chronic headache is rare. The inference from these considerations is that, despite severe brain trauma with meningeal damage and scarification, often associated with severe mental, motility, and sensory defects, persistent headache is uncommon.

Nonetheless, in a few instances intracranial structures are the source of the noxious stimuli that result in chronic post-traumatic headache. In this category, in addition to the headache associated with subdural hematoma, would be placed those headaches that are due to arachnoidal adhesions and the fibrotic organization of hemorrhage about pain-sensitive structures within the cranium. Penfield (1927) and Penfield and Norcross (1936) have studied a group of patients who exemplify this mechanism in operation.

Also, Penfield and Norcross have reported observations made during operative visualization upon four patients suffering from chronic post-traumatic headache. They found numerous adhesions between the dura and the arachnoidea. "Separation of these adhesions with a curved instrument produced pain—and the pain the patient likened to the pain he had habitually on coughing or sneezing." They inferred that the pain arose from the traction of these adhesions on the pain-sensitive dural arteries. Ross and McNaughton (1944) report that in two patients with chronic post-traumatic headache who had surgical exploration, traction upon such adhesions reproduced the patient's pain.

The fact that subdural adhesions occur after every craniotomy without producing headache was recognized by Penfield and Norcross and explained by stating that "in cases of traumatic headache there is shifting of the normal relationship of the brain to the overlying dura, so that traction is eventually exerted on the adhesions." Such a shift was produced experimentally in one of eight cats subjected to head injury. On the basis of these observations, Penfield introduced the procedure of subdural insufflation of air. He reported good results in the relief of most patients with post-traumatic headache. However, in a follow-up study of Penfield's patients undertaken some 20 years later, Ross and McNaughton were "able to report few cases in which the patient was cured or considerably improved several months to a few years after the procedure."

Ross and McNaughton also found that this type of post-traumatic headache was eliminated by the administration of ergotamine tartrate.

Watts *et al.* (1944) suggested that the headache and dizziness that follow head injury are sometimes due to contusion of the scalp and appear to be related to the scalp arteries. They found in a small group of patients that when headache was experienced at the site of injury, procaine infiltration around the scalp artery in the contused area temporarily relieved the headache, and that when a chronic headache could be completely relieved for several hours by procaine injection around the appropriate artery, resection of a piece of artery gave the patient "long-lasting relief." These authors described four cases of localized headache following trauma to the head, in which such resections were performed. One of these was completely relieved of head pain (8 months between operation and report); another obtained no relief; a third was free of pain for 11 months, when two headaches occurred at the site of the original pain; the fourth was very much improved by the operative procedure but had occasional spontaneous pain, and pain could be induced by tapping the forehead. It is likely that Watts was dealing with patients with the type 3 headache just described, and it is conceivable that some of those patients described by Friedman and Brenner (1944) as having their post-traumatic headache reproduced by histamine also had this type of headache.

Bues (1956) has made an additional study of the phenomenology of a large series of patients with post-traumatic headache. About 50% of his patients following head injury suffered headache. He described these headaches as occurring in attacks that began insidiously and gradually got worse during the course of an hour, but seldom lasted longer. They were recurrent from one to three times a week and often with long intervals between them. Sometimes their onset was related to season or other special circumstances. About three years after the accident about half of those who had had headaches initially still complained of recurrent episodes. Although the interval between headaches greatly increased, individual attacks were sometimes very severe. In his experience young persons were less likely to have headaches following head injury than were middle-aged individuals. The temperament of the individual was significantly related to the occurrence of headache. Scars on the outside of the head often assumed major importance and became extremely sensitive.

Bues' description of these headaches would suggest that many of his patients had vascular and muscle-contraction headaches, and some had very sensitive scars, observations in keeping with our own experiences.

A. E. Walker (1965) made a careful study and report on 739 men who had sustained head injuries in World War II and who were studied at intervals thereafter in four neurological centers in Baltimore,

New York, Boston, and Long Beach, California, six to nine years after injury. Headache, usually associated with other post-traumatic symptoms, occurred in 82% of the men, did not correlate with the severity of injury, but bore a much closer relationship to the neurotic type of personality and subnormal intelligence. Mental disturbances in the form of impaired judgment, mentation, memory, and alterations in personality could be correlated to severity of injury, but not with location of injury. Aphasia was conspicuous when the lesion in right-handed patients was in the left hemisphere, although 21% of such patients had major wounding on the right side. However, among the 47 left-handed patients who sustained head wounds, aphasia was associated only with left-sided lesions. Disturbances of the motor and sensory systems, commonly associated, in many instances improved. Some form of paroxysmal epileptic disorder occurred in 28% of the patients, but only 22.9% had more than one definite attack. The prognosis was more favorable in those patients who had their attacks soon after injury. In the social and economic rehabilitation of the head-injured patient the severity of injury played an important role, but perhaps even more important was the personality and intelligence of the head-injured men.

Walker *et al.* (1971) have reported on the life expectancy of head injured men with and without epilepsy. On the basis of a study of Bavarian veterans of World War I, made 50 years after the war, it has been found that life expectancy of men with head injuries, particularly those with post-traumatic epilepsy, is shorter than that of uninjured veterans and of the male population of similar age. This disparity becomes greater after the age of 50, and at age 75 is at least 3.3 years for the head injured, and 4.9 years for those with post-traumatic epilepsy.

Seven patients with post-traumatic epilepsy in addition to headache were divided into those who had had no attacks for two years or more and those continuing to have attacks. Although the numbers were small, there was no evidence that the brain waves were more often abnormal in the group with seizures than in the seizure-free group, thus suggesting that the encephalogram has a limited value in the prognosis of post-traumatic epilepsy.

The two features of special interest in this study are the observations that *(a)* the site of brain injury was not relevant to the amount of impairment of highest integrative functions—only the severity; and, *(b)* the occurrence of headache was related to factors other than brain damage.

It may not be inferred because a patient gives evidence of brain damage, such as motility and sensory disturbances, defects in mentation, or grossly abnormal CAT scans or operative visualization, that any associated headache is due to brain injury. In fact, in the New York Hospital patients, no relation existed between the presence or absence of such abnormalities and chronic post-traumatic headache. This is in accord with the inference of Friedman and Merritt (1945) who found no correlation between the occurence of headache and the severity of the injury as shown by the spinal fluid pressure or the presence of blood in the spinal fluid; and supports the opinion expressed by Brenner *et al.* (1944) that "it is doubtful if the degree of brain or meningeal injury is of significance in the genesis of the headache. Headache is related in some way to the fact of injury, not to any given feature of pathology demonstrable by the methods used,"

Also, Brenner *et al.* found no correlation between the duration of coma, disorientation, or amnesia and the incidence of post-traumatic headache. But they found the incidence of prolonged headache significantly high in patients who had a scalp laceration. There was no correlation between the incidence of prolonged headache, reflex changes, increased spinal fluid pressure, presence of blood in the spinal fluid, skull fracture, duration of hospital stay, or generalized electroencephalographic anomalies during the first week after the injury. There was close correlation between the duration of dizziness and the duration of headache. They found "a strikingly low incidence of prolonged headache in the group of recreational accidents, a suggestively low incidence among domestic accidents and a suggestively high incidence among industrial accidents."

From these various considerations it seems likely that noxious stimuli arising from within the head and causing pain either directly or reflexly are factors of relatively minor significance in the causation of chronic post-traumatic headache.

It may not be inferred that this type of headache has resulted from any direct damage to the cranial vasculature. Sustained resentment, tension, frustration, and exhaustion precipitated perhaps by the injury to the head were important to these patients, as are such states to other patients with vascular headaches and migraine.

The Pathophysiology of Scotomata Associated with a Sudden High-Intensity Head Pain

Six patients with post-traumatic headache complained of photophobia and of seeing bright flashes of light with sudden exacerbations of the headache. Also, two of these patients reported an intensification of light with photophobia during vertigo. In these patients and six normal subjects it was possible to induce a sudden intensification of light or bright flash and photophobia by deep painful pressure upon the soft structures of the occiput and neck, and in the six patients with post-traumatic headache by sudden painful movements of the head and neck. The induction of deep analgesia of the soft structures of the occiput and neck by the injection of 1% procaine hydrochloride made impossible experimental reproduction of headache and scotomata.

Comment. Various types of scotomata have different pathophysiology. Thus, scotomata associated with migraine headache are the result of vasoconstriction and ischemia usually within the cerebral cortex and sometimes possibly also in the retina. They characteristically precede the onset of headache but sometimes persist during the first part of the headache. Also, scotomata sometimes usher in a major epileptic seizure. Occipital lobe tumors may give rise to such visual disturbances. It is possible that the scotomata which are associated with a severe blow on the head result directly from cortical stimulation or damage. Also the sudden displacement of the eyeball by a blow, very much as when one rubs or presses upon the eyes, causes the retina and possibly the optic nerve itself to be mechanically stimulated.

Although ischemia within the cerebral cortex, direct cortical stimulation, or damage or mechanical irritation of the retina or the optic nerve may produce scotomata, another explanation for the intensification of light associated with post-traumatic headache seems more relevant. It has been shown that pain suddenly induced about the head may cause the subject to report that a constant light source appears brighter than before the onset of pain. It is inferred that a spread of excitation associated with a sudden high-intensity pain in the head may cause the subject to report a sudden flash of light. This would appear to be the explanation of seeing bright lights or stars with the precipitation of a painful muscle cramp or with painful pressure on a tender muscle in patients with headaches of types 1 and 2.

Neck Trauma and Vasodilating Headache

Vijayan (1977) has described a post-traumatic headache syndrome based on his observation of seven patients who suffered neck injury, Unilateral frontotemporal vasodilating headaches were associated with ipsilateral mydriasis and facial hyperhydrosis, followed by partial ptosis and miosis. Headache frequency ranged from two to three episodes per month to eight to twelve episodes per month. Pharmacologic studies showed that partial sympathetic denervation of the affected pupil had occurred during headache-free intervals. Vijayan did not find evidence of generalized autonomic dysfunction. He postulated that the third neuronal sympathetic pathway is partially damaged in the neck, so that the headache is in effect a form of dysautonomic pain. His patients responded to treatment with the beta adrenergic blocking agent, propranolol, in doses of 20–60 mg per day. They did not respond to ergotamine.

Whiplash Injury

In this litigious era, a modern cause of head and neck pain is said to be "whiplash injury." A rear-end automobile collision occurs, first hyperextending and then hyperflexing the cervical spine of the person(s) in the vehicle struck from behind. Most patients, shortly after the accident, complain of diffuse muscular soreness which is followed by neck and head pain. The neck pain is aggravated by movement. The head pain, particularly in the early stages of the injury, is considered to be a continuation of the neck discomfort, spreading upward from the neck, the occiput, over the vertex to the frontal regions, and often localizing behind the eyes. The pain is often dull and heavy but at times may assume a throbbing character. Almost never associated with nausea and vomiting, it is persistent and tends to last for days or weeks.

In many patients the pain syndrome abates before long, usually within the first month, though there may be recurrent episodes of "stiff neck." Unfortunately, the pain sometimes becomes chronic, especially when litigation is in progress.

Physical findings are few, nonspecific, and primarily related to the neck. There may be bilateral localized painful areas in the suboccipital and nuchal regions which are aggravated by deep pressure and palpation. Often the neck is held stiffly, and on cervical spine films an absence of normal lordosis is characteristic. Many of these patients have had pre-existing cervical osteoarthritis which may or may not be important. Almost none have cervical radiculopathy related to such an injury.

Treatment should be conservative. Often patients improve with simple reassurance; use of heat, hot packs, and massage; and flexion and extension exercises of the neck. A cervical collar used at night may be helpful. Use of a cervical support during the day may be indicated. Some may benefit from injection of local anesthetics and corticosteroids into tender and painful suboccipital areas. But many do not respond until the legal process has been concluded, and even then they may refuse to give up their symptoms.

The Pathophysiology of Vertigo That Accompanies Post-traumatic Headache

Observations were made on six of the New York Hospital patients with post-traumatic headache who had sudden exacerbation of pain accompanied by vertigo when they lifted their heads from the prone to the upright position. Vertigo was experimentally induced in these subjects when they were lying on a bed in the prone position by painful pressure upon tender regions in the deep tissues at the base of the skull and behind the ear. Sometimes the vertigo could be induced by stimulating with traction or pressure within the external auditory meatus. Two patients reported, during attacks of vertigo, intensification of light with photophobia. The induction of deep analgesia by the injection of 1% procaine

hydrochloride into deep tender areas of muscle at the base of the skull and behind the ear eliminated pain and giddiness and made their experimental reproduction impossible.

Comment. Vertigo as an accompaniment of head pain or post-traumatic headache probably does not stem from derangements within the semicircular canals. To explain such vertigo it is unnecessary to assume damage to the eighth cranial nerve or brainstem, or fundamental derangements in brainstem circulation. It is probable that noxious stimuli arising within muscles and their attachments cause a widespread excitation of the brain stem near the vestibular nuclei and thus produce the vertigo.

Campbell and Parsons (1944) induced head pain experimentally by injecting hypertonic salt solution into the scalp and neck. The pain was accompanied by giddiness, listing, pallor, sweating, nausea, and pulse changes. They, too, considered that these phenomena arose through spread of excitation among the cranial nerve nuclei and association tracts of the upper cervical cord and the brainstem. They also recognized that noxious stimuli arising in the periosteum, ligaments, connective tissue, blood vessels, and muscles of the upper cervical region could give rise to vigorous and sustained muscular contraction which augmented the original pain. They were able to eliminate both the local pain at the site of the experimental lesion in the neck and the referred pain about the head by procaine infiltration of the primary source of noxious stimulation.

Friedman and his co-workers (1945) found that 51% of 102 patients with head injury complained of dizziness or vertigo at some time after the injury. It was intermittent and of variable severity, duration, and frequency. Change in posture was the most common precipitating factor. There was little evidence that post-traumatic dizziness was related to damage to the vestibular end-organ.

The Psychodynamics of Post-traumatic Headache

So important do symbolic factors of, and aside from, the injury itself become to a patient with head trauma that their appraisal is necessary for a proper interpretation of the post-traumatic headache syndrome. The head has special symbolic significance in that injury of this part may do far more injury to the individual than the local tissue damage would, on superficial consideration, appear to justify. This topic, with an adequate bibliography, has been reviewed by Kozol (1945) and by Adler (1945).

To most anxious persons the use of the head, the wits, the ability to be ever on the alert, to apprehend danger and lurking forces of destruction, are the very bases of such meager security as they possess. To have an accident occur that involves the organ of these defenses is terrifying. The differences between civilian and military patients were not significant enough to justify special classification of data.

The Incidence of Psychoneuroses in Patients with Chronic Post-traumatic Headache

According to Brenner *et al.* (1944) the incidence of headache lasting longer than two months after injury was significantly high in those patients who were psychoneurotic prior to the accident; in those patients who without disturbance of consciousness were restless, excitable, apathetic, or particularly disturbed emotionally during the first week after the injury; in those patients who, after discharge, complained of fears, anxieties, fatigability, irritability, or concentration difficulties; and in those with unfavorable life situations, especially occupational difficulties and pending litigation.

The 63 patients of the New York Hospital series were examined by means of interview, the Shipley-Hartford Retreat Scale for Measuring Intellectual Impairment, and the Cornell Service Index.

Two-thirds of the patients were found to have some degree of intellectual impairment, and one-seventh were considered to have serious impairment of intellectual function.

As a result of the interview and the Cornell Service Index, Form S, which is intended to aid in the screening of "persons with personality or psychosomatic disturbance," it was revealed that two-fifths of the patients had serious disturbance. An

additional one-third had a moderate neuropsychiatric disturbance. Thus, almost three-quarters of the patients had anxiety feelings, concomitant bodily disturbances, and hypochondriasis as outstanding features. About four-fifths of the patients were psychoneurotic before they sustained head injury. Nearly one-half of the 37 subjects on whom data were available had a parent, usually the mother, who suffered from headache, and in addition almost one-third had evidence of neurosis or psychosis in some member of the family.

These facts about the occurrence of grave adaptive difficulties in some patients with chronic post-traumatic headache, make it extremely likely that delusional pain is a prevailing factor and that the peripheral elements are of incidental significance.

Kudrow and Sutkus (1979) have made a psychophysiological assessment of minimally injured patients with chronic post-traumatic headache. Twenty-nine patients having various types of chronic post-traumatic head pain were evaluated for cortical impairment by the Halstead-Reitin psychophysiologic test battery. When their scores were compared, moderately severely injured patients could not be distinguished from those with mild head injuries, although approximately half of all the patients had evidence of abnormal cortical function. In addition, eight patients with headache on the basis of a conversion reaction were tested and the results compared to those from the chronic post-traumatic group. A higher frequency of cortical impairment was noted in patients with headache on the basis of conversion reaction, although occurrence of depression was similar in both groups.

Kudrow and Sutkus suggest that cortical dysfunction, as determined by this test battery, is associated with both chronic post-traumatic headache and conversion cephalgia, but the extent of post-traumatic head pain cannot be correlated with the severity of the head injury. Since chronic post-traumatic headache may occur in the absence of serious head injury, it reflects instead a cerebral biochemical disorganization as a specific response to "an accident" and is similar to the chronic or emotional trauma seen in conversion cephalgia, rather than to any specific anatomic injury.

CLINICAL APPLICATION

To reduce the incidence of headache and the number and seriousness of other sequelae following head injury, it was formerly considered good practice to keep such patients in bed for many weeks after the accident. Eight to ten weeks of complete immobilization in bed was not unusual. In retrospect it seems likely that such prolonged bed rest produced many sequelae.

The Second World War and the Korean War, in renewing interest in manpower and in shortening convalescence, caused this attitude to be challenged. Patients were urged to get out of bed as soon as they desired and were pressed into active service within two to three weeks of the period of injury, assuming that mentation was not so disturbed as to impair military effectiveness. After such accelerated convalescence the usual sequelae of head injury were reduced or absent. This has been attributed in good part to the attitude of the physician who, in minimizing the significance of the head injury by getting the patient out of bed and urging him to take part in the ward routine, eliminated the unexpressed fears of the patient and convinced him as would no spoken word that the damage done had been insignificant.

If, on the other hand, after the accident the physician imposes long bed rest, is anxious about pain, vertigo, and lightheadedness; if he creates an atmosphere of uncertainty or impending catastrophe by his own doubts and anxiety, then these, too, are perceived and taken on as his own by the patient.

Akin to the anxious physician in his danger to the patient with head injury is the lawyer or advisor who, because of excessive caution or unscrupulousness, suggests that the head injury may be crippling or be followed by evil effects. Such persons may present the possibilities of subdural hematoma, brain abscess, convulsions, or other late sequelae of head injury, thus postponing legal and financial settlement and blocking the patient's return to work and domestic responsibilities.

Compensation conflicts should be quickly resolved by explanation of the dynamic factors involved; all financial arrangements settled, and court and other legal procedures promptly terminated. If this cannot be achieved, if court or other legal procedures are left pending, the symptoms, including headache, may be indefinitely prolonged. It is highly important that the patient understand his motivation in seeking compensation, and its cost to him in the creation and prolongation of his symptoms. Thus, a quickly settled, lesser reward is preferable to a higher one gained at the cost of prolonged litigation. In all events, whether adjusted early or late, in or out of court, the financial settlement should be fixed and final. Compensation must not be given for an indefinite period or until such future time as the prognosis is ascertained.

In the management of the post-traumatic headache, Jones and Brown (1944) are of the opinion that the injection of procaine hydrochloride into tender muscles is a valuable therapeutic device. Such procaine injections into the soft tissue of the painful area sometimes give temporary or long-lasting reduction in the intensity of headache. However, if such sustained local tenderness and steady aching headache have persisted for longer than six months, the likelihood of elimination by procaine injection is slight. There is little danger in the use of this method if the injections are not made near the foramen magnum and atlas. However dramatic the beneficial effects of the procaine injection procedure may sometimes be, the same end result can be achieved by the less painful and less dangerous procedures of massage and heat.

As mentioned above, occasionally the patient has, in addition to the steady, sustained headache, a pulsating headache that is strikingly reduced in intensity or eliminated by ergotamine tartrate given intramuscularly in 0.5 mg amounts.

But by far the most important component of the management is the consideration of the entire reaction to the head injury. Of prime importance is the recognition of a serious depression precipitated, or accentuated, by the head injury. Failure to make a diagnosis and evaluate this mood disorder may be followed by death through suicide.

Occasionally it is sufficient for a competent and respected physician to assure the patient that no major damage has been done, and even though discomfort or pain exist they do not mean irreversible defects. Also, for the physician to emphasize that the examination reveals that no serious sequelae will follow has important and constructive influence. These reassurances and interpretations often allay the anxiety of the patient so that his head sensations assume dwindling significance. Explanation of what it is that hurts, how the vertigo occurs, and something about the other bodily symptoms strengthen this formulation. Probably the most important reassurance is the attitude of the physician who gets his patient with head injury out of bed early and minimizes the significance of his symptoms.

An evaluation of the setting in which the accident occurred is very important. An appraisal of preaccident feelings such as anxiety, resentment, frustration, despair; a review of the entire life situation and the place of the accident in this setting, when understood by the patient, may make a basic difference in his attitude, emotional state, and bodily symptoms.

The prognosis for long-standing post-traumatic headache cannot be expressed in general terms, since much depends on the rapport between patient and physician. If the individual's history previous to the accident demonstrated long-standing and serious maladjustment, the prognosis is grave.

DISABILITY AFTER INJURY

The patient with long continued disability after injury presents a medical enigma. Patients with significant head injury may be particularly difficult to evaluate. The problem is further compounded by current economic and social pressures, especially the lure of large monetary awards which may be proffered by courts proceeding with elaborate and languorous speed toward decisions regarding remuneration for pain, suffering, and other indefinables.

What of the patient with chronic post-traumatic headache, with prolonged symptoms which defy treatment of whatever sort? Certainly these patients deserve the most careful and thorough study, which may serve to rule out organic disease. Yet it is rare to find any evidence of significant disease in a patient whose complaints extend over many years, especially if the initial injury was not severe. Individuals with chronic post-traumatic headache were demonstrated to have elevations in the hysterical, depressive, and hypochondriacal scales when psychologic testing was performed. Their headaches might then be interpreted as a manifestation of an inappropriate response to trauma, occurring in persons with an already vulnerable personality.

These concepts are supported by Miller and Stern (1965) regarding the late effects of head trauma. Briefly, the prognosis in severe trauma may not be as forbidding as it seems at the time of the initial injury, when the injury is severe. These authors dismiss prolonged disability, of the headache and dizziness sort, as a manifestation of neurotic behavior. One gets the impression that there may be an inverse relationship between the severity of the injury

and the eventual disability, in those with a susceptible personality structure. The English, with their long experience in compensation medicine, seem better disposed to call a spade a spade in such cases.

How then to classify patients with these symptoms? We would suggest that they be included in the general category of contemporary conversion reactions. This is a broad category of disease in which unconsciously simulated chronic illness may serve to obscure a serious emotional disorder. The patients complain of specific and relatively enduring physical symptoms, especially pain, for which no organic basis can be found. "Conversion" refers to the alternation of anxiety or depression produced by an emotional illness which, in a metaphorical sense, is thereafter converted into acceptable physical symptoms. The qualifying adjective 'contemporary' is necessary, since these reactions may vary considerably depending upon the structure and stresses engendered by the culture in which they occur. One no longer sees patients with the sort of hysteria demonstrated with such gusto by Charcot, for example. As the general level of education and sophistication rises, so also do the manifestations of conversion reactions become more subtle and complex.

Conversion reactions may thus be construed as conditions in which the patients enact sick role behavior, albeit subconsciously, since they are usually convinced of the somatic nature of their complaints. This is especially true in chronic headache related to previous trauma. The traumatic episode is or was tangible. There may well be permanent evidence in the form of scars, old fractures, or news clippings to support the patient's contention that his symptoms are related entirely to trauma. Furthermore, the patient may insist on some organic procedure calculated to allay his symptoms. In these circumstances, the various forms of physical therapy may be harmless and even effective. They have the merit of the laying on of hands. Often, however, more drastic surgical measures are employed, including nerve crushes and the like, cervical spinal fusions, and the removal of discs or spurs which may be centimeters away from the area of pain.

This might be called "Mt. Everest surgery"; the lesions are removed because "they are there." Whether these procedures are indicated must, of course, be carefully evaluated in the individual case. We suspect, however, that some of them represent placebo surgery, similar to the internal mammary artery ligations of angina pectoris.

The concept of prolonged disability in post-traumatic headache may thus need new scrutiny. Whether the headache is related to organic disease or to a conversion reaction, the patient is often nonetheless quite disabled. Indeed, those patients whose headache represents a conversion reaction are more likely to be seriously incapacitated than their brothers with organic disease. In recent years the psychiatric sequelae of trauma have become compensable; there is no good reason why patients with longstanding post-traumatic headache on the basis of a conversion reaction may not be included in this group.

SUMMARY

1. Post-traumatic headache is found to be of three varieties: (a) severe pain or circumscribed tenderness in a scar or site of impact; (b) a steady pressure sensation or aching pain in a circumscribed area, often in a band-like distribution; and (c) a throbbing and aching pain occurring in attacks, usually unilateral, and in the temporal, occipital, and frontal regions.

2. The first type is presented by those patients who have tender areas in the scalp, which may presist for years after the trauma.

3. The second type results from sustained skeletal muscle contraction. This is associated with tension and apprehension. In some instances these contractions represent unconscious protective immobilization of the head and neck.

4. The third type of headache is caused by recurrent episodes of distention of arterial walls. Such pain is reduced by compression of painful arteries and by use of ergotamine tartrate.

5. The pathophysiology of the pain following head trauma is therefore related to local tissue damage, sustained head or neck muscle contraction, and dilatation of the branches of the external carotid arteries.

6. Often the patient will exhibit more than one type of headache.

7. Nearly all patients studied harbored resentment related to the circumstances of their accident, or fear that they had sustained permanent damage to their brain. Such emotional reactions and attitudes were intimately related to the prolonged disability which often accompanies post-traumatic headache.

REFERENCES

Adler, A. (1945). Mental symptoms following head injury. *Arch. Neurol. Psychiat.* 53, 34.

Brenner, C., A. P. Friedman, H. H. Merritt, and D. E. Denny-Brown (1944). Post-traumatic headache. *J. Neurosurg.* 1, 379.

Bues, E. E. (1956). Formen des posttraumatischen kopfschmerze. *Der Neuralgische Schmerz*, p. 98. Georg Thieme Verlag, Stuttgart.

Campbell, D. G., and C. M. Parsons (1944). Referred head pain and its concomitants. Report of preliminary experimental investigation with implications for the post-traumatic "head" syndrome. *J. Nerv. Ment. Dis.* 99, 544.

Cyriax, J. (1938). Rheumatic headache. *Brit. Med. J.* 2, 1367.

Elliott, F. A. (1944). Tender muscles in sciatica. Electromyographic studies. *Lancet* 11, 47.

Friedman, A. P., and C. Brenner (1944). Post-traumatic and histamine headache. *Arch. Neurol. Psychiat.* 52, 126.

Friedman, A. P., C. Brenner, and D. Denny-Brown (1945). Post-traumatic vertigo and dizziness. *J. Neurosurg.* 2, 36.

Friedman, A. P., and H. H. Merritt (1945). The relationship of intracranial pressure and presence of blood in the cerebrospinal fluid to the occurrence of headaches in patients with injuries to the head. *J. Nerv. Ment. Dis.* 102, 1.

Jones, O. W., Jr., and H. A. Brown (1944). The measurement of post-traumatic head pain. *J. Nerv. Ment. Dis.* 99, 668.

Kozol, H. L. (1945). Pre-traumatic personality and psychiatric sequelae of head injury. *Arch. Neurol. Psychiat.* 53, 358.

Kudrow, L., and B. Sutkus (1979). Chronic post-traumatic headache: psychophysiologic assessment of minimally injured patients. *Headache 19*, in press.

Kunkle, E. C., B. S. Ray, and H. G. Wolff (1942). Studies on headache: the mechanisms and significance of headache associated with brain tumor. *Bull. N.Y. Acad. Med. 18*, 400.

Kunkle, E. C., B. S. Ray, and H. G. Wolff (1943).

Experimental studies on headache: analysis of the headache associated with changes in intracranial pressure. *Arch. Neurol. Psychiat. 49, 323.*

Merritt, H. H., A. P. Friedman, and C. Brenner (1944). Headache and the post-traumatic syndrome. *Trans. Am. Neurol. Assoc. 70, 57.*

Miller, H. (1961). Accident neurosis. *Brit. Med. J. 1, 919, 992.*

Miller, H., and G. Stern (1965). The long-term prognosis of severe head injury. *Lancet 1, 225.*

Penfield, W. (1927). Chronic meningeal (post-traumatic) headache and its specific treatment by lumbar air insufflation; encephalography. *Surg. Gynecol. Obstet. 45, 747.*

Penfield, W., and N. C. Norcross (1936). Subdural traction and post-traumatic headache: study of pathology and therapeusis. *Arch. Neurol. Psychiat. 36, 75.*

Ray, B. S., and H. G. Wolff (1940). Experimental studies on headache. Pain-sensitive structures of the head and their significance in headache. *Arch. Surg. 41, 813.*

Ross, W. D., and F. L. McNaughton (1944). Head injury. A study of patients with chronic post-traumatic complaints. *Arch. Neurol. Psychiat. 52, 255.*

Simons, D. J., E. Day, H. Goodell, and H. G. Wolff (1943). Experimental studies on headache: muscles of the scalp and neck as sources of pain. *Assoc. Res. Nerv. Dis. Proc. 23, 228.*

Simons, D. J., and H. G. Wolff (1946). Studies on headache: mechanisms of chronic post-traumatic headache. *Psychosom. Med. 8, 227.*

Vijayan, N. (1977). A new post-traumatic headache syndrome: clinical and therapeutic observations. *Headache 17, 19–22.*

Walker, A. E. (1965). Chronic post-traumatic headache. *Headache 5, 67.*

Walker, A. E., A. Luchs, H. Lechtape-Gruber, W. F. Caveness, and C. Kretschman (1971). Life expectancy of head injured men with and without epilepsy. *Arch. Neurol. 24, 95.*

Watts, J. W., W. B. Wiley, and R. H. Groh (1944). The relation of contusion of the scalp to post-traumatic headache and dizziness. *Assoc. Res. Nerv. Dis. Proc. 24, 562.*

Wolff, G. A., Jr., H. Goodell, and H. G. Wolff (1945). Prognosis of subarachnoid hemorrhage and its relation to long-term management. *JAMA 129, 715.*

17

INHERITANCE AND EPIDEMIOLOGY OF HEADACHE

RICHARD A. SMITH

INTRODUCTION

Migraine headache is a common disorder that often effects more than one member of a family. In 1873, Liveing observed that "megrim" appeared to be transmitted from parent to child. Although the subject of heredity and headache has received considerable attention, the role of inheritance is still unsettled because study of hereditary factors has been hampered by a number of methodologic problems. There is no biochemical or physiologic marker which can serve as a diagnostic test for headache. Lacking this, collection of data depends on the use of clinical criteria. Headache reports from patients, by necessity, constitute the data base. Although individuals and committees have proposed criteria for the diagnosis of migraine, when these are put to test they have proved inadequate to exclude all but the migraine sufferer. Most definitions of migraine stress the occurrence of unilateral head pain accompanied by nausea and visual disturbance. Some definitions include evidence for a positive family history of headache. Waters (1973) recently addressed the problem by comparing the expected and observed numbers of individuals with various combinations of symptoms commonly attributed to migraine. This study failed to document a "migraine syndrome." Ziegler (1976) came to a similar conclusion after studying the association of 27 headache variables. For example, nausea and unilateral headaches did not correlate. Further methodologic problems have been discussed by Dalsgaard-Nielsen (1970). He found that headache reports from patients are often inaccurate. This finding casts serious doubts on studies of family pedigrees which have been based on headache histories reported secondhand.

EPIDEMIOLOGY

Studies of migraine in office practice or hospital practice suggest that the prevalence of migraine ranges from 1 to 20% (Waters and O'Connor, 1971). A more direct and accurate estimate of the prevalence of migraine in the general population has been made by surveying communities. These pioneering studies were carried out in Wales by Waters (1970 and 1974; Waters and O'Connor, 1975). Not surprisingly, migraine was found to be more frequent in the general population than in defined groups. Prevalence was 23.2% for women age 21 and over, and 14.9% for men. Interviews of women selected from 12 American cities revealed an essentially similar prevalence (Markush *et al.,* 1975). In this group, migraine occurred with slightly greater frequency in blacks than whites. Social class was not seen as a significant headache variable in these American women or in subjects from Wales. Similarly, impressions that the patient with migraine is almost invariably intelligent were not borne out by this study (Waters, 1971).

Contrary to common belief, migraine is common among children. Bille (1962) found a 4% incidence in children age 7–15 in Uppsala, Sweden. In 62.5% headaches were one-sided. Approximately 80% of headaches were accompanied by nausea and 50% by visual aura. A positive family history was present in 78% of children. From age 7 to 9 the sex distribution was similar but above age 10 headaches were more frequent in girls. Recurrent headaches occurred in 6.3% of 7-year-old Finnish school children and 3.2% of these children were thought to have migraine (Sillanpää, 1975). Hemiplegic migraine is said to be common in children (Prensky, 1976). Basilar migraine, described by Bickerstaff (1961), is most common in adolescent girls—26 of 32 patients in the original series being of this age and sex. Although severe headaches usually start in the early decades of life, 23% of headache sufferers note the onset of headaches after age 40, and 4.1% after age 55 (Ziegler *et al.*, 1977).

FAMILY STUDIES OF MIGRAINE

Common Migraine

The patient with migraine headache commonly reports that other members of his family have similar headaches. The migraine syndrome has long been considered familial, and some investigators have presented familial occurrences as evidence of hereditary character. Tissot (1790) has been credited with first emphasizing the hereditary factor in migraine. In 1858 Symonds reported 44% of migrainous persons gave a history of headache in one or both parents. Figures of 50% positive parental history were reported by Liveing in 1873, 64% by Henke in 1881, 90% by Moebus in 1894, and almost 100% by Auerback in 1912. Allan (1928) who quotes these latter references, concluded a dominant mode of inheritance for migraine although his calculations were influenced by an unacceptably high estimate of the incidence (60%) of migraine in the general population. Balyeat and Rinkel (1931) stated that the factor of heredity in migraine was unquestioned, and presented four detailed family trees showing the occurrence of migraine in two and three generations. Lennox (1941) found 61% of a group of 425 patients with migraine headache at the Boston City Hospital, who were able to recall that a parent also had attacks of sick headache of a similar

nature. This contrasted with a group of nurses, medical students, and miscellaneous patients among whom 11% were able to recall a parent with migraine attacks. Graham (1954) in a study of 46 patients with migraine headaches, reported 80% of them gave a history of having relatives with migraine among immediate family of siblings, parents, aunts, uncles, and grandparents. Goodell, Lewontin, and Wolff (1954) analyzed 119 migraine patients who were selected by rigid clinical criteria including response of the headache to ergotamine tartrate. Pedigrees were constructed for each family based on information meticulously collected by personal interview, questionnaire, and review of correspondence among family members. It was found that the probability of migraine in offspring increased with the number of parents affected. It was concluded from these data that migraine was inherited as a "recessive gene" whose penetrance was obtained from the fact that of the 65 offspring of parents both of whom had migraine, only 45, or 69.2%, had headaches. In the first edition of this book a second interpretation of these data was suggested—"it is also entirely possible that a multifactorial inheritance related to several genes is responsible for the eventual expression of migraine." This interpretation is more in keeping with contemporary concepts of inheritance.

Friedman (1959) found an incidence of migraine in nearest relatives of 65% but he did not commit himself regarding the role of heredity and, in fact, felt environmental factors could play a dominant role. Friedman (1951) noted that migraine is more frequently seen in daughters than in sons of migrainous mothers. He reported further that familial incidence was 60% in patients who were refractory to therapy.

Selby and Lance (1960) reported a positive family history in 55% of 464 patients. Childs and Sweetman (1961) found that 37% of relatives of workers with migraine had a history of migraine, whereas relatives of healthy workers had a 6% incidence.

Reviewing three personal series of cases totaling 350 cases, Dalsgaard-Nielsen (1965) found a familial incidence of 90%. As expected, migraine occurred more frequently in maternal line than in paternal line in these series. The author concluded that "exogenic influences certainly play a very great part as the factors which precipitate headache but they must be considered to be secondary in relation to the actual disease of migraine which must be considered hereditary." He stated that "dominant heredity cannot be excluded," and "recessive heredity is improbable on account of varying manifestation and distribution of cases." However, Dalsgaard-Nielsen "considers it to be probable that the basis for heredity is complicated, possibly with an additive effect of numerous genes." Ziegler (1977) makes note that a positive family history of migraine has varied in the medical literature from 14 to 90%. He cautions that it would be unwise to compare reported series because varying diagnostic criteria for migraine have been used and only rarely was information obtained over an extended period. Further data regarding relatives have usually been obtained secondhand. This latter problem was a concern of Dalsgaard-Nielsen who observed "that it is not until several interviews that the patient can provide adequate information about, for example, actual dates, the nature of the headache, and the familial history of the migraine" (Dalsgaard-Nielsen *et al.*, 1970).

Complicated Migraine

Several varieties of vascular headaches are so striking in presentation that their identifying characteristics make them potential models for the study of hereditary patterns of headache. Both hemiplegic migraine and basilar migraine stand apart from the more common headache patterns from which they cannot be confused. They thus afford a unique opportunity for study when present in families. In 1910 Clarke published the history of a family in which three generations had suffered from the complaint of hemiplegic migraine. More recently, Glista *et al.* (1975) described a family in which 10 members experienced stereotyped migrainous attacks associated with motor, sensory, and language disturbances. None of the family had common migraine. The pedigree of

this family is diagrammed in Fig. 17-1. As can be readily seen, the mode of inheritance of hemiplegic migraine in this family excludes autosomal or dominant sex-linked inheritance.

This pedigree can be explained by either an autosomal recessive or multifactorial pattern of inheritance. It is of additional interest that at least one external factor was apparent in this family: 3 out of 10 afflicted members of the family experience their attacks in relation to minor head injury. More attention might profitably be given to these special cases of migraine in future research.

Twin Studies

Study of headache in identical and nonidentical twins offers an opportunity to assess genetic and environmental factors. Both members of a twin pair are concordant when they are affected similarly and discordant when only one member of the pair is affected. Since environmental factors are generally the same within families, data comparing the degree of concordance for headache among identical and nonidentical twins provide a clue as to the role of heredity in headache.

The most complete twin study was conducted by Ziegler *et al.* (1975). Twins were typed for blood grouping and several other biologic markers determined. The relative probability of monozygosity was calculated from these data and subjective measures such

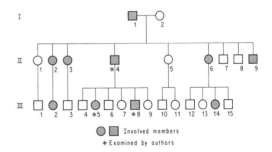

FIG. 17-1. Pedigree of a family with hemiplegic migraine. The circles are females, the squares are males; shaded symbols indicate affected members. Asterisks refer to patients examined by the authors. Reprinted by permission (Glista *et al.*, 1975).

as height and physical appearance were scored. Finally, the subjects themselves were queried for their opinion regardint the relatedness of their sibling. One hundred and six twin pairs were studied. It was concluded that 65 were dizygotic and 41 monozygotic. Approximately 11% of males and 22.5% of the females experienced severe headaches.

Analyzing concordance as to specific headache symptoms, the authors found that specific headache symptoms were no more concordant among twins than was the overall occurrence of headache.

In comparing the results of their study with previous twin studies, these authors make note of the fact that few of the earlier twin studies had exacting requirements for determination of zygosity. They also speculate that earlier studies were possibly at variance with their study because of difference in selection of patients. The authors studied a nonclinic population with severe recurrent headaches.

Juel-Nielsen (1964) reported concordance as to headaches in three of five pairs of monozygotic twins who were reared apart from each other. Lennox and Lennox (1960) found five sets of twins concordant for migraine. Three of these pairs also had seizures. Harvald and Hague (1956) in a survey of 1900 twins in Denmark found a 2.2% incidence of migraine. Six monozygotic twins were discordant, a concordance ratio of 33%. Fifty-four dizygotic twins were discordant for headache and three were concordant.

These results argue strongly against any simple pattern of inheritance, but the data have not generally been interpreted from the point of view of polygenic inheritance. In cases of polygenic inheritance concordance in twins depends on the population frequency of the disease as well as the heritability (Edwards, 1969). With a high heritability the concordance rate in identical twins may be quite low. This seeming paradox is illustrated by example of clubfoot. In this condition the incidence is 1 per 1000 and the heritability is approximately 70%. The concordance rate in monozygotic (MZ) twins has been determined to be 33%. This is roughly in agreement with the expected value.

The notion of heritability allows a prediction as to the relative influence of heredity and environment in cases of polygenic inheritance. It is calculated by comparing the known incidence of a condition in the general population with the incidence in relatives. Borrowing from the calculations of Smith (1970) it is possible to make an estimate of the heritability of migraine if data on the incidence of migraine in the general population and concordance rate in monozygous twins are known. As reviewed, these data are not consistent, but with reservations it can be speculated that the heritability for migraine is about 25%. This figure could be higher or lower. This estimate is arrived at by assuming a 20% incidence for migraine in the general population and by acepting the twin figures of Harvald and Hague (1956) as a minimal estimate of the concordance of headache in identical twins.

Conclusion

Progress has been made in the study of the epidemiology of headache. It is now established that headache occurs in the young with essentially equal distribution between the sexes until adolescence. After that, there is a disproportionate female preponderance. In nonclinic adult populations, headache prevalence is approximately 23% for women and 15% for men.

Confronted with conflicting statistics investigators have now come to appreciate that a history of migraine may not be clearly distinguished from other headaches. At the moment, the inability to clearly identify the family history of migraine precludes any progress toward defining the genetics of migraine. From the standpoint of the geneticist, it is extremely important to distinguish between similar conditions. Many conditions appear to be similar but are inherited quite differently. Other conditions (phenocopies) mimic genetic disorders but are determined by environmental factors. Until migraine can be better defined, the genetics of headache cannot be fruitfully investigated. For those that fancy such dry work, there is some cheer in that at least contemporary commentators, in contrast to earlier workers, consider the question of heredity and headache to be unresolved.

What lies ahead? Are the methodologic problems beyond solution? It is likely that some of the problems are artifacts of our system of analysis rather than nature. It may be more accurate to think of headache and its associated symptoms as part of a continuous process. Waters (1973) has suggested a similar hypothesis. Viewed differently, headache may yet be convincingly demonstrated to have an hereditary basis. Normal human traits such as stature and intelligence and abnormal traits such as hypertension are thought to have a multifactorial pattern of inheritance. They are distributed through the population in a Gausian manner (bell-shaped curve). It is likely that headache has a similar distribution, but proof of this hypothesis requires further study. Considering the methadologic obstacles, further progress in defining the role of heredity in migraine would seem to require a fundamental advance in our understanding of headache.

SUMMARY

1. Headache occurs in the young with essentially equal distribution between the sexes until adolescence.

2. Subsequently there is disproportionate female preponderance. In nonclinic adult populations, headache prevalence is 23% for women and 15% for men.

3. The genetics of migraine are difficult to state precisely because of our inability to clearly identify migraine in families, since data are based on patients' family history reports.

4. It is likely that migraine has a multifactorial pattern of inheritance, distributed through the population in a Gaussian manner. Nonetheless, pinpointing the role of heredity in migraine would seem to require a fundamental advance in our understanding of headache processes.

REFERENCES

Allan, W. (1928). The inheritance of migraine. *Arch. Intern. Med. 42*, 590-599.

Balyeat, R. M., and H. J. Rinkel (1931). Further studies in allergic migraine. *Ann. Intern. Med. 5*, 713.

Bickerstaff, E. R. (1961). Basilar artery migraine. *Lancet 1*, 15.

Bille, B. (1962). The frequency of migraine in children of school age. *Acta Pediatr. (Suppl. 136) 51*, 33.

Childs, A. J., and M. T. Sweetman (1961). A study of 104 cases of migraine. *Brit. J. Industr. Med. 18*, 234.

Clarke, J. M. (1910). On recurrent motor paralysis in migraine with report of a family in which recurrent hemiplegia accompanied the attacks. *Brit. Med. J. 1*, 1534-1538.

Dalsgaard-Neilsen, T. (1965). *Acta Neurol. Scand. 41*, 287-300.

Dalsgaard-Nielsen, T., H. Engberg-Pedersen, and Holger E. Holm (1970). Clinical and statistical investigations of the epidemiology of migraine; an investigation of the onset age and its relation to sex, adrenarche, menarche and the menstrual cycle in migraine patients, and of the menarche age, sex, distribution and frequency of migraine. *Dan. Med. Bull. 17*, 5.

Edwards, J. H. (1969). Familial predisposition in man. *Brit. Med. Bull. 25*, 58-63.

Friedman, A. P. (1951). *Modern Headache Therapy*, pp. 99-117. C. V. Mosby, St. Louis.

Friedman, A. P. (1959). *Headache, Diagnosis and Treatment*, p. 98. Davis, Philadelphia.

Glista, G. G., J. F. Mellinger, and E. D. Rooke (1975). Familial hemiplegic migraine. *Mayo Clinic Proc. 50 (6)*, 307-311.

Goodell, H., R. Lewontin, and H. G. Wolff (1954). Familial occurrence of migraine headache. *Arch. Neurol. Psychiat. (Chicago) 72*, 325.

Graham, J. R. (1954). The natural history of migraine: some observations and a hypothesis. *Am. Clin. and Climatological Assoc. Trans. 64*, 61.

Harvald, B., and M. Hague (1956). A catamnestic investigation of Danish twins. *Dan. Med. Bull. 3*, 150-158.

Juel-Nielsen, N. (1964). Individual and environment. *Acta Psychiat. Scand. 40 (Suppl. 183)*, 1-292.

Lennox, W. G. (1941). *Science and Seizures*, 2nd ed. Harper, New York and London.

Lennox, W. G., and M. A. Lennox (1960). *Epilepsy and Related Disorders*, Vol. I. Little, Brown., Boston.

Liveing, E. (1873). On megrim, sick-headache and some allied disorders. Churchill, London.

Markush, R. E., H. R. Karp, A. Heyman, and W. M. O'Fallon (1975). Epidemiologic study of migraine symptoms in young women. *Neurology 25*, 430-435.

Prensky, A. L. (1976). Migraine and migrainous variants in pediatric patients. *Pediatric Clinics of North America*, Vol. 23, No. 3, August.

Selby, G., and J. W. Lance (1960). Observations on 500 cases of migraine and allied vascular headache. *J. Neurol. Neurosurg. Psychiat. 23*, 23.

Sillanpää, M. (1976). Prevalence of migraine and other headache in Finnish children starting school. *Headache 15*, 288.

Smith, C. (1970). Heritability of liability and concordance in monozygous twins. *Ann. Hum. Genet. (Lond.)* *34*, 85.

Symonds, C. (1858). *Gulstonian Lectures*, p. 498. M. Times and Gaz.

Tissot, S. A. (1790). *Oevres de Monsieur Tissot*, Vol. 13, Grassel, Lausanne.

Waters, W. E. (1970). Community studies of the prevalence of headache. *Headache 9:* 178-186.

Waters, W. E. (1971). Migraine: intelligence, social class, and familial prevalence. *Brit. Med. J. 2:* 77-81.

Waters, W. E. (1973). The epidemiological enigma of migraine. *Intern. J. Epid.* 2, 189.

Waters, W. E. (1974). The Pontypridd headache survey. *Headache, 14,* 81-90.

Waters, W. E., and P. J. O'Connor (1971). Epidemiology of headache and migraine in women. *J. Neurol. Neurosurg. Psychiat. 34,* 148-153.

Waters, W. E., and P. J. O'Connor (1975). Prevalence of migraine. *J. Neurol Neurosurg. Psychiat. 38,* 613-616.

Ziegler, D. K. (1976). Epidemiology and genetics of migraine. *Pathogenesis and Treatment of Headache,* pp. 19-29. Spectrum, New York.

Ziegler, D. K. (1977). Genetics of migraine. *Headache 16,* 330-331.

Ziegler, D. K., R. S. Hassanein, D. Harris, and R. Stewart (1975). Headache in a non-clinic twin population. *Headache 14,* 213-218.

Ziegler, D. K., R. S. Hassanein, and J. R. Couch (1977). Characteristics of life headache histories in a nonclinic population. *Neurology 27,* 265-269.

18

RADIOLOGICAL INVESTIGATIONS IN THE
HEADACHE PATIENT*

STANLEY G. SEAT

Since headache may be a symptom of so many different diseases, its radiographic investigation has traditionally involved all of the neuroradiological procedures. Such investigations, however, have been dramatically altered by computerized tomography (CT), which was introduced to the medical community by Godfrey N. Hounsfield in 1973 (Hounsfield, 1973). Most radiologists consider this method one of the most important innovations in radiology since Roentgen discovered X-rays. It is especially valuable in intracranial evaluations and there have been exciting reports of successful CT examinations of the spinal structures (Nakagawa *et al.*, 1977). No other radiographic tool can diagnose or exclude as many different neurological diseases. Furthermore, except for the intravenous injection of iodinated contrast material with its well-known occasional adverse reactions, CT is a noninvasive procedure that can be performed, the patient's condition permitting, on outpatients. So dominant has this technique become that modern neurological diagnosis cannot be practiced without access to it.

While skull radiography, plain film tomography, angiography, pneumoencephalography, and radionuclide brain imaging still have roles to play, and in some instances are still the procedures of choice, their use is diminishing, and in the case of pneumoencephalography, has almost been eliminated.

*The author would like to thank Dr. Harvey A. Humphrey and Dr. Murray A. Warmath for providing the angiograms.

After 36 months of CT experience at the Mayo Clinic, the number of pneumoencephalograms had decreased by 80 to 90%, radionuclide brain scans about 50%, A-mode echoencephalograms around 75%, and angiograms only slightly (Baker, 1975). However, Baker also notes that the number of negative angiograms had decreased. These figures reflect the general experience in health facilities. Moreover, as more experience has been gained and referring physicians have developed confidence in CT scanning, the number of angiograms is also decreasing. This is reflected in community hospitals as well as academic centers. Reports from two community hospitals showed 60 and 66% decreases in the number of radionuclide scans being performed and indicated that angiography was being performed primarily for additional information in patients with positive CT examinations (Lurcke and Gilmore, 1977).

Thus, although it is conventionally said that various studies are complementary, brain CT excludes many others, the most frequently used complementary procedures being positive CT examinations and angiography. Even the traditional skull series is no longer felt to be necessary prior to CT (Weinstein *et al.*, 1977). Pneumoencephalography may follow a negative CT when a lesion in the cisterns or around the sella is strongly suggested clinically. When blood flow patterns are desired, a dynamic radionuclide study followed by static imaging remains the procedure of choice, since dynamic flow studies with CT are not possible with current equipment.

CT has been criticized because of its cost.

345

However, it has been shown that when cost effectiveness studies have taken into consideration the savings from elimination of other procedures, thereby reducing the hospitalization time (a saving for both patient and physician), CT has been deemed economical (Wartzman *et al.*, 1975; Evens *et al.*, 1977).

TUMORS

The detection of brain tumors by CT has been reported to have an accuracy as high as 98%, compared to 75–80% for radionuclide scans, by Knaus and Davis (1976). Christie *et al.* (1976) indicate about 90% for CT and

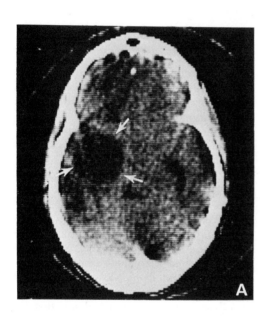

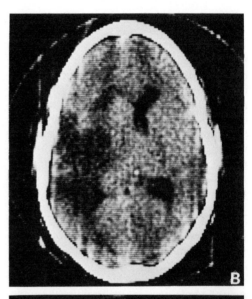

FIG. 18-1. A. Precontrast scan showing relatively round area of diminished radiodensity (arrows) with additional surrounding irregular area of diminished density secondary to edema.
B. Scan slightly superior to scan A shows extensive edema (irregular dark area), obliteration of the ventricles on the left, and marked deviation of midline structures.
C. Postcontrast scan shows irregular marginal enhancement (white appearance) of the round area demonstrated in scan A. This is frequently seen when the tumor has undergone central necrosis. This patient had an ependymoma. However, the findings of marked edema, distortion of anatomy, contrast enhancement, and frequently central necrosis are findings which may be associated with any neoplasm, especially glioma.

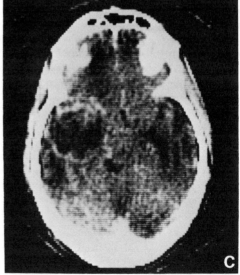

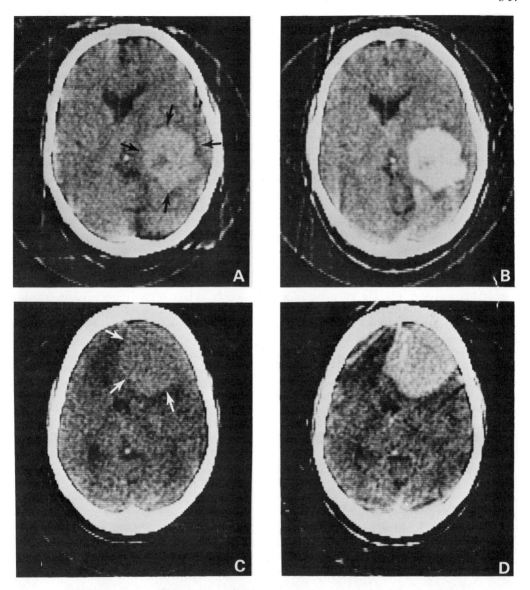

Fig. 18-2. A. Precontrast CT scan showing large meningioma (arrows) which is slightly more radiodense than surrounding normal brain tissue. The ventricles are shifted away from the lesion and distorted in configuration. Displacement of the septum pellucidum (thin line between lateral ventricles) away from the midline is also noted. The small rim of diminished density around the lesion indicates edema.

B. Postcontrast scan demonstrates increased density (enhancement) of the tumor following administration of intravenous iodinated contrast material.

C. Another patient with a large right-frontal meningioma (arrows). Density measurements were in the meningioma range but no calcifications could be seen on skull X-rays, which is not uncommon; CT is more sensitive in detecting calcifications. A rim of edema (dark area) surrounds the lesion and the lateral ventricles are compressed and displaced posteriorly and to the left.

D. Postcontrast scan demonstrates marked enhancement.

radionuclide scans, but note that some of the false negative CT examinations were performed prior to the use of contrast material and that their radionuclide studies were much more extensive and complex than those routinely performed. When data from several studies are taken into consideration, it appears that the detection rate for CT is about 95% and for radionuclide imaging slightly less. The additional advantage for CT is in determining more accurate anatomic information.

The size of the tumor is a determining factor in detection. Virtually all lesions greater than 2.5 cm are detected; but the smaller the neoplasm, the greater the rate of false negative results (Hirofumi *et al.*, 1977). Lesions, large or small, are detected by demonstrating a mass, surrounding edema, or displacement or distortion of adjacent structures—sometimes enhanced by contrast media (Fig. 18-1 and 18-2). The contrast material increases the density of some lesions because of the increased vascularity and/or breakdown in the blood-brain barrier. Therefore, this phenomenon is not confined to neoplasms. The location of tumors may cause obstructive hydrocephalus (Fig.

18-3). Metastatic lesions are readily detected by CT scan; marked surrounding edema with accompanying mass effect is the usual picture, and contrast enhancement is a constant finding (Fig. 18-4) (Davis, 1977).

Although CT is now the primary method of detecting intracranial neoplasms, this does not mean that a well performed and properly interpreted radionuclide examination will not detect the large majority of lesions and occasionally may detect a lesion not seen by CT. Therefore, it may be used as a second examination in case of a negative CT and continued strong clinical suspicion (Fig. 18-5).

Angiography gives highly specific information regarding the vascular supply to the tumor and has a very high degree of accuracy (Fig. 18-6). As previously noted, it is still frequently employed following positive CT scans prior to surgery, although the frequency is decreasing as confidence and knowledge about CT grows. Angiography also carries considerable risk and morbidity, which is the most important reason for eliminating it whenever possible. Patient anxiety may also be a problem. Statistics on complications are difficult to interpret since

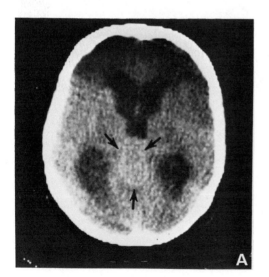 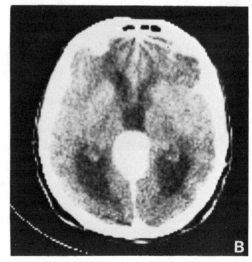

FIG. 18-3. A. A. vague oval mass of slightly increased density (arrows) is seen encroaching on the posterior third ventricle. The anterior third ventricle and lateral ventricles are greatly dilated.
B. Contrast enhancement dramatically confirms the tumor.

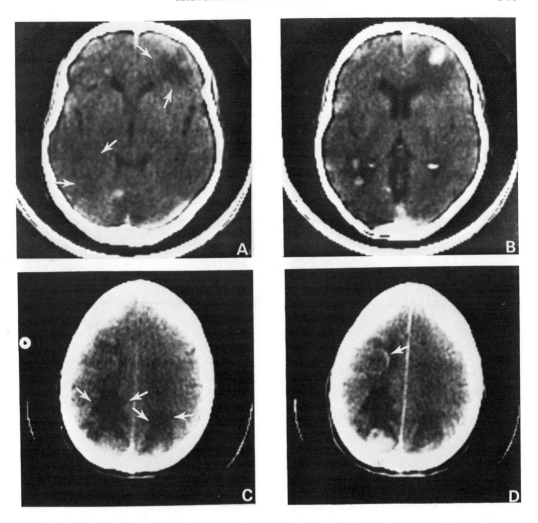

Fig. 18-4. A. Metastatic lesions with surrounding edema and associated mass effect on surrounding structures (arrows).
B. Enhancement of the lesions, but not the edema, is seen following contrast infusion. C. A second case of metastatic disease showing areas of diminished radiodensity secondary to edema (arrows).
D. Enhancement of the actual lesions is noted following contrast infusion. The ring configuration (arrow) is not unusual.

they vary considerably, especially when related to the patient's general health and underlying neurological condition. Miller *et al.* (1977) reported 0.7% severe and 5.5% mild complications for direct puncture of the carotids and 0.6% severe and 4.7% mild with retrograde brachial studies. Various series of studies with catheters are comparable. 0.5–1.0% severe and 5% mild complications are about average.

The yield from plain skull films is very low. In fact, the plain skull radiograph has one of the lowest yields of any diagnostic X-ray procedure. Except when sellar, petrous, or destructive bone lesions are suspected, many in-

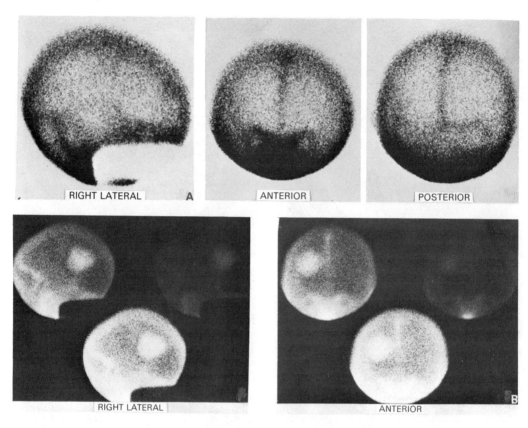

FIG. 18-5. A. Normal radionuclide brain scan utilizing technetium-99m pertechnetate. B. Scan showing isotope concentration in a meningioma. CT was not performed on this patient.

vestigators are bypassing plain film radiography in favor of CT (Weinstein *et al.*, 1977). Nevertheless, the skull X-ray does occasionally show displacement of normal calcified structures, abnormal calcifications (Fig. 18-7), reactive sclerosis (Fig. 18-8), bone erosion or destruction (Fig. 18-9), and sellar enlargement (Fig. 18-10); all such findings may be associated with intracranial neoplasms. Although all of the above findings are helpful in diagnosis, only bone destruction of the calvarium and sellar alteration are more consistently demonstrated with the plain skull X-ray than with CT, and even here the radionuclide bone scan is more sensitive to bone destruction than the conventional radiograph. Calcifications and meningiomas associated with reactive sclerosis

are demonstrated earlier and more consistently with CT examinations. Intrasellar lesions which are large enough to cause enlargement are also demonstrated readily with CT, although contrast enhancement is probably a necessity (Fig. 18-11). Some lesions too small to cause enlargement are still demonstrated by contrast-enhanced CT. Very small lesions are not usually seen by CT or plain skull X-rays. In these cases, small sellar erosions may occasionally be detected by tomography. At Montefiore Hospital and Medical Center in New York City, CT is the initial procedure for evaluating suspected sellar and suprasellar lesions, but is almost always correlated with skull films for more complete evaluation of sellar size and basal hyperostosis. When both are

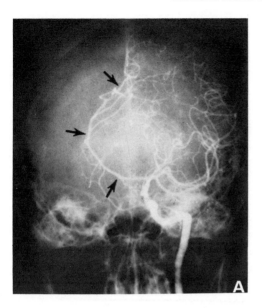
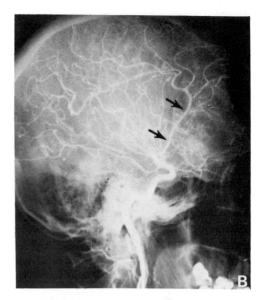

FIG. 18-6. A. Anterior-posterior projection of a carotid angiogram showing marked displacement of the anterior cerebral (arrows) across the midline secondary to a large tumor. B. The lateral projection shows the anterior cerebral (arrows) also to be displaced posteriorly by the frontal tumor. Numerous abnormal tumor vessels are seen in front of the anterior cerebral artery. This was a mixed type olfactory groove meningioma.

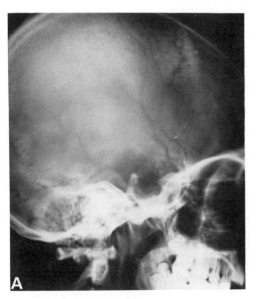
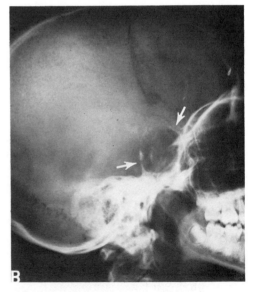

FIG. 18-7. A. Enlarged sella with mottled calcifications in the suprasellar area (not well reproduced). B. Later film shows progressive enlargement of the sella with partially calcified margin (arrows) of the suprasellar extension of the mass which was previously diagnosed as a craniopharyngioma.

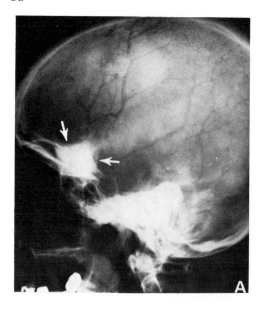
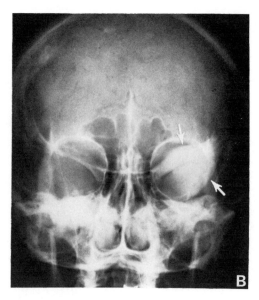

FIG. 18-8. A. Reactive bone production of left sphenoid and floor of anterior fossa (arrows) secondary to a meningioma. The appearance is quite typical.
B. Anterior-posterior X-ray showing same lesion (arrows).

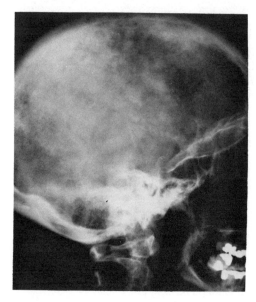

FIG. 18-9. Extensive bone destruction secondary to metastatic disease from the breast.

negative, polytomography is performed and, rarely, pneumoencephalography. However, pneumoencephalography is rarely positive when CT is normal. Patients with suprasellar lesions demonstrated by CT still have angiography prior to surgical intervention (Leeds and Thomas, 1977). This sequence seems typical for many centers.

ANEURYSMS AND VASCULAR MALFORMATIONS

CT examinations show aneurysms in most cases following contrast infusion; if the aneurysm is large, clotted, calcified (Fig. 18-12), or has hemorrhaged, it usually shows without contrast infusion (Lukin *et al.*, 1977). As newer equipment shows the vascular structures better, smaller lesions will be visualized and the exact location determined. For the present, however, the complete evaluation of an aneurysm is accomplished by angiography (Fig. 18-13). The remarks that concern

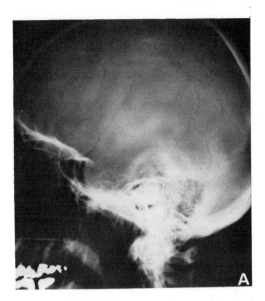

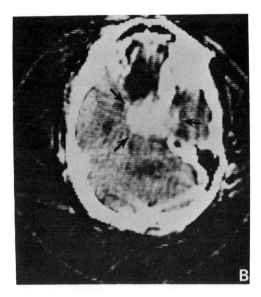

FIG. 18-10. A. Markedly enlarged sella. The posterior clinoids are destroyed.
B. CT scan following contrast infusion showing marked enhancement of the chromophobe
adenoma (arrows).

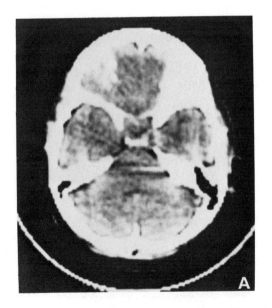

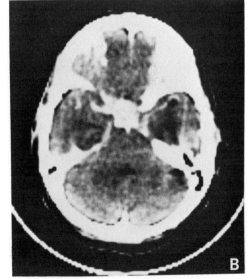

FIG. 18-11. A. Precontrast scan with no definite abnormality.
B. Postcontrast scan with profuse intrasellar enhancement in a chromophobe adenoma.

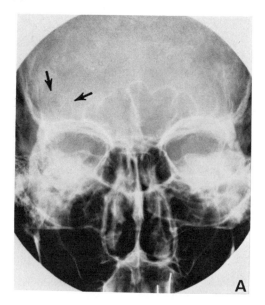
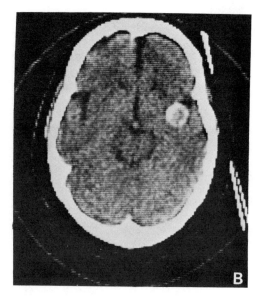

FIG. 18-12. A. Anterior projection of the paranasal sinuses shows a faint calcific ring in the approximate location of the middle cerebral artery (arrows). An aneurysm is suggested by the configuration.
B. CT clearly demonstrates the calcified aneurysm. CT is much more sensitive in detecting calcifications than conventional radiography.

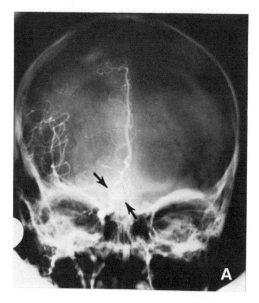
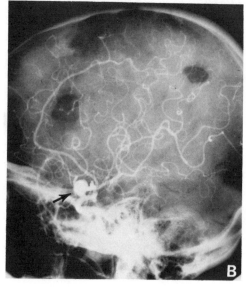

FIG. 18-13. A. Right carotid angiogram demonstrating an 11-mm aneurysm of the right anterior communicating artery (arrows).
B. Lateral projection demonstrating the same lesion (arrow).

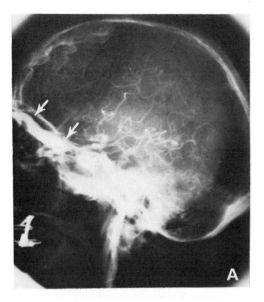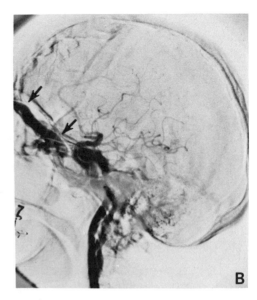

FIG. 18-14. A. Lateral projection of an angiogram showing large AV malformation in the floor of the anterior fossa and orbit (arrows).
B. Subtraction film of the same lesion demonstrates the malformation more clearly (arrows).

aneurysms also apply to AV malformations, but angiography is even more critical for complete evaluation prior to surgical intervention (Fig. 18-14).

CEREBROVASCULAR ACCIDENTS

Cerebral infarction is easily confirmed by CT, the size and location determined, and any associated hemorrhage demonstrated. Edema with secondary mass effect is seen early, variable patterns are seen during resolution, and later an area of decreased density becomes evident, frequently with enlargement of the adjacent ventricle and shift toward the lesion (Fig. 18-15). The pattern of infarction shows a more variable CT scan than do most other lesions and may mimic neoplasm, inflammation, and demyelinating disease (Lukin *et al.*, 1977). Therefore, clinical correlation is particularly important and serial studies are frequently necessary to determine the true nature of the abnormality.

Intracerebral hemorrhage has a characteris-

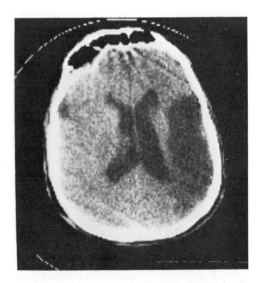

FIG. 18-15. Large area of diminished radiodensity conforming to the distribution of the right-middle cerebral artery. The slight enlargement of the ipsilateral ventricle, absence of shift of midline structures, and no contrast enhancement indicate the lesion is not recent.

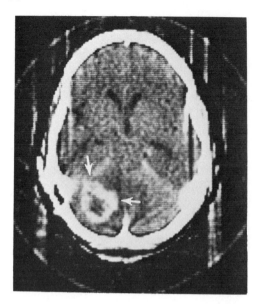

FIG. 18-16. Intracerebral hemorrhage. There is increased density in the left cerebellar area (arrows). Fresh clotted blood shows increased radiodensity which diminishes as lysis progresses.

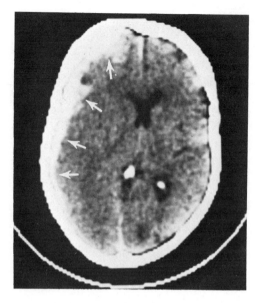

FIG. 18-17. Patient on anticoagulants with onset of headache followed by progressive neurological findings for 24 hr. The density (white) of the left subdural (arrows) indicates recent hemorrhage. There is marked shift to the right secondary to the mass effect of the hematoma.

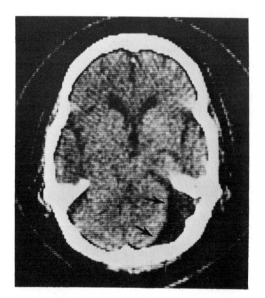

FIG. 18-18. Chronic subdural (arrows) is approximately the same density as CSF. There is less mass effect but some displacement and distortion of the quadrageminal cistern were demonstrated on scans at the appropriate levels.

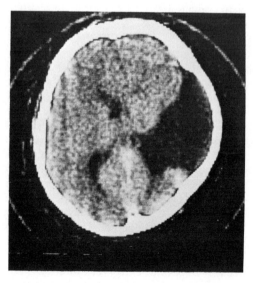

FIG. 18-19. Large right-sided porencephalic cyst. Note expansion of the adjacent skull and the communication with the ventricle.

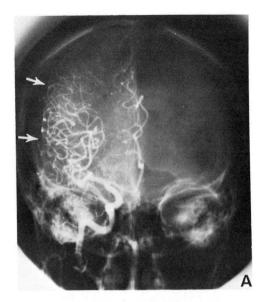 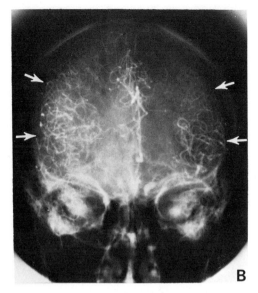

FIG. 18-20. A. Right carotid angiogram showing large subdural (arrows) displacing middle cerebral artery group away from the inner table but with relatively small displacement of the midline anterior cerebral artery group.
B. Bilateral opacification demonstrates bilateral subdurals which account for the minimal midline shift.

tic appearance and CT is the most specific and sensitive method of detecting both presence and extent of the hemorrhage (Fig. 18-16; Lukin *et al.*, 1977). The progress of an intracerebral hemorrhage is readily followed with CT.

EXTRACEREBRAL HEMORRHAGE

Extracerebral collections of blood, whether epidural or subdural, are usually demonstrated by CT, which is the initial procedure of choice. In recent extracerebral hemorrhages, as with intracerebral hemorrhages, the blood collection is denser than normal brain tissue (Fig. 18-17). This is felt to be secondary to the protein concentration in the hemoglobin (Davis *et al.*, 1977). However, this density decreases with time so that a subacute or chronic subdural presents as a lesion of low density (Fig. 18-18). Figure 18-19 has a somewhat similar appearance but is a large porencephalic

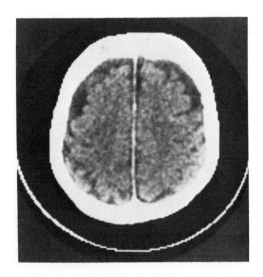

FIG. 18-21. Marked cortical atrophy has created large extracerebral spaces in both frontal areas. This should not be confused with bilateral subdural hematomas.

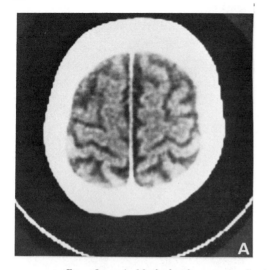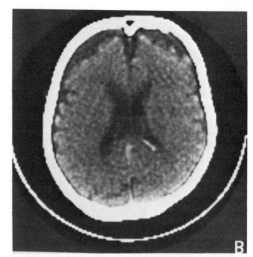

FIG. 18-22. A. Marked enlargement of sulci and interhemispheric space from cortical atrophy.
B. Mild ventricular enlargement is present but not to the same degree as the cortical atrophy. Same patient as in Fig. 18-21.

cyst. The patient had experienced severe trauma as a child. Angiography is highly specific for epidural and subdural hematomas (Fig. 18-20), but because of its much greater complication rate and morbidity, should be reserved for specific situations. Angiography is still required if the CT is negative, since at a certain time in the resolution process the hematoma may be isodense. Also, if the site of the bleeding (e.g., from an aneurysm) is to be

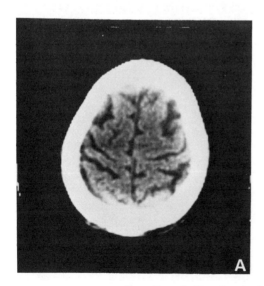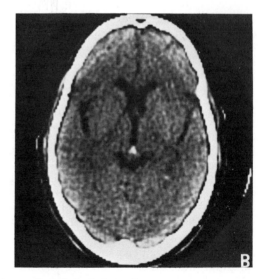

FIG. 18-23. A. Very large sulci secondary to cortical atrophy.
B. Probably normal ventricles for the patient's age.

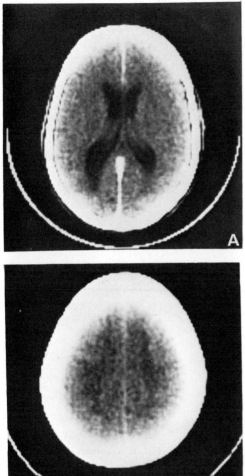
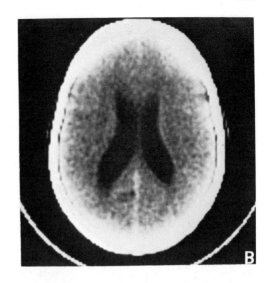

FIG. 18-24. A and B. Enlarged ventricles. C. Sections over vertex showing no sulci. None of the scans showed any evidence of an obstructing mass lesion.

determined, angiography must still be performed. Some care must also be exercised so that the large extracerebral space associated with cortical atrophy is not interpreted as being a chronic subdural (Fig. 18-21). However, this is rarely a real problem since the underlying gyri are not disturbed, there is no mass effect, and atrophy is more generalized.

CEREBRAL ATROPHY AND HYDROCEPHALUS

Cerebral atrophy and hydrocephalus, obstructive or communicating, are now easily diagnosed without the use of pneumoencephalography. CT clearly demonstrates cortical atrophy with marked enlargement of the sulci and, frequently, the interhemispheric fissures (Fig. 18-22). Whether the process involves the cortex, white matter, or both; and whether it is generalized or localized can usually be determined. Figure 18-23 shows marked cortical atrophy but with little if any change in ventricular size, whereas Fig. 18-22 shows some enlargement of the ventricles. When patients are found to have large ventricles but normal or even obliterated sulci (Fig. 18-24), a presump-

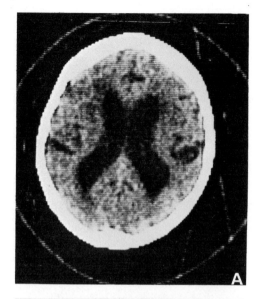

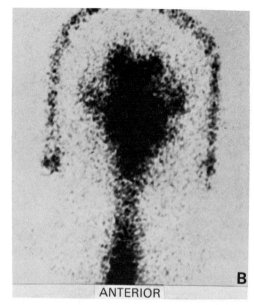

ANTERIOR

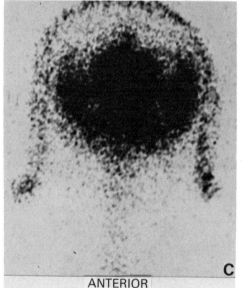

ANTERIOR

FIG. 18-25. A. CT demonstrating markedly enlarged ventricles.
B. Cisternogram 4 hr after radionuclide injection showing contrast in the basal cisterns and moving into the ventricular system. No activity is present in the subarachnoid space over the surface of the brain.
C. 24 hr after injection, the radionuclide persists in the ventricles with no activity over the surface of the brain, indicating extraventricular obstruction preventing passage of isotope over the surface of the brain.

tive diagnosis of hydrocephalus is made which may be verified by a radionuclide cisternogram (Fig. 18-25).

PAPILLEDEMA

The evaluation of the patient presenting with headache and papilledema without localizing neurological signs has been simplified by the use of CT. These patients may now bypass pneumoencephalography, angiography, radionuclide imaging, and skull X-rays and proceed directly to CT. When negative precontrast and postcontrast scans are obtained, it would appear to be safe to perform lumbar puncture to confirm the diagnosis of pseudotumor cerebri or benign intracranial hypertension (Weisberg and Nice, 1977). This conclusion was also reached by Huckman *et al.* (1976) except that they also obtained normal electroencephalograms and radionuclide scans in conjunction with the normal CT, but did bypass pneumoencephalography and angiography.

SUMMARY

Many organic causes of headaches can be diagnosed or excluded by radiographic or radionuclide procedures. Computerized Tomography has led to dramatically altered neurodiagnosis and is now the dominant procedure in our armamentarium. With a few exceptions, which have been noted, all other radiographic procedures are confirmatory or additive in diagnosing intracranial disease. Extracranial causes of headache such as sinusitis, temporal arteritis, and cervical spine problems are outside the realm of CT and are diagnosed by conventional radiography. At present, CT equipment is improving, and our experience with it expanding at such a fast pace that the diagnostic approach is changing almost monthly. Therefore, close cooperation between the clinician and neuroradiologist is more mandatory than ever to ensure that each patient receives the proper procedures in the proper sequence.

REFERENCES

Baker, H. L., Jr. (1975). Computed tomography and neuroradiology; a fortunate primary union. *Am. J. Roentgenol. 124,* 177–185.

Christie, J. H., M. Hirofumi, T. G. Raymundo, S. H. Corvell, and R. L. Shapiro (1976). Computed tomography and radionuclide studies in the diagnosis of intracranial disease. *Am. J. Roentgenol. 127,* 171–174.

Davis, D. O. (1977). CT in the diagnosis of supratentorial tumors. *Seminars in Roentgenology XII (2),* 97–108.

Davis, K. R., J. M. Taveras, G. H. Roberson, R. H. Ackerman, and J. D. Driessbach (1977). Computed tomography in head trauma. *Seminars in Roentgenology XII (1),* 53–62.

Evens, R. G., N. Rujanavech, and M. A. Mikhael (1977). Utilization, reliability and cost effectiveness of cranial computed tomography in evaluating pseudotumor cerebri. *Am. J. Roentgenol. 129,* 263–265.

Hirofumi, M., H. L. Chun, C. C. Lee, A. C. Pasquale, and J. H. Christie (1977). Reliability of computed tomography; correlation with neuropathologic findings. *Am. J. Roentgenol. 128,* 795–798.

Hounsfield, G. N. (1973). Computerized transverse axial scanning (tomography); Part I. Description of system. *Brit. J. Radiol. 46,* 1016–1022.

Huckman, M. S. (1976). Computed tomography in the diagnosis of pseudotumor cerebri. *Radiology 119,* 593–597.

Knaus, W. A., and D. O. Davis (1976). Computerized tomography versus radionuclide brain scanning in the diagnosis of brain tumor. Presented at the meeting of the American Federation for Clinical Research, Atlantic City, N. J.

Leeds, N. E., and N. P. Thomas (1977). Computerized tomography in the diagnosis of sellar and parasellar lesions. *Seminars in Roentgenology XII (2),* 121–137.

Lukin, R. R., A. A. Chambers, and T. A. Lemrick (1977). Cerebral vascular lesions; infarction, hemorrhage, aneurysm and arteriovenous malformation. *Seminars in Roentgenology XII (1),* 78–89.

Lurcke, D. A., and G. T. Gilmore (1977). Computed tomography's impact on nuclear medicine service in two community hospitals. *Applied Radiology 6 (3),* 149.

Miller, J. D., R. M. G. Grace, D. B. Russell, and D. J. Zacks (1977). Complications of cerebral angiography and pneumography. *Radiology 124,* 741–744.

Nakagawa, H., Y. P. Huang, L. I. Malis, and B. S. Wolf (1977). Computed tomography of intraspinal and paraspinal neoplasms. *J. Computer Assisted Tomography 1 (4),* 377–390.

Wartzman, G., R. C. Holgate, and P. P. Morgan (1975). Cranial computed tomography; an evaluation of cost effectiveness. *Radiology 117,* 75–77.

Weinstein, M. A., R. J. Alfidi, and P. M. Duchesneau (1977). Guest editorial. Computed tomography versus skull radiography. *Am. J. Roentgenol. 128,* 873.

Weisberg, L., and C. N. Nice (1977). Computed tomographic evaluation of increased intracranial pressure without localizing signs. *Radiology 122,* 133–136.

19

CERVICAL SPONDYLOSIS AND
MUSCLE CONTRACTION HEADACHES

CHARLES A. ROBINSON

INTRODUCTION

Cervical spondylosis is a degenerative disorder of the cervical spine, which when fully evolved is characterized by derangement of the intervertebral discs, apophyseal joints, vertebral bodies, and the supporting ligamentous structures of the cervical spine. Although the word "spondylosis" strictly refers to degenerative changes in the intervertebral discs, apophyseal joint and disc abnormalities usually coexist and such terms as cervical spondylosis, degenerative disc disease, discogenic disease, osteoarthrosis, and osteoarthritis are often used interchangeably.

Cervical spondylosis is encountered frequently in clinical practice and may be the cause of a variety of disturbing symptoms. Radiographic studies of patients age 50 and over have demonstrated a prevalence of spondylosis in the range of 75–85% (Pallis *et al.*, 1954; Lawrence, *et al.*, 1963; Brain, 1963). This fact assumes great clinical importance, in terms of headache, because it appears that headache may be the presenting and often the only symptom of spondylosis, occurring even in the absence of neck pain, radiculopathy, or myelopathy (Brain, 1963). Unfortunately, in such cases the patient may be subjected to unnecessary and costly diagnostic procedures, and ultimately may be cast off and mislabeled as a psychoneurotic while a potentially treatable disorder is overlooked.

Characteristics of Spondylotic Headaches

The spondylotic headache has many distinctive features that should alert the clinician to the possible diagnosis, particularly in the middle-aged or elderly patient. It is almost always occipital, whether unilateral or bilateral, and while pain often spreads to involve the frontotemporal regions as well, any headache that spares the occiput entirely is unlikely to be due to spondylosis (Brain, 1963).

The pain tends to be dull and nagging rather than throbbing, pulsating, or bursting. It is not unusual, however, particularly in longstanding cases, for pain to have an intermittent throbbing or lacinating component. Patients often describe their headaches as a feeling of tightness or as a band or vice-like, constricting sensation. Headache is often present upon awakening in the morning and may then subside after a period of minutes or hours, only to reappear or intensify later in the day under conditions of fatigue. Tension, depression, neck motion or position, arm use, automobile rides, desk work, watching television, and reading are often mentioned as exacerbating factors. Relief may be obtained by massaging the neck or scalp muscles, by standing under a warm shower or applying a heating pad to the neck or merely by resting quietly.

It is common for patients to complain of simultaneous pain in the neck, in or behind the ear, in the shoulder, periscapular regions, upper extremities, or supraclavicular or pectoral areas on the ipsilateral side—symptoms tending to wax and wane in concert. Intermittent or persistent upper extremity paresthesias often occur as part of the overall symptom complex and patients will frequently report restriction of neck motion and a cracking, popping or grinding sensation with movement of the neck. Vasomotor or autonomic symptoms may accompany the head and neck pain. Patients, for example, may complain of nasal congestion, lacrimation, photophobia, vertigo, or even syncope. The latter symptoms may occur because of involvement of the vertebral arteries or components of the sympathetic nervous system in the neck, but the pathophysiology is incompletely understood.

Anatomy of the Cervical Spine

A description of the anatomy, neural pathways, and pain-sensitive structures of the cervical spine will be given before considering the possible pathogenesis of headaches associated with cervical spondylosis. The osseous cervical spine is composed of seven vertebrae, each articulating with structures above and below by synovium-lined joints, the facet or apophyseal joints. The first two cervical vertebrae, the atlas (C-1) and axis (C-2) are unique in structure and are responsible for the major part of head motion in flexion, extension, and lateral rotation (Caillet, 1964). The ring-like atlas articulates with the occipital condyles of the skull and, under normal conditions, there is relatively little motion between the atlas and occiput, the two tending to move as one around the odontoid process (dens), the cephalic projection of the second cervical vertebrae. The axis has a large vertebral body and articulates by way of the superior facet joints with the inferior facets of the atlas. The odontoid process is stabilized in relation to the anterior arch of C-1 by a strong transverse ligament, the transverse cruciate ligament, and between the two is a synovium-lined bursa.

Each vertebral body from C-2 through C-7 is separated from the adjacent vertebrae by a fibrocartilaginous disc, the peripheral portions of which are composed of extremely strong concentrically and obliquely arranged collagen fibers which intertwine with one another and attach to the bony vertebral end plates. The central portion of the disc, the nucleus pulposus, is a gelatinous substance consisting of a matrix of water and proteoglycans (acid mucopolysaccharides, hyaluronate, chondroitin sulfate, keratosulfate) in a randomly oriented mesh-like networt of collagen fibers

(Eyring, 1969). The nucleus pulposus, a remnant of the fetal notacord, is deformable but incompressible (Wilkinson, 1971), and serves to keep the mechanical pressures that vary greatly with head and neck movement evenly distributed. The proteoglycan content of the nucleus pulposus increases to a maximum in about the third decade of life and then falls (Murayama, 1972) and, with aging, the nucleus becomes more fibrous. In the aged discs, the gel-like properties are lost and vertical loads are redistributed in an unequal fashion, so that localized points of high pressure develop, leading to rents or tears in the annulus.

The third through seventh cervical vertebrae are similar in structure with bodies that are concave superiorly, and convex inferiorly. The pedicles project laterally and posteriorly from the vertebral bodies and the laterally directed transverse processes provide the vertebral foramena through which the vertebral artery runs from C-6 cephalad: The laminae arise from the lateral masses and join posteriorly as the inferiorly directed spinous processes. The uncovertebral joints (neurocentral joints, joints of Von Luschka) are located on the posterolateral aspect of the vertebral bodies and at the anterior margin of the intervertebral neuroforamena. The uncovertebral joints are unique to the cervical spine and there is continuing debate concerning whether or not these structures are true synovium-lined joints or pseudoarthroses. Whatever the case, it is clear that these articulations are involved in degenerative and inflammatory conditions of the cervical spine and that such involvement is often of great clinical importance, Hypertrophic changes occurring at these joints may encroach upon the intervertebral neuroforamena and lead to compression of the emerging spinal nerves.

The ligamentous structures of the cervical spine include a strong anterior longitudinal ligament that continues cephalad from C-2 as the anterior atlanto-occipital ligament and a posterior longitudinal ligament that extends cephalad from C-1 as the tectorial membrane, which attaches above the anterior lip of the foramen magnum inside the posterior cranial fossa. The anterior longitudinal ligament is firmly attached to the anterior surfaces of the vertebral bodies and lightly to the annulus fibrosis while the posterior longitudinal ligament is firmly fixed to the disc margin and immediately adjacent bony surfaces, but not to the centers of the vertebral bodies where the nutrient blood vessels enter and leave the marrow cavity (Wilkinson, 1971). Other important ligamentous structures are the apical ligament, a fibrous remnant of the notacord that anchors the upper portion of the odontoid process to the anterior margin of the foramen magnum, the alar and cruciate ligaments of the occipito-atlanto-axial apparatus, the thick ligamentum flavum that extends between adjacent laminae and blends laterally with the anterior fibers of the (facet) articular capsule, the interspinous ligaments, and the ligamentum nuchae.

The spinal cord occupies the spinal canal, bounded anteriorly by the vertebral bodies, disks, and the posterior longitudinal ligament; anterolaterally by the uncovertebral joints, laterally and posterolaterally by the pedicles, articular processes, apophyseal articulations, laminae and ligamentum flavum; and posteriorly by the spinous process and interspinous ligaments. The segmental nerve roots exit the spinal cord through the intervertebral neuroforamena, each leaving above the corresponding numbered vertebra, except for C-8 which exits below the seventh cervical and above the first thoracic vertebra. The spinal cord is bathed in cerebrospinal fluid and enveloped by three membranes, the meninges, to which it is attached by the dentate ligaments. The meninges are comprised of an outer fibrous dura mater, a middle avascular, delicate, transparent arachnoid membrane, and an inner membrane, the delicate vascular pia mater. The epidural space, between the dura mater and the walls of the spinal canal, contains fat and a plexus of thin walled vessels. As each nerve root exits the vertebral canal, it carries with it for a short distance an extension of the dura meter, the dural sleeve.

The bony vertebral column is bounded anteriorly and anterolaterally by the scalenus (anterior, medius, and posterior), longus capitis, longus colli, and rectus capitis (anterior and lateral), muscles that act primarily as flexors, rotators, and, to a lesser extent, lateral benders of the head and neck. The muscles located posterolaterally and posteriorly serve primarily as extensors, lateral benders, and rotators of the head and neck and may be divided into deep (rectus capitis posterior major, rectus capitis posterior minor, obliquus capitis), middle (semispinalis capitis, longissiumus, splenius capitis), and superficial (levator scapula, trapezius) groups. The sternocleidomastoid muscles, acting in concert, flex the neck and, while acting singly, rotate the neck laterally and bend the head toward the shoulder.

Innervation

The cervical nerves are short, mixed spinal nerves formed by the union of the dorsal (sensory) and ventral (motor) nerve roots just distal to the dorsal root ganglia and proximal to the intervertebral neuroforamina. After providing a small recurrent meningeal branch (sinuvertebral nerve or nerve of Von Luschka), the cervical nerve almost immediately divides into dorsal (posterior) and ventral (anterior) rami, each carrying a mixture of sensory and motor fibers. The larger ventral rami communicate with the cervical sympathetic chain, some postganglionic sympathetic fibers traveling back through the foramen along the ventral root to communicate with the recurrent meningeal nerve, and then continue laterally and ventrally to supply the somatic structures of the trunk and upper extremities in a segmental fashion. The smaller dorsal rami divide into medial and lateral branches that innervate the paravertebral musculature and provide sensory innervation to the skin of the neck and scalp. The medial branch, additionally, supplies small nerve filaments to the facet joints at its level of origin and a descending branch continues caudally, providing muscular and cutaneous branches as well as several fine filaments to the superior aspect of the facet joints for one or two segments below (Mooney and Robertson, 1976).

The recurrent nerve of Von Luschka (the sinuvertebral nerve) appears to be of great clinical importance. While in the cervical region, the nerve is so small as to defy ordinary anatomical methods, physiologic studies in conjunction with the known anatomy of the sinuvertebral nerve in the lumbar region have allowed a formulation of its location and distribution in the cervical region (Cloward, 1960). The sinuvertebral nerve is formed by a junction of two roots, spinal and sympathetic. The spinal root takes origin from the ventral surface of the spinal nerve within the spinal canal. It is then immediately joined by sympathetic fibers which pass medially from the sympathetic chain and the nerve that is formed passes medially behind the vertebral body and, after a short course, divides into its terminal branches. These branches terminate in the anterior longitudinal ligament, posterior longitudinal ligament, posterior fibers of the annulus fibrosis, the longitudinal venous sinuses, epidural tissue of the vertebral canal, and the dura mater. The nerve is largely sensory, and appears to primarily subserve the function of pain. Receptors of the sensory nerve are located throughout the peripheral fibers of the annulus fibrosis of the intervertebral discs, including the attachment of these fibers to the margins of the adjacent vertebral body. It appears that the terminal fibers extend a short distance across the midline and decussate with those from the opposite side. It is likely that one sinuvertebral nerve may contribute to the nerve supply of the posterior surface of more than one cervical disc primarily by way of descending branches. When one considers the structures that receive their sensory innervation from the sinuvertebral nerve, the clinical relevance of this structure becomes apparent.

The posterior ramus of C-1, the suboccipital nerve, has no sensory distribution. The dorsal ramus of the second cervical nerve, the greater occipital nerve, passes between the atlas and axis, emerges below the obliquus capitis inferior muscle, ascends between the muscles of the suboccipital triangle, and the semispinalis capitis, and pierces the latter muscle and the trapezius close to their attachments to the occiput. The greater occipital nerve then continues into the scalp to supply cutaneous innervation for some distance lateral to the midline and as far superiorly as the vertex (Woodburne, 1965). Its lateral branches communicate with those of the lesser occipital nerve (a branch of the cervical plexus, containing fibers

from the anterior rami of C-2 and C-3) and branches also communicate with the occipitalis tertius, the medial branch of the posterior ramus of C-3. The greater occipital nerve, emerging between bony surfaces and powerful muscle groups, is particular vulnerable to trauma and pressure, a fact that is likely of great clinical importance, particularly when one considers that this nerve supplies sensation to a major portion of the scalp.

Head Pain Arising in the Cervical Spine

In addition to the cutaneous innervation provided by the greater occipital nerve, occipitalis tertius, and lesser occipital nerve, other neural pathways are likely involved in the production of head pain by disorders of the cervical spine. The most thoroughly investigated and perhaps most important is that dealing with the interaction of the trigeminal nerve complex with the afferent impulses ariving at the cord via the cervical spinal nerves. The forehead and face are supplied by pain fibers that travel with the ophthalmic (V-1), maxillary (V-2), and mandibular (V-3) divisions of the fifth cranial or trigeminal nerve. In general, the forehead and eyes are supplied by V-1, the cheeks, nose, upper lip, and teeth by V-2, and the lower lip, teeth and jaw by V-3. Additionally, a small area overlying the mandibular angle and parotid gland is supplied by the second and third cervical nerves (by the facial branches of the greater auricular nerve, a division of the cervical plexus).

Intracranially, sensory fibers of the trigeminal nerve supply the superior surface of the tentorium cerebelli, and all of the pain sensitive structures that lie above it. Many fibers of the maxillary and mandibular divisions of the fifth cranial nerve accompany the middle meningeal artery and its branches and form a network in the adventitia. Branches of the nerve have been seen to extend away from the artery out into the dura. There is less certainty about the nerve to the anterior meningeal arteries and the dura of the anterior fossa, but it is probable that the anterior meningeal branch of the internal carotid artery is accompanied by fibers that connect directly with the first division of the trigeminal nerve, the Gasserian ganglion (McNaughton, 1938). It is also probable that the meningeal branches of the ethmoidal arteries are accompanied by nerves that pass through the cribiform plate as branches of the infraorbital portion of the ophthalmic division. Studies on experimentally induced histamine headaches indicate that the fifth cranial nerve is undoubtedly the chief afferent nerve for headache arising from dilatation of the pial and cerebral arteries of the supratentorial fossae (Schumaker *et al.*, 1940).

The cell bodies of the trigeminal nerve are contained in the intracranial Gasserian (semilunar) ganglion from which the roots of the nerve proceed to the brainstem and enter it at the pontine level. The fibers carrying pain impulses do not synapse with their respective second-order neurons near their level of entry; instead, the nociceptive elements of all three divisions turn inferiorly within the brainstem as the descending tract of the trigeminal nerve and dip down past the cranial vertebral border to synapse with the second-order neurons within the upper cervical spinal cord (Kitahata *et al.*, 1974).

As the tract descends through the brainstem, it is joined by pain fibers traveling with branches of the seventh, ninth, and tenth cranial nerves so that, when it reaches the cervical cord, the tract also contains information from the deep facial structures, nasopharynx, oropharynx, deep middle and external ear, and dura mater of the posterior fossa (Pawl, 1977). Although fibers from V-1, V-2, and V-3 are discretely layered within the descending tracts of the trigeminal nerve, it is not known for certain whether fibers from each division peel off to synapse at separate levels within the upper cervical cord.

It is known that fibers from all three divisions are found as low as the second cervical segment (Kerr, 1961), and that fibers from the ophthalmic division are found as low as the fourth cervical segment. Furthermore, cervical afferent fibers from at least as low as C4 and probably C5 are found in the dorsal horn at the second cervical level (Kerr, 1963). After synapse with second-order neurons in the cervical cord, pain impulses cross the midline, ascend in the ventral secondary tract of V, rise through the brainstem to a secondary synapse within the thalamus, and from there, are projected to the parietal lobe cortex where discrimination of the quality and localization of pain occurs (Pawl, 1977).

Pain information arriving at the cervical spinal cord by way of the segmental nerves follows the pattern of the remainder of the cord. Nociceptive fibers are contained in the lateral portions of the posterior rootlets and penetrate the cord on its posterolateral surface, just peripheral to the dorsal gray horn. They do not immediately enter the gray matter to synapse, but rather ascend and descend as far as three segments from their point of entry in Lissauer's tract which is located adjacent to the dorsal gray horn. This tract mingles inperceptably with the descending tract of V in the upper four segments of the cervical cord (Pawl, 1977).

On leaving Lissauer's tract, pain fibers from cervical nerves penetrate the dorsal gray horn to synapse with second-order neurons. These second-order neurons are juxtaposed with second-order neurons of the descending tract V in the upper four cervical segments. Because of this complex pattern of sensory input to the upper cervical cord, pain information conveyed by cervical nerves as low as C-7 could, from a neuroanatomical standpoint, be distributed to the ventral ascending tract of V and be cataloged as headache, orbital pain, or even facial pain. In view of the numerous possibilities for overlap of pain from one afferent system to another centrally, it is, indeed, somewhat surprising that pain syndromes should remain as localized as they frequently do.

Pain Sensitive Structures in the Neck

Pain sensitive structures in the neck are, as noted above, innervated by the sinuvertebral nerves and the posterior primary rami of the spinal nerves and include the outer fibers of the annulus fibrosis; the vertebral periosteum; the ligamentum flavum; anterior longitudinal, posterior longitudinal, and interspinous ligaments; the posterior vertebral venous plexus;

the anterior dura mater; the facet articulations; and the paravertebral musculature and their enveloping fascia (Caillet, 1964; Mooney and Robertson, 1976; Edgar and Ghadially, 1976). The nucleus pulposus is generally considered to be devoid of nerve fibers, although, according to Shinohara (1970), in a degenerative disc, fine nerve fibers may accompany granulation tissue into the deeper layers of the disc. Although there is no firm evidence, many investigators have suggested that the autonomic plexus investing the vertebral arteries, primarily made up of sympathetic nerve fibers, contain nociceptive fibers (Pawl, 1977). While any or all of these pain sensitive structures may be affected by traumatic degenerative and inflammatory processes in the neck, their relative importance in causation of neck and head pain remains unclear.

Occipital Neuralgia

Hunter and Mayfield (1949) studied eleven patients who suffered recurrent attacks of severe hemicranial pain, who were treated either by avulsion of the greater occipital nerve or by intraspinal section of the sensory roots of C2 and/or C3. In eight patients, symptoms followed trauma and in the other three no history of trauma could be elicited. The symptoms were essentially identical. For the most part, pain was initiated in the suboccipital region and radiated to the vertex, temporal area, periorbital regions, and/or face, usually about the lower jaw. The authors observed that attacks of pain frequently occurred at night and were often associated with tearing, flushing of the face, alteration of sweating, and, at times, occlusion of the nasal passages on the side involved. Many patients also complained of vertigo and a sense of giddiness during a paroxysm of pain. When the patients were examined during attacks of pain, they appeared acutely ill and there was always exquisite tenderness over the course of the greater occipital nerve and at the point of emergence of the second and/or third cervical nerves on the side involved. Rotary movements of the neck, particularly hyperextension and rotation of the occiput to the painful side, exaggerated

the symptoms and manual traction on the head often provided transient relief. Pain abruptly ceased following infiltration of the greater occipital nerve or second and third cervical nerve roots with procaine.

Interestingly, patients with a history of trauma obtained lasting relief following avulsion of the greater occipital nerve or intraspinal section of the sensory roots of C-2 and/or C-3, but those without a history of trauma did not. The authors postulated that the patient's symptoms were a consequence of injury to the posterior primary ramus of C-2 caused by abnormal movement of C-1 in relation to C-2, the emerging posterior primary ramus of C-2 being compressed between the arches of the atlas and axis. They felt that injury to the second cervical nerve did not occur during normal neck range of motion, but did so if force were applied to the neck when it was already at the limits of its normal range and that, once damage had occurred, normal motion of the neck was capable of maintaining the nerve in a painful state. The authors attributed the occurrence of anterior head and facial pain to overlaping central neural pathways—i.e., between the cervical afferents and those of the trigeminal, pharyngeal, and vagus nerves.

The data on Hunter and Mayfield's patients were reported after a fairly brief period of follow-up, although subsequent studies suggested favorable long-term results following rhizotomy of the second and third cervical nerves (Chambers, 1954) or greater occipital neurectomy (Murphy, 1969). Many other studies, however, have reported unfavorable long-term results, a majority of patients reporting a recurrence of head pain with time, and the current consensus is that such surgical procedures are seldom indicated (Kerr, 1963; Pawl, 1977). It is suggested that recurrence of pain is related to the involvement of the many overlapping neural pathways in the upper cervical spine, that have been alluded to above.

Headache and Disorders of the Lower Cervical Structures

Brain (1963) observed that headache may be associated with a disc lesion at any level, but considered that the disc lesion itself was unlikely to be the cause of pain. Although no data were supplied, he stated that comparative X-ray studies of patients with and without headache showed that those with headache often had a predominant involvement of the upper cervical apophyseal joints. The systematic study needed to confirm the role of the facet joints in the production of headache has never been made, however. It should be noted that, in cervical spondylosis, radiographic abnormalities generally occur earliest and are most pronounced at lower cervical levels, particularly C-5 and C-6. In the absence of trauma, changes are infrequently observed at higher levels, and it is the opinion of this author that involvement of the upper cervical apophyseal joints is unlikely to be responsible for headache in the vast majority of patients with cervical spondylosis.

Raney and Raney (1948) noted the frequent appearance of headache and facial pain in patients with cervical spondylosis in whom the radiographic abnormalities were confined to mid and lower cervical levels. This observation has been made by many others, and many patient's have obtained relief or amelioration of headache following anterior cervical fusion at lower cervical levels (Pawl, 1977; Peterson *et al.*, 1975; White *et al.*, 1973). Cloward (1960) found that experimentally induced "disc pain" produced by the forceful injection of saline or contrast material into an abnormal disc caused pain that was felt in the neck, shoulder, and muscles along the medial scapular border, but never in the head, face, eye, or ear. Similar patterns of pain referral were observed following direct electrical or needle stimulation of the annulus fibrosis, anterior and posterior longitudinal ligaments. Cloward discounted the possibility that ruptured cervical discs per se were responsible for headache and facial pain. In the course of his studies, however, it was also observed that the pain that was experienced in the muscles along the vertebral border of the scapula was accompanied by muscle spasm and electromyographic evidence of increased muscle irritability; direct stimulation of the posterior disc surface or posterior longitudinal ligament caused pain in the neck that extended to segments above and below the stimulated level.

It is a common clinical experience that neck derangements are usually accompanied by spasm in the cervical paraspinous musculatures. Such spasm may be postulated to occur as a consequence of segmental reflex arcs, afferent impulses being conveyed to the cord by the sinuvertebral nerve, spinal nerve, and dorsal root. Within the dorsal gray horn, an internuncial neuron may then propagate the impulse to the anterior horn cell from whence it travels along the ventral root, spinal nerve, and posterior primary ramus to cause contraction of the paravertebral musculature.

We have previously seen that nociceptive impulses may ascend and descend within Lissauer's tract, that each cervical segment is supplied by fibers from more than one sinuvertebral nerve, and that there is considerable overlap of afferent impulses from the head and neck within the upper cervical cord. Therefore, chronic stimulation of a reflex arc, such as that postulated above, could give rise to a state of chronic contraction of both neck and head muscles, thereby giving rise to headache. In this sense, the mechanism of production of headache may be similar to that proposed for tension headaches (muscle contraction headaches). Support for this possibility is provided by the clinical similarities between spondylotic and tension headaches. Further evidence supporting the role of chronic muscle traction and the causation of headache will be presented below.

MUSCLE CONTRACTION HEADACHE (TENSION HEADACHE)

Although adequate epidemiologic data are lacking, "tension headache" in its varied forms is probably the most common type of headache in the general population. For most, fortunately, such headaches are relatively mild, transient, and infrequent. For many, however, they are intractable and often debilitating. It has been estimated that the incidence of tension headaches sufficiently severe and protracted to warrant neurologic referral is similar to that of migraine (Lance *et al.*, 1965; Kudrow, 1976). The terms "tension headache" and "muscle contraction headache" are often used synonymously and this practice will be followed here. The evidence that sustained contraction of the muscles of the neck and/or scalp, is, in fact, the mechanism of tension headache, will be presented below.

The pain in tension headache is most often described as dull, aching, nonpulsatile, and persistent. Additional descriptive terms include "tightness," "band-like," "cap-like," or "vice-like" sensations about the head; and "weight," "drawing," and "soreness." These sensations, while occasionally unilateral, are more often bilateral. Headaches may involve the occipital, parietal, temporal, and frontal areas, either singly or in any combination. Pain is often generalized. Patients commonly complain of associated pain, stiffness, or tightness in the neck. Often, there is soreness on combing or brushing the hair or when putting on a hat. While such headaches may be fleeting, with frequent changes in the site and intensity on recurrence, they are usually localized in one region and may be sustained with varying intensity for weeks, months, and even years. In its milder forms, tension headache may last for a period of only 1 or 2 hr and occur during, following, or in anticipation of a consciously stressful situation. In its more severe and chronic form, the pain may be virtually constant, the patient awakening with headache and pain continuing throughout the day without regard to the emotional content of the day's activities. A small percentage of patients may actually be awakened in the early morning hours by headache (Lance, 1978). The intensity of the headache may diminish if certain individually favored positions are assumed. The patient may limit the motion of the head, neck, and jaws to decrease discomfort, and pain may be less intense when the head is supported by the hands. Within the diffusely aching muscle tissues of the head, neck, and upper back, there may be found on palpation one or more tender areas or "nodules" which are sharply localized but which, when touched,

cause pain to spread to adjacent or even distant sites in the head. Additionally, pressure on contracted, tender muscles may elicit tinnitus, vertigo, and lacrimation, symptoms which also occur spontaneously.

Implicit in the description above is the fact that tension headache is almost invariably accompanied by spasm and/or tenderness of the muscles of the head or neck. This is borne out primarily by clinical experience, supported by a number of EMG (electromyographic) studies. Simons *et al.* (1943) demonstrated that experimentally induced head pain or spontaneous pain originating in or about the head, if sufficiently severe and sustained, can produce contraction in the neck and/or scalp muscles, which in turn, serves as a secondary source of pain. They induced head pain by several methods: intravenous administration of histamine phosphate, spinal drainage, injection of hypertonic saline into the temporal muscle, introducing an irritant into the conjectival sac, inducing abnormally sustained contraction of the external ocular muscles utilizing a vertical prism, and exerting continuous painful pressure on the head by means of a head screw apparatus.

Electromyograms were obtained prior to, during, and following experimentally induced head pain and the amount of muscle activity was estimated using a scale in which 10 represented the maximum of muscle potential. Subjects estimated their pain on the basis of an arbitrary scale, ten representing unbearable pain. It was observed that experimentally induced pain of brief duration was associated with neck muscle contraction and the subjective report of a momentary "tight ache" in the suboccipital region. Pain of short duration, however, did not maintain muscle contraction long enough to cause secondary symptoms of any significance in the head or neck.

When stimuli were applied to the head for sufficiently long periods of time, pain and tightness were experienced in the neck and were accompanied by marked contraction of the cervical musculature. In many instances, contraction was also observed in the scalp muscles. The induced muscle contraction was observed to outlast the initial pain stimulus as did the pain and stiffness which the patients experienced in the occiput and suboccipital regions. The secondarily induced pain was characteristically a deep, steady ache rather than a throbbing or sharp pain as might be expected were the pain of vascular or cutaneous origin. The authors noted that the involved head and neck muscles were tender, that massage of the muscles often relieved the pain, and that pain and stiffness were modified by head movement. They also demonstrated that procedures which increased the action potential increased the head pain, and conversely, procedures which diminished the action potentials also decreased the head pain. On the basis of their studies, the investigators reasonably concluded that the muscles were the actual source of pain.

In a related group of experiments, Simons *et al.* (1943) observed and performed EMG studies on patients with head pain secondary to frontal and maxillary sinusitis and in patients whose headaches seemed to be primarily related to anxiety and emotional tension. In both groups, pain, tenderness and muscle contraction could be identified in the neck and scalp muscles and the authors inferred that the actual cause of pain was chronic muscle contraction.

Many investigators have reported a positive correlation between resting frontalis muscle EMGs and the frequency of muscle contraction headaches (Budzynski *et al.*, 1973; Haynes *et al.*, 1975; Vaughan *et al.*, 1977). It is interesting, in this regard, that Neufeld and Davidson (1974) found that frontalis muscle tension was a more sensitive measure of the physiologic response to stress than was heart rate, skin conductance, or respiratory rate. Harper and Steger (1978) observed that frontalis muscle EMG activity was related to such complaints as tension, inadequacy, indecision, worry, depression, and anxiety, whereas, subjective reports of headache intensity correlated best with such personality (MMPI) measures as hypochondriasis, depression, and hysteria. It was concluded that muscle contraction headaches are, indeed, related to emotional and psycho-logical stress, but that EMG activity did not correlate well with headache intensity, perhaps because the primary determinants of headache pain per se are more related to the reported personality measures than to actual psychological stress.

Most EMG studies performed on patients with frequent tension headaches have demonstrated the presence of continuous action potentials in the frontalis, temporalis, and/or neck muscles, both during and between headaches (Budzynski *et al.*, 1973; Vaughan *et al.*, 1977; Peck and Kraft, 1977; Pozniak-Patewicz, 1976; Bakal and Kagnov, 1977). It has also been shown that in such patients the level of EMG activity, in certain but not all muscles tested, may be significantly greater during headache than when the patient is headache free (Haynes *et al.*, 1975; Tunis and Wolff, 1954); there is often a correlation between the headache level and EMG activity and biofeedback techniques, when successful, effect a reduction in the frequency and severity of tension headaches as well as a reduction in muscle tension as measured electromyographically (Budzynski *et al.*, 1973; Peck and Kraft, 1977; Bakal and Kagnov, 1977).

The studies alluded to above suggest that tension-related headaches are accompanied by and probably caused by sustained contraction of muscles of the scalp and/or neck. It also appears that muscle contraction may accompany and serve as a secondary source of pain in other types of headache. Wolff and his colleagues, for example, studied EMGs of the scalp and neck muscles in patients with migraine headaches and found evidence for considerable muscle contraction in these patients during and following an episode of migraine headache. Furthermore, Ergotamine tartrate given intravenously during the headache eliminated the pain within 15 min, but the neck and head muscle contraction persisted for some time thereafter (Simons *et al.*, 1973). Others have made similar observations. Bakal and Kagnov (1977) suggested that the distinction between muscle contraction and migraine headaches may, in some respects be more quantitative than qualitative. These authors compared muscle contraction (tension) headache and migraine patients for pain location, EMG activity (frontalis and neck muscles), and superficial temporal artery blood flow velocity; they found much overlap between the two groups with regard to all parameters studied. The pain locations were similar. Many migraine patients had headaches that were bilateral, dull, aching, and associated with discomfort and tightness in the neck. Conversely, many patient's with "muscle contraction headaches" reported that some of their headaches were unilateral, throbbing, and associated with nausea, vomiting, or visual disturbances. Furthermore, migraineurs had significantly higher frontalis muscle EMG activity between and during headaches than did either muscle contraction headache patients or nonheadache controls.

Pulse velocity results failed to statistically differentiate the groups, but similar patterns were found in migraine and muscle contraction patients. Frontalis muscle EMG biofeedback training was equally effective in reducing headaches in migraine and muscle contraction patients. Bakal and Kagnov did not feel that the results were a consequence of initial misdiagnosis. They suggested that muscle contraction and vascular factors may predispose to both types of headaches, although neither is a direct cause, and that in patients with longstanding headache histories, mixed patterns emerged. They noted a tendency, in both groups, toward increasing severity over the years and suggested that this may occur because of the individual patients inability to cope with less severe headaches, accompanied by an increasing physiological predisposition for headache.

Pozniak-Patewicz (1976) evaluated 183 patients with a variety of headaches and 51 nonheadache controls by EMG of scalp and neck muscles and found that the majority of headache patients, but not controls, had continuous electrical activity when voluntarily relaxed and headache free. This was true for all types of headache. During headache, the neck muscles were more involved than temporal muscles, and interestingly, the most intense

spasm occurred in patients with migraine headaches. It appeared that temporal muscle potentials actually dropped slightly during both migraine and muscle contraction headaches, while neck muscle potentials increased dramatically. The intensity of muscle spasm did not correlate with the duration or frequency of headache attacks or with the patients age, but it was observed that the intensity of neck muscle action potentials differed according to sex, the amplitude being three times higher in women. The author concluded that "cephalgic" spasm of head and neck muscles is a consequence rather than a cause of headache, and that the data obtained did not support the hypothesis that there is a specific type of headache of muscular origin.

Similarly, Majora et al. (1974) performed EMGs on the semispinalis muscles at the C4-C5 level on 57 patients with a variety of headache symptoms who were randomly selected from a larger population of headache patients. They encountered EMG abnormalities with considerable frequency in all types of headaches if the occipital region was involved. No relation was found between the EMG findings and age, sex, or degree of degenerative spondyloarthrosis. The authors concluded that an EMG examination of the cervical paraspinous muscles is warranted in headache of obscure etiology and that if the EMG is abnormal, even in patients with migraine, therapy directed only against the headache and not toward the cervical spine was likely to be unsuccessful.

The fact that clinical and EMG evidence of scalp and neck muscle contraction are found in a large proportion of patients with "tension" headache does not establish that muscle contraction per se is the cause of pain. Neither does the fact that scalp or neck muscle contraction may accompany other types of headache negate the possibility that some headaches are primarily a consequence of sustained muscle contraction. If it is accepted that increased muscle action potentials are an indication of muscle contraction, then the observations of Simons et al. (1943)—that experimentally induced or spontaneously occurring head pain, when accompanied by muscle spasm, is usually worsened by procedures that increase the muscle action potentials, and diminished by procedures that decrease the action potentials suggest that muscle contraction per se is a cause of pain.

The diagnosis of muscle contraction headache should be one of exclusion. Since it has been shown that many varieties of spontaneously or experimentally induced head pain may, if sufficiently sustained, cause neck and scalp muscle contraction, which in turn, serves as a secondary source of pain, the finding of muscle spasm or tenderness should not immediately lead to the conclusion that the headache is solely caused by chronic muscle contraction. A careful search for a primary source of pain, for example ocular, sinus, or temporomandibular joint disorders, should be undertaken. If such a primary source of pain cannot be found, it would then seem justified to infer that headache is primarily a consequence of chronic muscle contraction.

The findings of Pozniak-Patewicz (1976), Majora *et al.* (1974), and Bakal and Kagnov (1977) are not difficult to reconcile with the earlier observations and conclusions of Wolff and his colleagues. It would, indeed, be expected that a substantial proportion of chronic headache patients, whatever the initial "type" of headache, would have evidence of neck and/or scalp muscle contraction and that as headache becomes chronic, mixed patterns would emerge with pain (secondary to muscle contraction) serving as a common denominator. Thus, it is not surprising that patients with migraine and other types of head pain frequently complain of pain or tightness in the neck and occiput and that EMGs performed on the scalp and neck muscles of such patients are abnormal. It may well be that, in most if not all headaches, muscle contraction occurs as a secondary phenomenon, i.e., in response to fatigue, anxiety, stress, or posture, or in response to pain originating in other head or neck structures such as the eyes, teeth, paranasal sinuses, temporomandibular joints, and articulations or ligaments of the cervical spine. Simons *et al.* (1943) had suggested that neck muscle spasm may be analogous to that muscle spasm which occurs about a fractured bone or a perforated viscus, representing a protective fixation of the part. In some instances, they have suggested, the muscle contraction may be symbolic of withdrawing the head from noxious agents or of stabilizing the head and shoulders for a "charge against the threat."

Possible Mechanisms for Muscle Pain and the Role of Ischemia in Muscle Contraction Headaches

The mechanisms by which muscle contraction or spasm may cause pain are not known with certainty. It has been postulated that muscle contraction may cause pain by neural compression or by producing traction at the myofascial junction to periosteum. There has been no experimental substantiation for these claims. It is a common clinical experience to encounter pain in the neck and occiput, often extending anteriorly to the vertex or orbit, in patients who have occupations that require holding of the head and neck in a habitual posture for prolonged periods of time. This is true, for example, for stenographers, typists, pianists, violinists, microscopists, draftsmen, and writers. One might postulate that, when the head and neck are held rigidly for prolonged periods of time, the alternating contraction and relaxation that generally occur in muscle with varied movements of the head and neck may be lacking. It is known that sustained or repetitive voluntary contraction of skeletal muscle often gives rise to pain, stiffness, and tenderness. The novice weight-lifter, jogger, or skier may be virtually immobilized by pain for one or more days following the performance of unaccustomed exercise.

Lewis (1942) has remarked that muscles may be a source of pain and tenderness after steady voluntary contraction of 2 minutes' duration and that tenderness in a muscle that has continuously contracted for hours or days may outlast the actual contraction. Elliott (1944) demonstrated that, in patients with painful muscle contraction in the legs, needle electrodes placed in tender and painful "rheumatic nodules" will record vigorous action potentials, whereas electrodes placed in adjacent, painless, nontender muscles, will not record action potentials. Such painful "nodules" have been histologically examined by a number of investigators and, in general, no significant structural abnormalities have been found (see below).

It is known that skeletal muscle contains small, thinly myelinated A-delta fiber nociceptor units (Bonica, 1977). Hinsey (1928), in studying the blood vessels of skeletal muscle, observed afferent fibers in the adventitia of small arteries, veins, arterioles, and venules that extended to the terminal branches but not to the capillaries. He observed branches of such fibers in the adipose and connective tissue of the muscle surrounding these vessels and suggested that the afferent fibers and their fine-caliber nerve endings are probably the structures that convey impulses interpreted as muscle pain. Muscle contraction creates increased intramuscular pressure and the pressure is significantly greater in isometric than in isotonic contractions (Hill, 1948). Such contraction may cause compression of small blood vessels and result in ischemia.

Barcroft and Millen (1939) established the fact that human muscles are quite ischemic during strong contractions and hyperemic during weak contractions. They assumed that the suppression of the hyperemia during strong contraction is due to compression of the potentially dilated vessels by the taut muscle fibers, an inference borne out by the immediate appearance of hyperemia a few seconds after the muscle relaxes. It is, therefore, conceivable that muscle ischemia is a contributing or primary factor in the induction of pain in patients with headache accompanied by sustained scalp or neck muscle contractions. What remains uncertain is whether the contraction of the neck and head muscles is of sufficient magnitude to induce such ischemia.

Rodbard (1970) has studied the pain associated with muscle contraction and his findings are compatible with the hypothesis that contracting muscle produces a catabolote which generates local pain. In his experiments, the production of the pain catabolote varied with the magnitude of the tension developed in the muscle, the latter being related to the

number of contractions, the load, and the duration of contraction. Occlusion of the blood supply without contraction did not augment or produce muscle pain. Other investigators (Dorpat and Holmes, 1955; Perl et al., 1934) have also suggested that skeletal muscle pain may be a consequence of the accumulation of noxious metabolites in ischemic muscle, although the exact nature of the postulated metabolite(s) is not known with certainty.

It is a generally accepted physiological principal that every period of work (contraction) must be followed by a period of relaxation during which blood again flows through the capillary beds, supplying oxygen and removing accumulated waste products. Alternating contraction and relaxation generally permits painless, nonfatiguing muscle activity, whereas sustained muscle contraction upsets this normal cycle and results in ischemia, accumulation of waste products, and pain. Bonica (1977) suggested that emotional stress, tension, and depression, through psychophysiologic (corticofugal) mechanisms, may produce or augment skeletal muscle spasms, local vasoconstriction, and the liberation of pain-producing substances, thereby intensifying the associated pain. The emotional stimulus may be primary or a reaction to noxious stimulation. Through reflex responses and affective reactions, such peripheral noxious stimulation will, in turn, aggravate emotional stress and provoke more "psychophysiologic impulses" thus sustaining a "vicious circle" of pain. Bonica postulated that this is probably the mechanism of tension headache and pain due to spasm of the muscles of the shoulder girdle, low back, and chest.

There have been a number of observations that suggest that cranial artery (or at least scalp artery) vasoconstriction may play an important role in the production of muscle contraction headaches. Wolff and his colleagues observed that the administration of ergotamine tartrate, an agent that constricts the cranial arteries, often aggravates the muscle contraction headache, as does compression of the carotid artery on the side of the headache. Conversely, amyl nitrite, a cranial artery vasodilator, often transiently relieves headache of the muscle contraction variety. Tunis and Wolff (1954), employing measures previously used for the study of migraine headaches (Tunis and Wolff, 1952; Tunis and Wolff, 1953), compared temporal artery pulse waves of ten muscle contraction headache patients and ten nonheadache controls, the headache patients being studied both during headache and during intervals between headache. They found that, by all measures, headache patients were more vasoconstricted than controls and that, furthermore, vasoconstriction increased significantly during headache.

For example, the average pulse wave amplitude for control subjects was 12 mm. In headache patients the average pulse wave amplitude was 8.3 mm when they were asymptomatic and 4.6 mm during headache. In the headache patients, simultaneous EMG tracings from the area of the head pain demonstrated increased muscle contraction, often by tenfold as compared to EMGs obtained from the same area during a headache-free interval. From the observation that temporal headache was accompanied both by increased muscle contraction and by vasoconstriction, the authors concluded that head pain arose from sustained contraction of ischemic muscle. They suggested that skeletal muscle contraction itself, if sufficiently forceful and sustained, could be painful but that if there was, in addition, vasoconstriction of the relevant nutrient arteries, the amount and duration of muscle contraction necessary for pain production did not have to be as great and that the intensity of the resultant pain from a given degree of muscle contraction would be greater.

Subsequent studies on bulbar conjunctival ischemia in control and muscle contraction headache patients under a variety of circumstances (Ostfeld et al., 1957), demonstrated that (1) during frontal muscle contraction headache, bulbar conjunctival ischemia predictably occurred, (2) during life situations evoking anxiety, apprehension, and patterns of increased alertness and activity, bulbar conjunctival vasoconstriction predictably occurred, and (3) agents promoting extracranial ischemia intensified muscle contraction headaches while vasodilator agents alleviated

muscle contraction headaches. The authors also demonstrated, however, that induction of extracranial ischemia in persons subject to muscle contraction headaches during the headache-free intervals did not produce headache. The investigators concluded that increased skeletal muscle contraction about the head and humorally influenced extracranial vasoconstriction are parallel responses to certain life situations and that, acting together in the same persons, they induce muscle contraction headaches.

Bakal and Kagnov (1977) studied the superficial temporal artery blood flow velocity in patients with muscle contraction and migraine headaches using ultrasonic transducers. The transducers permitted recording of changes in blood flow velocity which were positively related to vasodilatation in the artery, the relationship being established by demonstrating an increased impulse velocity following the inhalation of amyl nitrate, a potent vasodilator. While their study did not provide an indication of the actual degree of vasoconstriction or vasodilatation in headache patients, they observed that both migraine and muscle contraction headache patients responded to a relatively nonaversive auditory stimulus (80 decibel white noise) with superficial temporal artery vasoconstriction, whereas control subjects responded with vasodilatation.

Other studies (Price and Tursky, 1976) have demonstrated that migraineurs exhibit stimulus-induced temporal artery vasoconstriction while control groups vasodilate. These studies suggest that both migraine and muscle contraction headache patients react to a variety of stimuli with vasoconstriction of scalp arteries. It would appear that in migraine patients such vasoconstriction gives way to rebound vasodilatation whereas in muscle contraction headache patients, there is sustained vasoconstriction.

Cohen (1978) described the difficulties in interpreting and comparing the existing studies on the relative roles of muscle contraction and vascular reactivity in migraine and tension headache patients because of procedural differences and the differences in the variables that were studied. He pointed out that many important points remain unanswered and aptly concluded that further studies are needed. He stated that such investigations should include careful and detailed descriptions of diagnostic criteria along with adequate demographic data and standardization of the measurements of physiologic variables.

REFERRED PAIN OF MUSCULAR ORIGIN

Pain associated with skeletal muscle spasm, when sufficiently severe to be of clinical importance, is often referred a distance from the muscle that is its source. The projected or referred pain depends on a small zone of hypersensitivity, commonly called the "trigger point" or "trigger area" located within a muscle in spasm (Travell, 1960). At this site, there is a lowered threshold to stimulation by pressure. Deep pressure on such a trigger area can reproduce the spontaneous pain at a distance and infiltrating it locally with procaine can eliminate the related reference zone of pain. Pain relief induced by the injection of such trigger points outlasts the pharmacologic effects of the injected agent. A trigger point in a skeletal muscle is identified by localized deep tenderness in a palpably firm band of muscle and by a positive "jump sign," a visible shortening of that part of the muscle which contains the band (Travell, 1976).

Induction of referred pain during sustained pressure on the trigger point is reported by the patient if the trigger point is actively causing episodes of referred pain and its threshold to mechanical stimulation is relatively low. It should be noted that skeletal muscle may contain "latent" trigger points which are clinically asymptomatic with respect to pain. Induction of referred pain is not reported during sustained pressure on the latent trigger point, but the point does exhibit deep tenderness and a positive "jump sign" on vigorous snapping (Travell, 1976). Normal muscle tissue does not contain latent trigger points and is not tender to ordinary pressure, but dormant trigger points may be readily activated by minor stress such as periods of immobility, overstretching of muscles, overuse and repetitive movement,

prolonged static effort, chilling or fatigue. Trigger points may develop as a consequence of discogenic disease causing nerve root compression, the trigger point occurring within the segmental distribution of the pain. Travell (1976) has suggested that this fact may explain the post-disc surgery syndrome of continuing pain—i.e., even when surgery was successful, the active trigger points remained.

Each skeletal muscle, and even each part of a given muscle, has a specific pattern of referred pain; that is, a trigger area at a particular site gives rise to essentially the same distribution of referred pain in one person as another. The referred pain patterns do not necessarily follow a simple neurosegmental distribution, but their constancy implies fixed anatomic pathways that link the trigger area with its reference zone. Furthermore, the relationship of the trigger area to its reference zone is the same, regardless of the activating stress.

Lewis (1938) found that pain produced by injecting noxious substances into muscle is identical with that resulting from muscle contracting under ischemic conditions, and noted that, as reported above, the resulting pain was often referred to a distance. Cyriax (1938) demonstrated that injections of 0.1 cc of a 4% solution of sodium chloride into the posterior cervical muscles close to their occipital insertion and into the occipitalis muscle itself gave rise to a pain that ran forward, forming a band that half encircled the head and reached its maximum intensity in the temple and forehead over the eye. Injections into an area between 2 and 5 cm below the occiput induced pain in the back of the head extending up to the vertex. Below this area, injections caused pain in the cervical region only. Campbell and Parsons (1944) later confirmed these observations.

Also using hypertonic saline as an irritant, Kellgren (1938) and later, Travell and her colleagues (Travell and Rinzler, 1952) were able to map various trigger points and their reference zones throughout the body. Trigger areas with remarkably constant zones of referral in the head and/or face were demonstrated in the trapezius, sternocleidomastoid, splenius capitis, occipitalis, temporalis, masseter, and external pterygoid muscles. They found that injecting various areas of these muscles not only gave rise to pain referred to sites at a distance in the head and neck, but also to referred deep tenderness in the same or similar distributions. Referred tenderness often persisted after the pain had subsided and could be abolished by procaine infiltrating of the original, but at that time, "dormant" trigger area. The degree of referred tenderness, in general, corresponded with the duration and severity of the induced pain. Injecting local anesthetic into the muscle or subcutaneous tissue in the reference zone abolished the referred tenderness, but not the referred pain, the latter only responding to infiltration of the original trigger point itself. Of particular interest was the finding that many nonpainful phenomena are also associated with muscle trigger points, particularly in the head and neck region. Travell (1960), for example, reported such nonpainful concomitants of the sternocleidomastoid muscle trigger points as blurred vision, lacrimation, coryza, postural light-headedness, and disequilibrium. Masseter muscle trigger points were found to mediate tinnitus and "stuffiness" of the adjacent ear, and temporalis muscle points were associated with extensive salivation and lacrimation. The nonpainful concomitants of these trigger areas were terminated by procaine infiltration of the trigger points. The mechanism underlying these associated phenomena has not been elucidated.

The anatomic or physiochemical nature of these muscle trigger points or so-called fibrocytic nodules, has never been adequately explained. Various studies have yielded inconclusive and often conflicting results. Travell (1954) demonstrated that a needle thermocouple inserted into a trigger area will record an elevated temperature (as compared to adjacent normal muscle) of 0.15 to 0.6 degrees and that a needle electrode inserted directly into a trigger area records 0.1 mV spike discharges of less than 3 or 4 msec at a rate of 10 to 90/sec for as long as 20 or 30 min (Travell, 1957). Brendstrup et al. (1957) found that biopsies obtained from fibrositic muscle showed an increased concentration of acid mucopolysaccharides, increased water content, increased

chloride content, and a slight accumulation of mast cells. They concluded that the firmer consistency of this portion of muscle is most likely due to edema. Awad (1973) reported that such biopsy specimens showed intercellular deposits of a *ground* substance believed to be mucopolysaccharides and that some have abnormally large myofilaments discharging mast cells and platelets. Fassbender and Wegner (1973), using electron microscopy, reported destructive changes in contractile structures, degenerating mitochondria, increased glycogen deposits, swollen, damaged endothelial cells, and focal areas of cellular proliferation. They inferred that the primary cause of such changes was hypoxia and did not feel that the lesions were inflammatory in nature. This is of particular interest in view of the possible contributing roll of ischemia in muscle pain that has been alluded to above. Of additional interest is Travell's observation (1957) that "vasoconstriction, pallor, sweating and coldness of the skin may be evident during intense referred pain; vasodilatation is observed at once after extinction of the responsible trigger points by local injection."

THERAPEUTIC CONSIDERATIONS

When intracranial pathology, and ocular, sinus, and temparomandibular joint disorders have been excluded and a diagnosis of muscle contraction headache can be made with relative certainty, empiric therapy can commence. In patients with underlying derangements of the cervical spine, appropriate pharmacologic management will often include the use of nonsteroidal antiinflamatory medications. Many such medications are currently available (eg., acetylsalicylic acid, indomethacin, naproxen, fenoprofen, ibuprofen, tolmetin, and sulindac). The use of such agents is largely empirical and the theraputic efficacy and toxicity may vary greatly among individual patients. Only one agent should be used at a time, but it may be necessary to try two or more medications sequentially before a successful agent is encountered. Such medications will certainly not benefit all patients and the side effects (which unfortunately for several nonsteroidal agents include headaches) may be limiting. Many medications are marketed as "muscle relaxants," but none appear to exert a direct relaxing effect on skeletal muscle. Most seem to act through central mechanisms and have tranquilizing and sedating properties. They are best used in short courses rather than continously over long periods of time and should be used cautiously, if at all, in patients who are depressed. Phenacetin-containing compounds are best avoided because of the possibility of analgesic nephropathy. There is no role for ergot alkaloids or anticonvulsant agents in the management of muscle contraction headaches, and narcotic analgesics should be avoided.

Various physical modalities may be helpful, whether or not there is an underlying disorder of the cervical spine. Local heat (moist or dry) may be useful in some patients, whereas ice packs may be more beneficial in others. Ultrasound, diathermy, and gentle massage of the tender neck muscles may also be of benefit. In many patients, particularly those with cervical spondylosis, intermittent cervical traction may be very helpful, and relatively inexpensive traction devices for home use are available. Skillful "manipulation" of the cervical spine may provide transient or long-lasting relief, but should be avoided when there is an underlying disorder that may be associated with instability of the cervical spine. Postural considerations are often of great importance. Patients are often unaware, until it has been pointed out to them, that their symptoms are exacerbated by positions they assume when, for example, watching television, reading, typing, speaking on the telephone, or sleeping. In patients who awaken in the morning with neck pain and/or headache, the appropriate use of a cervical pillow (e.g., the Jackson cervical pillow) is often useful. The judicious use of a properly made and fitted cervical collar, either hard or soft, for short periods of time is often helpful as adjunctive therapy. Rigid immobilization of the cervical spine is seldom necessary or indicated.

Additional adjunctive measures may include the skillful application of a vapo-coolant spray such as ethylchloride or fluoromethane (with the treated muscles maintained under passive stretch) or the injection of selected muscle "trigger points" with local anesthetic agents (Travell, 1976). It is common clinical practice to administer local anesthetic agents in combination with various corticosteriod preparations but the efficacy, if any, of corticosteroids has never been established. Other therapeutic modalities enjoying considerable success at the present time are transcutaneous electrical neurostimulation, acupuncture, acupressure, and Shiatsu massage. Surgical avulsion of the greater occipital nerve or of the intraspinal nerve roots of C2 and C3 are to be discouraged because of the high recurrence rates of headaches following such procedures. Such surgical measures may, however, be useful in a small percentage of carefully selected patients. A more recently described surgical technique has been the "radiofrequency denaturation" of neural and myofascia elements in the suboccipital region. The long-term efficacy of such procedures has yet to be established. In appropriately selected patients with degenerative disc disease limited to one or two levels, anterior interbody fusion may be considered (Peterson et al., 1975). Headache alone, however, is seldom an indication for the performance of anterior cervical fusion.

Life circumstances and associated psychopathology, whether considered a cause or a consequence of chronic headache, must always be taken into consideration. Some patients may benefit from the empiric initiation of a tricyclic antidepressant medication, preferably administered as a single dose at bedtime. Other patients may respond to counseling, relaxation techniques, or behavioral therapy, Formal psychotherapy may be considered, but there are no published results establishing its efficacy in the treatment of chronic headache. Biofeedback techniques hold a great deal of promise and will likely be more successful in the future as individual response patterns are recognized and therapy is applied on a more individualized basis.

SUMMARY

1. Cervical spondylosis, a degenerative disorder involving the intervertebral discs, articu-

lations, and supporting structures of the cervical spine, is a common and important cause of headache, particularly in the middle-aged and elderly population. Headache may be the presenting symptom in such patients.

2. Although neural pathways exist by which painful impulses arising in the neck may be cataloged as headache or facial pain, it is likely that the spondylotic headache is primarily a consequence of sustained contraction of the muscles of the scalp and neck.

3. Any painful stimulus in or about the head, if sufficiently severe and sustained, may cause contraction of neck and or scalp muscles which, in turn, may serve as a secondary source of head pain.

4. The clinical picture of muscle contraction headache may be highly variable, although pain is most often occipital, fronto-occipital, or generalized. Terms used to describe the quality of headache are tightness, band-like constriction, vise-like, and cap-like. The pain is characteristically sustained, persisting for days, weeks, months, or years.

5. Examination of the patient with muscle contraction headache discloses areas of muscle spasm and tenderness in the neck and, frequently, limitation of head and neck motion.

6. Mixed headaches, for example mixed vascular and muscle contraction headaches, are often observed in clinical practice, particularly in patients with headache of long-standing duration. Even when muscle contraction is considered to be a secondary phenomenon, it often requires treatment if headaches are to be successfully alleviated.

7. Therapy of muscle contraction headaches, whether associated with cervical spondylosis or not, is largely empiric, and successful treatment requires patience and perseverance on the part of the physician and his patient. Therapeutic measures may include the use of nonsteroidal antiinflammatory medications, Tricyclic antidepressants, non-narcotic analgesics, various physiotherapy modalities including intermittent cervical traction, the skilled use of vapor-coolant sprays and "trigger point injections," biofeedback and progressive relaxation techniques, behavioral therapy and, in highly selected patients, intensive psychotherapy.

8. Narcotic analgesics, ergot alkoloids, and phenacetin-containing compounds are to be discouraged.

9. Surgical procedures such as greater occipital neurectomy, intraspinal section of the spinal routes of the C2 and C3, radiofrequency denaturation, and anterior cervical fusion may be considered in a small, carefully selected group of patients.

REFERENCES

Awad, E. A. (1973). Interstitial myofibrositis, hypothesis of the mechanism. *Arch. Phys. Med. 54,* 449-453.

Bakal, D. A., and S. A. Kagnov (1977). Muscle contraction and migraine headache: psychologic comparison. *Headache 17,* 208-214.

Barcroft, H., and J. Millen (1939). The blood flow through muscle during sustained contraction. *J. Physiol. 97,* 17-31.

Bonica, J. J. (1977). Introduction to symposium on pain. *Arch. Surg. 112,* 749-761.

Brain, W. R. (1963). Some unsolved problems of cervical spondylosis. *Brit. Med. J. 1:*771-777.

Brendstrup, P., K. Jesperson, and G. Asboe-Hanson (1957). Morphologic and chemical connective tissue changes in fibrositic muscles. *Ann. Rheum. Dis. 76,* 438-440.

Budzynski, T. H., J. M. Stoyva, C. S. Adler, and P. J. Mullaney, (1973). EMG biofeedback and tension headache: a controlled outcome study. *Psychosom. Med. 35,* 484-496.

Caillet, R. (1964). *Neck and Arm Pain.* F. A. Davis, Philadelphia.

Campbell, D. G., and Parson, C. M. (1944). Referred head pain and its concomitants. Report of preliminary experimental investigation with implications for the post-traumatic "head" syndrome. *J. Nerv. Ment. Dis. 99,* 544.

Chambers, W. R. (1954). Posterior rhizotomy of the second and third cervical nerves for occipital pain. *JAMA 155,* 431-432.

Cloward, R. B. (1959). Cervical discography: a contribution to the etiology and mechanism of neck, shoulder and arm pain. *Ann. Surg. 150,* 1052-1064.

Cloward, R. B. (1960). The clinical significance of the sinu-vertebral nerve of the cervical spine in relation to the cervical disk syndrome. *J. Neurol. Neurosurg. Psychiat. 23,* 321-326.

Cohen, M. J. (1978). Psychological studies of headache: is there similarity between migraine and muscle contraction headaches? *Headache 18,* 189-196.

Cyriax, J. (1938). Rheumatic headache. *Brit. Med. J. 2,* 1367.

Dorpat, T. L., and T. H. Holmes (1955). Mechanisms of skeletal muscle pain and fatigue. *Arch. Neurol. Psychiat. 74,* 628-640.

Edgar, M. A., and J. A. Ghadially (1976). Innervation of the lumbar spine. *Clin. Ortho. 115*, 35–41.

Elliott, F. A. (1944). Tender muscles in sciatica. Electromyographic studies. *Lancet 1*, 47.

Eyring, E. D. (1969). The biochemistry and physiology of the intervertebral disk. *Clin. Orthop. 67*, 16.

Fassbender, H. G., and K. Wegner (1973). Morphologic and pathogenesis des Weichteilrheumatismus. *Z. Rheumaforsch. 32*, 355–374.

Harper, R. G., and J. C. Steger (1978). Psychological correlates of frontalis EMG and pain in tension headache. *Headache 18*, 215–218.

Haynes, S. M., P. Griffin, O. Mooney, and M. Parise (1975). Electromyographic biofeedback and relaxation instructions in the treatment of muscle contraction headaches. *Behav. Ther. 6*, 672–678.

Hill, A. V. (1948). The pressure developed in muscle during contraction. *J. Physiol. 107*, 518–526.

Hinsey, J. C. (1928). Observations on the innervation of the blood vessels in skeletal muscle. *J. Comp. Neurol. 47*, 23.

Hunter, C. R. and F. H. Mayfield (1949). Role of the upper cervical nerve roots in the production of pain in the head. *Am. J. Surg. 78*, 743–749.

Kellgren, J. H. (1938). Observations on referred pain arising from muscle. *Clin. Sci. 3*, 175–190.

Kerr, F. W. L. (1961). Structural relations of trigeminal spinal tract to upper cervical roots and solitary nucleus in cat. *Exper. Neurol. 4*, 134–138.

Kerr, F. W. L. (1963). Mechanisms, diagnosis and management of some cranial and facial pain syndromes. *Surg. Clin. N. Am. 43*, 951–961.

Kitahata, L., R. G. McAllister, and A. T. Taub (1974). Identification of central trigeminal nociceptors. *Adv. Neurol. 4*, 83.

Kudrow, L. (1976). Tension headache—scalp muscle contraction headache. In *Pathogenesis and Treatment of Headache* (O. Appenzeller, ed.). Spectrum, New York.

Lance, J. W. (1978). *Mechanism and Management of Headache*, 3rd ed. Butterworths, Boston.

Lance, J. W., D. A. Curran, and M. Anthony (1965). Investigation into the mechanism and treatment of chronic headache. *Med. J. Aust. 2*, 909.

Lawrence, J. S., R. DeGraff, and U. A. I. Laine (1963). Degenerative joint diseases in Random samples and occupational groups. In *Epidemiology of Chronic Rheumatism Vol. I.* (J. H. Kellgren, M. R. Jeffrey, and J. Ball eds.). Blackwell Scientific Publications, Oxford.

Lewis, T. (1938). Suggestions relating to the study of somatic pain. *Brit. Med. J. 1*, 321.

Lewis, T. (1942). *Pain.* MacMillan, New York.

Magora, F., A. Magora, O. Abramsky, and B. Gonen (1974). An electromyographic investigation of the neck muscles in headache. *Electromyogr. Clin. Neurol. Physiol. 14*, 453–462.

McNaughton, F. L. (1938). The innervation of the intracranial blood vessels and dural sinuses. *Assoc. Res. Nerv. Dis. Proc. 18*, 178.

Mooney, V., and J. Robertson (1976). The facet syndrome. *Clin. Orthop. 115*, 149–156.

Murayama, K. (1972). Biochemical studies of the age related variation of human intervertebral disks. *J. Jap. Orthop. Assoc. 46*, 81–104.

Murphy, J. P. (1969). Occipital neurectomy in the treatment of headache. *Md. State Med. S. 18*, 62.

Neufeld, R. W. J., and P. D. Davidson (1974). Sex differences in stress reponse: a multivariate analysis. *J. Abn. Psych. 23*, 178–185.

Ostfield, A. M., D. S. Reis, and H. G. Wolff (1957). Studies in headache: bulbar conjunctival ischemia and muscle contraction headache. *Arch. Neurol. Psychiat. 77*, 113.

Pallis, C., A. M. Jones, and J. D. Spillane (1954). Cervical spondylosis. Incidence and implications. *Brain 77*, 274–289.

Pawl, R. P. (1977). Headache, cervical spondylosis and anterior cervical fusion. *Surg. Ann. 9*, 391–408.

Peck, C. L., and G. H. Kraft (1977). Electromyographic feedback for pain related to muscle tension. *Arch. Surg. 112*, 889–895.

Perl, S., P. Markle, and L. N. Katz (1934). Factors involved in the production of skeletal muscle pain. *Arch. Intern. Med. 53*, 814–824.

Peterson, D. I., G. M. Austin, and L. A. Dayes (1975). Headache associated with discogenic disease of the cervical spine. *Bull. L. A. Neurol. Soc. 40*, 96–100.

Pozniak-Patewicz, E. (1976). "Cephalic" spasm of head and neck muscles. *Headache 15*, 261–266.

Price, K. P., and B. Tursky (1976). Vascular reactivity of migraineurs and nonmigraineurs, a comparison of responses to self-control procedures. *Headache 16*, 210–217.

Raney, A. A., and R. B. Raney (1948). Headaches: a common symptom of cervical disk lesions. *Arch. Neurol. Psychiat. 54*, 603–621.

Rodbard, S. (1970). Pain associated with muscle contraction. *Headache 10*, 105.

Schumaker, G. A., B. S. Ray, and H. G. Wolff (1940). Experimental studies on headache. Further analysis of histamine headache and its pain pathways. *Arch. Neurol. Psychiat. 44*, 701.

Shinohara, H. (1970). A study on lumbar disk lesions. *J. Jap. Orthop. Assoc. 44*, 553.

Simons, D. J., E. Day, H. Goodell, and H. G. Wolff (1943). Experimental studies on headache: muscles of the scalp and neck as sources of pain. *Assoc. Res. Nerv. Dis. Proc. 23*, 228–244.

Travell, J. (1954). Introductory remarks in *Connective Tissue: Transactions of the Fifth Conference*, pp. 12–22 (C. Ragan, ed.), Josiah Macy Jr. Foundation, New York.

Travell, J. (1957). *In* Symposium on the mechanism and management of pain syndromes. *Proc. Rudolf Virchow. Med. Soc. 16*, 128–136.

Travell, J. (1960). Temporomandibular joint pain referred from muscles of the head and neck. *J. Prosth. Dent. 104*, 745–763.

Travell, J. (1976). Myofascial trigger points: clinical review. *Advances in Pain Research*, Vol. 1, p. 919–

926. (J. J. Bonica and D. Albe-Fessard, eds.). Raven Press, New York.

Travel, J., and S. H. Rinzler (1952). The myofascial genesis of pain. *Post grad. Med.* 9, 425–434.

Tunis, M. M., and H. G. Wolff (1952). Analysis of cranial artery pulse waves in patients with vascular headache of the migraine type. *Am. J. Med. Sci.* 224, 565.

Tunis, M. D., and H. G. Wolff (1953). Studies on headache: long term observation of the reactivity of the cranial arteries in subjects with vascular headache of the migraine type. *Arch. Neurol. Psychiat.* 70, 551–557.

Tunis, M. D., and H. G. Wolff (1954). Studies on headache: cranial artery vasoconstriction and muscle contraction headache. *Arch. Neurol. Psychiat.* 71, 425–434.

Vaughan, R., M. H. Pawl, and S. N. Haynes (1977). Frontalis EMG response to stress in subjects with frequent muscle contraction headaches. *Headache* 16, 313–317.

White, A. A., W. O. Southwick, R. J. Deponte, J. W. Gainor and R. Hardy (1973). Relief of pain by anterior cervical spine fusion for spondylosis. A report of 65 patients. *J. Bone Joint Surg.* 55, 525.

Wilkinson, J. (1971). *Cervical spondylosis: its early diagnosis and treatment.* Saunders, Philadelphia.

Woodburne, R. T. (1965). *Essentials of Human Anatomy,* Oxford Univ. Press, New York.

20

THE TEETH AND JAWS AS SOURCES OF HEADACHE

FRANK V. HOWELL

INTRODUCTION

Both odontalgia and the broad area of motion-related disturbances referred to as temporomandibular joint (TMJ) syndrome, are of concern to the physician and the dentist. All too often, odontalgia or TMJ syndrome, also known as myofascial pain dysfunction syndrome, may in some stages mimic trigeminal or other neuralgias, or the patient may exhibit psychological disturbances which suggest to the clinician that the pain is not of local origin. Before anticonvulsant or antidepressant drugs are prescribed, and before surgical disruption of a peripheral nerve is considered, the possibility of local and reversible sources of nerve excitation must be ruled out. Ruling out dental disease and temporomandibular joint dysfunction is mandatory in the evaluation of headache and other head pain, particularly when it is monolateral.

Pain due to inflammatory and retrograde pulpal disease and to periodontal disease is relatively common and is not difficult to evaluate and eliminate, particularly if a specific lesion can be demonstrated clinically or radiologically. However, there are some atypical manifestations of pulpal disease and the TMJ syndrome in which a direct etiology is not evident. "Normal patterns" can be the exception rather than the rule.

The apprehension of impending dental procedures constitutes a real barrier to adequate diagnosis and may alter the pain pattern as well as affect the threshold of response of a patient to nerve testing, digital palpation, percussion, etc. In the TMJ syndrome, emotional factors are often of extreme importance and are an integral part of the painful condition because of nervous habits and bruxism.

ANATOMICAL AND PHYSIOLOGICAL CONSIDERATIONS

Impulses from the teeth and temporomandibular joint area are carried by branches of the second and third divisions of the fifth cranial nerve. Nerves enter the pulp through the apex and accompany the larger vessels to form an almost complete mantle around the arteries (Barkelbach, 1935). These nerve fibers form a complicated network between the odontoblasts and extend partially into the calcified portion of the dentinal tubule, permitting the surface of dentin, wherever exposed, to transmit pain as in caries or dentin fractures (Lewinsky and Stewart, 1935). Brashear (1936) found that more than half of the unmyelinated and small myelinated nerve fibers were less than 6μ with the remainder varying in size up to 10μ. Thermal, mechanical, and chemical stimulation of dentin in a normal tooth results only in pain with no other sensation. Sensations such as touch and pressure appear to be transmitted primarily to the nerve endings in the periodontal membrane and the alveolar bone.

A classic study by Robertson *et al.* (1947) demonstrated the distribution and pathophysiology of headache and other pain in the face and head resulting from afferent impulses originating in the teeth. Comparisons were made between experimental stimulation of the teeth and clinical situations in which morbid processes were present. In the study, two different electrical methods were employed: one, for inducing toothache well above the pain threshold, and the other, for inducing pain only at the threshold. For high-intensity toothache, a 60-cycle, 110 V stimulator was used with a step-down transformer giving a voltage from 0 to 25 V. A bipolar electrode was insulated to the tips. The handle of the electrode was held by the subject and the tips were placed securely against the tooth, utilizing small traumatic chips in the enamel and areas in which pit cavities were present. With the subject sitting in a chair, a rheostat was gradually advanced from zero to a voltage sufficient to induce toothache of 4 to 8+ intensity. Pain was estimated on an arbitrary basis of 1 to 10, with 10+ being extremely high intensity or the point at which patient experienced the "worst" pain. Toothache was held at the 4 to 8 intensity for a period of 10 min. In the lower ranges of intensity, initial current inducing toothaches had to be increased to continue to induce pain. Thus, the voltage was gradually increased and current was momentarily interrupted every 5 to 10 sec to keep the toothache in the 4 to 8+ range.

In the second method used to induce pain at its threshold, a "vitalometer" was employed as described by Ziskin and Wald (1938). This is a method similar to the pulp testing procedures performed clinically by most dentists. A single electrode is applied to the tooth and the circuit is completed through a coupling held in the hand of the subject. The pain threshold in this phase of the experiment was expressed as the smallest voltage which would elicit a painful sensation.

Description of Headache Resulting from Noxious Stimulation of the Teeth

In a study conducted at the New York Hospital, headache which occurred after experimental induction of toothache in the manner described above was divided into *Series 1, Noxious Stimulation of Teeth in the Upper Jaw*, and *Series 2, Noxious Stimulation of Teeth in the Lower Jaw*. In Series 1, the stimulation to a premolar or first molar tooth in the maxilla, pain of 4 to 8+

intensity and was manifested by pain in the tooth. However, following a break in the stimulating current, a jab of more intense pain was experienced as a "narrow column of pain which spread vertically into the eye, the orbital ridge, and the temple." With extremely intense toothache (10+), pain spread into adjacent teeth and along the maxilla. During the period of toothache, intense apprehension, profuse salivation, lacrimation, and flushing of the face on the side of stimulation were noted with generalized sweating. On termination of stimulation, pain decreased quickly to 1+ intensity with only a sensation of pressure between the teeth. After toothache completely diminished, there was a continuing sensation of tightness, slight numbness, and fullness over the cheek, and a tight, stiff sensation in the skin and deep tissues in the temporal region, the forehead, and scalp on the same side. Some stiffness in the temporomandibular joint and fullness in the ear was described. Within 5 to 10 min after all pain in the tooth was terminated, a steady aching and diffuse pain of 1+ intensity was experienced in the temporal region, along the zygomatic ridge, and for a short distance over the eye. Graphic demonstration of the pattern of head pain was expressed (Fig. 20-1) 5 min and 20 min after stimulation. Most headache persisted from 1 to 8 hr and in one instance for up t 24 hr with gradually diminishing intensity. Although the sensation of tightness, fullness, and numbness was rather short lived, during the period of diminishing intensity there was photophobia and injection of the conjunctiva, with tenderness to the temporal muscle and overlying tissues on palpation. Sensation to a pinprick was sharper.

In Series 2, a lower premolar or first molar tooth was stimulated in the same manner as in Series 1, maintaining the 4 to 8+ toothache for a period of 10 min. During the stimulation, there was intense aching pain in the tooth with a less intense pain throughout the lower jaw extending into the anterior wall of the ear canal. At the end of the stimulation, the high-intensity pain was quickly terminated, but a persistent sensation of pressure in the tooth was noted, often accompanied by a dull, diffuse, aching pain of low intensity throughout

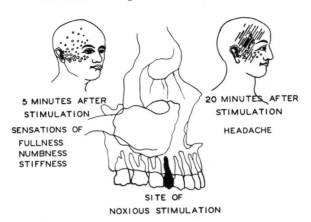

5 MINUTES AFTER
STIMULATION

SENSATIONS OF
FULLNESS
NUMBNESS
STIFFNESS

20 MINUTES AFTER
STIMULATION

HEADACHE

SITE OF
NOXIOUS STIMULATION

FIG. 20-1. The distribution of sensations of fullness, numbness, and stiffness, and the distribution of headache following noxious stimultion of a tooth in the upper jaw.

the lower jaw on the same side. Subsequently, there developed a sensation of fullness and heaviness, then a 2 to 3+ intensity of pain which extended throughout the upper and lower jaws into the zygoma and temporal area and extending over the top of the ear. There was also fullness and aching in the ear. This "lower half" headache was increased in intensity by biting and bending over. The pattern is well demonstrated in Fig. 20-2. Many of the same effects were noted as in Series 1—apprehension, lacrimation, salivation, flushing of the face, photophobia, and generalized sweating as well as stiffness of the masseter muscle. The quality of pain in response to aspirin was the same in Series 1 and in Series 2. In each series, the effects of noxious stimulation were completely reversible and no sequelae were noted. Results of this classic and extensive study are well documented by the clinical pattern of odontology due to retrograde and inflammatory odontalgia. In the same experiment, the effect of local anesthetic to the source of noxious stimulation adjacent to the tooth was applied in two phases. In the first, procaine injections, there was direct injection into the area of headache, and pain persisted in scattered fashion with greatest area of pain diminished. However, there was complete absence of pain following the local anesthetic injection by an infiltrative procedure (tuberos-

ity injection). Some pain returned following the cessation of anesthesia to the area; in some cases, the area remained free when normal sensation returned to the tooth.

In conclusion, it is obvious that the elimination of the headache after blocking the path of afferent impulses from the tooth and adjacent tissues allows one to assume that the experience was caused by afferent impulses arising from the stimulated tooth. These afferent impulses thus gave rise to excitatory processes in the brainstem which spread to exert effects on many trigeminal structures.

Practical Clinical Considerations

Although it can be demonstrated by the described experiments of toothache-induced headache and by clinical manifestation of odontalgia that the headache follows certain prescribed patterns, there is an obvious and practical clinical consideration. Only under unusual circumstances can this type of headache be seen without accompanying odontalgia from a diseased pulp or an inflamed periodontal condition. A relatively easy elimination of this pain by nerve blockage or infiltrative local anesthesia produces a fairly clear cut *cause and effect* relationship. Unfortunately, the observation made experimentally that the headache can return when the local

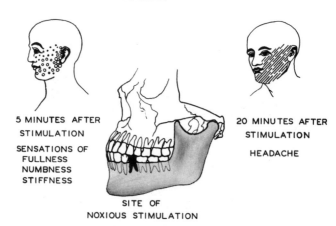

5 MINUTES AFTER
STIMULATION

SENSATIONS OF
FULLNESS
NUMBNESS
STIFFNESS

20 MINUTES AFTER
STIMULATION

HEADACHE

SITE OF
NOXIOUS STIMULATION

FIG. 20-2. The distribution of sensations of fullness, numbness, and stiffness, and the distribution of headache following the noxious stimulation of a tooth in the lower jaw.

anesthetic effect dissipates often leads, in a clinical situation, to discomfort for the patient. The present practice of using short-acting, local anesthetics for operative procedures should possibly be replaced by the use of longer-acting, local anesthetics, such as bupivacaine hydrochloride.

CRACKED-TOOTH SYNDROME

Odontalgia from the usual degenerative and inflammatory etiologies produces patterns of pain which become obvious when local anesthetic is utilized and the pain dissipates. The cracked-tooth syndrome (incomplete tooth fracture) is of considerable clinical significance to the physician as well as to the dentist in evaluating pain which does not follow the "usual" patterns of odontalgia-type, induced referred pain.

Incomplete tooth fracture, or cracked tooth syndrome, presents diagnostic problems which have been recognized in dental literature for a number of years. Gibbs (1954) termed the condition "cuspal fracture odontalgia." Sutton (1962) described the condition as "greenstick fracture of the tooth crown." Cameron (1964) coined the term "cracked tooth syndrome" and this appears to be the most commonly used designation. A subsequent report by Silvestri (1976) described the same condition as "the

undiagnosed split-root syndrome," but the term has not been generally adopted; Maxwell and Braly (1977) felt that all subsequent papers dealt with the same entity and thus coined the term "incomplete tooth fracture." In probably the most comprehensive study (Cameron, 1964) a significant series of cases was presented. From Table 20-1, it is obvious that more than half of all cracked teeth are mandibular molars with the second molar the most commonly involved. There has been considerable speculation as to the preponderance of involvement of the lower molar teeth, based upon the motion of the mandible and the posi-

TABLE 20-1   Locations of Cracked Teeth

TOOTH	No.	%
Mandibular		
second molars	17	34
first molars	9	18
third molars	1	2
bicuspids	1	2
Maxillary		
first molars	12	24
second molars	2	4
first bicuspids	6	12
second bicuspids	2	4
Totals	50	100

tion of the lingual cusps of the maxillary molars which produce a cleavage action. Molars most frequently involved have often been restored only in the central fossae and many of the teeth have no restoration whatsoever. Examination of prehistoric skulls does not reveal a significant incidence of cracked teeth, and it has been speculated that the popularity of hot liquids, such as coffee and soup, and the ready availability of cold and frozen foods, such as ice cream, combine to produce extensive expansion and contraction of the enamel and dentin, thus making the structure susceptible to fracture.

The symptomatology of cracked teeth is summarized in Table 20-2, from Cameron (1964). Typically, a patient will complain of pain radiating to the side of the head after biting on food which is compressible, such as nuts, meat, dried fruit, etc. Pain is often sudden and, after the initial impulse, localization of the specific tooth is sometimes difficult for the patient to determine. Following such an incident, the tooth is characteristically sensitive to cold. This sensation continues to be an important diagnostic consideration since the application of electric pulp testers often does not differentiate between a normal tooth and a cracked tooth, whereas a cracked tooth is extremely sensitive to cold.

The cracked tooth syndrome presents an unfortunate clinical situation since the patient experiences head pain. In the later stages, the odontalgia can become localized and severe with eventuation in actual pulpal death and usual sequelae. For this reason, when the condition is first discovered, coronal protection is indicated and, where possible, the vitality of the pulp is preserved in order to allow the odontoblasts to repair the fracture. It is obvious that extirpation of the pulp of a cracked tooth essentially condemns the tooth to eventual extraction since continued seepage of oral fluids will occur to the cracked areas making endodontic treatment unsuccessful.

TEMPOROMANDIBULAR JOINT SYNDROME (MYOFASCIAL PAIN DYSFUNCTION SYNDROME)

Costen's (1934) concept of occlusal disharmony with resultant damage to the temporomandibular joint with a wide variety of signs and symptoms has been totally discarded and replaced by concepts probably first delineated by Schwartz (1955). The term "temporomandibular joint pain dysfunction syndrome" was coined along with a plausible explanation of the pain patterns correlated with muscular and articular disturbances. The more popular term "myofascial pain dysfunction syndrome" is now frequently seen in the literature. Schwartz's studies replace the largely mechanical concept of an occlusal etiology with a broader concept of the entire masticatory apparatus. Schwartz particularly stressed that the psychological characteristics of the patient were often responsible for the occurence of the syndrome.

Although there are many diseases which affect the temporomandibular joint, most are not associated with the type of pain which is often associated with headache or confused with disturbances in the fifth nerve. Pain in the syndrome is felt to be due to spasm of the masticatory muscles and is often precipitated by an overextension of the jaw, stretching the muscle and producing a spasm upon contraction. This muscle overextension can be produced by an encroachment by prosthetic appliances or dental restorations on the space between the maxilla and the mandible or may result from overclosure as a result of loss of alveolar bone and/or the posterior teeth. Many oral habits, such as bruxism, have been implicated in producing the pain of the syndrome. Laskin

TABLE 20-2 Symptoms of Cracked Teeth

PAIN	NO. OF PATIENTS
Pressure	27
Cold	16
Heat	14
Ache	9
Cellulitis	5
Sweet	1
None reported	6

(1969) has described the "psychophysiological" characteristics of the syndrome.

Clinical Features and Diagnosis

There are varying clinical features, but four signs and symptoms must be present for a diagnosis of TMJ:

1. Muscle tenderness
2. Clicking or popping noise in joint
3. Limitation of jaw motion
4. Pain

To differentiate from organic diseases of the joint itself, two negative findings should be present:

1. No clinical, radiographic, or laboratory evidence of joint disease
2. Lack of tenderness in the joint to palpation through the external auditory meatus

Patients exhibit a median age of 32. A female majority of nearly 85% is seen in most studies. In a series Greene *et al.* (1969) found more than 80% of the patients had masticatory and cervical muscle tenderness. Specific muscles involved:

Lateral pterygoid	84%
Masseter	70%
Temporalis	49%
Medial pterygoid	35%
Cervical, scalp, and facial	43%

Clicking and popping occurred in 66% of the patients and limitation of movement, in 63%. Subluxations, vertigo, etc. occurred less frequently.

Because of the distribution of the fifth nerve, patients have described the pain as toothache, earache, sore neck, headache, sinus, and neuralgia.

Sudden onset is often described by patients, but in the Greene study only 48% of the patients could recall a specific incident related to the disease.

Intensification of pain often occurs as a distinctive feature because of the contralateral nature of the masticatory apparatus. Thus a patient with pain on the right side favors that side by chewing on the left, thereby increasing luxation and muscle spasm.

Treatment should be conservative and often is most effective when the masticatory apparatus is explained to the patient. Establishing a hinge relationship, and thus eliminating muscle spasm caused by luxation is paramount. This may require prostheses to provide posterior occlusal surfaces. Certainly conservative medications such as muscle relaxants are effective. Elimination or reduction of emotional factors is necessary. Myotherapeutic exercises and physiotherapy are adjuncts. Extensive occlusal equilibration or reconstruction can often lead to an intensification of the symptoms.

SUMMARY

1. By noxious stimulation of healthy and diseased teeth it is possible to analyze a variety of face and head pains that stem from the teeth.

2. Use of locally acting anesthetics to interfere with toothache-induced headache allows one to assume that the painful experience was caused by afferent impulses arising from the stimulated tooth.

3. The cracked-tooth syndrome (incomplete tooth fracture) may produce pain radiating to the head following mastication. Appropriate therapy will resolve the matter.

4. The temporomandibular joint syndrome represents a dysfunction of the entire masticatory apparatus. It is associated with muscle tenderness, clicking or popping noises in the joint, limitation of joint movement, and pain. Much of the pain is related to muscle spasm. Treatment should be invariably conservative.

REFERENCES

Berkelbach van der Sprenkle, S. (1935–36). Microscopical investigation of the tooth and its surroundings. *J. Anat.* 70, 233.

Brashear, A. D. (1936). Innervation of the teeth. *J. Am. Dent. Assoc.* 23, 662.

Cameron, C. E. (1964). Cracked tooth syndrome. *J. Am. Dent. Assoc.* 68, 405.

Costen, J. B. (1934). A syndrome of ear and sinus symptoms dependent upon disturbed function of the temporomandibular joint. *Ann. Otol. Rhinol. Laryngol.* 43, 1.

Gibbs, J. W. (1954). Cuspal fracture odontalgia. *Dental Digest* 60, 158.

Greene, C. S., M. D. Lerman, H. D. Sutcher, and

D. M. Laskin (1969). The TMJ pain-dysfunction syndrome: heterogeneity of the patient population. *J. Am. Dent. Assoc. 79*, 1168.

Laskin, D. M. (1969). Etiology of the pain-dysfunction syndrome. *J. Am. Dent. Assoc. 79*, 147.

Lewinsky, W., and D. Stewart (1935–36). The innervation of the dentine. *J. Anat. 70*, 349.

Maxwell, E. H., and B. V. Braly (1977). Incomplete tooth fracture. *J. Calif. Dental Assoc.*, October, pp. 51–55.

Robertson, H. S., H. Goodell, and H. G. Wolff (1947). Studies on headache: the teeth as a source of headache and other pain. *Arch. Neurol. Psychiat. 57*, 277.

Schwartz, L. (1955). Pain associated with the temporomandibular joint. *J. Am. Dent. Assoc. 51*, 394.

Silvestri, A. R. (1976). The undiagnosed split-root syndrome. *J. Am. Dent. Assoc. 92*, 930.

Sutton, P. R. N. (1962). Greenstick fracture of the tooth crown. *Brit. Dent. Jo. 112*, 362.

Ziskin, D. E., and A. Wald (1938). Observations on electrical pulp testing. *J. Dent. Res. 17*, 79.

21

THE EYES AS A SOURCE OF HEADACHE

REVISED BY DAVID M. WORTHEN

To the eye, as to the nasal and paranasal structures, there is incorrectly attributed a large number and variety of headaches. Although headaches in and about the eye are common, relatively seldom are they the result of noxious stimuli originating in the eye, the extraocular muscles, or the optic nerve. Similarly, although photophobia is a dramatic accompaniment of eye disease, it is most often a manifestation of noxious stimulation of head structures other than the eye.

Although headache and other pains due to disorders of the eye per se are numerically few, they may be intense and their implications sometimes ominous. Thus, errors of refraction, disturbances of extraocular muscular equilibrium, inflammation of extra- and intraocular structures, and increased intraocular pressure may cause headache. (Behrens, 1976; Behrens, 1978; Cogan, 1941). The investigations discussed in the following paragraphs were carried out to analyze the pathophysiology of such pain and to indicate principles for clinical application (Eckardt et al., 1943).

The sensory nerve fibers of the eye are derived chiefly from the ophthalmic division of the fifth cranial nerve, via the long ciliary nerves. These penetrate the eyeball in variable number around the optic nerve, and run forward in the sclerato enter the cornea circumferentially around the sclerocorneal junction. The nerve fibers innervating the cornea are in large part myelinated as they enter the corneal connective tissue, but lose their myelin sheaths as they pass from the periphery toward the center of the cornea. The unmyelinated ramifications of these fibers then form a plexus in the connective tissue with terminal twigs, knobs, loops, brushes, or fine skeins, and branches of this plexus penetrate into the epithelium where they may form a second plexus with free terminals. The cornea, therefore, contains a ramifying sensory innervation concerned in good part with the reception of pain, which is distributed both beneath and within the epithelial layer, and throughout the depth of the latter. Krause's end-bulbs, which are probably concerned with sensations other than pain, are found at the sclerocorneal junction (Strughold, 1924; Tower, 1943).

PAIN FROM OCULAR STRUCTURES

Sensitivity of Surface Ocular Structures

The modalities of touch, pain, and temperature were investigated on both the conjunctiva and cornea in normal subjects (Eckardt et al., 1943).

The recognition and localization of touch sensation was tested with cotton wisps. Temperature recognition was tested by applying small, smooth metal or glass rods at known temperatures. Finally, pain was investigated by pricking and pinching the conjunctiva. Throughout, the intensity of pain was estimated on the basis of 10 plus as maximum. The results of the investigation of these sensory modalities were uniform in five subjects.

CONJUNCTIVA

Cotton wisps applied to the conjunctiva produced the sensation of touch without pain. The area touched could be localized as below, above, right, or left. In testing temperature recognition on the conjunctiva, both bulbar and palpebral, it was found that applicators cooled to below 30° C were recognized as cool or cold, whereas above this temperature and up to 70° C, they were recognized only as touch. Application to the skin of the lid, however, caused the usual sensation of cold, cool, warm, and hot. Pricking or pinching the conjunctiva produced pain without definite radiation; and again, the experimental subject was able to localize the area stimulated as above, below, right, or left.

CORNEA

Application of cotton wisps to the cornea failed to produce any sensation of touch. Subliminal stimuli, in the form of a single cotton fiber applied lightly, produced no sensation at all, whereas stronger stimuli caused immediate pain with reflex blinking and withdrawal. Whether one or more such stimuli were applied, the sensation was pain without distinction between single or multiple pain sensations. Temperatures below 30° C were also recognized as cool or cold by the cornea, while between 30° and 70° C they produced only the sensation of pain.

On the conjunctiva touch, pain, and cold are perceived and localized. On the cornea, on the other hand, there has been found no recognition of warmth or heat up to 70° C. Only pain and cold are perceived, pain sensation being very intense and having a low threshold; touch and two-point discrimination are absent. It is possible that with other techniques touch could be perceived on the cornea.

Comment. Pain from injury or inflammation of the conjunctiva is of a steady, burning, and aching quality of minimal or moderate intensity. Pain from similar involvement of the cornea is usually of high intensity and there is tenderness of the eyeball. In neither instance is the pain related to the time of day. Photophobia with corneal lesions is of high intensity. The photophobia is characterized by its prompt reduction, or abolition, after the instillation of a topical anesthetic into the conjunctival sac. Much of the deep aching pain of corneal injury of infection is relieved by cycloplegia with 1% atropine or ¼% scopolamine. Patching the eye closed under pressure is also helpful. If an infection is present the patch must be removed frequently to apply antiviral or antibiotic agents.

Clinical Application. Definitive treatment of corneal lesions consists in removing the source of irritation. When immediate removal of the irritant is not feasible or possible, photophobia is diminished by reducing the light stimulus with dark glasses, eye shades and shields, and darkened rooms. Topical anesthetic should never be continually applied as it delays healing of the epithelium and leads to chronic pain and scarring of the cornea. Temporary relief for examination can be given with the use of 0.5% proparacaine hydrochloride (Ophthaine). Codeine sulfate (60 mg) by mouth and cold wet packs over the eyes may help. Such procedures are used only for temporary relief until the source of irritation can be removed. However, with chemical or ultraviolet burns and some infections, spontaneous recovery occurs with time alone. The irritation and pain resulting from the accumulation of exudate is eliminated by the use of warm physiologic saline. Antibiotic and antiviral ointments and drops may be indicated along with patching the eye and cycloplegia agents.

Recurrent Corneal Erosion. This syndrome is characterized by attacks of steady, burning, and aching pains of high intensity which is unilateral, and may be limited to the eyeball, but usually spreads over the distribution of the first division of the fifth cranial nerve. An attack may last for hours with a high-intensity pain beginning more often in the morning. It is associated with severe blepharospasm and photophobia, and may recur at intervals, sometimes of a year or more, for as long as six or seven years. The high-intensity pain is usually followed by minimal- or low-intensity pain, which may persist for days. The pain is greatly increased in intensity by opening the eyes, but may persist despite the tight closing of the eyelids. It is associated with redness of the conjunctiva and tear secretion. Examination of the cornea with fluorescine demonstrates that there is always a break in the epithelium, and there may be small scars or blebs. The syndrome usually is a sequel to injury to the eye or herpes simplex. It is best managed by keeping the eyelid closed and may be helped by the use of hyperosmotic (5% NaCl) drops or ointment to dehydrate the epithelium and allow the hemidesmosomes of the basal cells to seal to

Bowman's membrane. The history of recurrent attacks may sometimes superficially resemble that of migraine or other vascular, painful recurrent episodes. Removal of epithelium at the site of the lesion may be followed by healing and the elimination of pain. Fortunately this syndrome occurs rarely.

Increased Intraocular Pressure (Glaucoma)

In a New York Hospital patient with acute angle-closure glaucoma with an associated intraocular pressure above 90 mm Hg (four times the upper limit of normal), the pain experienced was localized in the eyeball with radiation to the homolateral frontal area up to the vertex (i.e., the area of distribution of the ophthalmic division of the trigeminal nerve). The pain was described as "terrible" couldn't be worse, and, at its height, nausea and vomiting ensued with inability to retain even water. Neither hot nor cold compresses, nor 60 mg of codeine phosphate by mouth had any effect, though 15 mg of morphine sulfate hypodermically did provide temporary relief. When intraocular pressure was reduced to 20 to 30 mm Hg by intensive miotic therapy, the pain was completely eliminated. A second patient with a less severe attack of acute glaucoma described the accompanying pain as a "bad aching pain." In this case the pain, while severe enough to cause nausea, remained localized in the eyeball itself. A third patient had an acute rise in intraocular pressure to 70 mm Hg following a vitreous hemorrhage. In this instance, the patient described a sharp pain in the eyeball and along the rim of the orbit as a bad ache extending throughout most of the area supplied by the ophthalmic division of the trigeminal nerve. Some patients have *no* pain with acute glaucoma and present only with the mid-dilated, fixed pupil, red eye, and nausea and vomiting.

That headache may be the most conspicuous feature of acute elevation of intraocular pressure was dramatically demonstrated in a closely observed group of patients in whom the sudden elevation of intraocular pressure was induced during the patients' reaction to stressful life circumstances. Thus in a group of 18 New York Hospital patients with glaucoma, the onset and exacerbation of eye symptoms and signs coincided frequently during reactions of anger, anxiety, and resentment and rarely with feelings of elation. Periods of tranquillity were associated with remissions.

The response to increased intraocular pressure was one of pain. This at first remained localized in the eyeball, but as intraocular pressure increased still further, it radiated so as to include the entire area of distribution of the ophthalmic branch of the trigeminal nerve. High pressures were accompanied by high-intensity pain, nausea, and vomiting.

Clinical Application. Though glaucoma may occur in young adults, its highest incidence is in persons between 40 and 60 years of age. Those with glaucoma of moderate degree complain of of aching in the globe and the area immediately around it. Since the intraocular pressure rise is commonly greater in the early morning hours, patients complain of headache on arising. Those with markedly increased intraocular pressure have dimness of vision, iridescent haloes around lights, and describe the experience of looking through a fog. These symptoms are accompanied by severe pain in the eye which spreads to involve the area of the first or the first and second branches of the trigeminal nerve. In the most severe cases generalized headache may be accompanied by nausea, vomiting, and malaise. There is striking tenderness of the eyeball accompanying such headache. Manual pressure on the eyeball accentuates the headache. Photophobia is also present. In angle-closure glaucoma the conjunctiva is red up to the cornea (limbus) and the pupil is mid-dilated, irregular, and not responsive to light.

For elimination of glaucoma headache, prompt reduction of intraocular pressure is necessary. It is self-evident that the patient should be referred immediately for ophthalmologic consultation, since relief of the glaucoma will relieve the headache. The most satisfactory classification of glaucoma is based on the appearance of the angle of the anterior chamber, and the treatment should be directed at the type of glaucoma present. Topical medications such as phenylephrine or atropine placed in the eye may induce angle closure and must be used with caution. Systemic medications usually produced minimal mydriasis and rarely evoke an angle-closure episode. Thus, fear of inducing glaucoma is not a sufficient reason for limiting systemic medications except for those few individuals with definitely narrowed angles. In this situation, 1% pilocarpine three or four times daily may be helpful prophylactically. Should acute glaucoma develop, intensive miotic therapy is indicated. The administration of carbonic anhydrase inhibitors lowers intraocular pressure strikingly in patients with glaucoma. Quick reduction in ocular pressure may be obtained by increasing serum tonicity using intravenous urea or mannitol, or oral glycerol. In rare instances, surgical decompression of the eyeball may be necessary.

IRIS

Incomplete anesthesia allowed observations on stimulation of the iris in four New York Hospital patients. Picking up this tissue with small-toothed forceps, or applying traction on it, produced high-intensity pain experienced in the eyeball; such pain was not further localized. This pain was promptly stopped by local applications of anesthetics or by retrobulbar injection of anesthetic.

Further observations were made in patients in whom iris adhesions were being broken with strong mydriatics or miotics. All these irides had been, or still were, the sites of local inflammatory disease. Traction on the iris tissue induced by chemical agents caused varying degrees of pain in the eyeball, which in some instances spread to the area supplied by the ophthalmic division of the trigeminal nerve on the same side. Local anesthesia by topical application or subconjunctival injection of cocaine or tetracaine lessened, but did not always stop the pain. Retrobulbar nerve block was not attempted. Morphine sulfate (15 mg) gave the patient some relief, but did not abolish the pain.

Clinical Application. The headache from intraocular inflammation is most intense in the eye itself. It may vary from dull or low-intensity aching in and around the globe to a high-intensity pain that radiates to involve the area supplied by the first brance of the trigeminal nerve. It is accompanied by marked photophobia. The pain is intense in the temporal region, is worse in the early hours of the morning, and may awaken the patient from sleep. The pain is continuous. Tenderness is present. Such headache is characterized by the reduction in intensity that follows the instillation into the conjunctival sac of atropine sulfate, 1% for cycloplegia of the ciliary body muscles.

Since the headache is due primarily to movement of the inflamed iris and ciliary body, atropine sulfate (2 drops, 1% solution) is instilled into the conjunctival sac sufficiently often to achieve and maintain full dilatation of the pupil (but not to exceed five times a day). This procedure is continued until the diseased structures have returned to their normal state. Hot, wet applications have additional therapeutic value. When adequate reduction of headache intensity is not achieved by these local measures, codeine phosphate (60 mg), or rarely, morphine sulfate (12 to 15 mg) is administered hypodermically at night.

Because of the importance of distinguishing the headaches from these major eye syndromes, the main points of difference are listed as follows.

1. In glaucoma, the pain is very intense, tension of the eyeball is greatly increased, tenderness of the eyeball is marked, vision is impaired, and there is photophobia and watery secretion. The cornea is "steamy," the conjunctiva and area near the cornea (limbus) are injected, the pupil dilated and sluggish, and the interior chamber shallow.

2. In iritis the pupil is small, sluggish, and often irregular, pain is moderatley intense, photophobia is marked, the eyeball is very tender, the iris is "muddy," and white cells may be seen in the aqueous humor on slit-lamp examination. The tension of the eyeball is normal or slightly low, the vision is moderately impaired, opacities may occur on the cornea and lens capsule, and there is vasodilatation deep within the tissue around the limbus.

3. In conjunctivitis the pupil is normal, vasodilatation is superficial, pain may be slight or absent, tenderness of the eyeball is rare, photophobia may be slight or absent or may be intense. Secretion is mucopurulent, vision is unaffected, tension is normal, the media are clear, the iris is normal, the aqueous fluid is normal, and the injection is only in the conjunctiva not the limbus.

A helpful reminder regarding the cases which should be referred to an ophthalmologist is "RSVP." Refer if there is: R—redness of the limbus, that part of the conjunctiva that rims the cornea; SV—sudden change in vision, in most of the serious conditions the vision changes over hours or days, not weeks or months; and finally, P—pain, and the type of pain that is severe, forcing the person to close their eyes and made worse by exposure of either eye to the light.

Headaches Associated with Refractive Errors and Extraocular Muscle Imbalances

STIMULATION OF THE EXTRAOCULAR MUSCLES

Opportunity for studying the effects of stimulating the extraocular muscles was afforded by patients on whom operations for strabismus were performed under local anesthesia. The muscles were exposed under light surface anesthesia and then stimulated in various ways. Pinching, pricking, or cutting the rectus muscles caused no sensation, but traction produced prompt exclamations of pain. The pain was always described as an aching sensation localized in the eye on the side of the stimulated muscle and deep in the orbit. There was no consistent radiation of the pain, and during these short periods of traction no pain was experienced in the back of the head or in the neck.

Clinical Application. Headaches from refractive error, hyperopia and astigmatism, and muscle imbalance usually begin with a feeling of heaviness in the head and pain in or around the eyes. They frequently occur both in the frontal and the occipital regions and the back of the neck. They are sometimes associated with diplopia or strabismus. Such headaches are commonly brought on by prolonged close application of the eyes as in reading or fine drawing. Less commonly they are precipitated by moving pictures. They nearly always diminish on less use of the eyes, as after a few hours of rest or a night's sleep, and vice versa, usually occurring in the afternoon or evening because of sustained use in the early part of the day. The headache is characterized by its occurrence or accentuation after use of the eyes in poor light or in close work.

Such headaches are steady and nonpulsatile in quality and are moderately intense. It is not usual for these headaches to be immediately relieved by closing the eyes, but attempts at near vision will increase the intensity. The eyeball is not tender and there is no increased pain on movement. There is more or less photophobia depending upon the intensity of the headache. These headaches are frequently accompanied by feelings of fatigue or strain in the eyes but not always with diminished visual acuity.

The explanation of such headaches is, first, that they are the result of the sustained contraction of intraocular muscles associated with excessive accommodative effort; and second, that they result from the unusually great and sustained extraocular muscle contraction associated with the effort to produce distinct retinal images and single binocular vision with fusion.

Simple myopia, in contrast to the ocular defects just mentioned, rarely produces headache. The reason for this is found in the fact that the myopic subject in attempting to improve his vision by the contraction of his eye muscles actually makes his vision worse and hence soon abandons the attempt.

Experimental Data. In order to study further their mechanism, these symptoms were reproduced by carrying out a number of experiments at the New York Hospital on individuals with no refractive error and no muscle imbalances. In one group of experi-

ments, attempts were made to induce excessive contraction of intraocular muscles by the subject's wearing various spherical and cylindrical lenses while proceeding with his ordinary day's work. The wearing of 5-diopter concave spheres (effect of hyperopia) resulted in the early development of a sensation of aching in and around the eyes; this sensation became more marked during and after prolonged reading. Cylindrical lenses produced similar results (effect of astigmatism). Convex lenses, however, produced only blurred vision without discomfort (effect of myopia). Thus, artificially induced hyperopia, astigmatism, and myopia reproduced accurately the symptomatology of the same conditions as they occur in patients.

Reproduction of extraocular muscle imbalances afforded consistent results. Maximal convergence with prisms caused a tense, drawn feeling in the forehead between the eyes, spreading to the temples. The sensation was one of tension rather than pain, but it became increasingly disagreeable. Occipital radiation did not occur.

Vertical prisms to the limit of fusion (effect of vertical muscle imbalance—hyperphoria) did not produce consistent symptoms in normal individuals. One subject wore a 1-diopter prism (base up) before the right eye with 1-diopter prism (Base down) before the left eye. This combination produced a vertical diplopia which was overcome in 5 min. For 30 min no symptoms were noted. Then slight dizziness and slight nausea began. An hour later the subject had become tense, irritable, and had difficulty in concentration. No definite headache was produced. Twenty minutes later the prisms were removed. An immediate inverse diplopia ensued, but disappeared in 5 min. The irritability immediately decreased and was gone in an hour. The same subject repeated the experiment twice: once for six hours, once for four. The second experiment was a duplication of the first. The third was similar, but was accompanied by a sensation of tightness in the head beginning 45 min after the prisms were put on.

In an attempt to explain the symptomatology in naturally occurring heterophoria, a patient with a pronounced convergence insufficiency was chosen. This patient had normal (20/15) vision in each eye and no refractive error. There was no vertical muscle imbalance. In distant vision (6 meters) there was an exophoria of 4 to 6 prism diopters while in near vision (⅓ meter) there was an exophoria of from 15 to 20 prism diopters. The near point of convergence was 16 to 18 cm. The subject was unable to read for even 15 min without developing severe frontal headache and burning of the eyes. The use of a pair of 6-diopter prisms (base in) completely relieved the symptoms by reducing the traction on extraocular muscles, the patient then being able to read in complete comfort.

Electromyographic recordings of this patient and of two normal individuals wearing vertical prisms were made. In each instance the symptoms that developed were accompanied by increased muscle potentials from the muscles of the head and the neck.

This work goes far to indicate that the sustained contractions of the muscles of the head and neck are the cause of a major part of the headaches associated with these extraocular muscle defects. Furthermore, it is apparent from these experiments that individuals subject to tension states and having some muscle imbalance or refractive error develop headaches of greater severity than do those individuals with the ocular defects alone. In other words, there is a cumulative effect of two separate factors, either one of which in itself will cause headache.

Pain in the back of the head from noxious stimulation of the structures within the eye was not obtained by experimental stimulation during short periods. But more prolonged stimulation, as indicated above, through the use of lenses that induced sustained intra- and extraocular muscle contraction did result in headache in the back of the head that could be demonstrated to be the result of prolonged contraction of skeletal muscle. Moreover, it is extremely likely that prolonged noxious stimulation of any structure in the eye will cause sustained muscle contraction and pain especially in the back of the head and in the neck, where the largest muscles are attached. This view is supported by the observation that procaine injected in the region of the greater occipital nerves in patients with severe occipital headache associated with glaucoma and iridocyclitis eliminated the pain for an indefinite period (Papiliam et al., 1943). As in other instances of headache from sustained contraction of the muscles of the head and neck in association with disorders of the head, the phenomenon is most evident in anxious, tense persons, in whom pre-existing or readily induced muscle contraction is augmented by the effect of noxious stimulation from the eye.

Patients with greater occipital neuralgia frequently consult an ophthalmologist because of pain in the eye, orbit, and temple (Knox and Mustonen, 1975). In a group of patients described by Knox and Mustonen, 27 women and 3 men aged 17–72, most had been given anesthetic injections. Tenderness to pressure is the key to the diagnosis. After applying pressure to control areas pressure is applied just beneath the occipital protuberence. Pain may be felt into the eye, orbit, frontal, and temporal areas.

The headaches that are caused by muscle imbalance (heterophoria) are eliminated by proper alignment of the visual axes. Prescribing of lenses may be helpful. Use of muscle exercises (orthoptic training) or muscle surgery may be necessary. Since the headaches are related to excessive muscular effort in an attempt to produce single binocular vision and fusion, occlusion of one eye will usually stop the headache so long as that occlusion is maintained. If the headache is not eliminated by this procedure, it is evident that muscle imbalance cannot be the etiologic factor and no amount of muscle correction can be expected to abolish the headache. Prescribing lenses for the relief of headaches solely on the basis of refractive errors is likely to be unproductive unless the history of eye strain is clear.

Headaches associated with ocular neuroses are common. Individuals with this type of complaint usually have good visual acuity and describe severe headaches with even momentary use of the eyes, a most unlikely circumstance. Such headaches should probably be interpreted as a type of conversion reaction and psychiatric referral may be necessary.

Headache from Aniseikonia

Whether unequal retinal images (aniseikonia) per se are a cause of headache and other ocular symptoms is at present a subject of debate. It is said that such a mechanism for headache does not exist and that the correction of the defect through "size-difference" lenses eliminates the headache. Final evaluation of the question awaits further evidence.

An unpublished study made at the Wilmer

Clinic, Johns Hopkins Hospital, Baltimore, is pertinent to the question whether aniseikonia is important as a cause of headache. It was found from the study of several hundred medical students that aniseikonia existed in an appreciable number, but headache did not occur in this group. On the other hand, patients with aniseikonia and headache who were given lenses aimed to correct their defect in most instances had less headache for varying periods thereafter. It is possible that reduction in the contraction of ocular and other head muscles is a factor in this improvement; however, that the effect of such lesions is not always at the simple physiological level is indicated by one patient who was given a correction lens over the wrong eye through an optician's error in mounting and reported complete elimination of headache, although, in fact, the error was doubled instead of corrected. The use of lenses designed to equalize retinal size differences in order to relieve persistent headaches is not recommended. It is suggested that many individuals with this problem are, in fact, manifesting another form of ocular neurosis.

Improperly prepared or fitted lenses in patients without aniseikonia can also produce headache. The onset of headache associated with a new prescription for glasses or contact lenses should raise suspicion of the obvious etiology, which can be readily corrected.

Retrobulbar (Optic) Neuritis

The primary symptoms of retrobulbar neuritis are blurring and dimming of vision but, in addition, pain may occur, sometimes preceding the visual symptoms by several days, localized behind or close to the eye. Frequently there is pain on movement of the eye and there may be associated tenderness of the globe. The visual problems are often self-limited, may progress over several weeks, may persist from weeks to months, but usually eventually disappear, leaving a disc which appears pale to inspection.

On examination there is frequently decreased pupillary response to light in the affected eye in contrast to the normal eye, and color vision may be impaired. Most commonly one finds a central scotoma, but other field defects involving nerve fiber bundles may occur. Visual acuity may itself be normal in approximately 20% of cases (Chamlin, 1953).

At the time of retrobulbar neuritis, the optic nerve head usually appears normal or there may be some slight blurring of the disc. On occasion, acute inflammation of the optic nerve head itself will be seen, and is termed papillitis.

Approximately ⅓ of patients with retrobulbar neuritis will progress, eventually, to multiple sclerosis, though the interval may literally be measured in years (Percy et al., 1972). The majority of cases of retrobulbar neuritis are, however, idiopathic, although occasionally they are attributed to orbital or intraocular inflammation, sinusitis, meningitis, or sarcoidosis.

Corticosteroids are employed by almost all physicians and surgeons who treat this problem, but their precise value is still unresolved. There is no question that corticosteroids will reduce pain and decrease edema which is probably enough reason for their use, but it is not clear whether they preserve vision (Gould et al., 1977).

Pseudotumor

Head pain may be caused by orbital tumor or pseudotumor. Pseudotumor is defined as an inflammatory space-occupying painful orbital lesion with associated ophthalmoplegia, proptosis, and visual loss; it is usually responsive to steroids (Jellinek, 1969). Most cases of this type are self-evident, and if they are not, careful eye examination usually suggests such a lesion. The CAT scan has proved invaluable in the diagnosis of orbital tumor and pseudotumor, since it allows one to look directly at the orbital and retro-orbital structures in a quick and painless manner. Occasionally unilateral thyroid ophthalmopathy may occur but it should be emphasized that exophthalmos is almost never painful unless it is extreme, in which case, again, the diagnosis will be self-evident.

Referred Ocular Pain

Ocular pain may be referred from multiple diseases and disorders of nonocular origin.

These are discussed in detail in the appropriate sections. The reader is therefore directed to the discussions of ocular pain associated with herpes zoster (Chapter 11), tumors (Chapter 13), aneurysms (Chapter 7), cranial arteritis (Chapter 10), cluster headache (Chapter 6), papilledema (Chapters 13, 14), and arterial hypertension (Chapter 8).

PHOTOPHOBIA

Photophobia (literally, fear of light) is the commonest reaction accompanying damage to the eye. It is of two general varieties. First, in the eye in which there is inflammation of the iris and ciliary body, light via reflex induces direct pull on, displacement of, or injury to the diseased structures, resulting in high-intensity pain. Such painful reaction to light is always allayed by immobilization of the diseased iris and ciliary body, even though cycloplegia results in a greater amount of light entering the eye. This type of photophobia is obviously the result of direct mechanical trauma of the inflamed structures induced by movement via the light reflex.

The second type of photophobia, and the one which will be the topic of further investigation here, occurs in individuals with healthy irides, and is elicited by abnormal amounts of light or by normal amounts of light if there be noxious stimuli arising from the eye or adjacent structures inside or outside the head. This type of photophobia has two major components: (1) a motor component that involves skeletal muscle (winking), smooth muscle (vasodilatation), and gland (lacrimation); and (2) a sensory component, i.e., a person on looking into a given light source experiences the light as momentarily brighter and the noxious stimuli as causing more pain. In studying the mechanism of this type of photophobia, a group of normal individuals at the New York Hospital were first exposed to excessively bright lights to ascertain the sensations aroused, which were described as uncomfortable, disagreeable, and unpleasant. There was increased lacrimation and frowning, with difficulty in keeping the eyes open, and involuntary winking was increased. On prolonged exposure there was an ache of 1 to 2 plus intensity in

the eyes and temples. Following such exposure the usual afterimages were experienced. Having made these preliminary qualitative observations, a series of quantitative experiments was carried out on normal subjects, using various chemical and mechanical procedures, to elucidate this type of photophobia still further.

In these experiments the rate of involuntary winking on direct exposure to a standard bright light for a measured period of time was chosen as the most satisfactory index of photophobia.* The subject was seated in a room lighted by a diffuse overhead light giving 2-candle-power intensity in his vicinity, before a standard experimental light of 23-candle-power intensity, from which, however, he was shielded. Then, by means of a shutter mechanism, each eye was exposed individually to this standard light for a period of exactly 20 sec, and the number of involuntary closures or winks counted. One eye, in each experiment, was stimulated with the mechanical or chemical agent being tested, while the other eye served for comparison.

Experimental Data

SERIES 1

In one experiment surface irritation from a foreign body (a small silk thread) was found, under the experimental conditions, to cause photophobia after an initial period had elapsed in which the subject was allowed to adjust to the presence of the foreign body in his eye. The winking response rose from the basic level of 4 to 5 per 20 sec to 10, and throughout the period of the experiment was at a consistently higher level in the irritated eye than in the other eye (Fig. 21-1).

Similarly, surface irritation from 2% ethylmorphine hydrochloride (an agent that produces local vasodilatation and ultimate acute conjunctival edema) likewise resulted in photophobia, repeated experiments with this drug giving a three- to fourfold increase in the winking response (Fig. 21-6, top curve). If, on the other hand, surface anesthesia was produced in an unirritated eye with 1% tetracaine, there resulted an immediate reduction in

---

*The increased winking rate associated with photophobia was the only accurately measurable component. However, in all instances it was associated with the experiences that the standard light was brighter, and that the noxious stimulus caused higher-intensity pain.

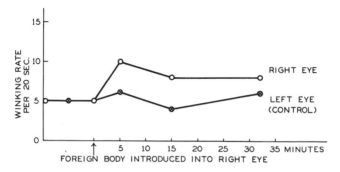

FIG. 21-1. Photophobia with a mechanical irritant.

the normal winking response, which was obtained on exposure to the standard light. Figure 21-2 illustrates such an experiment, showing a fall in the blinking response from the basic level of 4 to 6 per 20 sec of exposure, to 0 to 1.

SERIES 2

Cycloplegia, as noted previously, reduces photophobia in the eye with a diseased iris by virtue of immobilization of the iris. In the normal eye, in contrast, cycloplegia increases photophobia because of the increased amount of light entering through the dilated pupil. This relation between increased pupillary area and photophobia is shown in Fig. 21-3, which summarizes an experiment in which 5% eucatropine was used as a mydriatic in one eye while the normal fellow served for comparison. As the curve shows, the blinking response was maintained at a higher level in the eye with the greater pupillary area.

When a surface irritant, such as ethylmorphine hycrochloride, was introduced in one eye after both

eyes had been treated with homatropine, there was produced the typical photophobia from a surface irritant superimposed on that resulting from a cycloplegic (Fig. 21-4).

SERIES 3

Irritation of the surface of one eye, as above demonstrated (Series 1), kept the wink level of that eye above the wink level of its unirritated fellow eye. In experiments in which such irritation was produced by foreign bodies or by ethylmorphine hydrochloride, there always resulted some vasodilatation and conjunctival edema, and the question arises whether or not these reactions played a role in photophobia.

To answer this question surface irritation was produced in both eyes by instilling 2% ethylmorphine hydrochloride; this resulted in the usual increased winking response, the rate per 20-sec exposure jumping from below 10 to the neighborhood of 25. Epinephrine (1-1000) was then instilled in one eye.

Under these circumstances the vasodilatation and

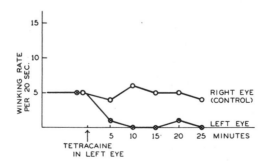

FIG. 21-2. Surface sensitivity and photophobia (no irritant).

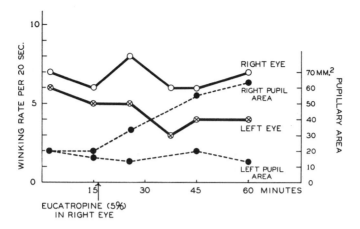

FIG. 21-3. Pupillary area and photophobia.

edema were rapidly reduced in the eye with epi-nephrine without there being an appreciable effect on the photophobia, the winking response subsiding not more rapidly in the eye treated with epinephrine than in the other eye.

SERIES 4

However, when light surface anesthesia was pro-duced in the irritated eye there was a prompt and significant reduction in photophobia, as shown in Fig. 21-5. In this experiment a patient with a small particle of glass in the left eye was exposed to the standard bright light for 20-sec periods, each eye

being so exposed separately. The unaffected right eye maintained a consistent wink response of 7 per 20 sec, whereas the wink response in the left eye was 30 or above per 20 sec; this response was not altered by the instillation of epinephrine. However, when surface anesthesia was produced in the left eye with 0.5% tetracaine, there resulted, within 30 sec, a pre cipitous fall in the wink response of this eye from the previous level of 30 to a level of 4 (Fig. 21-5), the particle of glass remaining in the eye throughout the period of the experiment.

That surface sensitivity is necessary to experience photophobia is shown in still another experiment in which one eye was anesthetized with 0.5% tetracaine, following which ethylmorphine hydrochloride was

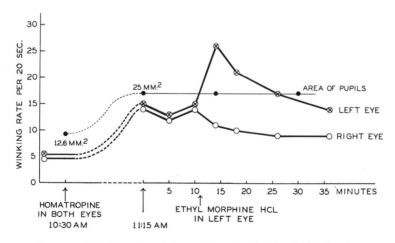

FIG. 21-4. Relation of pupil size to photophobia (chemical irritant).

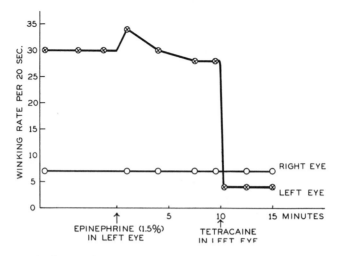

FIG. 21-5. Surface sensitivity and photophobia (mechanical irritant, left eye).

instilled in both eyes. Under these circumstances (Fig. 21-6) the unanesthetized eye had a four- to fivefold increase in the winking response, while that of the anesthetized eye did not rise above the original base line. The same result was obtained in a patient who had had a complete section, on one side of the sensory trigeminal for tic douloureux; the insensitive eye, in this case, had no increase in the wink response following the instillation of ethylmorphine hydrochloride.

SERIES 5

It would thus seem that photophobia is the product of the reaction between an irritant, on the one hand, and light reception on the other. The question then arises as to whether the requisite irritant could not be anywhere within the distribution of the ophthalmic division of the trigeminal, and photophobia still result? To answer this question the following experiments were made: 0.3 cc of 6% sodium

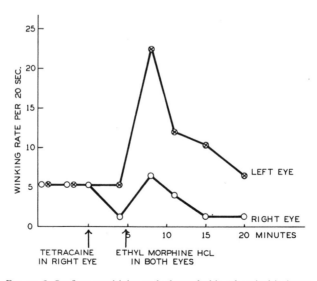

FIG. 21-6. Surface sensitivity and photophobia (chemical irritant).

chloride was injected into the frontalis muscle of one side just above the supraorbital margin. This procedure caused pain of moderate severity which radiated chiefly to the temporal region, but to some extent to the upper and lower jaws as well. With irritation produced in this manner there resulted a four- to fivefold increase in the wink response of the eye on the affected side when it was exposed to the standard light for 20 sec; the winking rate gradually subsided as the pain decreased, and finally returned to the baseline only when the pain was eliminated.

The photophobia that often accompanies the headache of meningeal irritation and migraine is additional evidence that noxious stimulation anywhere within the region supplied by the ophthalmic division of the trigeminal nerve may operate, with a light stimulus, to produce photophobia.

SERIES 6

Siegwart (1920) has shown conclusively that a blind eye never experiences photophobia on direct stimulation by light, a fact that we have been able to substantiate. However, is this because of the absence of the cortical connections of the optic nerve, or is it due to the destruction of those fibers that pass to the pretectal nuclei (whence connections with the midbrain and lower centers are established)?

Evidence that it is the latter fibers that are concerned in the winking component of photophobia is afforded by subjects with Argyll Robertson pupils in whom there is no pupillary response to light, presumably because there is a breakdown in the reflex mechanism between the pretectal nuclei and the effector nerves. Repeated experiments on such patients have shown that there is no increased winking response on exposure to the standard light for 20-sec intervals, even though surface irritation is first produced by the instillation of ethylmorphine hydrochloride. Yet they did experience intensification of light and pain. That the absence of increased winking was not due to insufficient light entering the eye through the constricted Argyll Robertson pupil was shown in experiments in which these pupils were dilated maximally with 5% eucatropine. Under these circumstances there was still no increased winking response on exposure to the standard light in the presence of surface irritation with ethylmorphine hydrochloride. Moreover, it was found that if maximal constriction of the normal pupil was effected with pilocarpine, the same winking response on exposure to the standard light followed the instillation of ethylmorphine hydrochloride as was obtained in the identical experiment without pilocar-

pine (cf. Series 1). Therefore, the absence of an increased winking response in the Argyll Robertson pupil is not the result of a decreased amount of light entering the eye because of pupillary constriction.

It is likely, therefore, that absence of photophobia in the blind eye is due both to missing cortical and pretectal connections, accounting respectively for lack of pain and light sensations, and lack of motor responses.

General Discussion

It becomes apparent, from the foregoing experiments, that photophobia is a product of light stimulus and trigeminal (ophthalmic) irritation. If either of these sensory mechanisms is sufficiently depressed, photophobia disappears. The side actions developing in surface irritation, the principal one being vasodilatation, are not prerequisites for photophobia, nor does their reduction diminish photophobia. This is in direct contradistinction to Lebensohn (1934) who concluded that local vasodilation was a necessary prerequisite for photophobia.

It is likely though not conclusively demonstrated that the entire central mechanism of the sensory trigeminal nerve, including mesencephalic root and nucleus as well as the hindbrain nucleus, is involved in photophobia.

Corbin and Harrison (1940) have shown that the majority of the fibers of the mesencephalic root pass, by way of the mandibular nerve and its branches, to the muscles of mastication, and that many of them enter the inferior alveolar nerve as well. He has further demonstrated that the only representation of the mesencephalic root in the ophthalmic division of the trigeminal consists of a moderate number of fibers going to the ethmoidal nerve, that the maxillary nerve contains fibers from the root only in its superior alveolar and and sphenopalatine branches. His observations are based on the experimental destruction of the mesencephalic nucleus and its root in cats by means of the Horsley-Clarke stereotaxic instrument. Sections of the animals' cranial nerves and their branches were then studied for the presence of degenerating fibers demarcated by means of osmic acid technic. In a later experiment, Corbin and Harrison (1940) demonstrated, by picking up action potentials in the mesencephalic root of the trigeminal, that these root fibers, which are contained within the masticator, alveolar, and palatine nerves, constitute the afferent limbs (proprioceptive) of masticator reflex arcs, coordinating and controlling chewing movements. No attempt was made by these workers to pick up action potentials in the mesencephalic root upon stimulating the ophthalmic division of the trigeminal or its branches, nor were they able to assign any function to the mesencephalic root fibers which Corbin had previously found in the ethmoidal branch of the ophthalmic.

In contradistinction to Corbin, van Valkenberg (1911) demonstrated that many fibers in the ophthalmic division of the trigeminal in the human come from cells of the mesencephalic nucleus. He describes a case in which the first division of the trigeminal was destroyed by a tumor which spared, however, the second and third divisions. Subsequent study of the mesencephalic nuclei revealed a marked diminution in the number of cells on the side of the tumor as compared with the healthy side; this loss of cells, moreover, was most striking in the cephalic portion of the nucleus.

While the observations of Corbin (1940) are of extreme importance, they may very well represent only a part of the picture, since they were designed to demonstrate only myelinated nerve fibers. Sheinin (1930) has shown that approximately 50% only of the total number of cells in the mesencephalic nucleus of the dog are of the type giving rise to large myelinated fibers (his type A cells); and in Corbin's work, the majority of the degenerating fibers were of the medium- to large-sized variety. Hence, they might be assumed to arise from the type A cells of Sheinin. About 40% of the total cell count of the mesencephalic nucleus consists, according to Sheinin, of small cells (his type C); these cells, reasoning by analogy with the small cells of the spinal ganglions (Ranson 1912), may give rise to unmyelinated fibers (in addition to association fibers). Further, it is the generally accepted belief that pain fibers are often unmyelinated, at least in the spinal nerves, and that these unmyelinated fibers are distributed chiefly in the cutaneous nerves,

Ranson (1915). It seems reasonable, therefore, to postulate that the pain fibers to the anterior segment of the eye, a structure derived embryologically from the ectoderm, are unmyelinated fibers and that they may in part arise from small cells in the mesencephalic (sensory) nucleus.

The topic of sensation of the eye is subject to ever on-going investigations, but many of the issues are still unresolved. Although there is no general agreement, G. Weddell (1959) one of the most active investigators, has drawn the following conclusions.

Relatively few (if any) sensory terminals in the cat's cornea, served by myelinated axons 6 to 12 mm in diameter, are strictly modality-specific. On the other hand, a cursory examination of the action potential records shows that the distribution in time of the various spikes evoked by each of the non-injurious stimuli differs. For example, direct current stimuli always evoke rhythmic, sometimes synchronous spikes, which can never be confused with, say, the activity evoked by brushing. Again rhythmic pairing and dispersion of spikes is more prominent following heat exchange than it is following brushing. Finally, injurious stimuli gave rise to rhythmic high-frequency outbursts resembling those evoked by strong direct current stimuli. Thus, although at present no definite temporal configuration of spikes can be related to stimuli having particular physical characteristics, there is every reason to believe that such a relationship may exist.

The territories of cornea served by different myelinated axons overlap extensively. This means that the profuse interweaving terminal network of fine nerve filaments in any given area of the cornea is served by axons having diameters spread throughout the 6- to 12-mm range.

This, however, certainly does not represent the total neural structural arrangement involved in photophobia. It is known that impulses from noxious stimulation of the trigeminal area, including the cornea, are mediated by the spinal tract of the trigeminal and its nucleus. This fact was substantiated in a patient in the New York Hospital with platybasia. He had, as a result of this congenital bony deformity, pressure on the lower end of the posterior hindbrain. There was not only diminution in pin prick and temperature on the left side of the head and face in the distribution of all three branches of the trigeminal nerve, but also a diminished corneal reflex on the same side.

Since the descending root of the trigeminal does carry fibers for pain from the cornea, it, too, must play a role in photophobia. However, since connections between the optic tectum and lower centers are abundantly established by the tectobulbar and tectospinal tracts, this need not alter our concept of the mechanism of photophobia.

Patients with the Argyll Robertson pupil (indicating midbrain disease) had faulty or absent wink responses when a strong light was projected onto the retina, yet they experienced intensification of light and pain. These observations support the thesis that the motor components of photophobia involve chiefly the brainstem.

In short, from the experimental data cited in this chapter the author's explanation of photophobia is as follows. At the segmental level the afferent impulses from light entering the colliculus through the retina, exert by spread an excitatory influence on the facial nerve nucleus causing the increase in winking frequency. The spread of excitation from the site of noxious stimulation in the eye involves much of the trigeminal nerve nucleus. After spreading throughout the trigeminal nuclei, these afferent impulses exert additional excitatory influence on the facial nerve nucleus so as to augment further winking frequency. The spread of excitation both caudad and cephalad, in addition to causing contraction of facial, cervical, masseter, and temporal muscles, induces vasodilatation and lacrimation. To explain the mutual intensification of noxious and light stimuli, a different neural apparatus must be involved. Afferent impulses from light on the retina entirely separate from those that go to the colliculus enter the external geniculate body. There through a synapse secondary disturbances are conveyed to the cerebral cortex. At neither the brainstem nor thalamic level is it possible for neurones involved in vision to be influenced or modified by spread of excitation from neurones involved with noxious stimuli. Such phenomena can take place only at the level of the cerebral cortex.

SUMMARY

1. Through the conjunctiva are perceived touch, pain, and cold; there is the ability to localize fairly accurately. There is no mechanism, on the other hand, for recognizing warmth or heat up to 70°C.

2. Through the cornea are perceived, under the conditions of our experiments, only pain and cold; touch is absent, and warmth and heat up to 70°C are not recognized as such.

3. Increase in intraocular pressure produces pain. When this pressure is sufficiently high, the pain radiates to the entire distribution of the ophthalmic branch of the trigeminal and may be accompanied by nausea.

4. Pinching, sticking, or cutting the extraocular muscles does not cause pain. Traction on them, however, produces immediate pain which is localized deep in the orbit.

5. Pain from the iris is likewise produced only by traction. In this instance the pain is referred to the eyeball itself and, if of sufficient intensity, to a part of the area of distribution of the ophthalmic division of the trigeminal as well.

6. Artificially induced hyperopia and astigmatism cause headache, while induced myopia usually does not.

7. Induced extraocular muscle imbalances cause tenseness and irritability, and eventually headache with abnormal electromyograms from the muscles of the head and neck. Clinically occuring muscle imbalances produce same symptoms and the same type of myograms.

8. Photophobia is of two kinds: (a) that resulting from movement of an inflamed iris, and (b) that resulting from the central interaction of afferent impulses from light stimulation of the retina, with afferent impulses from noxious stimulation of adjacent tissues, mainly those supplied by the first division of the fifth cranial nerve.

9. The central neural mechanisms involved in photophobia represent functional disturbances at two levels: the one within the brainstem, the other within the cerebral cortex.

10. Although headaches in and about the eye are exceedingly common, rarely are they the result of noxious stimuli originating in the eye, the extraocular muscles, or the optic nerve. Similarly, although photophobia is a dramatic accompaniment of eye disease, it is most often a manifestation of noxious stimuli arising in head structures other than the eye.

REFERENCES

Behrens, M. M. (1976). Headaches and head pains associated with diseases of the eye. In *Res. Clin. Stud. Headache* (M. Granger and G. Poch, eds.), Vol. 4, pp. 18–36. S. Karger, Basle.

Behrens, M. M. (1978). Headache associated with disorders of the eye. *Med. Clin. N. Am. 62*, 507–521.

Chamlin, M. (1953). Visual field changes in optic neuritis. *Arch. Opthalmol. 50*, 669.

Cogan, D. G. (1941). Popular misconceptions pertaining to ophthalmology. *N. Engl. J. Med. 224*, 462.

Corbin, K. B. (1940). Observations on the peripheral distribution of fibers arising in the mesencephalic nucleus of the fifth cranial nerve. *J. Comp. Neurol. 73*, 153.

Corbin, K. B., and F. Harrison (1940). Function of the mesencephalic root of the fifth cranial nerve. *J. Neurophysiol. 3*, 423.

Eckardt, L. B., J. M. McLean, and H. Goodell (1943). Experimental studies on headache: the genesis of pain from the eye. *Assoc. Res. Nerv. Dis. Proc. 23*, 209.

Gordon, B. L. (1934). Importance of cephalgia in ocular diagnosis. *Arch. Ophthalmol. 11*, 769.

Gould, E. S., A. C. Bird, P. K. Leaver, and W. I. McDonald (1977). Treatment of optic neuritis by retrobulbar injection of triamcinolone. *Brit. Med. J. 1*, 1495.

Jellinek, E. H. (1969). The orbital pseudotumor syndrome and its differentiation from endrocrine exophthalmos. *Brain 92*, 35.

Knox, D. L., and E. Mustonen (1975). Greater occipital neuralgia: an ocular pain syndrome with multiple etiologies. *Trans. Am. Acad. Ophthalmol. Otolaryngol. 79*, 513–579.

Lebensohn, J. E. (1934). Nature of photophobia. *Arch. Ophthalmol. 12*, 380.

Papiliam, V., I. G. Russu, and I. Pacurariu (1943). Treatment for ophthalmic headache with procaine hydrochloride infiltration of greater occipital nerves. *Wien. Med. Wschr. 93*, 77.

Percy, A. K., F. Nobrega, and L. Kurland (1972). Optic neuritis and multiple sclerosis. *Arch Ophthalmol. 87*, 135.

Ranson, S. W. (1912). The structure of the spinal ganglia and of the spinal nerves. *J. Comp. Neurol. 22*, 159.

Ranson, S. W. (1915). Unmyelinated nerve fibers as conductors of protopathic sensation. *Brain 38*, 381.

Ruedemann, A. D. (1940). Headache and head pain of ocular origin. *Med. Clin. N. Am. 24*, 335.

Sheinin, J. J. (1930). Typing of the cells of the mesencephalic nucleus of the trigeminal nerve in the dog based on Nisslgranule arrangement. *J. Comp. Neurol. 50*, 109.

Siegwart, K. (1920). Zur frage nach dem vorkommen und dem wessen des blendungschmerzen. *Schweiz. Med. Wchnschr. 50*, 1165.

Strughold, H. (1924). Uber die dichte und schwellen der schmerzpunkte der epidermis in den verschiedenen korperregionen. *Z. Biol. 80*, 367.

Tower, S. (1943). Pain: definition and properties of the unit for sensory reception. *Assoc. Res. Nerv. Disc. Proc. 23*, 16.

VanValkenberg, C. T. (1911). Zur vergleichenden anatomie des mesencephalen trigeminusteils. *Folia Neurobiol. 5*, 360.

Weddell, G., E. Palmer, and D. Taylor (1959). The significance of the peripheral anatomical arrangements of the nerves which serve pain and itch. *Pain and Itch: Nervous Mechanisms.* Ciba Foundation Study Group No. 1. (In honor of Y. Zotterman, G. E. W. Wolstenholme, and Maeve O'Connor, eds.) Little, Brown, Boston.

22

THE RELATION OF LIFE SITUATIONS, PERSONALITY
FEATURES, AND REACTIONS TO THE MIGRAINE SYNDROME

REVISED BY RICHARD W. ANDERSON

The role of suppressed anger as a precipitant of headache has long been known. In 1743 D. Junkerius wrote that the primary cause of migraine is anger, especially when it is tacit and suppressed [*ira, in primis tacita et suppressa*] (Jonckheere, 1971). This theme appears regularly in case studies of migraine patients. Fromm-Reichman (1937) concluded from experience with eight patients that "they could not stand to be aware of their hostility against beloved persons; therefore, they unconsciously tried to keep this hostility repressed, and finally expressed it by the physical symptoms of migraine." Her patients repressed hostility, fearing they would be deprived of the protection of their families. Their envious desire to destroy their rivals' brilliance was turned inward, resulting in symptoms within the patients' heads.

Wolff's subsequent study of the life histories, and sustained feelings and attitudes of migraine patients provided rich documentation of this theme, although he did not hold anger to be pathognomonic of headache. Various "pernicious emotional reactions" were cited as precipitants of attacks.

Material and Method. Awareness of the potential importance of the psychobiologic aspects has prompted the study of the personality functions of 46 subjects with migraine (Wolff, 1940; Wolff, 1937). These functions were systematically investigated, although no free association or far-reaching analysis was undertaken. Among the subjects in this group certain features were found to occur with striking frequency. Many degrees of the same personality quality were encountered, and no subject demonstrated every one of the characteristics to be described. The subjects studied presented common personality features that are in no sense pathognomonic of migraine, nor are they associated with migraine alone. However, these personality features in certain life situations are especially prone to call forth pernicious emotional reactions. In subjects predisposed to migraine, attacks often occur during such reactions; hence the personality functions of these persons become important.

These subjects gave detailed descriptions of their attacks and were familiar with the march of symptoms that were personally characteristic. They had periodic pains in the head, usually unilateral in onset but commonly becoming generalized. The headaches were associated with nausea and sometimes with vomiting, constipation, and diarrhea. Not infrequently the attacks were ushered in by scotomata, hemianopia, unilateral paresthesia, and speech disorders. Other bodily accompaniments were sensations of abdominal distention, cold, cyanosed extremities, tremors, pallor, dryness of the mouth, and excessive sweating, even though there was a feeling of being chilled. The attacks lasted from a few hours to several days. After an attack most patients experienced a period of especial buoyancy and well-being. At such times talkativeness, witty conversation, quick perception, and more than even the usual drive were common. In the interval between attacks of migraine, gastrointestinal disturbances, notably constipation, occurred in about half the patients. Diarrhea was less frequent. In most instances the attacks of migraine had recurred since childhood or adolescence with variable intensity and frequency. No social, intellectual, or economic group predominated. All but one of the patients was under

50 years of age. In the series there were 25 women and 21 men. Usually the subjects had forebears with similar syndromes.

Outstanding Personality Features and Their Development; Childhood Adjustment

The accounts of the childhood of these persons revealed that more than half were "delicate" (or treated as such), shy and withdrawn, and usually extremely obedient to the desires of their parents. They were commonly sober, polite, well-mannered children who did their school work conscientiously. This docility was often contrasted in the same person, however, with an unusual stubbornness or inflexibility provoked by particular situations. Moreoever, several, as children, had been obstinate, argumentative, and disobedient, a few were actually sullen and hostile, while others were characterized as singularly independent. These apparently contrasting qualities of character were often a prominent feature of the child's personality. Courteous, gracious, polite, and accommodating behavior was associated in the same person with obstinacy, open defiance, or even rebellion. Sensitiveness was associated in the main with restrained "proper" social relations, but it was on occasion expressed in frank pugnacity and defensive "chip on the shoulder" deportment. Temper tantrums occasionally resulted when these children were frustrated or pushed. Though most of them were not pugnacious, one child was unusually militant, taking offense at fancied slights and insults and precipitating fights and quarrels. Most of them did not participate in adolescent "hoodlumism."

Although parents and teachers found it difficult to change the pace and manner of conduct of these sensitive children, they found them trustworthy and energetic and, on the whole, respected and admired them. Consequently, these children were given responsibilities at an early age. Also they were given special privileges by adults and were considered unusually thoughtful and responsive to the wishes and needs of their elders.

Exceptional attachment to the mother was sometimes, but not universally, noted. Commonly this relationship was nothing deeper than that expressed by one mother as "John seems closer to me than do the other children," although in two instances pathologic accentuation of this relationship occurred.

The children took good or even excessive care of their toys, protecting them from destruction and from other children. Some found it difficult to part with toys of the past. They were careful of their clothes, and their lockers were usually in order. They were generally neat and clean, obediently washing their hands and teeth. One migrainous woman said, "I was extremely careful with my toys; in fact, I have most of my dolls from my childhood at home. Also, I was very neat with my clothes. My mother used to say that I stayed clean all day."

During adolescence and later these children were even more than usually preoccupied with moralistic and ethical problems, particularly concerning sex. In their relations with their fellows they were likely to be disappointed that others did not share their moralistic preoccupation.

Outstanding Personality Features and their Development; Adult Adjustments

Ambition and Success

In adults the qualities of character described took more definite form and were sometimes even accentuated to an exceptional degree. Nine-tenths of the migrainous subjects were unusually ambitious and preoccupied with achievement and success. Almost all attempted to dominate their environments—the less successful merely by the force of their demands and the tyranny of their moods, and the more successful through the acquisition of power, money, or distinction. Many of these individuals said they had lost the ability to feel tired. With perhaps two exceptions they were conscientious, persistent, and exacting, attempting to arrange or bring order wherever possible. They were meticulous, the surroundings in which they placed themselves reflecting their neatness and fastidiousness, yet most of them were efficient.

Perfectionism and Efficiency

On the whole they were a well-dressed group, including those in the most distressing financial circumstances. Their clothes were rarely 'fashionable' or conspicuous, but were conservative, with neatness rather than attractiveness as the prevailing effect. Among the men polished shoes, pressed trousers, and neatly arranged neckwear and hair were conspicuous. The women sometimes even sacrificed a degree of attractiveness for austerity or severe neatness.

These subjects usually made a feature of their 'perfectionism' and efficiency and thence gained much praise and personal satisfaction. Because of and through these qualities many responsibilities descended upon them, which they gladly accepted. About a fourth of them, owing to their characteristic qualities, had been made secretaries again and again of the various social or professional organizations of which they were members. In general, these men and women were extremely hard working and were endowed with a great deal of energy and striving. According to their friends they seemed to be tireless in pursuing their goals. In intellectual and creative work this revealed itself through endless effort to attain the perfect result of flawless data; in others, less sophisticated, in the attitude that "everything must be just so." Thus, one housewife called herself a "Dutch cleanser" and her husband jokingly referred to her as a "fanatic with a dust brush," suggestively remarking, "If you would throw away that mop you would probably feel better." A migrainous hair dresser expressed it: "If I give a wave and it doesn't come out just right, it annoys me frightfully." Several subjects said, "I take things too hard."

Despite their efficiency they often allocated responsibility poorly, fussing, worrying, and following up their instructions or directions to see that they were properly carried out, commonly preferring to do tasks themselves rather than to assume the risk of allowing others to do them. In one instance this was expressed as, "I feel as though no one can do things as well as I do them"; in another, "If I tell the housemaid to do something, I like to follow her up to see that it is properly done," and again, "I fuss and bother and worry about matters that I have turned over to someone else." These qualities were illustrated further in an able and ambitious research worker who, in addition to her full-time laboratory pursuit, conducted a home for herself and her husband. She said: "I had a maid once a week to clean house, but I couldn't let her wash the dishes. It irritated me too much to watch her. She would not change the water several times, as I instructed her to do, and I felt that the dishes were not clean. When I wash dishes, I change the water and rinse each dish thoroughly until I know it's clean."

The intensity with which these subjects attacked their work, their determination to "see a thing through," and their tireless persistence made interruptions extremely distressing. They often found it difficult to stop until a task was completed. This commonly meant long, irregular hours or periods of intense application. Despite apparent success, several subjects harassed themselves with the conviction that they had not done enough with their lives and opportunities and that at their age they should be further advanced.

Ambition and striving made work extremely important in the life pattern of these subjects, and frustration in work was particularly hard to bear. To be away from the workbench deprived them of the satisfaction of achievement, so that vacations were often periods of headache.

The anxiety and tension associated with interruption in work appeared to be connected in some subjects with headaches on Sundays and holidays. However, headaches had other components. The let-down, or release of tension or anxiety, also appeared to be a factor. The "let-down" headache was not necessarily associated with boredom, with frustration at not being at work, or with apparent tension. In fact, with some of these migrainous subjects 'letting down' became an elaborately developed ritual. This type of headache was noted also on the first day of a vacation, immediately after final examinations, and during the first few days of a long sea voyage. Each of these situations was immediately preceded by forced activity and the strain of preparation or packing. In short, any sudden change of program, release from discipline, tension, restraint, or sudden slowing down in pace was commonly accompanied by an attack of migraine.

Attacks followed failure but not only failure, since success sometimes precipitated them. Thus, on two occasions one subject observed that headache came on after the successful conclusion of tedious experiments which she had believed would demonstrate nothing. A distinguished investigator noted after a prolonged, severe, and successful "grind," the time that he allowed himself for relaxation and recreation would often be a period of headache. These attacks were perhaps akin to the aforementioned "let-down" episodes.

In the following instance the anticipation of criticism precipitated an attack of migraine:

A perfectionistic pathologist submitted a much belabored communication to a scientific periodical and eagerly awaited word of its acceptance. Several weeks later he was confronted by an envelope containing his returned and supposedly rejected article. He was deeply humiliated and disappointed. An hour passed before he opened the envelope, and during this period a severe headache developed. The attack was not arrested despite the fact that the envelope contained not only his manuscript but the 'proof' and a letter of commendation from the editor.

Time-Bound Factors

An outstanding feature of the migraine attack is its occurrence in relation to the period of "let down," as mentioned above. Headache attacks commonly occur on week ends, the first days of a holiday, Sundays, and on the occurrence of a planned social engagement or travel. The almost predictable relation in some instances of the headache attack to such periods bewilders patients, who then point to the fact that their headaches occur not with tension, but when they are relaxed. The "let down" is a serious biologic readjustment especially in those who are in a sense, "stress addicted."

Orderliness

The love of order, lists, headings, titles, subtitles, and card index systems was prevalent among these persons. Several had treasured stamp collections which were elaborately classified. In addition to his stamp collection, which was meticulously arranged, one migrainous medical student, six nights in the week, typed the lecture notes of each day. This he had done for seven school years. At the end of each course these edited notes were bound and placed on a shelf with other similar volumes to be turned to with pride and satisfaction.

In the contributions of the migrainous scientists, arrangement, classification, enumeration, statistical manipulation, and detailed analysis played the major part. Theoretical considerations other than those that flowed directly from a mass of exact data were rare, and the free expression of scientific fantasy in philosophic correlation was not common.

Several migrainous subjects who had orderly habits of work were indifferent about their personal appearance and households. Their preoccupation with orderliness and arrangement did not always extend over all departments of life. Apparently, if their major concern had become one of ambition, centered primarily on distinction, money, or power, they were less meticulous or even indifferent about their homes and dress.

In creative and esthetic effort the love of formalism and nicety of detail were also commonly shown. Most cultivated persons were fond of contrapuntal music and were particularly partial to Bach, Haydn, and Mozart. They were unsympathetic to less formal and more voluptuous expression. In the plastic arts, notably painting, lithography, and etching, the same enthusiasm for the formal or architectural was observed.

Doubts and Repetitions

Repetition and persistence in many instances appeared to fill the needs of special character traits and therefore afforded satisfaction. That is to say, in some subjects pleasure resulted from these perfectionistic activities, perhaps in the same sense that a child secures pleasure from repeating some act again and again. Occasionally, however, repetitions gave less satisfaction and, in a few, actual dissatisfaction and boredom. The fear of being found wrong or open to criticism was given by several in explanation of apparently unnecessary reviewing and repetition of some act of responsibility. Possibly also correlated with the fear of being found wrong was the difficulty in making a decision. Procrastination, delay, and avoidance in taking a stand or making a judgment were occasionally outstanding. Usually, as already mentioned, the orderly or repetitious behavior was socially acceptable as an expression of extreme cleanliness, neatness, or carefulness.

Resentments

About two-thirds of the subjects harbored strong resentments, a quality that seemed to be linked with inelasticity. They found it difficult to forgive or accept the foibles of their fellows. In several this was associated with the desire to be "well thought of;" that is, rather than "talk through" or overtly express resentment against a fellow human, they remained ostensibly friendly, nevertheless harboring deep feelings of resentment against those who injured them. This reaction of resentment and inability to forgive was often turned on the subject himself, so that personal deviations from set standards resulted in devastating self-accusation and flagellation.

Attitude Toward Bodily Inadequacy

The attitude of most of the subjects toward the headaches was strikingly similar. In the intervals between attacks they blatantly disregarded loss of sleep and common-sense limits of work in pursuit of their goals. They were outspoken and stoical in waiving reasonable restrictions. Furthermore, they were often unduly sensitive at such times even to being reminded of their headaches. Yet, on the other hand, with the onset of an attack many of these same subjects enthusiastically welcomed inquiry about their health and often dominated their environment and tyrannized over their families with their distress and needs. As a result of these bodily disturbances these already anxious subjects experimented with dietary regiments, particularly in the elimination of certain foods. These restrictions were either prescribed by physicians or elaborated by themselves.

The subject's attitude toward the attacks appeared to be part of his attitude toward his body in general; that is, these people usually had a disregard for the body as long as it functioned well, but they reacted with resentment when the body interfered with the attainment of their ends. This appeared to be a further expression of an unwillingness on the part of the subject to adapt himself in this case to the limitations of his organism.

Caution and Economy

By no means miserly or penurious, these subjects made every effort to obtain the most for their money and were fully aware of the disposition of their means. Making a good bargain, often at considerable sacrifice of time and energy, afforded great satisfaction. Waste or extravagance was revolting, and they were averse to gambling or rash investment. Orderly bookkeeping and budgeting were characteristic. Cautious spending was associated with the purchase of goods of full and lasting value. Ephemeral or transient returns were less commonly sought. Extravagance, however, was notable in one woman who bought expensive gifts for her mother. In fact, there was sometimes noted, side by side with the meticulous accounting for each penny, extreme beneficence as regards larger sums. Also, money was desired as a means to power. Another apparent contradiction resulted from the conflict between cautious spending and the strong impulse to "have a thing right away." This strong desire overcame the caution of one person and led her to buy on the installment plan.

More than two-thirds of the subjects were much interested in time. The desire to "get the most" for their money and the desire to get as much done as possible in a given time were linked. There was concern about being on time, doing several things at the same time, and the use of spare time. Thus, "When I have free time, I like to have something in my fingers, something to do." Impatience was characteristic, and efficiency was held at a premium. Thus, "I get crazy when I can't get action;" or again, "I am bothered by the fact that things do not move faster than they do." To get behind with work produced great distress in several. In one instance the time problem was expressed: "I get irritable when I have to wait for things; I like everybody on time. If I make an appointment, I expect people to be there." Another subject said: "Time is my worst enemy. It seems to me that I am always working against it, not because my thoughts and movements are slow, but because they are directed toward a perfect result which not only must be accurate when approximations would be adequate but also must be neatly recorded. A letter to a friend or the framing of a picture receives as much respect as my occupational pursuit, although less important tasks are seldom undertaken because of lack of time."

Social Relations

The social relations of these migrainous persons were usually of a cautious, circumscribed nature, permitting intercourse only on impersonal subjects. Almost without exception they cultivated a courteous gracious manner which further enabled them to conduct their social relations at arm's length and likewise protected them from intimacy that might engender friendly criticism. As a result, many of them gave the impression of being cold, aloof, politic, and detached, despite an astutely developed charm and *savior faire* and a frankly demonstrated desire to be thought well of.

Anxious anticipation of social intercourse was a common percursor of migraine in many subjects. In some few unmarried women headaches were brought on by anticipation of a social evening in the company of men; others had them when they were about to make new contacts with perhaps unsympathetic persons. A few avoided meeting new people as far as possible, especially when "off their own soil," unless they could be admittedly in the dominant position.

Sexual Adjustments

Sexual dissatisfaction existed in more than four-fifths of the women. There had been inadequate preparation for menstruation and for the sexual role, and overreaction to the discomfort with each menstrual period. Courtship and marital relations were made difficult by the somewhat arbitrary and inelastic notions concerning sex. Sexual contact was as infrequent as once a month and in one instance only once in two months. Orgasm was seldom attained, and the sex act was accepted as, at best, a reasonable marital duty. In several instances it was deemed frankly unpleasant and was resented. Notwithstanding, such persons expressed devotion to their mates and maintained ostensibly satisfactory domestic relations.

A subject who had been in love with her husband at the time of marriage became aware of unacceptable defects in his character toward the end of the first year of married life. After the birth of a child she lost all respect and devotion for him and became sexually frigid. Migraine began at this time, and the attacks were frequent and severe during the next three years, with the exception of three months when her husband was away on business.

It is doubtful whether any underlying structural or physiologic defect was responsible for the dissatisfaction with sexual experience. This was particularly so since in all the men orgasm was successfully achieved. The failure on the part of the women seemed to be linked with the general personality problem and inflexible standards, and also with the inability to "let themselves go." More plasticity in all relationships is perhaps expected of women, and consequently the same character qualities of rigidity, or "not letting go," seemed to create even greater difficulties for the women than for the men.

The fear of pregnancy, sometimes expressed, was shown on investigation to have a similar basis. There was an unwillingness to lose body form, to be forced to retire from social and industrial life, and to meet the limitations imposed by caring for a child; in other words, the person was reluctant to accept and adjust herself to the consequences of maternity, rather than fearful of the risks to life involved in pregnancy and delivery.

A woman who frankly feared pregnancy, several times had a nightmare in which she dreamed that she was delivering herself of a baby. On such occasions she cried out in her sleep and awoke with an attack of migraine headache.

Attacks in women just before or during menstruation were not uncommon. Several women were physically uncomfortable during this period, and this, added to the burden of domestic routine, precipitated attacks.

In one woman, who frequently had attacks just before menstruation, an interesting correlation was observed. This subject had noted variation in the intensity of her sex urge, which was more active during the first week following the cessation of menstruation and declined thereafter until she was frigid just preceding the next menstrual period. She declared that sexual intercourse during the post-menstrual week was pleasant and satisfied her, but during the premenstrual period it was always unpleasant and was followed within 24 hours by an attack of migraine.

Specific Emotional Reactions

More than nine-tenths of the subjects with migraine were unusually ambitious and preoccupied with success, had personalities with perfectionism and a desire to have things "just so" as outstanding characteristics. This basic inelasticity was often covered by a smooth surface of poise and social grace. They gravitated naturally into positions of responsibility but found it difficult to modify their standards and to adjust themselves to the variable and uncertain factors of their life situations. In reaction to the experience that other human beings and environmental conditions were not "just so," pernicious emotional reactions were developed and sustained. These were chiefly tension, dissatisfaction, and resentment. The severity of the reactions depended on the degree of the subject's inflexibility and the demands of the environment.

The manifestations of tension, such as restlessness, adventitious movements, or tics, were common but by no means universal. Many of the subjects "looked alert" and "at attention," expressed by one patient as "I'm always on the go. I want to do this, I want to do that." There was sometimes noted, particularly in men, the quality of studied poise, most often accompanied with a tense facial expression with furrowed foreheads, contraction between the eyebrows, quick moving eyes, and perhaps uneasy laughter. One such person referred to himself as "temperamental and apt to fly off the handle," and another said, "When things don't go smoothly, I go right up in the air." One woman referred to herself as a "spitfire—I flare up and boil over." Yet superficially these men and women might be regarded as well poised. One subject's handwriting during periods of extreme tension became unreadable, one became overtalkative, another spoke more rapidly and articulated poorly. In some, quick and excessive movements were observed, while others acted as though they suffered from ennui or boredom; still others seemed to be completely relaxed, except when alone or at work. High-speed automobile driving was a manifestation in several cases, heavy smoking and coffee drinking in others.

Genuine relaxation was seldom attained, and only a few subjects achieved resting points of satisfaction in their work. The intensity of drive noted in these persons suggested that they did not enjoy the actual "doing" and that the goal was the important source of their satisfaction. Accomplishment seldom brought more than the most transient pause, one task quickly following the next until the attack of migraine interrupted the procession of activity for hours or days. After such a period of enforced and detachment from responsibility and work, these persons returned to their labors with renewed vigor.

There was variety not only in the types of emotional reactions but also in their intensity and duration. As already indicated, sustained emotional states of anticipation, anxiety, resentment, and tension were common. Of particularly long duration were anxiety and tension. The depth of the emotional responses was not profound, save in a few instances. Most common was a long-sustained and superficial pervasive uneasiness or anticipation of unto-ward events which periodically merged into a slightly deeper reaction of anxiety with ten-sion. Less common but sometimes important were short-lived intensely moving reactions of rage. In fact, the most intense emotional re-sponses were those of resentments and rage which, when prolonged, as only occasionally happened, were associated with revenge and spiteful reaction. Most of the subjects in this group had failed to correlate their attacks of migraine with life situations or their reactions to the latter. Many recognized, however, the existence of their tension states, although more than half expressed no dissatisfaction with them and a few even obtained pleasure from the feeling that they were "alert and striving."

Demonstration of the Specific Nature of the Stress Related to Migraine Headache Attacks

Two American Protestant missionaries had mi-graine attacks at frequent intervals for many years. One was stationed in Korea, the other in China. Both were conscientious, perfectionistic, ardent, tireless workers, and successful in their missions. With the invasion of the Japanese military forces into their respective missionary fields, both were made pris-oners of war. Prison life was routine, but coupled with hard labor, disciplinary difficulties. malnutri-tion, illness, deprivation, and separation from family and friends. During this entire prison stay of almost three years, neither of these men had migraine headache attacks.

With liberation and restoration of proper diet and return to their work life, migraine headache attacks recurred at irregular intervals in both individuals.

Even though these individuals were subjected in prison to extremely adverse circumstances, these stress-inducing situations did not create feelings per-tinent to the migraine syndrome by imposing per-sonal responsibility and the opportunity for frustra-tion in work. Also, feelings of guilt were assuaged. In the words of one such guilt-laden subject, "The major tragedy of prison life was that one got to like it."

Vascular headaches were of less frequent occur-rence during the adverse circumstances coupled with the occupation of Holland by the Germans during World War II. Shortly after the liberation, headache attacks recurred in practically all persons subject to them before (Smitt, 1953).

The fact that migraine headache attacks in those with the migraine syndrome are rarely precipitated during hospital stays is analogous. Even though hospital life imposes limitation of activity, deprivations, curtailing of creative effort, incarceration, and perhaps discomfort and pain, the stress is not of a nature rele-vant to migraine attacks. It induces no serious conflict asnd tension such as result from the challenge of home and work life, where the patient is called upon to perform in terms of self-imposed standards.

In general, sustained tension with excessive striving and frustrated ambition and anxiety about family, financial, or personal security, to which might be added an unsatisfactory sex life, appeared to furnish optimal conditions in these subjects for the precipitation of attacks of migraine.

EXPERIMENTAL INDUCTION OF MIGRAINE HEADACHE

In the endeavor to crystallize understanding of the particular type of situation that can trigger a headache, the following study was made (Marcussen and Wolff, 1949). A detailed history was obtained from 20 patients of the events of the 24 hours preceding a given headache. In almost every instance there oc-curred an episode to which the patient reacted with rage and resentment to which he was unable to give full expression. This type of blocked reaction took place during a short period of a high degree of anxiety and tension, or following a longer period of gradually ac-cumulating tension. The pertinent point in these patients is the observation that in many instances the precipitating event was in itself trivial and under other circumstances would not have disturbed these individuals. In the setting in which it did occur, however, it was, in effect, "the straw that broke the camel's back," the final insult. Each of these individuals had been accumulating hostility, resentment, and tension for varying periods before they were exposed to the event which precipitated the headache. The following protocols are representative.

A 30-year-old Italian housewife presented herself at the New York Hospital with a history of almost daily unilateral vascular headache of varying intensity and duration for about two months. Prior to this series of attacks she had had typical migraine headaches every few weeks since adolescence. The present series of headaches paralleled the development of a progressively severe feeding problem in her 4 ½-year-old daughter. The patient stated that her headaches followed meals with monotomous regularity. The child refused to eat despite the patient's every effort to induce her to do so. At this persistent refusal, the mother would become angry and berate the child violently. Often she would attempt to force food between the child's clenched teeth. Failing this, the mother became so enraged several times, that she assaulted her daughter so violently that the child was left stunned and bruised. Within an hour after such an encounter the patient would develop a high-intensity headache, usually unilateral, which required opiates or ergotamine tartrate for relief. Later this woman realized that she might seriously injure her daughter during one of these assaults and would therefore storm out of the room before she gave way to physical violence. Under such circumstances the subsequent headache would be more intense. The mother felt extremely

guilty about her failure as a parent and was humiliated by the comments of neighbors who overheard her outbursts and observed the child's progressive weight loss.

During her first clinic visit the patient confessed her story to a friendly and sympathetic physician. She displayed considerable emotion during the interview and felt appreciably relieved at the end. She had no further headache during the following week, the first remission in months. At her next visit, the same physician adopted a stern and unsympathetic attitude. He scolded the patient for her behavior and criticized her for her failure to control herself in dealing with the child, pointing out the damage which she was doing to the child and to herself. All this the patient seemed to accept well, smiling and agreeing with the physician. The interview terminated after an hour, but 10 min later she developed a high-intensity bitemporal and frontal throbbing headache accompanied by blurring of vision and nausea. The headache disappeared within 30 min after the intramuscular injection of ergotamine tartrate (Fig. 22-1).

A 57-year-old widow whose husband had recurrent manic attacks during the ten years of their marriage noted that her migraines occurred only after she had seen her husband through a manic episode. During these he was overactive, critical, verbally abusive, socially irresponsible, and financially unwise. She managed to have his internist prescribe clorpromazine and was able to persuade

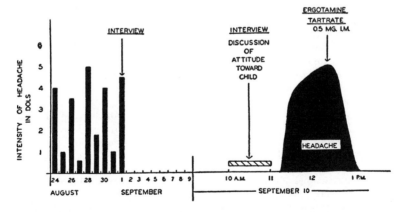

FIG. 22-1. Experimental precipitation of a migraine headache attack in a setting of mounting tension by the introduction of a topic arousing conflict, anger, and guilt. Attack terminated by the intravascular administration of ergotamine tartrate. Initial interview on September 1, by dispelling guilt and conflict, reduced the frequency and intensity of attacks. The subsequent interview, intensifying these feelings, precipitated the headache.

him to take the drug, which terminated the attacks within several weeks. Only then did she experience a week of nausea and scintillating scotomata, followed by eight or nine days of incapacitating, throbbing unilateral headache. She had had these attacks since she was 16 and did not believe that their frequency was greater during her marriage; their timing was, however, directly related to her husband's manic behavior.

Effects of Situations or Procedures That Dispel Tension and Anxiety

Inversely, situations that dispel tension, relieve anxiety, and dissipate the effects of frustration and resentment, modify the course of a patient with migraine headache attacks.

A less dramatic and destructive personality change may occur at the menopause in women and at a comparable period in the life of men. At such a time the relentless pursuit of perfection and approval may cease, and instead a more rational attitude be adopted which does not have such costly sequelae. On the other hand, the climacteric may see the beginning of migraine. When an individual, who has previously been able to meet his excessive energy demands, begins to slow down as the accompaniment of aging, the resultant conflicts may lead to headaches.

Groen (1951) described a patient with Addison's disease who had had a history of attacks of migraine headache through much of his life. The headaches ended with the onset of Addison's disease (weakness, vomiting, and fatigue). But in one respect the patient's state was improved. He said, "I feel better. I am no longer troubled by headache." When after treatment the evidence of Addison's disease diminished he again began having attacks of migraine headache.

A study was made, in collaboration with Dr. H. Gold of the Cornell University Medical College, of a 40-year-old teacher and investigator who had attacks of hemicrania. These had begun ten years previously, and occurred during times of stress fatigue, and tension about five times a year. He was an exceedingly conscientious, meticulous, hard worker. In six attacks during two years headaches were eliminated by codeine and did not recur, when, with continued administration of the agent at 5-hr intervals during four days he could remain in bed and be protected from important decisions, discrimina-

tions, and responsibilities. During these two years, however, in four experiments with the same amounts and intervals of medications for four days, the subject was denied bed rest and protection from his duties. The codeine produced in him minor toxic effects; and in this state of impaired energy and initiative, he was asked to assume his usual daily load of work, to be performed according to his usual standards of excellent performance and high speed. To carry on work during this state of depleted energy, memory loss, and difficulty in thinking, concentration, attention and retention, was onerous and distressing. The results of his efforts were poor and the outcome of long hours of faulty attention and concentration unsuccessful. Because of his temperament the patient could not accept slow or imperfect performance. The energy expenditure necessary, coupled with the poor product, created considerable resentment, anxiety, and tension.

During this phase headache began. It was usually unilateral in onset but then sometimes became generalized. It was of extremely high intensity, and of a deep aching quality. Throbbing occurred at first and was followed by a steady headache which persisted for hours. There was concomitant abdominal distress and nausea. The headache was in all regards a vascular headache of the migraine variety. When work was abandoned and sleep attempted, the headache became gradually less intense and after several hours was gone.

The significance of these experimental data is apparent for those patients with intractable headaches who take frequent and large amounts of medications in futile attempts to free themselves of pain so as to "keep going" at their usual responsibilities and duties. Continued medication adds to their depletion, and leads to further frustration, failure, tension, and stress.

The qualities of character which occurred so frequently among the migrainous subjects included in this study resemble those described by Abraham (1925) and further elaborated by Fenichel (1934) in his discussion of the patient with compulsions. Fenichel mentioned migraine as one of the accompaniments of this particular personality constitution. Meyer (1930) has described a group of persons characterized by difficulty with decisions, by doubts, rituals, and fears, and with anticipation of panic should fulfillment fail to be achieved. Anxiety and depression were common accompaniments. Such malfunctions were designated by him as 'obsessive remunative tension states.' The tension and anxiety and the compulsive and repetitive behavior in the subjects studied at the New York Hospital may ally them with the "neurotic" patients in these groups. However, these studies are not inclusive enough to establish definitely whether the personality features described are the forerunners of a neurosis of the obsessive-compulsive type. Furthermore, and possibly also owing to the method, no data were obtained that allowed these personality features to be correlated genetically with infantile anal attitudes.

Ross and McNaughton (1945) made Rorschach records of 50 individuals with migraine headaches, comparing them with the records of 149 persons without migraine. The personality features that stand out according to these studies are: rigidity, persistence toward success, difficulty in sexual adjustment, perfectionism, conventionality, intolerance, and, in general, obsessive-compulsive features. The authors concluded that patients with migraine are not essentially more "neurotic" or more closely allied to subjects with brain disease than an unselected group even though some have shown features in common with psychoneurotics, and others in common with individuals suffering from brain disease.

Alvarez (1947) made a study of the personality features and attitudes of more than 500 patients, most of them women with migraine, and was impressed by the closeness of his own independently made observations to those described above. His case notes admirably exemplify the behavior and mood disorder (the socalled twilight spells, dysphrenia hemicrania transitoria, or *dämmerzust÷ande*) characterized by depression and apathy, and a dazed, confused, or detached state, which may occur independently of the headache attack.

The number of subjects in the New York Hospital series numbered several hundred; nevertheless, to infer that all persons with migraine will be found to have the personality features and reactions mentioned here is unjustified. However, since these subjects were *unselected*, they form in all likelihood a representative group of persons with migraine. It may therefore by postulated that some other persons with migraine have similar personality features and reactions.

Personality features and reactions dominant in individuals with migraine are feelings of insecurity with tension, manifested as inflexibility, conscientiousness, meticulousness, perfectionism, and resentment. These temperamental features lead to frustration; to dissatisfactions about family, financial, or personal status; and to intolerance of periods of low energy in themselves, or of relaxed standards in themselves and others.

The elaboration of a pattern of inflexibility and perfectionism for dealing with feelings of insecurity begins early in childhood. The individual with migraine aims to gain approval by doing more and better than his fellows through "application" and "hard work," and to gain security by holding to a stable environment and a given system of excellent performance, even at high cost of energy. This pattern, as mentioned before, brings the individual increasing responsibility and admiration with but little love, and greater and greater resentment at the pace he feels obliged to maintain. It usually works moderately well through adolescence, or even later, but with increasing pressure and decreasing energy it becomes harder to maintain. Then the tension associated with repeated frustration, sustained resentment, and anxiety, often followed by fatigue and prostration, becomes the setting in which the migraine attack occurs.

In short, certain individuals have a predisposition and psychobiologic equipment which makes them prone to sustained and pernicious emotional states. During such states labile physiologic mechanisms set off the chain of events constituting the attack of migraine.

This medley of personality features and reactions so often found in those with vascular headache of the migraine type is an aggregate of adaptive pattern, largely of a defensive nature.

RECENT STUDIES

Jonckheere (1971) noted that 11 of 16 typical migraine patients were obsessional, aggressive, or both, and that their aggression, along with their headaches, had a tendency to disappear when psychotherapy permitted its expression.

Using detailed histories and three psychomatric tests in a controlled study of 100 migrainous individuals, Henryk-Gutt and Rees

(1973) found significantly greater "N" (neuroticism) scores on the Eysenck Personality Inventory, higher hostility scores on the Buss Scale, and more psychological symptoms in the migraine sufferers than in the control subjects. On an abbreviated Minnesota Multiphasic Personality Inventory, female migraine patients showed higher anxiety and somatization scores. Emotional stress was found to be important; over half the subjects had suffered their first migraines during a period of emotional stress. During a two-month period of observation, over half of the 120 attacks recorded by 43 subjects were related in time to a stressful event. However, there was no objective evidence that the subjects had experienced greater stress then the controls. These findings suggested increased reactivity of the autonomic nervous system as a predisposing factor for the development of migraine attacks. Women in all groups reported headaches twice as frequently as men, and female migraine clinic patients had attacks four times more often than women migraine sufferers found in a random sampling of the Civil Service Register. The authors concluded that migraine subjects are predisposed, by constitutional and not by environmental factors, to experience a greater than average reaction to a given quantity of stress. The authors were unable to confirm that migraine subjects are especially obsessional or ambitious and suggested that previous studies were insufficiently comprehensive since the groups studied were self-selected and not fully representative or migraine subjects in general. However, all the traits described in previous studies were seen as aspects of the above average "N" scores observed.

Rogado (1974) gave the Minnesota Multiphasic Personality Inventory to 150 selected outpatients: 50 with migraine, 50 with cluster headache, and 50 controls; sexes were equally represented in each group. Both headache groups reported more psychopathology than the control group, and the profiles of both migraine and cluster patients indicated the presence of obsessive-compulsive traits. Elevations on the hysteria scale were consistent with the dissociative behavior often observed in headache patients. Both headache groups scored higher on the hypochondriasis and low back pain scales. The headache groups did not differ significantly from the control group on a scale indicating uncertainty in sexual identification.

In a review of the studies of Waters and O'Connor (1970), Howarth (1965), Maxwell (1966), and Henryk-Gutt and Rees (1973), Philips (1976) concluded that there was only minimal support for the view that migraine sufferers were more neurotic than age-matched normals. In a random sample of 1500 patients in a general practice all of whom were given the Eysenck Personality Questionnaires, he found among the respondents 39 migraine patients, 24 tension headache patients, and five with migraine and tension headaches. No significant group differences were found in neuroticism, extraversion, or psychotic behavior, and only slightly elevated lie scores in female migraine patients. These cases, collected from a community sample *without* reference to a headache complaint, cannot be distinguished from normal subjects. Prevailing views of the personality of headache sufferers have been formed only from the study of those who seek our help, and may not be representative of headache sufferers in the general population.

In a study of 1300 identical twins, Lucas (1977) found migraine concordance rates of 26% in monozygotic and 13% in dixygotic twins. When the personality profiles of twins discordant for migraine were compared, no significant differences between pairs on the P, E, N, and L scales of the Maudsley Personality Inventory were found. This finding refuted previous reports of increased neuroticism scores in patients with migraine. The overall incidence of migraine in this sample was 15%. Family histories were positive for migraine in 60% of the cases where both twins were affected. When only one twin was affected, 45% of the family histories were positive; when neither had migraine, only 31% of family histories were positive. Only 50% of the subjects with common migraine and 38% of those with classical migraine had consulted a doctor for their symptoms. Childhood vomiting, eczema, and travel sickness were linked with migraine; epilepsy was not.

Several of the psychological studies of headache have focused on patients with cluster and tension headaches, and consequently are not reviewed in this chapter. In his review Harrison (1975) noted that four MMPI studies (Steinhilber *et al.*, 1960; Martin *et al.*, 1967; Martin, 1972; and Rogado *et al.*, 1974) on 325 subjects (50 migraine, 100 cluster, 125 tension, and 50 "other" headaches) showed a common profile, characterized by a "conversion V" (elevation of the hypochondriasis and hysteria scales with more moderate scores on depression), suggesting that the patient's anxiety is bound by somatic complaints, as well as being held in check by compulsive defenses. A number of studies of patient self-reports on various scales and inventories led Harrison to conclude that headache patients describe themselves as more anxious, overwrought, tense, vulnerable, forgetful, and moralistic than do controls. He reports three studies using Rorschach protocols which yielded no positive findings that would replicate from one study to the next. Although psychological factors may be a cause of or a predisposition to headache, it is possible that the neuroticism observed in headache patients may be a consequence of the risk of sudden intense pain, or of adaptation to being a patient.

Information about headache was collected by Markush *et al.* (1975) from a nonclinical sample of 451 women, aged 15 to 44, in 12 major U.S. cities. Twenty-three percent of them had experienced headaches with two or more migraine characteristics (throbbing, aura, vomiting, or distress affecting daily activities) during the year preceding the interview. The frequency of such symptoms was significantly greater in women who smoked, or had in the past smoked cigarettes, in those with lower incomes and poor education, and in those with a history of hypertension, stomach ulcer, and fainting. Complaints of tension and depression were significantly more frequent in those reporting headaches. Age, race, marital status, number of living children, and use of oral contraceptives were not found to be significant. This study plainly indicates that migraine is not limited to the elite and affluent.

In general, the nonclinical psychological studies and interviews with migraine patients do not support the widely held view that the migraine patient is likely to be compulsive, inhibited in the expression of anger, attached to neurotic defenses, and dependent. It is probable that selection biases prevent clinicians from seeing a representative sample of migraine sufferers, and that the neuroticism discovered during the treatment of these patients is actually a function of the patient state itself. Certainly, the possibility of experiencing the sudden, sometimes disabling, pain could generate responses of irritability, anxiety, or dependency in the strongest of us. Since nonclinical studies show that only 50% of migraine sufferers consult physicians, it is possible that the traits we have considered as causes of or predispositions to migraine may be nothing more than characteristics that correlate highly with the seeking of medical attention. Epidemiologic studies and psychological samplings are to date far outnumbered by clinical accounts. It is from these that we have acquired a picture of the "migraine personality."

As physicians, we are concerned primarily with the relief of suffering. The relationship of migraine to stress has not been disproved by any existing data. Views of migraine from vantage points broader than the clinical suggest that many stresses—social, economic, and psychological—may activate the unique vascular responses known as migraine. In the management of migrainous patients we can do no less than counsel in such a manner as to ameliorate responses to external stresses and reduce internal conflict concerning dependency and suppressed hostility where our unique relationship with the patient makes this possible.

FORMULATION OF THE DYNAMICS OF THE BEHAVIOR PATTERN OF PATIENTS WITH MIGRAINE HEADACHE

In broad terms the migraine headache represents a vascular mechanism for coping with life situations which are stressful to the individual. Up to a certain point the patient is able to deal with the accumulating tension and hostility resulting from the stress which he faces. Beyond this he cannot continue, and there ensues a period of disabling pain during which he is forced to a halt, (Knopf, 1935).

In these individuals, the cranial vascular apparatus is a major participant in one of the protective patterns shown by various systems of the body (Graham and Wolff, 1938). In common, these reactions serve to remove the individual from the threat or the threat from the individual.

A person with migraine deals with his life situations in a way which expensively depletes his reserve of energy. The rate at which this energy is expended is dependent on his reactions to the circumstances. Beyond a certain point he is no longer able to continue the costly and extravagant adjustment he has been making. He exhausts his bodily capacity to continue to deal with his situation in this extravagant way. When he reaches this point there is a collapse of his adaptive or protective apparatus. At that time, a cranial vascular reaction supervenes which becomes so painful that he must withdraw from his frustrating and threatening life situation. During the period of retreat and withdrawal there is apparently a restoration of the energy reserves which then permits a repetition of the whole pernicious cycle.

SUMMARY

1. Migraine is strongly related to stress. Half the attacks reported are associated with responses to external or intrapsychic stresses. Although only half of those who suffer migraine consult physicians, those who do so are, according to individual case reports and psychological studies, to be characterized as having feelings of insecurity and tension manifested in inflexibility, conscientiousness, meticulousness, perfectionism, and resentment. These features of temperament lead to frustration, to dissatisfactions with family, financial, or personal status, and to intolerance of periods of low energy in the self, or of relaxed standards in the self and others.

2. The elaboration of a pattern of inflexibility and perfectionism for dealing with feelings of insecurity often begins early in childhood. The individual with migraine aims to gain approval by doing more and better than his fellows through application and hard work, and to gain security by holding to a stable environment and to a given system of excellent performance, even at a high cost of energy.

3. This behavioral pattern brings the individual increasing responsibility and admiration with but little love, and greater and greater resentment at the pace he feels obliged to maintain. Often he is able to maintain himself through adolescence or even later, but with increasing pressure and decreasing energy it becomes harder to comply with his own standards.

4. When the tension associated with repeated frustration, sustained resentment, anger, and anxiety builds to a critical level, the setting is created in which the migraine attack occurs. From a dynamic point of view it is wise to view these personality features and reactions as adaptive arrangements elaborated by those with proclivities to evoke such responses under the circumstances of duress, rather than to consider them as primary features of personality structure or the cause of headaches.

5. Certain individuals have a disposition and psychobiological equipment which predisposes them to sustained pernicious emotional states. During such states labile physiologic functions set off the chain of events constituting the vasomotor crisis characteristic of vascular headaches of the migraine type. In broad terms the migraine headache may be seen as a vascular mechanism for coping with life's situations which are stressful to the individual patient.

6. Awareness of personality characteristics and of the stresses that provoke or aggravate the migraine response is essential to the effective treatment of these patients. The physician has a unique opportunity not only to assist the patient in modifying his responses to the external factors he considers stressful, but what is more important, to change the patient's reaction to unrealistically rigid internal demands. The impaired performance usually accompanying a migraine attack provokes depression, which often can be ameliorated in an understanding discussion. It is also possible to effect limited modification of excessively strin-

gent internal standards, particularly those responsible for the suppression of angry feelings.

7. Long-term management of the migraine patient is based on judicious drug therapy and systematic attention to the psychological factors described above.

REFERENCES

Abraham, K. (1925). Erganzungen zu Lehre von Analcharacter. *Internationalen Psychoanalytischen Verlag.*

Alvarez, W. C. (1947). The migrainous personality and constitution. The essential features of the disease: a study of 500 cases. *Am. J. Med. Sci. 213,* 1.

Fenichel, O. (1934). *Outline of Clinical Psychoanalysis,* Trans. Betram D. Dewin and Gregory Zilboorg. Norton, New York.

Fromm-Reichman, F. (1937). *Psychoanal. Rev. 14(1).*

Graham, J. R., and H. G. Wolff (1938). Mechanism of migraine headache and action of ergotamine tartrate. *Assoc. Res. Nerv. Dis. Proc. (1937) 18,* 638; *Arch. Neurol. Psychiat. 39,* 737.

Groen, J. (1951). (Amsterdam, Holland). Personal communication. Harrison, R. H. (1975). Psychological testing in headache: a review. *Headache 13,* 177–185.

Henryk-Gutt, R., and W. L. Rees (1973). Psychological aspects of migraine. *J. Psychosom. Res. 17,* 141–153.

Howarth, E. (1965), Headache, personality and stress. *Brit. J. Psychiat. 119,* 1193.

Jonckheere, P. (1971). The chronic headache patient. *Psychother. Psychosom. 19,* 53–61.

Knopf, O. (1935). Preliminary report on personality studies in thirty migraine patients. *J. Nerv. Ment. Dis. 82,* 270.

Lucas, R. N. (1977). Migraine in twins. *J. Psychosom. Res. 20,* 147–156.

Marcussen, R. M., and H. G. Wolff (1949). A formulation of the dynamics of the migraine attack. *Psychosom. Med. 11,* 251.

Markush, R. E., H. R. Karp, A. Heyman, and W. M. O'Fallon (1975). Epidemiologic study of migraine symptoms in young women. *Neurology 25,* 430–435.

Martin, M. J. (1972). Muscle contraction headache. *Psychosomatics 13,* 16–19.

Martin, M. J., H. P. Rome, and W. M. Swenson (1967). Muscle contraction headache; a psychiatric review. *Res. Clin. Stud. Headache 1,* 184–204.

Maxwell, H. (1966). *Migraine: Background and Treatment.* J. Wright, Bristol, Pa.

Meyer, A. (1930). Outline of Psychopathology for Use at Henry Phipps Psychiatry Institute, Baltimore, unpublished.

Philips, C. (1976). Headache and personality. *J. Psychosom. Res. 20,* 535–542.

Rogado, A. Z., R. H. Harrison, and J. R. Graham (1974). Personality profiles in cluster headache, migraine, and normal controls. *Arch. Neurobiol. (Madr) 37 (Suppl.),* 227–241.

Ross, W. D., and F. L. McNaughton (1945). Objective personality studies in migraine by means of the Rorschach method. *Psychosom. Med. 7,* 73.

Smitt, W. G. S. (1953). Pathogenesis and general symptomatology of headache. *Folia Psychiat., Neurol., Neurochirurg. 56,* 107.

Steinhilber, R. M., J. S. Pearson, and J. G. Rushton (1960). Some psychological considerations of histamic neuralgia. *Proceedings of the Staff Meetings of the Mayo Clinic 35(24),* 691–699.

Waters, W. E., and P. J. O'Connor (1970). The clinical validation of a headache questionnaire. In *Background to Migraine* (A. L. Cochrane, ed.) Heinemann, London.

Wolff, H. G. (1937). Personality features and reactions of subjects with migraine. *Arch. Neurol. Psychiat. 37,* 895.

Wolff, H. G. (1940). "Migraine," *Modern Medical Therapy in General Practice,* p. 2068. Williams and Wilkins, Baltimore.

23

THE BIOCHEMISTRY OF AFFECTIVE DISORDERS AND THEIR RELATIONSHIP TO HEADACHE

EDWARD B. MOHNS

INTRODUCTION

Within the past fifteen years there has been an exciting growth of interest in the biochemistry of both the affective disorders and headache. Severe depression and mania were once thought to be of purely intrapsychic origin, and the treatment of choice was held to be psychodynamic psychotherapy. Without discounting the etiologic importance of psychosocial and developmental factors, recent work in genetics and psychopharmacology has shifted much of the focus. Similarly, headache at one time was considered by many to be simply a "psychosomatic" illness affecting those with compulsive, depressive, or otherwise neurotically encumbered characters. More recent studies have not confirmed this belief, though many headache patients may be psychological and physiological overreactors. Evidence in the areas of genetics, pathophysiology, and treatment offer increasing promise of eventual understanding of these heterogeneous syndromes.

This discussion will summarize some of our present knowledge of the biochemistry of affective disorders, the biochemistry of headache, and some hypotheses concerning interrelationships. The section on affective disorders is relatively more detailed, since these data both permit and restrict the conclusions which can be drawn concerning possible relationships to headache. Discussion of the biochemistry of headache will be restricted to vascular headache since this is virtually the sole focus of the biochemical headache literature.

There is a large body of literature, and many studies are a challenge to interpret, are hard to compare, or report contradictory results. Throughout this review, it should be kept in mind that both depression and headache are highly heterogeneous syndromes. Also, in looking at the specific biochemical system changes, it is generally unknown if such changes are primary or secondary, are specific or nonspecific for a given condition (most are not), or are pathological or compensatory. A further methodologic difficulty is our inability to study the human brain *in vivo*, and the consequent limitations of second-order or inferential data. Finally, physiologic systems are far more interdependent and complex than we can yet grasp.

BIOCHEMISTRY OF AFFECTIVE DISORDERS

A. Neuroendocrine Systems

1. INTRODUCTION

Marked changes in mood, appetite, sleep, libido, arousal level, and activity level may be produced by alteration in hypothalamo-pituitary-adrenal (HPA) function, and such changes are often noted in depressed and manic patients. A depressed patient with diencephalic Cushing's syndrome may be difficult to diagnose, and the mood changes associated with steroid administration are well known. It is now known that portions of the hypothalamus produce factors or hormones which act to either release or inhibit release of pituitary hormones (Harris, 1972; Harris, 1948). Three hypothalamic factors have been isolated or synthesized; these include thyrotropin-releasing factor (TRF) (Schally *et al.,* 1973), Luteinizing-hormone-releasing factor (LHRF) (Matsuo *et al.,* 1971), and growth-hormone-release-inhibiting factor (GRIF, or somatostatin) (Brazeau and Guillemin, 1974). The evidence suggests that these factors are under the control of the biogenic amines (Ettigi and Brown, 1977). Schildkraut (1965) first hypothesized an abnormality of biogenic amines in the etiology of affective disorder. Neuroendocrine abnormalities have been shown in patients with affective disorder (Sachar and Coppen, 1975), and these may well be a function of neurotransmitter or neurotransmission abnormality.

2. ADRENOCORTICOTROPIC HORMONE (ACTH)

Available evidence may suggest a central catecholamine (CA) mechanism inhibiting ACTH secretion and a central serotonergic stimulatory mechanism of ACTH release in man (Ettigi and Brown, 1977). A number of reports suggest abnormal HPA function in depressed patients. Most workers have found elevated plasma cortisol and 17-hydroxy-corticosteroids (Carroll, 1976; Corroll, 1972a), and this does not appear to be a function of a non specific factor such as illness, anxiety, or hospitalization (Caroll, 1972b). Plasma cortisol elevations in some depressed patients are not suppressed by administration of dexamethasone, suggesting persistently elevated ACTH secretion in these patients (Carroll, 1976; Stokes, 1972). Such patients have shown flattening of the normal diurnal variation in secretion of cortisol, with secretory peaks increased in frequency and magnitude over a 24-hour period (Sachar *et al.,* 1973a).

Cerebrospinal fluid (CSF) cortisol levels have been studied in depressed patients, but conflicting results will require further studies for resolution (Ettigi and Brown, 1977). The studies of cortisol secretion in mania also report conflicting results.

3. GROWTH HORMONE (CGH)

Dopamine (DA), norepinephrine (NE), and serotonin (5-HT) appear to exert positive control on GH release (Frohman and Stachura, 1975). Many factors influence GH regulation and secretion including stress, sleep, prolonged fasting, arginine infusion, altered protein intake, changes in plasma glucose, fatty acid concentration, gender, oral contraceptive medication, and phase of menstrual cycle (Ettigi and Brown, 1977). 5-Hydroxytryptophan (5-HTP), the amino acid precursor of 5-HT, has been reported to cause a rise in plasma GH levels in normals (Imura *et al.,* 1973), and one study of depressed patients reported an inadequate GH response to 5-HTP (Takahashi *et al.,* 1974). In a study of five manic-depressive patients in the manic state, no significant difference in GH response to 5-HTP was found in comparison to controls (Takahashi *et al.,* 1974).

Postmenopausal unipolar depressed females have been reported to show a clearly reduced GH response to insulin hypoglycemia (Gruen *et al.,* 1975), and another study reported a lower GH response to hypoglycemia during acute depression than after recovering (Endo *et al.,* 1974). Peak GH release after a single intravenous administration of amphetamine sulfate was significantly lower in nine endogenous depressives than in controls (Langer *et al.,* 1976).

4. THYROID HORMONE

Production and release of thyroid hormone depends on thyroid-stimulating hormone (TSH), which in turn depends on thyrotropin-releasing factor (TRH). It is believed likely that noradrenergic neurons stimulate TRH secretion and serotonergic neurons inhibit TRH secretion (Ettigi and Brown, 1977). DA may well also be involved. Administration of TRH to depressed patients seems to transiently lessen the depressed mood, but whether or not this may be a placebo response remains controversial. Both TSH and L-tri-iodothyronine (T₃) are reported to accelerate or potentiate the response of depressed female patients to tricyclic antidepressants (TCA) (Cohen, 1975). Hypothyroidism in humans may produce insomnia and ruminative depression. Emlen *et al* (1972) have shown this state to be associated with increases in brain tyrosine hydroxylase in rats and therefore with an increase in the brain CA biosynthetic potential. However, there is no evidence of abnormal thyroid function in depressed or manic patients.

5. PROLACTIN

In a recent review, Ettigi and Brown (1977) suggest that a reduction in CA activity and an increase in 5-HT activity stimulate the release of prolactin. Both bipolar and unipolar depressed patients showed an elevated basal prolactin concentration compared with normal controls (Sachar *et al.*, 1973b). Further work to clarify prolactin secretion in affective disorder remains to be done.

6. LUTEINIZING HORMONE (LH) AND FOLLICLE-STIMULATING HORMONE (FSH)

It has long been noted that alterations in sex hormone function affect mood. Perhaps partly because of hereditary factors, depression is more common in females and is more likely to occur premenstrually, postpartum, menopausally, or in association with oral contraceptives. Thus far the biochemistry of such conditions has not been extensively studied. The relationship of neurotransmitters to LH and FSH secretion in humans remains to be established. One study reported lower plasma LH in depressed postmenopausal women compared with controls (Altman *et al.*, 1975). Measurement of plasma testosterone in 14 depressed males before and after recovery showed no change (Sachar *et al.*, 1972). Estrogens and progesterone are reported to affect monoamine oxidase (MAO) (Janowsky, *et al.*,

1971), but the clinical significance of this is not yet clear. Other than at a speculative level, better biochemical understanding in these arenas awaits future research.

Depression is associated with sodium retention, water retention, and increase in body weight. Studies with NA²² confirm this as well as the release of sodium ion during recovery. There is some evidence that in mania there is even greater retention of sodium ion than in depression (Kety, 1975). The location of the retained sodium may be intracellular, but this remains to be confirmed. In any case the pathophysiology and significance of these changes is unclear. Mendels *et al.*, (1976) indicated in a review that intracellular sodium is characteristically higher in bipolar patients, whether symptomatic or not, suggesting a trait rather than a state variable. They have also suggested that there is a subgroup of depressed patients with a genetically determined abnormality of some aspects of cell membrane properties which regulate the movements of electrolytes across the plasma membrane. Exemplary data include (1) differential distribution of the lithium ion across the erythrocyte membrane (seemingly under genetic control) in depressed patients responsive to lithium, as compared to nonresponders, (2) lower active transport of sodium in erythrocytes in psychotic than in neurotic depressives, and (3) reduced rate of entry of Na²² from plasma into lumbar spinal fluid of depressed patients.

C. Biogenic Amines

1. INTRODUCTION

Early work demonstrated that reserpinized animals showed increased 5-hydroxy-indoleacetic acid (5-HIAA) excretion and decreased brain 5-HT. Reserpine was shown to deplete brain NE and DA as well. Subsequently it was noted that iproniazid had antidepressant properties related to its action as a monoamine oxidase inhibitor (MAOI), and a variety of less toxic MAOIs were developed for the treatment of depression. The observation was made that administration of

L-dihydroxyphenylalanine (L-DOPA), the major DA precursor, was capable of reversing reserpine-induced depression in animals, whereas 5-HTP, the 5-HT precursor, was not. This led to greater interest in the CAs, primarily DA and NE, and further evidence was developed that amphetamine and single doses of TCAs increased the concentration of NE at central synapses. The CA hypothesis states that endogenous depressions are due to a functional deficiency of central CAs, particularly NE, whereas mania is associated with an excess of amine (Schildkraut, 1965). 5-HT is also believed to be involved in the affective disorders (Coppen, 1972a).

An overview of the literature indicates that the biogenic amine hypotheses, while productive heuristic devices, are in themselves marked oversimplifications at best. Research thus far has developed some interesting early leads, which I will briefly review. However, an eventual comprehensive formulation of the biochemistry of affective disorders will need to consider the simultaneous alteration of a variety of biogenic amines, feedback mechanisms, postsynaptic receptor activity, enzymes, hormones, ions, and membrane functions.

2. PRECURSOR ADMINISTRATION

NE is formed by conversion of the amino acid L-tyrosine through L-DOPA and DA. 5-HT is synthesized from L-tryptophan through 5-HTP and decarboxylation of 5-HTP to 5-HT. L-DOPA and tryptophan cross the blood-brain barrier, hence the rationale for trying these amino acids as antidepressants. The CSF concentration of tryptophan has been reported to be lower in depressive patients than in controls (Coppen et al., 1927b); free plasma tryptophan concentrations are reported to be reduced in female depressives but increasing to normal on clinical recovery (Coppen et al., 1973). In contrast, Ashcroft al., (1973) did not observe altered CSF tryptophan in depressed patients. Garfinkel et al. (1976) found no baseline difference between depressed patients and controls in free or total plasma tryptophan, but found an alteration in tryptophan metabolism in depressives, uncovered by carbidopa administration. Garfinkel et al. (1976) cite four articles which reported antidepressant properties of tryptophan, and five articles which did not.

There are several reports suggesting effectiveness of 5-HTP in mania (Prange et al., 1974). More recently, L-tryptophan has been proposed as a specific and physiologic hypnotic (Hartmann, 1977).

Generally, treatment with L-DOPA has yielded poor or confusing results in depressed patients. Henry et al. (1976) cite two reports in which less depression was found following L-DOPA administration in some retarded depressives but five reports in which L-DOPA was followed by an increased degree of depression in Parkinsonian patients. Hypomanic behavior has been produced with L-DOPA in bipolar depressed patients (Godwin et al., 1970; Murphy et al., 1971; Murphy, 1972). However the magnitude or significance of changes in brain NE resulting from increased brain DA are not yet understood.

3. BIOGENIC AMINE DEPLETION

Alpha-methylparatyrosine (AMPT) and parachlorophenylalanine (PCPA) pass the blood-brain barrier and inhibit the synthesis of NE and 5-HT, respectively (Spector et al., 1965; Koe and Weissman, 1966). Reserpine depletes the brain of 5-HT, NE, and DA nonselectively. The biogenic amine hypotheses have been studied by administration of these drugs, on the assumption that alteration in the functional availability of neurotransmitter would be expected to alter affective symptomatology.

An association between reserpine treatment and depression is widely known. However, it has been estimated that only about 6% of patients treated with reserpine for long periods of time develop depressive illness which appears to be endogenous (Goodwin and Bunney, 1971). These authors also conclude that the likelihood of the reserpine syndrome resembling endogenous depression is proportional to the likelihood of the patient having a past history of depression. Therefore, reserpine may precipitate depression in a small number of susceptible people, rather than universally causing depression in man. Bernstein and Kaufman (1960) did the only known prospective study of reserpine on mood in 50 patients, over a period of 12 to 18 months. They found no significant depression, but 12 patients developed a "pseudodepression," or "a reaction of excessive tranquilization with diminished psychomotor activity." Mendels and Frazier (1974) hypothesized that behavioral changes in man attributed to reserpine are at least partially due to the "sedative-motor" effect of DA depletion.

AMPT competitively inhibits tyrosine hydroxylase, the rate-limiting enzyme in CA biosynthesis, and depletes both brain and peripheral CAs. In a review of human and animal studies, Mendels and Frazier (1974) concluded that while AMPT may produce sedation and various behavioral effects, there is relatively little evidence that it has a direct effect on mood in either normal or psychiatrically disturbed persons. Shopsin *et al.* (1975) showed that AMPT did not prevent or reverse the antidepressant response to imipramine in depressed patients, but that PCPA did.

PCPA inhibits brainstem tryptophan hydroxylase, reducing the conversion of tryptophan. Interpretation of studies using PCPA are complicated by the fact that PCPA causes some reduction of NE stores (Welch and Welch, 1967; Welch and Welch, 1968). Also, PCPA does not appear to inhibit tryptophan hydroxylase equally in all tissues, *e.g.*, it does not inhibit tryptophan hydroxylase in the pineal (Deguchi and Barchas, 1973). In a review, Mendels and Frazier (1974) concluded that healthy volunteers, patients with carcinoid syndrome, and migrainous patients develop behavioral side effects from PCPA but not significant depression. In animals, PCPA produces behavioral changes reminiscent of mania, e.g., hypersexuality, insomnia, increased aggression, and irritability. Hyperalgesia is also noted. However, Shopsin *et al.* (1976) were able to reserve the antidepressant action of the MAOI tranylcypromine sul-

fate in bipolar and unipolar endogenously depressed patients with PCPA.

The amine-depletion data generally suggest an aminergic role in mood regulation, particularly for 5-HT, but do not support the simplistic notion of a primary depletion in aminergic function in depression.

4. BIOGENIC AMINE METABOLITE CONCENTRATIONS

A further research strategy has been the measurement in CSF and urine of amine metabolites. The concentration of 5-HIAA in urine probably provides no useful information about 5-HT turnover in brain. However, urinary 3-methoxy-4-hydroxyphenylglycol (MHPG) is believed to be a useful index of brain NE turnover. Both MHPG and 5-HIAA have been extensively studied in CSF, with interesting although somewhat controversial results.

Urinary MHPG levels may be lower, the same, or greater than normal in depressed patients. Low pretreatment MHPG levels correlate with favorable response to imipramine or desipramine and failure to respond to amitriptyline (Fawcett *et al.*, 1972; Maas *et al.*, 1972; Beckmann and Goodwin, 1975; Schildkraut, 1973). Conversely, normal or high pretreatment levels of urinary MHPG in depressed patients have been found to correlate with favorable response to amitriptyline and failure to respond to imipramine (Maas, 1975). It has further been shown that "low-MHPG" patients given dextroamphetamine (which inhibits MAO, favors release of NE, and inhibits reuptake of NE at the presynaptic nerve terminal while having relatively weak effects on 5-HT) showed temporary brightening of mood; however normal or high-MHPG patients given dextroamphetamine showed no change or became more depressed (Fawcett *et al.*, 1972; Fawcett and Siomopoulous, 1971).

In view of these data, and since imipramine *in vivo* primarily blocks the reuptake of NE and has relatively weak effects on 5-HT systems, Maas (1975) suggested that in one subgroup of depressives there is biochemical and pharmacologic evidence for an abnormality of NE but not of 5-HT. He also raised the possibility of another subgroup of depressives in which there is an abnormality of 5-HT but not of NE or DA, noting that amitriptyline blocks 5-HT reuptake, but is not effective in blocking NE uptake.

Coppen et al. (1972a) found CSF 5-HIAA reduced in both depressed and manic patients. This persisted after clinical recovery, raising the question of a trait rather than state variable. Other studies of CSF 5-HIAA have yielded conflicting results. (Goodwin and Post, 1975). There is also general disagreement as to whether the CSF 5-HIAA level correlates with severity of depressive illness or psychosis. However, Van Praag and Korf (1974) report that depressed patients with evidence of reduced CNS 5-HT turnover show an antidepressant response to 5-HTP. Of interest is the report from Asberg et al. (1973) in which depressed patients with low pretreatment levels of CSF 5-HIAA failed to respond to nortriptyline (somewhat more potent in blocking NE reuptake than in blocking 5-HT reuptake), whereas patients with higher CSF 5-HIAA levels had favorable responses to nortriptyline. Those with lower CSF 5-HIAA respond to chlorimipramine, which strongly blocks 5-HT reuptake but not NE reuptake (Mendels et al., 1976). The concept of a "5-HT depression" subgroup within the affective disorders has been given further support by Asberg et al. (1976), who found a bimodal distribution of CSF 5-HIAA concentrations in 68 depressed patients. 5-HIAA concentration was correlated with the severity of depression in the lower, but not in the upper, mode. They further reported preliminary findings that a negative correlation may exist between CSF MHPG and severity of illness, but only in those patients in the upper 5-HIAA mode. Future studies in this area should be of great interest.

Though controversy exists at this early stage of development, evidence is beginning to accumulate for the practical value of reclassifying depression according to biogenic amine metabolite activity. Clearly, the affective disorders are heterogeneous both biochemically and clinically.

5. TREATMENT EFFECTS

Following release into the synaptic cleft, the physiologic activity of NE and 5-HT is largely terminated by reuptake into the presynaptic neuron. TCAs inhibit reuptake after acute administration of these drugs, thereby presumably potentiating and prolonging neurotransmitter function. This mechanism, although consistent with the biogenic amine hypotheses, is too quick to be the basis for the antidepressant effects of the TCAs. Clinically, the efficancy of these drugs becomes evident only after days or weeks. Amphetamine and other direct CNS stimulants are not effective antidepressants, and TCAs do not produce a "high" in normal volunteers. Oswald et al. (1972) pointed out that depression may actually worsen during the first week on imipramine and reported that imipramine 75 mg daily made 12 nondepressed volunteers rate themselves as depressed in the first week but not in the third week on the drug. These data again suggest that depression is a complex biologic state rather than a simple exaggeration of normal physiology, and that the original model of transmitter deficiency or excess is not adequate.

An alternative model of affective disorder is postsynaptic hypersensitivity. Ghose et al. (1975) reported that depressive patients require significantly lower doses of intravenous tyramine to elevate the systolic blood pressure by 30 mm Hg, than do controls. Depressed patients also appear to metabolize tyramine differently. (Sandler et al., 1975). Goodwin et al. (1975) found that chronic treatment of depressed patients with tricyclics did not reverse the low level of CSF amine metabolites; rather it reduced the rate of amine synthesis further. Segal et al. (1974) reported decrease in regional rat brain tyrosine hydroxylase activity after eight days of administration of desmethylimipramine, but no change in enzyme activity 24 hours after a single dose of the same drug. Chronic reserpine induced a delayed increase of tyrosine hydroxylase activity. These authors posit that the depression-prone patient has CA receptors with heightened responsiveness and that the therapeutic response to TCA may be related to a further decrease in CA biosynthesis. Their model is experimentally and intuitively intriguing, and deserves further emphasis and investigation.

There is some evidence that the enzyme adenylate cyclase serves as the adrenergic receptor, catalyzing the formation of cyclic AMP from ATP, which then acts as a postsynaptic intracellular "second messenger." Urinary cyclic AMP has been reported to be low in depression and elevated in mania by some, but not all, investigators (Mendels *et al.*, 1976). Studies of CSF cyclic AMP are still too preliminary to assess.

Mania and depression, in addition to the more obvious differences, have a number of important features in common (Mendels *et al.*, 1976) For example, lithium administration has been shown to be of therapeutic value in both mania and selected cases of depression (Baastrup *et al.*, 1970; Schou, 1973), suggesting a biochemical similarity, perhaps a common ionic imbalance, in these clinical states. The actions of lithium are complex, and not yet well understood. Mendels and Frazier (1975) have proposed that some membrane properties regulating movement of electrolytes across the plasma membrane, in a subgroup of affective disorder, may be abnormal. If so, this could provide a bridge between electrolyte and biogenic amine factors in the pathophysiology of affective disorders.

Cathechol-o-methyltransferase (COMT) is a parasynaptic enzyme that inactivates both NE and DA. Low levels of COMT have been reported in the red cells of some manic and depressed patients (Dunner *et al.*, 1971; Mendels *et al.*, 1976), and the abnormality is stable regardless of the clinical or treatment status of the patient. Davidson *et al.* 1976) found that in 15 unipolar depressed women erythrocyte COMT levels linearly correlated with response to imipramine (best outcome occuring at low COMT). How best to integrate this information into the larger framework is not yet clear,

and adequate data on COMT in males is not yet available.

Since MAOI is useful in some depressed patients, a limited number of studies have attempted to clarify MAO activity in affective disorder. Evidence suggests that clinical efficacy is proportional to actual MAO inhibition, as measured in platelets. Several types of MAO occur, and a classification into A and B forms has been widely accepted. Human platelets appear to contain solely the B form (MAOB) (Murphy and Donnelly, 1974). Relatively little information is available as yet regarding the forms and distribution of MAO in the human brain. From the few studies available, it is not clear if platelet MAO is decreased, normal, or increased in affective disorder. Gershon *et al.* (1977) found no difference in plasma MAO activity between patients with primary affective illness and control patients. It should also be noted that clinically effective MAOIs may also act as potent inhibitors of reuptake (Hendley and Snyder, 1968).

A cholinergic-adrenergic hypothesis of mania and depression has been suggested by Janowsky *et al.* (1972), with mania representing adrenergic predominance and depression representing a predominance of cholinergic systems. The notion of cholinergic activity playing some role is supported by the reports that the anticholinesterase physostigmine reduces some manic behavior (Janowsky *et al.*, 1973), and that some patients report transient signs and symptoms of depression after physostigmine. However, the clinical efficacy of TCAs does not vary with the differences in anticholinergic potency (Snyder and Yamamura, 1977). The role of acetylcholine in affective disorders remains to be clarified.

D. Trace Neurotransmitters

The accumulation of structural analogs of normal synaptic neurotransmitters (substitute, or "false" neurotransmitters) can have profound behavioral and neurologic consequences. There has long been speculation as to whether such metabolic abnormalities may mediate psychiatric syndromes, including the affective disorders. Thus far there has been a paucity of research interest. Baldessarini and Fischer (1977) have provided a provocative discussion of this topic.

E. Pain Research

It has long been recognized that physical or hypochondriacal complaints occur commonly across the full spectrum of psychiatric diagnoses. Pain is perhaps the most frequent physical complaint and depression the most frequent primary psychiatric disgnosis in a population of patients initially categorized as hypochondriacal (Kenyon, 1976). Significant physical abnormality will be found in approximately half of such patients. Ziegler et al. (1960) reviewed the cases of 100 randomly chosen patients with a primary diagnosis of depression, and found that 28 patients demonstrated conversion symptoms of pain. Cassidy et al. (1957) found headache to be the most common somatic symptom in a group of 100 patients with manic-depressive illness, but they did not specify the type of headache. Probably many or even most such headaches are of the muscle contraction type, though Serry and Serry (1965) commented that migraine was one of the most frequent symptoms of "masked depression."

It can be reasonably stated that depression causes pain, and it is also true that pain causes depression. Sternbach (1975) suggested that acute pain is associated with anxiety, but persistent pain often with the development of increasing depression and endogenomorphic signs. It has been suggested that chronic pain patients seem to have 5-HT-type depression (Sternbach et al. 1976), and these authors reported that chlorimipramine, a TCA which blocks reuptake of 5-HT but not NE, reduces chronic pain more effectively than does amitriptyline, which affects both 5-HT and NE reuptake. Bradley (1963) has suggested that the coincident onset of pain and depression is associated with relief of pain when the depression is treated with electric convulsive therapy (ECT). Mandel (1975) reported remarkable improvement in four of six patients treated

with nondominant hemispheric unilateral ECT for chronic pain (without demonstrable physiologic basis) and associated secondary affective disorder (depression). However, it is not clear whether or not ECT is useful in intractable pain in which there is not a significant associated depression.

The CNS mechanisms of analgesia are under intensive study. There is compelling evidence for a 5-HT-mediated pain inhibitory mechanism in the CNS, with additional evidence that NE may normally function to reduce the activity of the CNS analgesia system and that DA is necessary for the normal functioning of the system (Mayer and Price, 1976). Dietary or chemical depletion of brain 5-HT increases sensitivity to pain, and administration of tryptophan and 5-HTP returns both 5-HT levels and pain thresholds to normal. It has been shown that brain opiate receptors depend on the same 5-HT system (Snyder, 1977; Mayer and Price, 1976), and indeed a major research strategy has been the model of morphine-induced analgesia.

The recent discovery of morphine-like endogenous polypeptides, termed endorphins or enkephlin, which bind stereospecifically to brain opiate receptors, has given rise to enthusiasm of bandwagon proportions, much current research, and the usual early phase of overinterpretation of some results. These polypeptides are potent analgesics, produce complex behavioral changes when administered to experimental animals, and can be blocked or reversed with naloxone, an opiate antagonist (Goldstein, 1976; Guillemin, 1977; Snyder, 1977; Bloom et al., 1976). Other naturally occuring brain peptides have been reported to be endorphin antagonists (Guillemin et al., 1976). Naloxone administration has not proven useful in schizophrenia or affective disorders (Davis et al., 1977; Kurland et al., 1977), or naltrexone in chronic schizophrenia (Mielke and Gallant, 1977). Kline et al. (1977) have reported that intravenous beta-endorphin produces euphoria and clinical improvement of some duration in both schizophrenic and depressed patients. In one study, Terenius et al. (1976) reported that reduced symptoms of schizophrenia after neuroleptic treatment are associated with a decreased level of endorphin in the CSF, and they also found elevated endorphin levels in the CSF of manic patients. Segal *et al.* (1977) pointed out that beta-endorphin produces periods of hyperactivity resembling the behavioral response to amphetamine, both of which are to some extent antagonized by naloxone, and therefore speculated that psychological disturbances similar to those produced by amphetamine may be due to excessive endorphin receptor activation.

The physiology and pathophysiology of these newly-discovered transmitters remain to be worked out, but are clearly of great importance.

F. Prostaglandins (PGs)

This unique group of cyclic fatty acids has a broad range of physiologic activities, including effects on endocrine and reproductive glands, gastrointestinal motility and gastric secretion, hematopoietic function, cardiovascular and renal function, inflammatory tissue responses, and water and electrolyte movement across a variety of membranes (Coceani, 1974; Wolfe, 1975). In the nervous system, PGs are thought to function postsynaptically by inhibition or facilitation of neurotransmission through cyclase inhibition or activation, and by means of a negative feedback loop to inhibit further release of neurotransmitter from the presynaptic nerve (Gross *et al.*, 1977). PGs interact with CAs and 5-HT, though the interactions are not well understood. Psychotropic drugs exert a variety of effects on PG synthesis and catabolism. There are few reports of PGs in psychiatric illness as yet, but future work in this area may prove to be of great usefulness.

BIOCHEMISTRY OF HEADACHE

A. Cluster Headache

Nearly all of the biochemical literature on headache has focused on vascular headache, particularly migraine and cluster headache. Their cause is not yet known. Cluster headache is considered by most authors to be a biochemically and clinically distinct entity, rather than simply a migraine variant, though both are vascular disturbances and perhaps of related or similar neurogenic origins.

Whole blood histamine levels rise quickly during the attack of cluster headache, but minimally and late in migraine. Plasma 5-HT levels do not change significantly after a cluster headache, but decrease during migraine (Anthony and Lance, 1971). However, Sjaastad (1975a) found that measurement of whole blood histamine permits no meaningful statements about a possible relationship to the symptoms of cluster headache, and he summarized the literature as indicating that the concept of a histamine-cluster headache interrelationship had not yet been adequately investigated. Sjaastad and Sjaastad (1977a) have more recently found that the inconsistency of attack-related increase in urinary histamine excretion makes it unlikely that histamine is a causative agent in cluster headache, and suggest that histaminuria is more likely a consequence of attacks. They have also found no defects of histamine catabolism in vascular headache patients (Sjaastad and Sjaastad, 1977b). The failure of antihistaminic drugs in the treatment of cluster headache is well known. Veger *et al.* (1976) H_2 receptor antagonist, as not useful in the treatment of cluster headache.

The defect in cluster headache may be a locally liberated vasodilator, and treatment with vasoconstrictor agents and agents which interfere with the activities of vasoactive amines is frequently helpful.

B. Migraine Headache

1. THE NEUROGENIC CONCEPT OF MIGRAINE.

Migraine is a heterogeneous group of syndromes usually characterized by episodes of throbbing headache, unilateral or bilateral, believed by most authors to be associated with characteristic cranial vascular changes. The principal feature is not always pain, since neurologic, psychiatric, gastrointestinal, chest, renal, and peripheral vasomotor changes may occur with or without the headache. The clinical course is often subject to major and unexplained fluctuations. There appears to be a genetic predisposition in some patients and not in others. The range of provoking stimuli is vast, including dietary factors, emotional stress, bright or flickering lights, changes in the weather or in altitude, hormonal factors, mild hypoglycemia, allergens, etc.

Though the etiology of migraine is unknown, the pathophysiology has been somewhat more accessible. Most authors agree that cranial vasoconstriction and vasodilatation are usually involved and that this neurovascular reaction, possibly a hypersensitive cerebral protective mechanism, occurs in response to changes in either the internal or external environment. The neurogenic concept of vascular headache of the migraine type (see pp. 124–125) suggests that noxious factors, as perceived by the brain, may induce cerebral vasodilatation or vasospasm via an integrative disorder of the central vasomotor centers, the intracranial and extracranial blood vessels, and the microcirculation. This model included both central and peripheral vasomotor reaction, as well as a sterile inflammatory reaction, evoked by activity of the nervous system. At the level of pathophysiology local sterile inflammation is presumed to be mediated in part by vasoactive amines such as histamine, 5-HT, NE, tyramine, the slow-reacting substance (SRS), as well as kinins, prostaglandins, heparin, acetylcholine, and perhaps others (Dalessio, 1974; Dalessio, 1976b). Platelets may be a major source of these vasoactive substances, and lung tissue may contribute as well.

2. DATA REGARDING POSSIBLE IMMUNE AND PLATELET-MEDIATED PATHOPHYSIOLOGY

Immune complex deposition may also be a factor in the inflammatory response, and drugs used in prophylaxis of migraine such as methysergide, antihistamines, cyproheptadine, and corticosteroids are experimentally effective in limiting the deposition of immune complexes (Dalessio, 1976b). In support of this thesis, Lord and Duckworth (1977) demonstrated complement breakdown products in migraine patients several hours before headache onset and elevated immunoglobulin levels associated with migraine. Their data suggest a late-onset immune reaction of short duration; this in turn might partially explain some features of migraine such as platelet release of 5-HT, basophil and mast cell degranulation, increased whole blood histamine during attacks, fluid retention, increased thrombotic tendency, and increased CSF lactate and gamma-aminobutyric acid (GABA). Confirmation and clarification of such immune data will be required, particularly in view of the methodological problems involved in studying these mediators.

With an eye to the early immune data, however, it is of interest that Anthony (1968), noting the fall in plasma 5-HT at the beginning of migraine attacks, incubated "headache-free platelets" with "migraine plasma" from the same patient. This produced a drop in platelet 5-HT comparable to that of "migraine platelets." On this basis, Anthony postulated the presence of an "endogenous 5-HT releasing factor" in plasma during migraine. More recently, Sandler (1977) has also proposed that platelet 5-HT release is secondary to an unknown humoral substance, and that the reduced activity of platelet MAOB shown in both symptomatic and asymptomatic migraine patients is a secondary manifestation of platelet damage rather than a direct contributor to the headache, Complement activation and IgG immune complexes cause platelet release of 5-HT (Pfueller and Luscher, 1974), and, were there a known mechanism for acute and rapid neurogenic complement activation, it would be tempting to consider this as the unknown plasma factor of Anthony and Sandler. Perhaps increased immunoglobulin levels and complement activation, if confirmed, are another facet of a hypersensitive cerebral protective mechanism in at least some patients.

Recent evidence suggests that migraine patients show platelet hyperaggregation during the headache-free period and headache prodrome, and subsequent decrease in platelet aggregation during the headache phase (Deshmukh and Meyer, 1976; Couch and Hassanein, 1976a; Deshmukh and Meyer, 1977). A model is proposed for the pathogenesis of migraine, in which the cyclic changes in platelet dynamics play a primary role (Deshmukh and Meyer, 1977). The use of platelet antagonists in the treatment of migraine has recently been emphasized by Dalessio (1976b). The model of Deshmukh and Meyer usefully organizes a number of clinical and biochemical findings but does not clearly indicate whether the platelet abnormality is primary or secondary. Why a generalized biochemical abnormality would preferentially affect the cerebral vasculature is not addressed. Correlation of data regarding platelet aggregation with the available data regarding immunoglobulins and complement as well as platelet MAOB in migraine would be of great interest.

3. BIOGENIC AMINE DATA

Intuitive observations, treatment data, and a wealth of inferential experimental data all point to some contribution to migraine via alteration of CA and indoleamine physiology, whether central and/or peripheral. Acute reserpine administration has been reported to precipitate migraine-like headache in susceptible individuals, and this may be reversed by intravenous administration of 5-HT (Kimball et al., 1960). The frequency and severity of migraine may be decreased by reserpine administration (Genefke et al., 1975; Fog-Moller et al., 1976). A decreased frequency of migraine after chronic administration of L-tryptophan has been reported by Poloni et al. (1973). Similar success with chronic administration of 5-HTP is also reported (Sicuteri, 1973). A single oral dose of L-DOPA is reported to increase headache pain and induce vomiting in migraine patients (Sicuteri, 1977). However, L-DOPA may sometimes benefit migraine attacks (McDowell, 1970; Horrobin, 1973a).

Amitriptyline has been found effective both in chronic muscle contraction headache (Lance and Curran, 1964) and in the prophylaxis of migraine (Gomersall and Stuart, 1973; Couch et al., 1976). Noone (1977) reported chlorimipramine to have beneficial effects in prevention of migraine. MAOIs have been reported to be useful in migraine prophylaxis (Anthony and Lance, 1969). Chronic lithium administration

may be of prophylactic benefit in some patients with cluster headache (Kudrow, 1977). Propranolol and prindolol (beta-adrenergic receptor antagonists) are reportedly of prophylactic value in migraine (reviewed in Ekbom, 1975). Ghose et al. (1977) suggested therapeutic usefulness of a selective alpha-adrenergic blocker, indoramin. Laitenen (1975) reported significant prophylactic benefit of acupuncture in migraine, and other work shows that acupuncture analgesia in humans is reversible by naloxone (Mayer and Price, 1976) and may well be mediated by endorphins (Pomeranz, 1977). Methysergide has been extensively used in prophylaxis of migraine, possibly by functioning as a 5-HT receptor agonist (Dalessio, et al., 1961) or perhaps by an unknown independent effect on the cerebral vasculature (Saxena, 1972). Ergotamine is also a 5-HT antagonist, though its direct vasoconstrictor action may be more relevant to its use in migraine. Clonidine has been used in prophylaxis of migraine in doses low enough to preclude any antihypertensive action. The CNS effects of clonidine are complex and are not yet understood.

Dietary phenylethylamine may precipitate migraine attacks in some patients, and patients with migraine are reported to have a phenylethylamine oxidizing defect (Sandler et al., 1974), which may possibly be related to MAOB deficiency. Subsequently, Sandler (1975) has discussed these findings in relation to reportedly high activity of MAOB in human pineal (Goridis and Neff, 1972), as one possible pathophysiologic mechanism which awaits further study. Dietary tyramine may be related to migraine attacks in some patients. Altered tyramine metabolism is reported in migraine patients (Youdim et al., 1971), similar to the deficit found in depressive patients (Sandler et al., 1975). Ghose et al. (1977) have reported increased blood pressure sensitivity to intravenous tyramine in migraine patients, closely paralleling their findings in depressed patients.

CSF studies are few, and have mostly concentrated on 5-HIAA as an indicator of CNS 5-HT turnover. Hyyppa and Kangasniemi (1977) reviewed previous conflicting reports of minor variations in CSF 5-HIAA levels in migraine patients, and they presented current work in which they correlated free plasma tryptophan, of particular importance in CNS 5-HT metabolism, with CSF 5-HIAA levels in migraine patients with and without headache. Both CSF 5-HIAA and plasma free tryptophan rose significantly with headache measured 4 hours after onset, though in 4 of 18 patients, CSF 5-HIAA decreased during migraine attack. The authors suggest that CSF 5-HIAA levels during migraine reflect changes of plasma-free tryptophan and are not of primary pathogenetic significance. Welch *et al.* (1976) found elevated CSF levels of GABA and cyclic AMP in patients with stroke and in migraine patients studied during an attack. These authors suggest that in both conditions the biochemical changes are secondary to ischemia. It has also been reported that transient cerebral ischemia in animals produces homolateral and contralateral hemispheric 5-HT depletion (Welch *et al.*, 1977).

4. OTHER PATHOGENETIC PROPOSALS

It has been hypothesized that migraine is the manifestation of a central congenital biochemical dysfunction of pain perception (Sicuteri, 1972), with postulated brain 5-HT deficiency and central denervation hypersensitivity. This model would be analogous to pain of the thalamic syndrome type. Many of the difficulties in characterizing migraine as a "low-serotonin syndrome," whether central or peripheral, have been cogently argued by Sjaastad (1975b). In reviewing the case for 5-HT, Sandler (1975) states that its role in the pathogenesis of migraine has yet to emerge, and that the 5-HT hypothesis has not yet proven particularly useful at either a research or clinical level. More recently Sicuteri (1976, 1977) has expanded his hypothesis to include possible CNS DA and NE abnormalities of the postsynaptic hypersensitivity type. There are aspects of his argument which have appeal, but experimental confirmation is lacking.

Another pathogenetic hypothesis, that of "impaired central inhibition," has been advanced by Appenzeller (1975). He argues from the documented peripheral platelet MAOB deficiency in migraine patients to a theoretical central MAOB deficiency which could lead to a periodic accumulation of vasoactive substances in the brain. This in turn might contribute to disinhibition of the 5-HT-mediated raphe neurons with subsequent excessive autonomic discharge, and/or produce change in the cranial vasculature. Appenzeller does not present his model as all-encompassing and advocates extensive research to test the hypothesis.

5. ELECTROLYTE METABOLISM

Migraine is often associated with decreased rates of excretion of water, sodium, potassium, and creatinine prior to and during the early phases of an attack, and with increased rates of excretion during the subsiding phase of an attack. The available evidence suggests that these changes do not bear a causal relationship to headache, and are probably a nonspecific concomitant (see pp. 92–98 and Greene, 1973). The pathophysiology remains unclear but may represent a parallel response to perceived stress. As yet there are no data suggesting a trait variation in sodium metabolism or cell membrane function in migraine.

6. ENDOCRINOLOGY OF HEADACHE

Several lines of indirect evidence favor a significant association between reproductive hormonal changes and migraine. The sexual prevalence of migraine is about equal in children, but greatly favors women among adults. There is some association between menses and exacerbation of migraine. Epstein *et al.* (1975) reported significantly higher plasma estrogen and progesterone levels during the luteal phase in women with migraine as compared to controls, whether migraine was of mentstrual or nonmenstrual type. Of precautionary importance, however, is the report from Kashiwagi, *et al.* (1972a) that headaches of all types are equally likely to be worse in association with the menstrual cycle and that hysteria is associated with reported exacerbation of headache in relation to the menstrual cycle.

Approximately 70% of women with migraine improve during pregnancy, particularly after the first trimester, but the physiology mediating this improvement remains unclear. It has commonly been believed that many migraine patients improve with the onset of menopause, but evidence to the contrary has been presented (Klee, 1968: Whitty and Hockaday, 1968). Oral contraceptives, particularly the low-estrogen variety, have been noted to be associated with either onset or exacerbation of migraine (Whitty et al., 1966; Carrey, 1971; Kudrow, 1975), but they may also temporarily improve migraine (Grant et al., 1974). Replacement estrogen therapy is associated with increased incidence of migraine, and the effect may be ameliorated by decreasing the dose of estrogen by 50% and giving the drug daily instead of cyclically (Kudrow, 1975). Of considerable interest are the reports that both estrogen and oral contraceptives increase platelet aggregation (Mettler and Selchow, 1972; Kalendovsky et al., 1975) as well as increasing blood coagulability and roughening the vascular endothelium. Migraine is associated with increased risk of vascular disease and early mortality (Leviton et al. 1974). Several authors have discussed a possible role of prolactin in migraine, though no clear abnormality of prolactin has been shown (Horrobin, 1973b' Hockaday et al., 1976).

Since hormonal changes are associated with a broad spectrum of other physiologic changes, the possibilities with respect to the pathophysiology of migraine are obviously numerous and complex. Biogenic amine physiology is one such variable, and, for example, the associations between hormonal changes, platelet and uterine MAOB activity, and migraine may eventually prove quite valuable in helping to elucidate some aspects of pathophysiology in at least a subgroup of migraine patients. The minimal experimental data available have led to some interesting speculation, which will hopefully be followed by the necessary clinical and basic research. The reader is referred to Greene (1973), Kudrow (1976), Grant et al. (1974), Hockaday et al. (1976), Appenzeller (1976), and elsewhere in this volume for further general discussions in this area.

BIOCHEMICAL RELATIONSHIPS BETWEEN AFFECTIVE DISORDERS AND HEADACHE

Vascular headache and depression are common disorders. On a statistical basis the occurrence of both disorders in the same patient would not be a rare event, even if there were no common etiologic or pathophysiologic factors. The prevalence of both disorders in women and in association with hormonal changes is frequently commented upon, if not mechanistically understood. A further theoretical basis for overlap between these populations is suggested by the idea that both disorders may be primitive protective mechanisms which become diseases by activating spontaneously, too easily, too greatly, or in a biologically maladaptive context.

It appears that there is a greater than expected frequency of both migraine and muscle contraction headache among primary depressive patients, and prominent, if transient, mood alteration as well as a significantly increased incidence of affective disorder in migraine patients (Kashiwagi et al., 1972b; Diamond, 1964; Cassidy, et al., 1957). Unfortunately, few systematic studies have been done regarding the overlap between the affective disorder and vascular headache populations. Some data are difficult to interpret due to uncertainty as to exactly what types of headache have been included. Others appear to consider depression to be a single disgnostic entity. Also, it is striking to note that the neurologic literature on headache is replete with descriptive references to affective disorders, whereas the psychiatry literature is virtually silent on the topic of coexisting migraine.

Couch et al. (1975) studied the presence of depression in 236 outpatients who presented to a headache clinic with severe or disabling migraine. Headache severity was studied quantitatively, and the Zung Self-rating Depression Scale was used to measure depression. The results suggest a weak but significant relationship between migraine and depression, and this prompted the authors to consider that the population under study might be composed of several subgroups. Further data analysis revealed that there was a striking correlation of migraine and depression in those patients who had focal neurologic symptoms of migraine (paresis, sensory disturbance, difficulty with speech, and loss of consciousness). The authors raised the possibility of a shared or overlapping CNS monoaminergic dysfunction in this latter group of patients. If this possibility is to be evaluated, data regarding diagnostic subtype of depression, family history, sequential CSF MHPG and 5-HIAA levels, and differential treatment response to amitriptyline versus imipramine or nortriptyline would be essential. Also to be addressed would be the question of whether a similar incidence of depression occurs in any population sustaining repeated and significant neurologic insult.

More recently, Ziegler et al. (1977) reported further investigation of the association of headache and anxiety and depression in a nonclinic volunteer population. In both sexes, in most age groups, subjects reporting disabling headaches had mean anxiety and depression scores in excess of those subjects reporting a history of mild or no headache. This difference was more striking in the youthful, and for all age groups more consistent in women. The strongest association was between depression and headache severity in women. In both sexes depression scores peaked in the youngest and in the oldest age groups sampled. A strong association was found between frequency of disabling headache and both depression and anxiety in both sexes in the youthful, with some association between headache frequency and depression in older women, and with a weaker association between duration of headache and degree of anxiety and depression. These data are of interest, but in the absence of diagnostic information they permit no conclusions to be drawn about possible overlap between vascular headache and primary affective disorder.

Studies of amitriptyline prophylaxis of migraine suggest that there is a weak predrug correlation between depression and severity of migraine, again suggesting a nonhomogeneous population with respect to these variables (Couch et al., 1976: Couch and Hassanein,

1976b). A weak relationship was found between improvement in migraine and improvement in depression, and these authors suggest that the effectiveness of amitriptyline in the prophylaxis of migraine is not mediated by its antidepressant properties. The doses of amitriptyline ranged from 50 to 100 mg per day. Gomersall and Stuart (1973) deliberately permitted selection of a dose of amitriptyline which had no appreciable side effects (10 to 60 mg per day), found it effective in prophylaxis of migraine, but reported improvement percentages somewhat lower than those reported by Couch et al. (1976). Whether amitriptyline is acting centrally or peripherally (or more likely both), and in what way, awaits experimental data. These same questions hold concerning the mechanisms of action of MAOIs, reserpine, 5-HTP, lithium, and adrenergic blockers in the prophylaxis of vascular headache.

With the exception of the data regarding CSF GABA and cyclic AMP (Welch et al., 1976), solid evidence of physicochemical abnormality in migraine is thus far restricted to the periphery. It seems unlikely that in vascular headache there will prove to be a permanent CNS biochemical abnormality measurable by currently available techniques. In affective disorder there is strongly suggestive evidence of CNS abnormalities of both NE and 5-HT neuronal function in at least some subgroups of patients.

Populations of patients with vascular headache and with primary affective disorder appear to overlap biochemically in the areas of abnormal tyramine metabolism and abnormal blood pressure sensitivity to administration of intravenous tyramine. The prevalence and relationship between these abnormalities in either patient population remains to be established, and we do not yet know if the affected subgroup of migraine patients might be a contributing source to the increased incidence of depressive illness in migraine, or vice versa. The genetics, pathophysiology, and CNS implications of a common fundamental defect in tyramine metabolism are not yet known. The heightened blood pressure sensitivity to intravenous tyramine is compatible with a variety

of possible central and/or peripheral alterations of noradrenergic function, including
biosynthesis, storage, release, degradation, receptor responsiveness, or some combination.
In migraine, the blood pressure sensitivity is
mechanistically consistent with the reported
platelet MAOB deficiency, but there are no
studies showing a correlation between variation in MAOB function and blood pressure
sensitivity to intravenous tyramine. A corresponding subgroup of depressives with abnormal MAO function has not yet been clearly
defined.

Of the various possibilities, the concept of a
shared postsynaptic noradrenergic receptor
hypersensitivity seems particularly plausible
and, perhaps more fundamentally, there may
be a shared genetic predisposition toward abnormality of receptor membrane transport
which need not necessarily be limited to NE
systems alone. As discussed earlier, there are
several early lines of evidence to suggest a
defect of this type in at least a subgroup of the
affective disorders.

Considering this tenuous extrapolation for
a moment, there is no intrinsic reason why
a heritable defect of this kind, having perhaps evolved from originally adaptive neu-
roregulatory mechanisms, could not occur
as a spectrum varying both as to expressivity
and regional distribution. In migraine, the
primary defect might be relatively mild and
hence more easily reversible or compensated,
compatible with the paroxysmal nature of the
disorder. The distribution might be primarily
in CNS areas of vasomotor control, but
perhaps in other areas of brain as well, compatible with the observable clinical heterogeneity
and with the vast number of seemingly
nonspecific triggers. In both the vascular
headache and affective disorder populations,
the distribution of postsynaptic defect could
conceivably include the central pain inhibitory
mechanisms. In affective disorder such a defect might be more consistent and severe, compatible with an illness of insidious onset, longer
duration, and greater accessibility to biochemical investigation. The regional distribution in
affective disorder would be largely different as
compared to migraine, but with the apparent

potential for distributional overlap. Thus, of
those inheriting a spectrum postsynaptic
hypersensitivity or receptor membrane transport defect, some would develop one of the
migraine or vascular headache syndromes,
some would develop one of the affective disorder subtypes, and relatively few would fully
develop both. Any or all of the CNS neurotransmitter systems may be involved, varying
from subgroup to subgroup.

A speculative model of this kind is admittedly nonspecific, but has the advantage of
synthesizing the little concrete information
presently available regarding overlap between
the affective disorders and headache. There
are already an ample number of specific
hypotheses, and there are more than an ample
number of good research questions in search
of an investigator.

SUMMARY

1. For the purposes of this discussion, review
of the biochemistry of affective disorders has
been largely limited to depression. Biochemistry of headache is confined to discussion of
vascular headache, since this is virtually the
sole focus of the biochemical headache literature.

2. Both depression and vascular headache
are clinically and biochemically heterogeneous. In neither is the etiology known. The
literature in both areas is in an early stage of
development, and permits few definite conclusions.

3. Psychological and physiological abnormalities are associated with abnormal
hypothalamo-pituitary-adrenal function. Such
changes are also often noted in patients with
affective disorders. These functions are under
the partial control of biogenic amines. Some
depressed patients show elevated plasma cortisol levels, evidence of persistently elevated
ACTH secretion, and flattening of the normal
diurnal variation in secretion of cortisol.
Growth hormone release is impaired in some
patients. Both thyroid-stimulating hormone
and T_3 may potentiate the response of depressed female patients to tricyclic antidepressants, but there is no evidence of abnormal

thyroid function in affective disorder. Some unipolar and bipolar depressed patients show an elevated basal prolactin secretion. Sex hormone function affects mood, but the biochemistry involved has not been extensively studied.

4. Sodium and water retention occurs in both depression and mania. Apparently there is a subgroup of depressives with genetically determined abnormality of cell membrane regulation of electrolyte movement. Adenylate cyclase may serve as the adrenergic receptor. Urinary cyclic AMP has been reported to be low in depression and elevated in mania by some, but not all investigators. These data may eventually provide a bridge between electrolyte and biogenic amine factors.

5. The biogenic amine hypotheses have generated considerable research data supporting abnormality of NE and 5-HT-mediated pathways in the affective disorders, but are not adequate or evidently correct models at present. Postsynaptic hypersensitivity may be a more viable general etiologic hypothesis than that of transmitter deficiency or excess. Data suggesting practical value of reclassifying depression according to biogenic amine metabolite activity is presented ("NE depression" and "5-HT depression" subgroups). The mechamisms of action of antidepressant drugs and lithium are not yet clear.

6. Low levels of erythrocyte catechol-o-methyltransferase (COMT) have been reported to exist in some depressed and manic patients. In some unipolar depressed females low erythrocyte levels may correlate with response to imipramine. Abnormal MAO function in affective disorder has not been clearly defined.

7. Depression may be associated with abnormal metabolism of tyramine and tryptophan. Abnormalities of plasma free tryptophan have not been established in affective disorder. Some depressives show abnormally heightened blood pressure responsiveness to intravenous tyramine.

8. Primary depression is very commonly associated with complaints of pain, and chronic pain quite often results in depression with endogenomorphic signs and symptoms. Depres-

sion which develops in association with chronic pain may be primarily of the 5-HT type. 5-HT mediates a pain inhibitory pathway in the CNS. NE may normally function to inhibit the activity of this pathway, and DA to enhance it. Opiate receptors and endorphins, or enkephalin, depend on the same 5-HT system. Endorphins are neurotransmitters whose functions are not yet well understood but appear to include a role in regulation of mood and cognition.

9. Prostaglandins interact with CAs and 5-HT, and are affected by psychotropic drugs. Their role in psychiatric illness is not yet known.

10. The neurogenic concept of vascular headache of the migraine type is briefly reviewed.

11. A fall in plasma and platelet 5-HT is associated with migraine but not with cluster headache attacks. This is consistent with the tendency toward platelet hyperaggregation shown by migraine patients. Reported abnormalities of platelet MAOB function in migraine may be secondary to platelet damage as well, though MAO function may be affected by many other factors including estrogen and progesterone levels. It is not yet known if alterations in MAO function play a pathophysiologic role in vascular headache, either peripheraly or centrally. The significance of peripheral serotonin changes is not clear. Other vasoactive amines including NE may also serve to mediate the peripheral sterile inflammatory response in migraine. Complement activation and immunoglobulin data suggest that a late-onset immune reaction of short duration may be involved in some patients.

12. Successful prophylaxis of migraine in some patients with 5-HT precursors, L-DOPA, reserpine, amitriptyline, chlorimipramine, MAOIs, alpha and beta adrenergic receptor blockers, clonidine, methysergide, and acupuncture argues powerfully for a pathophysiologic and perhaps etiologic role of NE and 5-HT. The mechanisms of action of these agents in migraine, and whether central or peripheral or both, remains to be determined.

13. Dietary phenylethylamine and tyramine may be related to migraine attacks in some

patients. A phenylethylamine oxidizing defect is described, and some migraine patients show altered tyramine metabolism similar to that found in depressed patients. Increased blood pressure sensitivity to intravenous tyramine has been reported in migraine patients, closely paralleling the findings in depressed patients.

14. CSF GABA and cyclic AMP may be elevated both in patients with stroke and patients with migraine during an attack, in both instances attributed to ischemia. There is no solid evidence for other CSF biochemical abnormalities in vascular headache thus far.

15. The amine-specific CNS pathogenetic hypothesis of congenital biochemical dysfunction of pain perception and that of impaired central inhibition are briefly reviewed.

16. Fluid and electrolyte shifts associated with migraine are apparently nonspecific concomitants, perhaps as a function of perceived stress. As yet there are no data suggesting variation in sodium metabolism or cell membrane function in migraine.

17. Reproductive hormonal changes influence vascular headache by mechanisms not yet known. Migraine may be associated with menses, oral contraceptives, or estrogen replacement. Better understanding of the relationships between hormonal changes and biogenic amine physiology awaits future research.

18. There appears to be a greater than expected frequency of both vascular and muscle contraction headache among patients with primary affective disorders, and increased incidence of affective disorder in vascular headache patients. Available data are presented concerning the clinical overlap between these two patient populations. Both affective disorder and vascular headache may represent primitive protective mechanisms which become diseases by activating spontaneously, too easily, too greatly, or in a biologically maladaptive context.

19. It can generally be said that both the vascular headache syndromes and the affective disorders utilize mechanisms involving CA and 5-HT-mediated pathways. However, experimental data regarding more specific biochemical overlap between these populations is lim-

ited to abnormal tyramine metabolism and heightened blood pressure sensitivity to intravenous tyramine in some patients from both populations. The central implications, genetics, pathophysiology, and other ramifications of these defects await future research.

20. Extrapolating from the limited concrete data available, the proposal is made that vascular headache and the affective disorders might have in common a heritable defect in postsynaptic receptor hypersensitivity, or perhaps more fundamentally a shared genetic predisposition toward abnormality of receptor membrane transport which need not be limited to any specific neurotransmitter system alone. Thus, of those inheriting such a defect, some would develop one of the migraine or vascular headache syndromes, some would develop one of the affective disorder subtypes, and relatively few would fully develop both.

REFERENCES

Altman, N., E. J. Sachar, P. H. Gruen, F. Halpern, and S. Eto (1975). Reduced plasma LH concentration in post-menopausal depressed women. *Psychosom. Med.* 37 274–276.

Anthony, M. (1968). Plasma serotonin levels in migraine. *Adv. Pharmacol. 6,* 203.

Anthony, M., and J. W. Lance (1969). Monoamine oxidase inhibition in the treatment of migraine. *Arch. Neurol. 21,* 263–268.

Anthony, M., and J. W. Lance (1971). Histamine and serotonin in cluster headache. *Arch. Neurol. 25,* 225–231.

Appenzeller. O. (1975). Pathogenesis of vascular headache of the migrainous type: the role of impaired central inhibition. *Headache 15,* 177–179.

Appenzeller, O. (1976). Monoamines, headache and behavior. In *Pathogenesis and Treatment of Headache* (O. Appenzeller, ed.), pp. 43–48. Spectrum, New York.

Asberg, M., L. Bertilsson, D. Tuck, B. Cronholm, and F. Sjöqvist, (1973). Indoleamine metabolites in the cerebrospinal fluid of depressed patients before and during treatment with nortriptyline. *Clin. Pharmacol. Ther. 14,* 277–286.

Asberg, M., P. Thoren, and L. Traskman (1976). "Serotonin depression"—biochemical subgroup within the affective disorders? *Science 191,* 478–480.

Ashcroft, G. W., I. M. Blackburn, D. Eccleston, A. I. M. Glen, W. Hartley, N. E. Kinloch, M. Lonergan, L. G. Murray, and I. A. Pullar (1973). Changes on recovery in the concentrations of tryptophan and the biogenic amine metabolites in the cerebrospinal fluid of patients with affective illness. *Psychol. Med. 3*, 319-325.

Baastrup, P. C., J. C. Poulsen, M. Schou, K. Thomsen, and A. Amdisen (1970). Prophylactic lithium: double-blind discontinuation in manic-depressive and recurrent depressive disorders. *Lancet 2*, 326-330.

Baldessarini, R. J., and J. E. Fischer (1977). Substitute and alternative neurostransmitters in neuropsychiatric illness. *Arch. Gen. Psychiat. 34*, 95-964.

Beckmann, H., and F. K. Goodwin (1975). Antidepressant response to tricyclics and urinary MHPG in unipolar patients. *Arch. Gen. Psychiat. 32*, 17-21.

Bernsten, S., and M. R. Kaufman (1960). A psychological analysis of apparent depression following Rauwolfia therapy. *J. Mt. Sinai Hospital 27*, 525-530.

Bloom, F., D. Segal, N. Ling, and R. Guillemin (1976). Endorphins: profound behavioral effects in rats suggest new etiological factors in mental illness. *Science 190*, 630-632.

Bradley, J. J. (1963). Severe localized pain associated with depressive syndrome. *Brit. J. Psychiat. 109*, 741-745.

Brazeau, P., and R. Guillemin (1974). Somatostatin: new-comer from the hypothalamus. *N. Engl. J. Med. 290*, 963-964.

Carrey, H. M. (1971). Principles of oral contraceptives: 2. Side effects of oral contraceptives. *Med. J. Aust.2*, 1242-1250.

Carroll, B. J. (1972a). Plasma cortisol levels in depression. In *Depressive Illness: Some Research Studies* (B. Davies, B. J. Carroll, and R. M. Mowbray, eds.), pp. 69-86. C. C. Thomas, Springfield, Ill.

Carroll, B. J. (1972b). The hypothalamic-pituitary axis: functions, control mechanisms, and method of study. Op. cit., pp. 23-68.

Carroll, B. J. (1976). Psychoendocrine relationship in affective disorders. In *Modern Trends in Psychosomatic Medicine, Vol. 3* (O. W. Hill, ed.), pp. 121-153. Butterworths, Boston.

Cassidy, W. L., N. B. Flanagan, and M. F. Spellman (1957). Clinical observations in manic-depressive disease. *JAMA 164*, 1535-1546.

Coceani, F. (1974). Prostaglandins and the central nervous system. *Arch. Intern. Med. 133* 119-129.

Cohen, R. A. (1975). Manic-depressive illness. In *Comprehensive Textbook of Psychiatry-II* (A. M. Freedman, H. I. Kaplan, and B. J. Sadock, eds.), pp. 1012-1024. Williams and Wilkins, Baltimore.

Coppen, A., A. J. Prange, Jr., P. C. Whybrow, and R. Noguera (1972a). Abnormalities of indoleamines in affective disorders. *Arch Gen. Psychiat. 26*, 474-478.

Coppen, A., B. W. L. Brooksbank, and M. Peet (1972b). Tryptophan concentrations in the cerebrospinal fluid of depressive patients. *Lancet 1*, 1393.

Coppen, A., E. G. Eccleston, and M. Peet (1973). Total and free tryptophan concentration in the plasma of depressive patients. *Lancet 2*, 60-63.

Couch, J. R., and S. Hassanein (1976a). Platelet agregability in migraine and relation of aggregability to clinical aspects of migraine. *Neurology 26*, 34.

Couch, J. R., and R. S. Hassanein (1976b). Migraine and depression: effect of amitriptyline prophylaxis. *Trans. Am. Neurol. Assoc. 101*, 234-237.

Couch, J. R., D. K. Ziegler, and R. S. Hassanein (1975). Evaluation of the relationship between migraine headache and depression. *Headache 15*, 41-50.

Couch, J. R., D. K. Ziegler, and R. Hassanein (1976). Amitriptyline in the prophylaxis of migraine. *Neurology 26*, 121-127.

Dalessio, D. J., W. A. Camp, H. Goodwell, and H. G. Wolff (1961). Studies on headache. The mode of action of UML-491 and its relevance to the nature of vascular headache of the migraine type. *Arch. Neurol. 4*, 235-240.

Dalessio, D. J. (1974). Vascular permeability and vasoactive substances: their relationship to migraine. *Adv. Neurol. 4*, 395-401.

Dalessio, D. J. (1976a). Disorders of immune mechanisms and headache. In *pathogenesis and Treatment of Headache* (O. Appenzeller, ed.) pp. 125-129. Spectrum, New York.

Dalessio, D. J. (1976b). Use of platelet antagonists in the treatment of migraine. *Headache 16*, 129-130.

Davidson, J. R. T., M. N. McLeod, H. L. White, and D. Raft (1976). Red blood cell catechol O-methyl-transferase and response to imipramine in unipolar depressive women. *Am. J. Psychiat. 133* 952-955.

Davis, G. C., W. E. Bunney, Jr., E. G. De Fraites, J. Kleinman, D. Van Kammen, R. Post, and R. Wyatt (1977). Intravenous naloxone administration in schizophrenia and affective illness. *Science 197*, 74-77.

Deguchi, T., and J. Barchas (1973). Comparative studies on the effect of parachlorophenylalanine on hydroxylation of tryptophan in pineal and brain of the rat. In *Serotonin and Behavior* (J. Barchas and E. lsdin, eds.), pp. 33-47. Academic Press, New York.

Deshmukh, S. V., and J. S. Meyer (1976). Platelet dysfunction in migraine and effect of self-medication with aspirin. *Stroke 7*, 11.

Deshmukh, S. V., and J. S. Meyer (1977). Cyclic changes in platelet dynamics and the pathogenesis and prophylaxis of migraine. *Headache 17*, 101-108.

Diamond, S. (1964). Depressive headaches. *Headache 4*, 255.

Dunner, E. L., C. K. Cohn, E. S. Gershon, and F. K. Goodwin (1971). Differential catechol-O-methyltransferase activity in unipolar and bipolar affective illness. *Arch. Gen. Psychiat. 25*, 348-353.

Ekbom, K. (1975). Adrenergic beta-receptor blockers. In *Vasoactive Substances Relevant to Migraine* (S. Diamond, D. J. Dalessio, J. R. Graham, and J. L. Medina, eds.), pp. 19–24. C. C. Thomas, Springfield, Ill.

Emlen, W., D. S. Segal, and A. J. Mandel (1972). Effects of thyroid state on pre-and post-synaptic central adrenergic mechanisms. *Science 175*, 79–82.

Endo, M., J. Endo, and M. Nishikubo, (1974). Endocrine studies in depression. In *Psychoneuroendocrinology* (N. Hatatoni, ed.), pp. 22–31. S. Karger, New York.

Epstein, M. T., J. M. Hockaday, and T. D. R. Hockaday (1975). Migraine and reproductive hormones throughout the menstrual cycle. *Lancet 1*, 543–547.

Ettigi, P. G., and G. M. Brown (1977). Psychoneuroendocrinology of affective disorder: an overview. *Am. J. Psychiat. 134*, 493–501.

Fawcett, J., and V. Siomopoulous (1971). Dextroamphetamine response as a possible predictor of improvement with tricyclic therapy in depression. *Arch. Gen. Psychiat. 25*, 247–255.

Fawcett, J., J. W. Maas, and H. Dekirnenjian (1972). Depression and MHPG excretion. Response to dextroamphetamine and tricyclic antidepressants. *Arch. Gen. Psychiat. 26*, 246–251.

Fog-Moller, F., T. Dalsgaard-Nielsen, I. K. Genefke, and G. Nattero (1976). Therapeutic effect of reserpine on migraine syndrome: relationship to blood amine levels. *Headache 16*, 275–278.

Frohman, L. A., and M. E. Stachura (1975). Neuropharmacologic control of neuroendocrine function in man. *Metabolism 24*, 211–234.

Garfinkel, P. E., J. J. Warsh, H. C. Stancer, and D. Sibony (1976). Total and free plasma tryptophan levels in patients with affective disorders. *Arch. Gen. Psychiat. 33*, 1462–1466.

Genefke, I. K., T. Dalsgaard-Nielsen, B. Bryndum, F. Fog-Moller, and J. A. P. Jensen (1975). Concentration of serotonin in blood platelets: effect of reserpine in migraines. *Headache 15*, 136–138.

Gershon, E. S., R. H. Belmaker, K. Ebstein, and W. Z. Jonas (1977). Plasma MAO activity unrelated to genetic vulnerability to primary affective illness. *Arch. Gen. Psychiat. 34*, 731–734.

Ghose, K., P. Turner, and A. Coppen (1975). Intravenous tramine pressor response in depression. *Lancet 1*, 1317–1318.

Ghose, K., A. Coppen, and D. Carroll (1977). Intravenous tyramine response in migraine before and during treatment with indoramin. *Brit. Med. J. 1*, 1191–1193.

Goldstein, A. (1976). Opioid peptides (dorphins) in pituitary and brain. *Science 193*, 1081–1086.

Gomersall, J. D., and A. Stuart (1973). Amitriptyline in migraine prophylaxis. Changes in pattern of attacks during a controlled clinical trial. *J. Neurol. Neurosurg. Psychiat. 36*, 684–690.

Goodwin, F. K., H. K. H. Brodie, D. L. Murphy, and W. E. Bunney, Jr. (1970). L-DOPA,

catecholamines and behavior: a clinical and biochemical study in depressed patients. *Biol. Psychiat. 2*, 341–366.

Goodwin, F. K., and W. E. Bunney, Jr. (1971). Depression following reserpine: a re-evaluation. *Semin. Psychiat. 3*, 435–448.

Goodwin, F. K., and R. M. Post (1975). Studies of amine metabolites in affective illness and schizophrenia. A comparative analysis. In *The Biology of the Major Psychoses. A Comparative Analysis* (D. X. Freedman, ed.), pp. 299–332. Raven Press, New York.

Goodwin, F. K., R. L. Sack, and R. M. Post (1975). Clinical evidence for neurotransmitter adaptation in response to antidepressant therapy. In *Neurobiological Mechanisms of Adaptation and Behavior* (A. J. Mandell, ed.). Raven Press, New York.

Goridis, C., and N. H. Neff (1972). Evidence for specific, monoamine oxidase in human sympathetic nerve and pineal gland. *Proc. Soc. Exp. Biol. Med. 14*, 573–574.

Grant, E. C. G., J. D. Carroll, and J. Pryse-Davies (1974). Monoamine-oxidase and migraine. *Lancet 2*, 1449.

Greene, R. (1973). The endocrinology of headache: the Sandoz lecture. In *Background to Migraine* (J. N. Cumings, ed.), pp. 82–92. Heinemann, London.

Gross, H. A., D. L. Dunner, D. Lafleur, H. L. Meltzer, H. L. Muhlbauer, and R. R. Fieve (1977). Prostaglandins. A review of neurophysiology and psychiatric implications. *Arch. Gen. Psychiat. 34*, 1189–1196.

Gruen, P. H., E. J. Sachar, N. Altman, and J. Sassin (1975). Growth hormone responses to hypoglycemia in post-menopausal depressed women. *Arch. Gen. Psychiat. 32*, 31–33.

Guillemin, R., N. Ling, R. Burgus, and L. Lazarus (1976). Abstract, 10th International Congress of Biochemistry, Hamburg, Germany.

Guillemin, R. (1977). Endorphins, brain peptides that act like opiates. *N. Engl. J. Med. 296*, 226–228.

Harris, G. W. (1948). Electrical stimulation of the hypothalamus and the mechanism of neural control of the adenohypophysis. *J. Physiol. (Lond). 107*, 418–429.

Harris, G. W. (1972) Humours and hormones. *J. Endocrinol. 53*, 2–23.

Hartmann, E. (1977). L-tryptophan: a rational hypnotic with clinical potential. *Am. J. Psychiat. 134*, 366–370.

Hendley, E. D., and S. H. Snyder (1968). Relationship between the action of monoamine oxidase inhibitors on the noradrenaline uptake system and their antidepressant efficacy. *Nature (Lond.) 220*, 1330–1333.

Henry, G. M., M. Buchsbaum, and D. L. Murphy (1976). Intravenous L-DOPA plus carbidopa in depressed patients: average evoked response, learning, and behavioral changes. *Psychosom. Med. 38*, 95–105.

Hockaday, J. M., K. M. S. Peet, and T. D. R. Hockaday (1976). Bromocriptine in migraine. *Headache* 16, 1109-1114.

Horrobin, D. F. (1973a). Prevention of migraine by reducing prolactin levels. *Lancet 1*, 777.

Horrobin, D. F. (1973b). *Prolactin: Physiology and Clinical Significance.* Medical and Technical Lancaster, England.

Hyyppa, M. T., and P. Kangasniemi (1977). Variation of plasma free tryptophan and CSF 5-HIAA during migraine. *Headache 17*, 25-27.

Imura, N., Y. Nakai, and T. Yoshimi (1973). Effect of 5-hydroxytryptophan on GH and ACTH release in man. *J. Clin. Endocrinol. Metab. 36*, 204-206.

Janowsky, D. S., W. E. Fann, and J. M. Davis (1971). Monoamines and ovarian hormone-linked sexual and emotional changes: a review. *Arch. Sex. Behav. 1*, 205-218.

Janowsky, D. S., M. K. El-Yousef, J. M. Davis, and H. J. Sekerke (1972). A cholinergic-adrenergic hypothesis of mania and depression. *Lancet 2*, 632-635.

Janowsky, D. S., M. K. El-Yousef, J. M. Davis, and H. J. Sekerke (1973). Parasympathetic suppression of manic symptoms by physostigmine. *Arch. Gen. Psychiat. 28*, 542-547.

Kalendovsky, Z., J. Austin, and P. Steele (1975). Increased platelet aggregability in young patients with stroke. *Arch. Neurol. 32*, 13-20

Kashiwagi, T., J. N. McClure, Jr., and R. D. Wetzel (1972a). The menstrual cycle and headache type. *Headache 12*, 103-104.

Kashiwagi, T., J. N. McClure, Jr., and R. D. Wetzel (1972b). Headache and psychiatric disorders. *Headache 12*, 659-663.

Kenyon, F. E. (1976). Hypochondriacal states. *Brit. J. Psychiat. 129*, 1-14.

Kety, S. S. (1975). Biochemistry of the major psychoses. In *Comprehensive Textbook of Psychiatry/II* (A. M. Freedman, H. I, Kaplan, and B. J. Sadock, eds.), pp. 178-187. Williams and Wilkins, Baltimore.

Kimball, R. W., A. P. Friedman, and E. Vallejo (1960). Effect of serotonin in migraine patients. *Neurology 10*, 107-111.

Klee, A. (1968). *Clinical Study of Migraine.* Munksjaard, Copenhagen.

Kline, N. S., C. H. Li, H. E. Lehmann, A. Lajtha, E. Laski, and T. Cooper (1977). B-Endorphin-induced changes in schizophrenic and depressed patients. *Arch. Gen. Psychiat. 34*, 1111-1113.

Koe, K. B., and A. Weissman (1966). Parachlorophenylalanine: a specific depletor or brain serotonin. *J. Pharmacol. Exp. Ther. 154*, 499-516.

Kudrow, L. (1975). The relationship of headache frequency to hormonal use in migraine. *Headache 15*, 36-40.

Kudrow, L. (1976). Hormones, pregnancy, and migraine. In *Pathogenesis and Treatment of Headache*

(O. Appenzeller, ed.), pp. 31-41. Spectrum, New York.

Kudrow, L. (1977). Lithium prophylaxis for chronic cluster headache. *Headache 17*, 15-18.

Kurland, A. A., O. L. McCabe, T. E. Hanlon, and D. Sullivan (1977). The treatment of perceptual disturbances in schizophrenia with naloxone hydrochloride. *Am. J. Psychiat. 134*, 1408-1410.

Laitinen, J. (1975). Acupuncture for migraine prophylaxis: a prospective clinical study with six months' follow-up. *Am. J. Clin. Med. 3*, 271-274.

Lance, J. W., and D. A. Curran (1964). Treatment of chronic tension headache. *Lancet l*, 1236-1239.

Langer, G., G. Heinze, B. Reim, and N. Matussek (1976). Reduced growth hormone responses to amphetamine in "endogenous" depressive patients. *Arch. Gen. Psychiat. 33*, 1471-1475.

Leviton, A., B. Malvea, and J. R. Graham (1974). Vascular diseases, morality and migraine in the parents of migraine patients. *Neurology 24*, 669-672.

Lord, G. D. A., and J. W. Duckworth (1977). Immunoglobulin and complement studies in migraine. *Headache 17*, 163-168.

Maas, J. W., J. A. Fawcett, and H. Dekirmenjian (1972). Catecholamine metabolism, depressive illness, and drug response. *Arch. Gen. Psychiat. 26*, 252-262.

Maas, J. W. (1975). Biogenic amines and depression. Biochemical and pharmacological separation of two types of depression. *Arch. Gen. Psychiat. 32*, 1357-1361.

Mandel, M. R. (1975). Electroconvulsive therapy for chronic pain associated with depression. *Am. J. Psychiat. 132*, 632-636.

Matsuo, H., A. Arimura, R. M. G. Nair and A. V. Schally (1971). Synthesis of the porcine LH- and FSH-releasing hormone by the solid phase method. *Biochem. Biophys. Res. Commun. 45*, 822-827.

Mayer, D. J., and D. D. Price (1976). Central nervous system mechanisms of analgesia. *Pain 2*, 379-404.

Mayer, D. J., D. D. Price, J. Barber, and A. Rafii (1976). Acupuncture analgesia: evidence for activation of a pain inhibitory system as a mechanism of action. In *Advances in Pain Research and Therapy, Vol. 1* (J. J. Bonica and D. Albe-Fessard, eds.), pp. 751-754. Raven Press, New York.

McDowell, F. H. (1970). Changes in behavior and mentation. In *L-DOPA and Parkinsonism* (A. Barbeau and F. H. McDowell, eds.), pp. 321-325. Davis, Philadelphia.

Mendels, J., and A. Frazier (1974). Brain biogenic amine depletion and mood. *Arch. Gen. Psychiat. 30*, 477-451.

Mendels, J., and A. Frazier (1975). Lithium distribution in depressed patients: implications for an alteration in cell membrane function in depression. In *The Psychobiology of Depression* (J. Mendels, ed.), pp. 101-122. Spectrum, New York.

Mendels, J., S. Stern, and A. Frazier (1976).

Biochemistry of depression. *Dis. Nerv. Syst. 37,* 2-9.

Mettler, L., and B. M. Selchow (1972). Oral contraceptives and platelet function. *Thrombos. Diathes. Haemorrh. 28,* 213-220.

Mielke, D. H., and D. M. Gallant (1977). An oral opiate antagonist in chronic schizophrenia: a pilot study. *Am. J. Psychiat. 134,* 1430-1431.

Murphy, D. L., H. K. H. Brodie, F. K. Goodwin, and W. E. Bunney, Jr. (1971). Regular induction of hypomania by L-DOPA in "bipolar" manic depressive patients. *Nature 229,* 135-136.

Murphy, D. L. (1972). L-DOPA, behavioral activation, and psychopathology. *Res. Publ. Assoc. Res. Nerv. Ment. Dis. 50,* 472-493.

Murphy, D. L., and C. H. Donnelly (1974). Monoamine oxidase in man: enzyme characteristics in platelets, plasma and other human tissues. In *Neuropsychopharmacology of Monoamines and Their Regulatory Enzymes* (E. Usdin, ed.), p. 71. Raven Press, New York.

Noone, J. F. (1977). Psychotropic drugs and migraine. *J. Intern. Med. Res. 5,* 66-71.

Oswald, I., V. Brezinova, and D. L. F. Dunleavy (1972). On the slowness of action of tricyclic antidepressant drugs. *Brit. J. Psychiat. 120,* 673-677.

Pflueller, S. L., and E. Luscher (1974). Studies of the mechanisms of human platelet release reaction induced by immunologic stimuli, 1. Complement-dependent and complement independent reactions. *J. Immunol. 113,* 1201-1210.

Poloni, M., G. Nappi, A. Arrigo, and F. Savoldi (1974). Cerebrospinal fluid 5-hydroxy-indoleacetic acid level in migrainous patients during spontaneous attacks, during headache-free periods and following treatment with L-tryptophan. *Experientia 30,* 640-641.

Pomeranz, B. (1977). Naloxone blockade of acupuncture analgesia: endorphin implicated. *Life Sciences 19,* 1757.

Prange, A. J., Jr., I. C. Wilson, C. W. Lynn, L. B. Alltop, and R. A. Stikeleather (1974). L-tryptophan in mania: contribution to a permissive hypothesis of affective disorder. *Arch. Gen. Psychiat. 30,* 56-62

Sachar, E. J., F. Halpern, R. S. Rosenfeld, T. F. Gallagher, and L. Hellman (1973). Plasma and urinary testosterone levels in depressed men. *Arch. Gen. Psychiat. ,28,* 15-18.

Sachar, E. J., L. Hellman, H. P. Roffwarg, F. S. Halpern, D. Fukushima, and T. Gallagher (1973a). Disrupted 24-hour patterns of cortisol secretion in psychotic depression. *Arch. Gen. Psychiat. 28,* 19-24.

Sachar, E. J., A. G. Frantz, N. Altman, and J. Sassin (1973b). Growth hormone and prolactin in unipolar and bipolar depressed patients: responses to hypoglycemia and L-DOPA. *Am. J. Psychiat. 130,* 1362-1367.

Sachar, E. J., and A. J. Coppen (1975). Biological

aspects of affective psychoses. In *Biology of Brain Dysfunction,* Vol. 3 (G. E. Gaull, ed.). pp. 215-245. Plenum, New York.

Sandler, M., M. B. H. Youdim, and E. Hanington (1974). A phenylethylamine oxidising defect in migraine. *Nature 250,* 335-337.

Sandler, M. (1975). Monoamines and migraine: a path through the wood? In *Vasoactive Substances Relevant to Migraine* (S. Diamond, D. J. Dalessio, J. R. Graham, and J. L. Medina, eds.), pp. 3-18. C. C. Thomas, Springfield, Ill.

Sandler, M., C. S. Bonham, M. F. Cuthbert, and C. M. B. Pare (1975). Is there an increase in monoamine-oxidase activity in depressive illness? *Lancet 1,* l045-1046.

Sandler, M. (1977). Transitory platelet monoamine oxidase deficit in migraine: some reflections. *Headache 17,* 153-158.

Saxena, P. R. (1972). The effects of antimigraine drugs on the vascular responses by 5-hydroxytryptamine and related biogenic substances on the external carotid bed of dogs: possible pharmacological implications to their antimigraine action. *Headache 12,* 44-54.

Schally, A. V., A. Arimura, and A. J. Kastin (1973). Hypothalamic regulatory hormones. *Science 179,* 341-350.

Schildkraut, J. J. (1965). The catecholamine hypothesis of affective disorders: a review of supporting evidence. *Am. J. Psychiat. 122,* 509-522.

Schildkraut, J. J. (1973). Norepinephrine metabolites as biochemical criteria for classifying depressive disorders and predicting responses to treatment: preliminary findings. *Am. J. Psychiat.130,* 695-698.

Schou, M. (1973). Prophylactic lithium maintenance treatment in recurrent endogenous affective disorders. In *Lithium: Its Role in Psychiatric Research and Treatment* (S. Gershon and B. Shopsin, eds.), pp. 253-267. Plenum, New York.

Segal, D. S., R. Kuczenski, and A. J. Mandell (1974). Theoretical implications of drug-induced adaptive regulation for a biogenic amine hypothesis of affective disorders. *Biol. Psychiat. 9,* 147-159.

Segal, D. S., R. G. Browne, F. Bloom, N. Ling, and R. Guillemin (1977). B-Endorphin: endogenous opiate or neuroleptic? *Science 198,* 411-413.

Serry, D., and M. Serry (1965). Masked depression and the use of antidepressants in general practice. *Med. J. Aust. 1,* 334-338.

Shopsin, B., E. Friedman, M. Goldstein, and S. Wilk (1975). The use of synthesis inhibitors in defining a role for biogenic amines during imipramine treatment in depressed patients. *Psychopharmacol. Commun. 1,* 239-249.

Shopsin, B., E. Friedman, and S. Gershon (1976). Parachlorophenylalamine reversal of tranylcypromine effects in depressed patients. *Arch. Gen. Psychiat. 33,* 811-819.

Sicuteri, F. (1972). Headache as possible expression

of deficiency of brain 5-hydroxytryptamine (central denervation supersensitivity). *Headache 12*, 69–71.

Sicuteri, F. (1973). The ingestion of serotonin precursors (L-5-hydroxytryptophan and L-tryptophan) improves migraine and headache. *Headache 13*, 19–22.

Sicuteri, F. (1976). Migraine, a central biochemical dysnociception. *Headache 16*, 145–159.

Sicuteri, F. (1977). Dopamine, the second putative protagonist in headache. *Headache 17*, 129–131.

Sjaastad, O. (1975a) Is histamine of significance in the pathogenesis of headache? In *Vasoactive Substances Relevant to Migraine* (S. Diamond, D. J. Dalessio, J. R. Graham, and J. L. Medina, eds.), pp. 45–66. C. C. Thomas, Springfield, Ill.

Sjaastad, O. (1975b). The significance of blood serotonin levels in migraine. *Acta Neurol. Scand. 51*, 200–210.

Sjaastad, O., and O. V. Sjaastad (1977a). Urinary histamine excretion in migraine and cluster headaches: further observations. *J. Neurol. 216*, 91–104.

Sjaastad, O., and O. V. Sjaastad (1977b). Histamine metabolism in cluster headache and migraine: catabolism of C histamine. *J. Neurol. 216*, 105–117.

Snyder, S. H. (1977). Opiate receptors and internal opiates. *Sci. Am. 236*, 44–56.

Snyder. S. H., and H. I. Yamamura (1977). Antidepressants and the muscarinic acetylcholine receptor. *Arch. Gen. Psychiat., 34*, 236–239.

Spector, S., A. Sjoerdsma, and S. Udenfriend (1965). Blockade of endogenous norepinephrine synthesis by alphamethyl-tyrosine, an inhibitor of tyrosine hydroxylase. *J. Pharmacol. Exp. Ther. 147*, 86–95.

Sternbach, R. A. (1975). Psychophysiology of pain. *Intern. J. Psychiat. Med. 6*, 63–73.

Sternbach, R. A., D. S. Janowsky, L. Y. Huey, and D. S. Segal (1976). Effects of altering brain serotonin activity on human chronic pain. *Adv. Pain Res. Therapy 1*, 601–606.

Stokes, P. E.(1972). Studies on the control of adrenocortical function in depression. In *Recent Advances in the Psychobiology of the Depressive Illnesses*, U. S. DHEW Publication 70-9053. (T. A. Williams, M. M. Katz, and J. A. Shield, Jr., eds.), pp. 199–220. U. S. Government Printing Office, Washington.

Takahashi, S., H. Kondo, and M. Yoshimura (1974). Growth hormone responses to administration of L-5-hydroxytryptophan (L-5-HTP) in manic depressive psychosis. In *Psychoneuroendocrinology* (N.

Hatatoni and M. Tsu, eds.), pp. 32–38. S. Karger, New York.

Terenius, L., A. Wahlstrom, L. Lindstrom, and E. Widerlöv (1976). Increased CSF levels of endorphins in chronic psychosis. *Neuroscience Letters 3*, 157–162.

Van Praag, H. M., and J. Korf (1974). Serotonin metabolism in depression: clinical application of the probenecid text. *Intern. Pharmacopsychiatry 9*, 35–51.

Veger, T., D. Russell, and O. Sjaastad (1976). Histamine H^2 antagonists and cluster headache. *Brit. Med. J. 2*, 585.

Welch, A. S., and B. L. Welch (1967). Effect of p-chlorophenylalanine on brain noradrenaline in mice, letter to editor. *J. Pharm. Pharmacol. 19*, 632–633.

Welch. A. S., and B. L. Welch (1968). Effect of stress and para-chlorophenylalanine upon brain serotonin, 5-hydroxyindoleacetic acid and catecholamines in grouped and isolated mice. *Biochem. Pharmacol. 17*, 699–708.

Welch, K. M. A., E. Chabi, J. H. Nell, K. Bartosh, A. N. C. Chee, N. T. Mathew, and V. S. Achar (1976). Biochemical comparison of migraine and stroke. *Headache 16*, 160–167.

Welch, K. M. A., R. Gaudet, T. P. F. Wang, and E. Chabi (1977). Transient cerebral ischemia and brain serotonin: relevance to migraine. *Headache 17*, 145–147.

Whitty, C. W. M., J. M. Hockaday, and M. M. Whitty (1966). The effect of oral contraceptives on migraine. *Lancet 1*, 856–859.

Whitty, C. W. M., and J. M. Hockaday (1968). Migraine: a follow-up study of 92 patients. *Brit. Med. J. 1*, 735–736.

Wolfe, L. S. (1975). Possible roles of prostaglandins in the nervous system. In *Advances in Neurochemistry* (B. W. Arganoff, ed.), pp. 1–49. Plenum, New York.

Youdim, M. B. H., C. S. Bonham, M. Sandler, E. Hanington, and M. Wilkinson (1971). Conjugation defect in tyramine-sensitive migraine. *Nature (Lond.) 230*, 127–128.

Ziegler, F. J., J. B. Imboden, and E. Meyer (1960). Contemporary conversion reactions: a clinical study. *Am. J. Psychiat. 116*, 901–909.

Ziegler, D. A., R. S. Hassanein, and J. R. Couch (1977). The association of headache with anxiety and depression in non-clinic population. Report from the annual headache symposium of the Research Group on Headache and Migraine of the World Federation of Neurology, 11th World Congress of Neurology, Amsterdam.

24

BEHAVIORAL THERAPIES AND HEADACHE

RICHARD A. STERNBACH

BEHAVIORAL ANALYSIS OF PAIN

Because there is no purely objective measure of pain, behavioral signs are very important. Pain may be thought of as a symptom of an underlying disease, as is fever, and thus a nonspecific symptom. But whereas a thermometer can give accurate and repeated readings of the fever, in conscious or unconscious animals and in humans, there is nothing comparable for pain. We depend upon behavior to assess pain.

If a patient says, smilingly, that he is in pain, we are not overly impressed with its severity. If a patient, restless and perspiring, tells us his pain is not severe, we are more likely to believe our eyes than our ears. Thus, there are three major kinds of pain behaviors we attend to: verbal; motor; and physiological, especially autonomic. All three kinds are easily susceptible to conditioning or learning procedures, and so neither words, nor motor behavior, nor autonomic patterns will bear a perfect relationship to "real" pain, since all will reflect sociocultural influences as well as "pure" neurological activity (Lang et al., 1972).

Fordyce (1976) has pointed out that pain behaviors of all three kinds may be thought of as either *respondent* or *operant*. Respondents are *elicited* by antecedent noxious stimuli, and thus are usually reflexive: the sudden withdrawal, vocalization, and increased pupillary diameter and pulse rate, for example. Such respondents are conditioned in the classical or Pavlovian manner; any stimulus regularly paired with the noxious stimulus will itself acquire the ability to elicit similar responses—the dentist's office, or a parent's angry voice, for example.

In contrast, operants are *emitted* behaviors which are governed by the reinforcers which follow them: moaning behavior, rewarded by attention from the family; taking analgesics, rewarded by a decrease in pain; being bedridden, rewarded by respite from unpleasant work, but punished by a decline in income. These operants are conditioned in the Skinnerian manner; any behavior followed by a favorable consequence (positive reinforcer) is more likely to recur—it will increase in frequency. Any behavior followed by an aversive consequence (negative reinforcer, punishment) will be less likely to recur, and it will similarly show a decrease in frequency if there are no positive consequences. It should be noted that a decrease of pain is usually a positive reinforcer, and whatever diminishes pain is likely to be repeated (or sought after).

In practice, one usually encounters chronic pain patients who show a mixture of respondent and operant behaviors. This is usually reflexive behavior to antecedent pathogenic stimulation, and operant behavior maintained by contingent environmental consequences. The analysis of any patient's pain may not be advanced by questions as to "psychogenic" versus "somatogenic," but it may be furthered a great deal by attention to both reflexive respondents and contingent-controlled operants.

Such an analysis of pain abandons the disease model for a learning model. The disease

440

model views pain as a symptom of underlying pathology, and the appropriate treatment is therefore directed to the presumed cause, which can be diagnosed by appropriate tests. The learning model, on the other hand, views the pain behavior itself as the pathology to be modified, and attention is directed specifically to the operants (Fordyce *et al.*, 1968). Although this may seem to be missing the point, to those accustomed to the traditional approach, and merely a technique to teach stoicism while leaving "underlying" pain untreated, in fact measures of subjective pain show improvement in follow-up studies of operant treatment for chronic pain (Fordyce *et al.*, 1973; Ignelzi *et al.*, 1977).

Since much if not most treatment of headaches is empirical rather than directed at "pathology," it follows that a systematic operant conditioning approach should be compatible with such treatment. Certainly for many of the muscle contraction and vascular headaches, the pain *is* the disease, and its elimination constitutes an effective treatment.

Operant Conditioning

If a person has a site of tissue injury or similar source of noxious stimulation, then respondent pain behaviors are quite likely to be elicited. There is adequate stimulation and automatic responses. Respondents are thus controlled by antecedent stimuli. However, if there is little or inadequate noxious stimulation, it is still possible for pain behaviors to be emitted, because they are receiving effective reinforcement. They are now occurring because of the reinforcing conditions which follow them.

Operant pain behaviors such as moaning, limping, and the like occur as a direct and automatic response to noxious stimulation, as with respondents, but in addition the operants come under the control of environmental consequences. Operant pain behaviors are more likely to occur when followed by positive or reinforcing conditions, or when healthy behaviors are punished or not rewarded. Pain behaviors are less likely to occur when they are

not followed by positive reinforcement, or when they are punished, and healthy behaviors are rewarded.

Conditioning of behaviors is temporary, and can be maintained only by periodic reinforcement. However, once a behavior is in a person's repertoire, the reinforcers need not be frequent. In fact, they may be quite intermittent, and some of the behaviors most resistant to change are those which receive relatively infrequent reinforcement, such as gambling behavior and payoffs, or polysurgical addiction and the desired surgery.

Conditioning effects are usually specific to the conditions under which they take place, but then may generalize. Being ill in bed may bring temporary respite from unpleasant drudgery, and thus be reinforced, but the behavior recurs only in the setting of such drudgery. However if other needs are met simultaneously by other effects, such as attention from an otherwise negligent spouse, then the sick behavior may occur again when attention is needed, or when the spouse is present.

There is a variety of operant pain behaviors which are troublesome to the patients, their families, and the health care personnel involved. These include limitations of physical activities, work disability, irritability at home, withdrawal from social interactions, hypochondriacal preoccupations, doctor-shopping, polysurgical addiction, and polypharmacy and drug dependence. Most of these represent operants which are reinforced by the satisfaction of dependency needs, but the drug problem is an especially involved one which requires separate consideration.

ANALGESIC USE AND ABUSE

Experience suggests that analgesic overuse is a problem in at least 50% of chronic pain patients in general, and headache patients in particular. In addition to the well-recognized associated problems of addiction, habituation, and toxicity, there is the central problem that the pain can be drug dependent. Many patients' *constant* and daily muscle contraction or vascular headaches are drug dependent. Andersson (1975) has shown that vascular headaches can become ergotamine dependent.

It is a truism that even non-narcotic analgesics are not entirely benign when used frequently in large amounts: aspirin causes bleeding, phenacetin causes renal damage, acetaminophen liver damage. When these agents are combined with narcotics, as they frequently are, significant physiological as well as behavioral pathology may result.

Fordyce (1976) has shown, by an analysis of the usual medication regimen for pain, how respondent pain can become operant pain. That is, the headache, which may initially occur because of a somatic pain generator, may come under environmental control from the use of medications prescribed for the pain. The result is that the pain is maintained by the analgesic designed to relieve it.

Typically, analgesics are prescribed on an "as needed" (*prn*) basis. This is particularly true for intermittent pain problems, such as recurrent headaches. The intent is to limit the amount of analgesic ingested in order to avoid the problems just noted. The effect,however, can be the opposite, because of the reinforcing properties of the analgesics on the behaviors they follow (pain; associated affect such as anxiety or depression; other pain behaviors).

All that is necessary for any medication to be a powerful positive reinforcer is that it make the patient feel better. One of the most obvious ways it can make him feel better is by reducing his pain. Anything that reduces pain is a positive reinforcer; it increases the likelihood that the immediately preceding behaviors (pain, taking medication) will be repeated. The contingency is established that a feeling of well being can follow the experience of pain and the expression of pain behaviors.

The effect of the analgesic is not limited to pain relief, however; it may relieve anxiety, counter depression, or treat insomnia. This is particularly important when the patient finds it easier to tolerate physical pain than emotional pain. He is likely to interpret or perceive his distressing affect as pain.

In addition to reinforcing (and maintaining) pain, analgesic use also reinforces the physician's prescription writing. The patient in pain is a person who usually demands relief. He can be insistent and even obnoxious, challenging the physician's self-image as a competent healer. Inasmuch as it may be impossible to treat the (assumed) underlying pathology, the physician can prescribe the analgesic the patient demands and thus satisfy part of his self-concept ("to comfort always"). This is a positive reinforcement. At the same time he escapes the unpleasant interaction with the patient, which is another positive reinforcer. Thus the physician is rewarded for writing the script, as the patient has been for requesting it, and the interaction is therefore more likely repeated.

Such doctor-patient transactions are relatively common and subtle; physician and patient frequently manipulate each other in a variety of ways without mutual awareness, playing "pain games" (Sternbach, 1974). These transactions have not been adequately studied, although a beginning has been made. Bond and Pilowsky (1966) found that in patients with advanced cancer, their subjective rating of the severity of their pain did not always generate a proportionate request for analgesics; requests, when made, did not consistently lead to the administration of analgesics; and the strength of the medication was not proportionate to pain levels. In a follow-up study, Pilowsky and Bond (1969) performed a factor analysis on such interactional data. They found that nursing staffs tended to withhold the stronger drugs from patients who had greater self-concepts of invalidism; but when such patients were women, the nurses more frequently took the initiative and medicated them with stronger analgesics. Older patients were likely to be given weaker medications.

From such data as these, it is obvious that requests for pain relief are not determined solely by the severity of the pain, and the administration of analgesics is influenced by a number of perceptions and motivations.

Managing Pain Medications

The patient who overuses medications probably has operant pain, or medication-dependent pain. He probably also is physically dependent upon the drug, would show withdrawal symptoms if the medication were abruptly discontinued, and has habituated to the effects of the drug (initial doses no longer sufficing to reduce pain severity). In addition, there are probably obvious and subtle pain behaviors associated with the ingestion of analgesics. Such a patient needs to be withdrawn from the analgesics and any associated drugs of abuse, such as sedatives, hypnotics, and psychotropics. This process almost invariably requires inpatient status, with good nursing supervision.

THE WITHDRAWAL PROCESS

It is not enough merely to detoxify the patient. That could be done by withholding medications, and monitoring withdrawal symptoms over a week or two, allowing the patient to go "cold turkey." Only part of the problem is solved this way; no lasting behavior change results. The process should be gradual and systematic, not merely for the patient's physical comfort, but to extinguish the pain behaviors which led to analgesic use, and to permit the acquisition and reinforcement of pain-incompatible behaviors.

There are several principles which experience has shown must be followed, without exception, for the withdrawal process to proceed smoothly and to have good long-term effects:

1. *There must be NO injections of ANY distress-relieving medications—analgesics, hypnotics, sedatives, or tranquilizers.* Patients develop a "fix on the needle," or psychological dependence on the injection process, probably because of the very rapid and marked effect of the drug administered this way, which is a potent reinforcer.

A corollary of this principle is that all such medications must be given orally. Rarely, if nausea and vomiting make this impractical, as in some migraine episodes, the drug must be administered *per rectum*. The needle should never be used.

2. *Drugs must be given on a fixed time schedule, and never PRN.* This breaks up the contingent relationship between the pain and the medication. It makes it unnecessary for the patient to have an increase in pain severity to get the reinforcing substance. Furthermore, by following a regular clock schedule strictly, the pain is not permitted to increase to severe levels, nor fluctuate widely in severity, as frequently happen on a *prn* schedule. Consequently, the patient is kept comfortable, while the reinforcement of pain increments by the analgesic is extinguished.

3. *Multiple drug usage should be reduced to the minimum and combined into one "pain cocktail."* Patients frequently have been taking several analgesics, such as codeine, propoxyphene, and occasional meperidine. They often are taking several sedatives as well, such as diazepam and phenobarbital. Such combinations are unnecessary, and may be reduced to a single agent for each class, representing analgesics, sedatives, and hypnotics.

Analgesics can be converted into an equivalent dose of methadone, e.g., 5 mg every 4 hr (not to exceed 40 mg), sedatives represented by a sedating antihistamine such as hydroxyzine, etc. (Halpern, 1974). These agents can be combined into a single mix masked by cherry syrup or orange drink with a total volume of 10 cc, given every 4 hr around the clock. As the amount of the active ingredients is decreased each day, the amount of the masking vehicle is increased proportionately, to keep the volume constant (Fordyce, 1976).

If the patient is depressed, and has a sleep disturbance, an antidepressant with hypnotic qualities can be added to the nighttime mixture. Amitriptyline or dosepin, 75 mg, is an appropriate starting dose. If depression is not a problem, but insomnia is, oxazepam 30 mg can be added to this cocktail.

4. *Starting levels and decrements should be set in a manner which keeps the patient comfortable.* It is unreasonable to expect analgesics to eliminate pain completely, especially with chronic use, but they should "take the edge off," at least. The initial dosage level for 24 hr should be equal to or slightly higher than the amount the patient has actually been taking in a 24 hr period previously, at fixed 3 or 4 hr intervals.

Doses should be reduced daily by a rate of 10% of the initial daily dose. Thus, if methadone is given the first day at an adequate total daily amount of 30 mg in six divided doses, it is reduced each day by 3 mg. This should be done on the second day by reducing every other divided dose by 1 mg, on the third day the remaining doses are reduced to 4 mg, etc.

The purpose of this, in addition to keeping the patient comfortable, is to make the daily reductions in strengths small enough, and yet the interval and amounts reliable enough, that the patient need not be preoccupied with the medication issue, or the withdrawal process, and can turn his attention to more useful matters. Although the patient knows that withdrawal is taking place, the masking vehicle and fixed volume prevent his knowledge of the rate, and the fact that he is not uncomfortable with the withdrawal prevents his being alarmed.

5. *The patient should be kept as busy as is practical, in activities which simulate his usual daily activities as much as possible.* Merely lounging about in bed or in the hospital room is not satisfactory, because it does not give much opportunity for the production of pain-incompatible behaviors which can be reinforced. Physical therapy, occupational therapy, even volunteering a few hours each day at a work station, permit the shaping of healthy behaviors.

If the patient's pain is activity-related, then he must learn how to pace himself to take a rest break before the pain increases. Waiting for an increase in pain severity, then resting, tends to reinforce the pain just as taking analgesics does, because rest is also a positive reinforcer for most persons. Consequently, rest breaks should also be on a fixed time schedule, and the patient can use the time in the hospital to learn an appropriate schedule.

6. *An explicit understanding as to what is being done, and why, is essential to success.* The patient must agree to the goals and methods of the withdrawal process. If this agreement is not absolutely clear and explicitly stated, it is likely to be doomed to failure, as the patient may sabotage the effort. He may do so by not taking his medications when delivered, because of absence of severe pain, then request the next dose early, etc. Or he may simply leave the hospital, remain in bed all the time, etc.

Similar explicit understandings with the nursing staff are essential. Unless they understand the goal and methods of the program, they may sabotage it. They may do so by not delivering the pain cocktail on time, waiting for the patient to ask for it, as they are used to *prn* orders. Or they may not awaken the patient at night. Or they reinforce pain behaviors by acting sympathetic to complaints of pain, instead of praising active healthy behaviors, etc. All this can be prevented by writing clear and specific orders, and also by conferring frequently with the nursing staff on each shift.

BIOFEEDBACK TECHNIQUES

A particular form of operant conditioning is that which uses the methodology of biofeedback. This consists of detecting, transducing, amplifying, and and displaying one of the subject's physiological functions immediately and continuously. This may be his pulse rate, skin temperature, muscle tone, peripheral blood flow, or electro-encephalogram. If the subject is appropriately motivated or rewarded, he can learn to increase or decrease the rate or amplitude of the displayed function "at will."

Miller (1969) summarized many carefully controlled animal studies which demonstrate that laboratory animals can learn visceral and glandular responses for appropriate reinforcements. Normal human subjects are reinforced in the laboratory by monetary rewards for, say, raising skin temperature above a resting baseline. Patients presumably find the procedure intrinsically rewarding when advised that acquiring such "voluntary" control over a function may enable them to avoid a headache or other symptom.

Clinical experience suggests that most headache patients can acquire the desired response relevant to their symptom in a dozen or so laboratory training sessions. Those who then practice the technique regularly have good long-term results, while those who fail to practice do not.

Biofeedback for Muscle Contraction Headaches

Budzynski *et al.* (1973) assigned 18 muscle contraction headache patients to one of three groups: EMG frontalis muscle biofeedback; a similar group which received false feedback; and a control (no training) group. Auditory feedback was used, and there were 16 sessions of training each of 20-min duration. The first group showed a significantly lower EMG tension level after three-month follow-up than the second. Four of six patients in the first group experienced significant improvement in headaches, compared to one in the second group and none in the third. After 18 months, three of four patients contacted from the first group continued improved.

Wickramasekera (1973) gave five patients verbal relaxation training, with a very modest improvement in frontalis muscle EMG activity and headache frequency and intensity. This was followed by EMG biofeedback, which result in dramatic decreases in EMG readings and headache activity, maintained in nine-week follow-up.

McKenzie et al. (1974) reported a clinically significant reduction in headaches in eight patients given ten training sessions in EEG alpha biofeedback. They showed greater improvement than eight patients who only listened to relaxation tapes. Results were sustained two months later. In a larger study with longer follow-up, two of these authors (Montgomery and Ehrisman, 1976) show that 13 of 22 patients who completed alpha training responded to questionnaires six months to three years later. They continued to report a statistically significant reduction in frequency and severity of headache.

Warner and Lance (1975) used only relaxation training, one 20-min training session per week for four weeks, and instructed patients to practice daily. Of 17 patients, 13 had daily headaches, and four had headaches almost every other day. At six-month follow-up, four were free of headache, four had one headache per month, three had less than one headache per week, and three had headaches as frequently as before, but much less severe. There were similar significant reductions in medication usage.

Bakal (1975) has pointed out that although such empirical studies may be promising, in fact there is little evidence to relate psychological tension and muscle contraction headaches. He notes that most of these studies have not specified the critical psychological and physiological changes underlying the reduction of the headaches.

Biofeedback for Vascular Headaches

Learned relaxation techniques have been applied to vascular headaches as well as muscle contraction headaches. The rationale, aside from purely empirical results, has been that pain responses and relaxation responses are incompatible, and that the latter could prevent the former. Gannon and Sternbach (1971) showed that a patient with post-traumatic vascular headaches could prevent these by entering a learned high-alpha state, although he could not stop a headache already present by this method.

Strictly behavioral nethods, without biofeedback methodology but similar effects, have been reported by Mitchell and Mitchell (1971). Seventeen migraineurs were assigned to either a relaxation training group, a combined desensitization-relaxation-assertiveness group, or a no-treatment control group. The combined treatment group showed a significant reduction in frequency and duration of migraine episodes, whereas the other two groups did not. In a second study, 20 migraineurs were assigned to either a desensitization-relaxation group, a combined desensitization-relaxation-assertiveness group, or a no-treatment control group. The combined desensitization group showed a significant reduction in frequency and duration of attacks, whereas the desensitization group alone was not different from the control group. However, Warner and Lance (1975) reported that simple training in relaxation techniques enabled 8 to 12 patients to reduce migraine episodes more than 50% and nine of the patients were able to reduce their medication by over 30%.

Sargent et al. (1972, 1973) have shown that using autogenic training combined with biofeedback for learning hand warming has resulted in improvement in approximately 75% of 62 migraineurs. Solbach and Sargent

(1977) reported on a follow-up survey of 110 patients more than three years after treatment. Seventy-four patients completed 270 days of training and follow-up; 76% of this group could be contacted. Thirty-six patients failed to complete the program, and only 33% of this group could be contacted. Those who completed training showed a greater decrease in headache intensity and duration and use of medications.

The concept of using hand-warming techniques rests on the assumption that migraineurs have a vasomotor instability, such that the headache episode is associated with peripheral vasoconstriction and cephalic vasodilatation; by increasing the blood volume in the extremities, there should be a reduced flow and dilatation in the cephalic vasculature, and thus less or no headache.

Elliott et al (1974) have shown that in fact there is impaired reflex vasodilatation in the extremities of migraineurs as compared with controls, confirming an earlier report of Appenzeller et al. (1963). In addition, Rickles et al. (1977) used psychophysiological techniques and multivariate statistical analysis on 13 migraine patients compared with matched controls, and demonstrated individual response stereotypy in the patients. This consisted of cardiovascular variables showing the greatest responses to stimuli, even during headache-free periods, which was different from the response of headache-free controls.

However, although patients may learn to acquire voluntary control of blood flow, it would appear that temperature biofeedback would not be an efficient technique, since surface temperature is a sluggish response to vasomotor activity, and other variables such as pulse volume would permit faster learning. Actually Koppman et al. (1974) have shown that seven of nine patients rapidly learned to constrict or dilate the superficial temporal artery, using feedback of the pulse volume.

Another problem complicating the whole application of such treatment methods to those with vascular headaches, is the assumption of a uniform pathophysiology. Not all with such headaches are true migraineurs, and certainly not all have peripheral vasomotor changes be-fore or during their attacks. Mixed patient groups may give mixed results to such biofeedback training. Mitch et al. (1976) used autogenic instructions and hand-warming biofeedback on 20 patients, and found that 65% improved on 2 or more of 4 measures, and 35% improved on one or none. Ten of the patients were contacted at six-month follow-up and in general maintained their improvement; however, the authors observed that those with mixed vascular and muscle contraction headaches were not helped.

Similarly, Medina et al. did a one-year follow-up study of 27 patients with migraine or mixed migraine and muscle contraction headache. Patients were trained in both EMG and skin temperature methods, and assessment was made of severity and frequency of headaches and medication usage. Thirteen patients (50%) showed a significant improvement.

What precisely occurs with successful biofeedback treatment? Kentsmith et al. (1976) found a decrease in plasma levels of dopamine-B-hydroxylase activity. Sovak et al. (1976) found that with the application of heat to the hands, vasodilatation occurred in the superficial cephalic arteries as well as in the extremities. However with voluntary (biofeedback-learned) dilatation of the hands, there was a constriction of the superficial arteries of the head. This may serve to correct the response stereotypy noted by Rickles et al. (1977).

It thus appears that biofeedback may be helpful in some vascular headache therapies, particularly those associated with peripheral vasomotor changes. When biofeedback is combined with other behavioral treatments, success rates go up: Adler and Adler (1976) note that they combined biofeedback and psychotherapy in three-quarters of the 58 patients they followed-up five years after treatment. They found a persistent reduction of headache frequency of 70—100% in 86% of the patients followed. However, as Bakal (1975) as noted, when several treatment modalities are combined in this fashion, it is not possible to specify which of them is responsible for observed improvement, nor the relative weight to assign to the several simultaneous treatments.

HYPNOSIS

We have already described hypnotic-like training procedures associated with biofeedback: relaxation training, desensitization, autogenic suggestions, and assertiveness training all involve the giving of instructions or suggestions to patients in order to produce responses incompatible with pain responses. The same can also be said of hypnosis, which has a longer history.

Unfortunately, the clinical research literature in hypnosis is quite sparse, particularly with respect to headaches. This is surprising, considering the number of years hypnosis has been used, and the large number of quite good experimental studies with normal subjects. For some reason, most of the clinical papers on this subject fail to use controls, or objective data, and usually consist of general statements and anecdotal case examples (Blumenthal, 1963; Kroger, 1963). However, Hilgard and Hilgard (1975) have written an excellent review of both the clinical and experimental literature on hypnotic relief of pain. Their review shows that hypnosis may indeed be an effective treatment for headache.

Harding (1961, 1967) reported first on a group of 25 chemotherapy-resistant migraineurs treated by hypnosis. Five had complete relief on follow-up ½ to 2-½ years later, and six had 25 to 75% reduction in severity or frequency. He described his method in detail (Harding, 1961). Later, he reported on 90 such patients, with ½ to 8 year follow-up. Thirty-four reported complete relief, and 29 reported 25–75% reduction in the frequency, duration, or intensity (Harding, 1967). Later, he reported the same 70% success rate for 200 patients (Hilgard and Hilgard, 1975).

Anderson et al. (1975) reported on 47 patients, randomly assigned to hypnotherapy (N =23) or to chemotherapy with prophylactic prochlorperazine (N=24). Monthly evaluations were made for one year, using as measures the number of attacks per month, the number who had grade-4 attacks, and the number

experiencing complete remission. For those receiving hypnotherapy, the number of attacks and the number of blinding attacks were significantly lower than those of the prochlorperazine group, which did not improve on these two measures. Ten of 23 patients on hypnotherapy obtained complete remission during the last three months of the trial, as compared with only 3 of 24 on the drug.

Thus a clinical series, and a controlled clinical study, show hypnosis to be effective in migraine. Is it merely suggestion that is effective, or relaxation? Stacher et al. (1975) used four subjects and four experimental conditions: (1) waking and hypnotic relaxation suggestions, (2) waking and hypnotic analgesic suggestions, (3) measuring pain threshold, (4) and measuring pain tolerance to electric shock. They found suggestion of analgesia more effective in raising threshold and tolerance than suggestion of relaxation, in both waking and hypnotic states; and suggestions of both relaxation and analgesia were more effective in raising threshold and tolerance in the hypnotic than in waking state. Thus hypnotic analgesia can most effectively raise pain threshold and pain tolerance.

An interesting comparison was made in a study of the mechanisms of acupuncture analgesia (Mayer et al., 1976). Acupuncture raised pain thresholds to electric shock by 27%, on the average, and its analgesic effects were reversed by the narcotic antagonist naloxone; hypnotic analgesia raised pain thresholds an average of 85%, and its effects were not reversible by this means.

Although the effectiveness of hypnotic analgesia seems fairly certain, its mechanism of action is not clear, and is still the subject of much debate. The technique of such hypnosis for migraine, however, is well described by a number of authors. Harding (1961) and Anderson et al. (1975) both suggest control over vasomotor activity. Barber (1977) uses an indirect suggestion of comfort for all pain problems, and Maher-Loughnan (1975) uses intensive, prolonged, and indirect hypnotherapy on resistant cases. It appears that, over the years, there has been a tendency for clinical hypnosis techniques to be less authoritarian and more permissive, and less magical and more rational in explanations to the patients. This seems to lower patient resistance and increase the rate of success.

Although the number of good clinical studies of hypnosis for headaches is small, the results to date suggest that it may be a useful treatment. Like biofeedback, it should certainly be tried on those resistant to chemotherapy. And considering their benign nature, both hypnosis and biofeedback may well be thought of as the first line of treatment, rather than the last (Finer, 1974).

Summary

1. Patients with chronic pain usually show a mixture of respondent and operant behaviors. Usually they exhibit reflexive behavior to antecedent pathogenic stimulation, and operant behavior maintained by contingent environmental consequences.

2. Operant pain behaviors are more likely to occur when followed by positive or reinforcing conditions, or when healthy behaviors are punished or not rewarded.

3. Experience suggests that analgesic overuse is a problem in at least 50% of chronic pain patients in general, and headache patients in particular.

4. Managing pain medications should include withdrawal, avoidance of injections, provision of drugs on a fixed time schedule, when possible, reduction of multiple drug usage, and attempts to increase the patient's activity. The patient must agree to the goals and methods of the withdrawal process.

5. A particular form of operant conditioning is that which uses the methodology of biofeedback. Electromyographic feedback may be useful for muscle contraction headaches. Autogenic training with associated hand warming has been shown to improve patients with migraine.

6. Hypnosis may also be an effective treatment for headache, but control studies have not been done.

References

Adler, C. S., and S. M. Adler (1976). Biofeedback psychotherapy for the treatment of headaches: a 5-year follow-up. *Headache 16*, 189-191.

Anderson, J. A. D., M. A. Basker, and R. Dalton (1975). Migraine and hypnotherapy. *Intern. J. Clin. Exp. Hypn. 23*, 48-58.

Andersson, P. G. (1975). Ergotamine headache. *Headache 15*, 118-121.

Appenzeller, O., K. Davison, and J. Marshall (1963). Reflex vasomotor abnormalities in the hands of migrainous subjects. *J. Neurol. Neurosurg. Psychiat. 26*, 447-450.

Bakal, D. A. (1975). Headache: a biopsychological perspective. *Psych. Bull. 82*, 369-382.

Barber, J. (1977). Rapid induction analgesia: a clinical report. *Am. J. Clin. Hyp. 19*, 138-147.

Blumenthal, L. S. (1963). Hypnotherapy of headache. *Headache 2*, 197-22.

Bond, M. R., and L. Pilowsky (1966). Subjective assessment of pain and its relationship to the administration of analgesics in patients with advanced cancer. *J. Psychosom. Res. 10*, 203-208.

Budzynski, T. H., J. M. Stoyva, C. S. Adler, and D. J. Mullaney (1973). EMP biofeedback and tension headache: a controlled outcome study. *Psychosom. Med. 35*, 484-496.

Elliott, K., D. B. Frewin, and J. A. Downey (1974). Reflex vasomotor responses in the hands of patients suffering from migraine. *Headache 13*, 188-196.

Finer, B. (1974). Clinical use of hypnosis in pain management. In *Advances in Neurology*, Vol. 4 (J. Bonica, ed.), pp. 573-579. Raven Press, New York.

Fordyce, W. E. (1976). *Behavioral Methods for Chronic Pain and Illness*. C. V. Mosby, St. Louis.

Fordyce, W. E., R. S. Fowler, Jr., J. F. Lehmann, and B. J. DeLateur (1968). Some implications of learning in problems of chronic pain. *J. Chronic Dis. 21*, 179-190.

Fordyce, W. E., R. S. Fowler, Jr., J. F. Lehmann, B. J. DeLateur, P. L. Sand, and R. B. Trieschmann (1973). Operant conditioning in the treatment of chronic pain. *Arch. Phys. Med. Rehab. 54*, 3998.

Gannon, L., and R. A. Sternbach (1971). Alpha enhancement as a treatment for pain: a case study. *J. Behav. Therapy Exp. Psychiat. 2*, 209-213.

Halpern, L. M. (1974). Psychotropic drugs and the management of chronic pain. In *Advances in Neurology*, Vol. 4 (J. Bonica, ed.), pp. 539-546. Raven press, New York.

Harding, H. C. (1961). Hypnosis and migraine or vice versa. *Northwest Med. 6n*, 168-172.

Harding, C. H. (1967). Hypnosis in the treatment of migraine. In *Hypnosis and Psychosomatic Medicine* (J. Lassner, ed.), pp. 131-134. Springer-Verlag, New York.

Hilgard, E. R., and J. R. Hilgard (1975). *Hypnosis in the Relief of Pain*. Kaufmann, Los Altos, Calif.

Ignelzi, R. J., R. A. Sternbach, and G. Timmermans (1977). The pain ward follow-up analyses. *Pain 3*, 277-280.

Kentsmith, D., F. Strider, J. Copenhaver, and D. Jacques (1976). Effects of biofeedback upon suppression of migraine symptoms and plasma dopamine-B-hydroxylase activity. *Headache 16*, 173-177.

Koppman, J. W., R. D. McDonald, and M. G. Kunzel (1974). Voluntary regulation of temporal artery diameter by migraine patients. *Headache 14*, 133-138.

Kroger, W. S. (1963). Hypnotherapeutic management of headache. *Headache 3*, 50-62.

Lang, P. J., D. G. Rice, and R. A. Sternbach (1972). The psychophysiology of emotion. In *Handbook of Psychophysiology*, (N. S. Greenfield and R. A. Sternbach, eds.), pp. 623-643. Holt, Rinehart and Winston, New York.

Maher-Loughnan, G. P. (1975). Intensive hypno-autohypnosis in resistant psychosomatic disorders. *J. Psychosom. Res. 19*, 361-365.

Mayer, D. J., D. D. Price, J. Barber, and A. Rafii (1976). Acupuncture analgesia: evidence for activation of pain inhibitory system as a mechanism of action. In *Advances in Pain Research and Therapy*, Vol. I. (J. Bonica and D. Albe-Fessard, eds.), pp. 751-754. Raven Press, New York.

McKenzie, R. E., W. J. Ehrisman, P. S. Montgomery, and R. H. Barnes (1974). The treatment of headache by means of electroencephalographic biofeedback. *Headache 13*, 164-172.

Medina, J. L., S. Diamond, and M. A. Franklin (1976). Biofeedback therapy for migraine. *Headache 16*, 115-118.

Miller, N. E. (1969). Learning of visceral and glandular responses. *Science 163*, 434-445.

Mitch, P. S., A. McGrady, and A. Iannone (1976). Autogenic feedback training in migraine: a treatment report. *Headache 15*, 267-270.

Mitchell, K. R., and D. M. Mitchell (1971). Migraine: an exploratory treatment application of programmed behaviour therapy techniques. *J. Psychosom. Res. 15*, 137-157.

Montgomery, P. S., and W. J. Ehrisman (1976). Biofeedback alleviated headaches: a follow-up. *Headache 16*, 64-65.

Pilowsky, I., and M. R. Bond (1969). Pain and its management in malignant disease: elucidation of staff-patient transactions. *Psychosom. Med. 31*, 400-404.

Rickles, W. H., M. J. Cohen, and D. L. McArthur (1977). A psychophysiology study of ANS response patterns in migraine headache patients and their headache free friends. Paper presented at 19th annual meeting of the American Association for the Study of Headache, San Francisco.

Sargent, J. D., E. E. Green, and E. D. Walters (1972). The use of autogenic feedback training in a pilot study of migraine and tension headaches. *Headache 12*, 120-124.

Sargent, J. D., E. D. Walters, and E. E. Green (1973). Psychosomatic self-regulation of migraine headaches. *Seminars in Psychiatry 5*, 415-428.

Solbach, P., and J. D. Sargent (1977). A follow-up evaluation of the Menninger pilot migraine study using thermal training. Paper presented at 19th annual meeting of the American Association for the Study of Headache, San Francisco.

Sovak, M., A. Fronek, R. Doyle, and D. R. Helland (1976). Some hemodynamic observations during biofeedback vasomotor training. *Proceedings, San Diego Biomedical Symposium, 15*, pp. 363-367. Academic Press, New York.

Stacher, G., P. Schuster, P. Bauer, R. Lahoda, and D. Schulze (1975). Effects of suggestion of relaxation or analgesia on pain threshold and pain tolerance in the waking and in the hypnotic state. *J. Psychosom. Res. 19*, 25-265.

Sternbach, R. A. (1974). *Pain Patients: Traits and Treatment*. Academic Press, New York.

Warner, G., and J. W. Lance (1975). Relaxation therapy in migraine and chronic tension headache. *Med. J. Aust. 1*, 298-301.

Wickramasekera, I. (1973). The application of verbal instructions and EMG feedback training to the management of tension headache—preliminary observations. *Headache 13*, 74-76.

25

CLINICAL OBSERVATIONS ON HEADACHE

REVISED BY DONALD J. DALESSIO

Incidence

The most common headaches are those associated with mood disorders, particularly depression, anxiety, and emotional tension. Next most commonly encountered are vascular headaches of the migraine type and associated variants including cluster headache. The headaches provoked by fever and septicemia probably rank next in frequency, and then come those due to nasal and paranasal, ear, tooth, and eye disease. The headaches of meningitis, intracranial aneurysm, brain tumor, and brain abscess, though most important and singularly dramatic, are less common.

Intensity

The most intense headaches are those due to ruptured intracranial aneurysm, meningitis, fever, migraine, and those associated with arterial hypertension. The subarachnoid hemorrhage resulting usually from ruptured intracranial aneurysm produces a headache that is sudden in onset, reaches great intensity in a very short time, and may be associated with feelings of faintness or with unconsciousness. The onset of pain is soon followed by the development of a stiff neck and the presence of blood in the lumbar spinal fluid. The very intense headache of meningitis is accompanied by a very stiff neck which prevents passive flexion of the head on the chest. The spasm of the muscles of the neck associated with the intense headaches of migraine inhibits flexion of the neck.

The intensity of the headaches associated with brain tumors, brain abscesses, 'sinus-disease, and tooth and eye disease is usually only moderately severe. Hemorrhage into the parenchyma of the brain may not cause headaches unless the hemorrhage breaks through into the ventricular or subarachnoid spaces; then intense headache may result. Also, hemorrhage into a brain tumor causing additional and serious displacement of the brain may result in moderately severe headache.

Brain abscess may be a painless disorder unless associated with circumscribed meningitis or periostitis. However, when of long standing, brain abscess may produce headache because of generalized brain displacement and traction on pain-sensitive structures.

One rare form of very intense headache is encountered in patients in the terminal phase of brain tumor. This headache is generalized, paroxysmal, and agonizing, and often ends in stupor. The pain may last for 3 sec to a half hour and then disappear as quickly as it came, leaving the patient exhausted. With such headache the patient may pass into coma and die.

Quality of Headache

The headaches of fever, migraine, hemangiomatous tumors, and those associated with arterial hypertension are characteristically throbbing or pulsating in quality. Headache associated with emotional tension or resulting from secondary muscle contraction from eye or sinus disease has the quality of tightness or external pressure or may be band-like, cap-like, or vise-like. The headache of brain tumor and of meningitis, though occasionally pulsating, is usually of a steady aching quality.

Site

Vascular headaches of the migraine type may occur anywhere in the head and face. Most common site of migraine headache is the temple. Migraine headache at some time involves both right and left sides, although any one attack may be strictly unilateral. The headache of tooth, sinus, or eye disease, shortly after its onset, is usually in the front of the head, roughly in the region near the site of stimulation; subsequently, the pain may be predominantly in the back of the head and neck due to secondary muscle contraction. Headaches associated with pituitary adenomas and parasellar tumors are often bitemporal.

The headaches of posterior fossa tumors, early in the development of the tumor and before the beginning of general brain displacement, are usually over the occiput or behind the ear. Headaches from supratentorial tumors, before serious brain displacement occurs, are usually in the front or on the top of the head. Occasionally, if the tumor involves the dura and the bone, the headache may be near or over the site of the leasion. Early in the course of the tumor or before general displacement of the brain has occurred, the headache is usually on the side of the tumor.

Subdural hematoma produces a headache of considerable intensity, usually localized over or near the site of the lesion, most commonly over the frontoparietal areas. The headache may be intermittent but is present, usually, some time each day, for weeks, months, or longer. A history of almost continuous headache from the date of injury is characteristic; there is no long 'silent period" immediately after the injury.

The headaches associated with tumors of the cerebellopontine angle and acoustic neurinoma are often localized in the postauricular region. Like other brain tumor headaches, they are intermittent and of moderate intensity. They are associated with hyperalgesia of the postauricular region on the same side as the tumor. Headache is one of the earliest manifestations of acoustic neurinoma. Headache is a later manifestation of cerebellopontine angle tumors.

The headache or pressure sensations associated with emotional tension are usually first evident and most intense in the neck, shoulders, and occiput, but later spread to include the frontal region. They may be unilateral or bilateral.

Disease involving the dome of the diaphragm or the phrenic nerve causes pain high in the shoulder and neck. Similarly, in rare instances coronary occlusion and myocardial insufficiency cause pain in the lower jaw, high in the neck, and in the occiput. Disease and dysfunction of structures below the diaphragm do not induce headache except indirectly through fever, sepsis, or bacteremia.

Tenderness

Tenderness in the region of the dilated cranial arteries on the outside of the head and sometimes diffusely over the slightly edematous and aching side of the head may be conspicuous during vascular headache of the migraine type and for some hours thereafter. Also, there may be tenderness of the skin of the face as a result of inflammation of the nasal and paranasal spaces, of the teeth, and of the ear. Muscle in a state of sustained contraction, secondary to pain anywhere in the head, may become tender on palpation. Thus, brushing and combing the hair may be a painful experience during or after migraine headache. With myositis and myalgia there may be tender areas in the muscles of the head and neck. Because of the hyperalgesia, percussion of the head may cause pain over or near an underlying brain tumor.

Periostitis secondary to frontal, ethmoid, or sphenoid sinus disease or mastoiditis produces a pain of moderate to severe intensity associated with local tenderness at the site of disease. If the pain is sufficiently severe and continuous it may become generalized. If the mastoid or sinus disease is limited to the bone (osteomyelitis) it is painless. The tenderness or hyperalgesia associated with mastoid disease with periostitis is far greater than the hyperalgesia associated with posterior fossa brain tumor.

Tenderness at a site of head injury, and often associated with a scar, may persist for many years. Also, in post-traumatic headache there often occur tender muscles or nodules in parts of the head remote from the site of injury. Headache of the vascular type akin to migraine with tenderness over the arteries may be initiated by head injury.

Effects of Manual Pressure

Pressure upon the temporal, frontal, supraorbital, postauricular, occipital, and common carotid arteries often reduces the intensity of migraine headache and that associated with arterial hypertension. Support of the head makes any patient with headache feel more comfortable. The pain of chronic muscle contraction headache may be intensified by firm manipulation of tender muscles or regions of tenderness. Conversely, gentle massage and simple measures of physical therapy including heat and hot packs not infrequently will produce muscular relaxation and relieve this form of headache.

Effect of Position of the Head

In many instances vascular headache of the migraine type is made worse by assuming a horizontal position and is relieved by an erect position. It is often made worse by ascending stairs, by moving about rapidly, or by lifting objects. Sitting quietly in an upright position often proves to be most comfortable. The lying-down position may at first make the headache associated with nasal and paranasal disease more intense, but subsequently the headache subsides. A sudden change in position, usually from the lying down to the sitting up, and less frequently from the sitting up to the lying down, may make the headache of brain tumor more intense. Unlike the migraine

headache, the headache of brain tumor is often worse when the patient is in the upright position. The head-down position aggravates most headaches, except those due to spinal drainage and occasionally those associated with brain tumor. Muscle tension headache is usually reduced in intensity by movements of the head and neck which extend the contracted muscles.

Straining at stool and coughing increase all but muscle contraction headaches and those due to spinal drainage. Sharp flexion or extension of the head often reduces the intensity of post puncture headache, whereas jugular compression increases the headache.

The Effect of Head Jolt

Headaches known to arise primarily from dilatation of pain-sensitive intracranial vessels, particularly arteries (i.e., the headache that follows the intravenous administration of histamine, that induced by hypoglycemia and the headaches of fever, systemic infection, 'hangover," postpuncture reaction and the early postconcussion state) are easily aggravated by even mild head jolting. Patients having headaches known to arise primarily from inflammation of pain-sensitive intracranial arteries and veins and their adjacent structures (i.e., the headaches accompanying meningitis and those following ventriculography or pneumoencephalography) are particularly sensitive to head jolting. The threshold of jolt headache during these states may be depressed 2.0 to 3.0 g or more. In patients with intracranial masses (i.e., subdural hematoma or brain tumor) the threshold of jolt headache is usually depressed and the location of the headache induced by jolting may indicate the side of the lesion. The threshold of jolt headache may be lowered in relatively infrequent instances of vascular headache of the migraine type that have a portion of their orgin within the cranial cavity.

On the other hand, headaches arising from structures on the outside of the head (i.e., muscle tension headache, most migraine headaches, and the headache induced by the injection of hypertonic saline into the temporal muscle) are not significantly intensified by head jolting, and the threshold to jolt headache is not lowered.

Chronological Features

Vascular headaches may be as brief as 20 or 30 min, or it may last for days, or, rarely, for weeks. The usual headache is terminated within 24 hours. A striking feature of migraine is the freedom from headache between prostrating attacks. The headaches of brain tumor are intermittent but usually occur during part of every day and vary in intensity from time to time. Headache associated with chronic sinus disease is intermittent-but quite predictable; it may occur during the working hours of each day for weeks or even months. Muscle contraction headache or pressure sensations associated with sustained tension and anxiety may persist for days, weeks, or even years.

Headaches associated with hypertension and migraine most commonly have their onset in the early hours of the morning so that the patient awakens with the pain. Such migraine headaches characteristically diminish in intensity in the evening. Headaches of the cluster type very commonly occur during the sleeping hours from midnight to two o'clock in the morning. The headache of brain tumor, if it be connected in any way with the time of day, is more severe in the early part of the day, though not in the early hours of the morning. The headache associated with nasal and paranasal disease usually begins and is worst in the morning and improves toward the late afternoon or when the patient retires. Headache associated with eye disease usually begins in the latter part of the day or evening. Muscle contraction headache or pressure sensations are usually worse at the end of the working day.

Vascular headaches of the migraine type are common during week ends, during the first period of vacation holidays, and immediately after vacation. They are very common just before the onset of menstruation. Patients with migraine-type headache often have fixed days of the week when their headaches occur.

Headache associated with nasal and para-nasal disease is usually more common during periods when the upper respiratory infections prevail, namely, the darker months of the year. Migraine headache occurs during periods of increased conflict, tension, or stress for the individual; for example, during early fall for the schoolteacher, during rush or holiday seasons for the merchant, during very hot or humid weather for those who feel ineffective and prostrated during such climatic states. Exacerbations of tic douloureux are common in the spring and fall, notably March and October.

Headaches that begin in childhood or at puberty and recur especially with menstruation and at certain fixed intervals during many years, are in all likelihood of the migraine variety. The migraine variety of headache often stops at menopause. On the other hand, they may occasionally begin at this time.

Sustained Contraction of Muscle

Contractions of the muscles of the head and neck occur with all headaches. If the contractions are of sufficient duration, they themselves become a cause of headache. Headache and a very stiff neck accompanied by Kernig's sign are associated with widespread meningitis. The Kernig sign may be absent even late in the course of a carcinomatous invasion of the meninges at the base of the brain. Headache and stiff neck are common with tumors of the posterior fossa, but the stiff neck may be overcome by persuasion and the passive movements of the head by the examining physician.

Contraction of the muscles of the neck, head, and back may become so great with meningitis that it cannot be relaxed and the patient assumes the position of opisthotonus. With posterior fossa tumors muscle spasm may cause tilting of the head or lifting of the shoulder. The muscle contraction headache associated with prolonged anxiety and tension may cause backward tilting of the head and half closing of the eyes. Muscle contraction is always an accompaniment of migraine headache and is one explanation of the slow relief afforded by ergotamine tartrate to some patients in whom this component is major.

Mucous Membrane Injection

Redness and swelling of the mucous membrane of the nose with or without nosebleeds may occur with migraine. Also injection of the conjunctiva may be seen. The mucous membrane injection and engorgement may be conspicuous and give rise to headache in those with allergic sensitivities to inhaled dusts and pollens and in those in whom the nasal mucous membranes are involved during periods of major adaptive difficulties. With the rare exception of headache due to neoplastic invasion of paranasal structures and antral infection via the dental route, no headache associated with disease of the nasal and paranasal sinuses occurs without obvious congestion of the turbinates and nasal mucous membranes.

Gastrointestinal Disturbances

Anorexia, nausea, and vomiting, though most commonly associated with vascular headache of the migraine type, may be associated with any headache, and the more intense the headache the more likely they are to occur. Vomiting without nausea may occur with brain tumors, especially those of the posterior fossa. Nausea and vomiting with little or no headache may occur in persons with migraine. The headache associated with sinus or eye disease is seldom associated with vomiting. Constipation is commonly associated with migraine, although diarrhea also occurs. Distention and flatulence are common in migraine and tension headaches but are seldom associated with other headaches.

Polyuria

Polyuria is commonly associated with migraine headache attacks and, with the exception of the headache associated with third ventricle tumors, seldom occurs with other headaches. Tension states with headaches may be linked with frequency of urination.

Visual Disturbances

Both scintillating scotomata and visual field defects, such as unilateral or homonymous hemianopia, may occur with migraine headaches. Such defects in vision may occur with brain tumor headaches when the tumor is due to a lesion of the of occipital lobes or is adjacent to the visual pathways. The visual disturbances of migraine, with the exception of blurred vision and diplopia, seldom occur with the headache but usually precede it. They are usually short-lived, i.e., under one hour. Enlarged pupils and lacrimation may cause faulty vision during a migraine headache, but when defects in visual acuity or in the fields of vision outlast the headache attack, it is likely that a cerebral vascular accident or brain tumor is the cause. Defects in color vision and colored rings about lights may occur with headache associated with glaucoma. Ptosis of the eyelid may be an accompaniment of the headache of brain tumor or of a berry aneurysm of the circle of Willis, especially in the latter case when linked with a fixed and dilated pupil. Ptosis also occurs with ophthalmoplegic migraine, a symptom complex involving paresis of the muscles supplied by the third cranial nerve, and occasionally also of those supplied by the fourth and sixth cranial nerves. It usually has its onset late in the headache attack, persists for days or weeks, and is due to edema of tissue near or about the affected cranial nerves. Partial closure of the eyes due to edematous lids or to muscle contraction may lead to the complaint of faulty vision.

Horner's syndrome may appear as a manifestation of cluster headache. Photophobia is associated with any headache experienced chiefly in the front or top of the head. It is commonly noted in patients with meningitis, migraine, nasal and paranasal disease, eye disease, brain tumor, and muscle contraction headache. Injection of the sclera and conjunctiva may accompany such photophobia. If the intensity of the pain is very great, photophobia, lacrimation, and sweating of the homolateral forehead and side of the face also occur.

When headache is linked with papilledema, it is in most instances due to an expanding intracranial mass. However, in patients with brain tumor, headache often occurs without papilledema, and papilledema without headache. In the advanced phase of hypertensive encephalopathy, headache and papilledema are usual. Ruptured aneurysm and subdural hematoma may cause intense headache without papilledema. Ruptured intracranial aneurysms are sometimes accompanied by retinal hemorrhages, which when unilateral are usually on the side of the rupture. Meningitis does not affect the eye grounds except possibly to induce slight suffusion. During migraine headache unilateral arterial and venous dilation in eye grounds may occur.

Vertigo and Other Sensory Disturbances

Vertigo may be a forerunner of a migraine headache attack. Vertigo is sometimes associated with the headaches of brain tumors, although feelings of unsteadiness are more common. Fleeting vertigo with sudden movement or rotation of the head often accompanies the post-traumatic headache and muscle-tension headache.

Ménière's or the labyrinthine syndrome is occasionally associated with headache. Other sensory disturbances such as paresthesias of the hands and face may occur as a forerunner of the migraine headache. However, paresthesias that persist during or outlast the headache attack are more common in patients with brain tumors and in those with epilepsy.

Mood

The wish to retire from people and responsibilities, a dejected, depressed, irritable, or negativistic mental state bordering on prostration or stupor is a dominant aspect of the migraine attack and may in some instances be more disturbing than the pain in the head. Apathy, listlessness, or even euphoria may be associated with brain tumor headache.

The headache associated with muscle tension may occur in a tense, irritable person, but the patient is usually more willing to accept attention, massage, or medication in contrast to the patient with a migraine headache attack who commonly expresses the wish to be left alone. Exaltation or feelings of especial well-being are common sequels to the migraine headache attack. The suffering experienced with the headache of fever, meningitis, or ruptured aneurysm may be very great, but the mental state is that of reaction to severe pain. Headache and other head pain of a delusional nature may occur in depressed, hypochondriacal, or hysterical patients.

Sleep

Vascular headaches of the migraine type, even of the most severe type, do not disrupt sleep entirely, except for short periods. Those of brain tumor, sinus disease, and muscle contraction permit sleep. Therefore, when an individual complains of long periods of sleep loss because of headache, it is well to consider anxiety or depression as the dominant aspect of the illness. The headache of meningitis usually interrupts sleep. Migraine headaches of the vascular type may also occur after periods of excessively prolonged, or very deep sleep.

Cluster headache often occurs during REM sleep.

Family History

The headache of migraine and that associated with arterial hypertension are the only familial headaches.

The Effect on Headache of Local Analgesic Action

The local infiltration of procaine hydrochloride into the source of noxious stimuli about the head, which are responsible for headache at a near or remote site, promptly terminates the headache, usually for a period of 1–2 hr. Thus the application of procaine to the inflamed nasal mucous membranes, the turbinates, or about the ostium of the frontal nasal duct promptly eliminates headache that stems from the nose and 'sinus disease.' The infiltration of procaine into the tissues around an inflamed tooth speedily terminates headache arising from such a source. The injection of procaine into a tender nodule or primary site of muscle pain eliminates headache due to myalgia or sustained muscle contraction. The application of cocaine to the cornea terminates headache arising from this source. The infiltration of procaine about a tender pulsating artery during a migraine or vascular headache obliterates that portion of the headache which has its source in that artery: for example, the temporal, postauricular, frontal, occipital, supraorbital, or sphenopalatine artery, etc.

On the other hand, infiltration of procaine into areas of referred headache, i.e., skin and muscle, causes appreciable reduction but seldom complete elimination of headache. The infiltration of procaine about a major nerve eliminates the headache if this nerve be the specific pathway for afferent impulses giving rise to pain in the periphery: for example, the inferior and superior maxillary nerves from inflamed teeth, the occipital nerve in occipital myalgia and occipital migraine, and the first division of the fifth cranial nerve for frontal or temporal migraine, etc. Procaine infiltration of the 'trigger zone' or area of pain, i.e., the skin, subcutaneous tissue, and muscle, or procaine infiltration about the specific afferent nerve temporarily obliterates pain of major trigeminal neuralgia. Methysergide (Sansert) may be effective in preventing headaches of the migraine type.

Other Chemical Agents That Modify Headaches

The effectiveness of analgesics with central action is dependent entirely upon the intensity of pain and not at all on the site of origin or the particular mechanism inducing the pain. Thus, 60 mg codeine sulfate or 15 mg morphine sulfate may be necessary for the high-intensity headaches of meningitis, ruptured aneurysm, and of certain fevers such as typhus and typhoid fever; whereas agents such as acetylsalicylic acid in 0.3—to 0.6-gm amounts are effective against other types of

headache. Fortunately the headache of brain tumor is seldom so intense as to require the opiates. Ergotamine tartrate if given parenterally and in sufficient amounts will usually modify or abolish the headache of migraine.

Other Factors that Modify Headache

Decompression of skull and removal of brain tumors very commonly afford relief of headache due to such tumors. This is not universally true, since headaches caused by pituitary adenomas often persist after the tumor has been removed.

The evacuation of pus from beneath the periosteum and from the adjacent paranasal sinuses and mastoid cells often affords prompt elimination of the headache associated with empyema of these regions. However, the persistence or development of frontal headache after simple sinusotomy is evidence of the presence of extradural infection, and possibly of subdural infection. Similarly, the persistence or development of post-or preauricular headache after simple mastoidectomy is good evidence for the existence of adjacent extra— and possibly subdural infection.

CLINICAL PATHOLOGICAL ABNORMALITIES AND HEADACHE

Slight elevations in body temperature are common during migraine headache attacks. Fever may be associated with the headache of carcinomatous meningitis and brain tumor. It occasionally occurs with the headache of carcinomatous meningitis and brain tumor. It occasionally occurs with the headache linked with nasal and paranasal infection.

Any fever, especially that during the onset of an infection, may be associated with headache. Unusually intense during this phase are the headaches of typhoid and typhus fever and "grippe." Headache may be the earliest manifestation of an infection.

The combination of headache, fever, and a very stiff neck is common with meningitis, meningismus, and blood in the subarachnoid space.

Chilly sensations and hot flashes without

change in body temperature are common in patients with migraine attacks and the headache associated with muscle contraction. The headache of brain abscess is commonly accompanied by periodic elevations of temperature.

The headaches of bacterial meningitis and subarachnoid hemorrhage are usually associated with leukocytosis. Headache and stiff neck with slight if any leukocytosis is noted in luetic meningitis and sometimes in tuberculous meningitis. The headaches of typhoid fever, influenza, or "grippe" may be associated with leukopenia.

The headache following severe convulsions or a series of convulsions may be associated with leukocytosis. The headache associated with brain tumor, particularly if it be in the frontal region, is rarely accompanied by leukocytosis. Headache and leukocytosis coupled with fever most commonly are associated with brain abscess. An elevated sedimentation rate may be striking with cranial arteritis.

BETA BLOCKERS

Propranolol has been proposed as prophylactic treatment for migraine by many investigators since the original suggestion was made by Weber and Reinmuth in 1972. It is theorized that beta blocking drugs such as propranolol prevent cranial vasdilatation and in this way provide headache prophylaxis. Usually a starting dose of 20 mg twice or three times daily is given, increasing by 20–40 mg every third or fourth day until control is achieved. The peak plasma levels of propranolol are reached approximately 90 min after oral intake. Some of the reports from Scandinavia suggest that very large doses of the drug need to be employed, up to 240 mg per day. These reports give no account of serious side effects with propranolol, but the experienced clinician will recognize that the drug has widespread effects, and should be employed with extreme caution in patients with cardiac disease, particularly conduction defects, congestive heart failure, and in those atopic individuals who may be predisposed to bronchial asthma. One can monitor the effect of propranolol by observing the pulse rate. The pulse rate should not be depressed below 60 beats per min. in a healthy individual with migraine with this medication.

Computerized Axial Tomography (the CAT scan) and Headache

Most authorities agree that the CAT scan is the greatest advance in diagnostic medicine in the last several decades. This noninvasive technique uses a computer coupled with a special X-ray device to produce vividly detailed cross-sectional pictures of the body's interior. A narrow X-ray beam scans the patient's head in a series of 1-cm-wide slices. A total of 28,800 absorption readings are produced in 5 min. The readings are processed by a minicomputer that calculates 6400 absorption values of the material in each slice from the simultaneous 28,800 equations. The technique discloses variations in tissue density which aid in detecting many pathological conditions.

The technique gives information about the brain and its appendages which could previously not be obtained, or was obtained only with the greatest difficulty, using techniques such as pneumoencephalography, cerebral angiography, ventriculography or radioisotope scanning. In many cases hazardous procedures such as pneumoencephalograms and cerebral arteriograms can now be avoided.

The CAT scan makes it possible to differentiate hemorrhage from tumor, to follow multiple brain lesions, and to monitor chemotherapy; the accuracy in diagnosing supratentorial lesions is above 90%. Furthermore, the testing can almost always be done on an outpatient basis, is rapid, and does not overexpose the patient to radiation.

The CAT scan is of particular value in evaluating the patient with headache. It allows the rapid differentiation of conditions such as brain tumor, chronic subdural hematoma, arteriovenous malformation, aneurysm, and hydrocephalus which result in chronic recurrent headaches that at times simulate migraine. Also, for the first time, the CAT scan has enabled us to recognize transient morphological changes, such as cerebral edema in the cerebral parenchyma, caused by an acute attack of migraine, especially complicated migraine of the hemiparetic variety.

In a small percentage of patients with complicated migraine, transient abnormalities such as cerebral edema that last only a few days, will appear in CAT scans. In addition, in patients with repeated severe attacks, enlargement of the cerebral ventricles and cerebral cortical atrophy have been reported.

The indications for the use of the CAT scan in patients with recurrent headache are as follows: a. if the neurological exam or clinical history makes one suspect an intracranial lesion, b. in cases of complicated migraine including hemiparetic and vertebral basilar varieties, where there is a question of a structural lesion, c. in patients with brain tumor phobia, as a method of reassurance.

SOME OLD CLINICAL SAWS THAT NEED COMMENT

Unilaterality

If headache is always on the same side, should one suspect an aneurysm? What does it mean to have a persistent focal headache? Does a unilateral headache suggest aneurysm? Should the patient be studied? Are angiograms indicated?

The patient's history must be taken seriously, but is the patient providing the diagnosis, or is the history confusing both patient and physician? Focal headaches imply focal disease. The clinician should be alert for local infection such as sinusitis or inflammation (cranial arteritis) or diseases of the facial organs including the eyes and nose. He should also be concerned about endocrine and metabolic diseases, especially diabetes.

But if the headache is typically migrainous, or suggests cluster headache, then it should be accepted as such. Aneurysms are, by and large, nonpainful entities. Angiomas do not often produce pain. Angiomas may rupture, bleed, clot, calcify, provoke seizures, and eventually inhibit learning, but they do not usually hurt.

Many patients with migraine always have their headache on the same side, and there isn't any requirement that the headache must shift from side to side. This first maxim, then, has produced many unnecessary angiographic studies and evoked much needless worry amongst clinicians. If focal disease is not present, the clinician should accept the persistent repetition of unilateral throbbing head pain as compatible with vascular headache of several types, including migraine and cluster headaches.

Association of Vascular Lesions and Migraine

Are aneurysms common in patients with migraine? Migraine is a common disease and aneurysms are also common, so it is reasonable to assume that the two entities may occasionally appear in the same patient. But there is little evidence that the two syndromes are related. Asymptomatic aneurysms are asymptomatic. If an aneurysm begins to expand rapidly, it will produce a particularly severe localized pain which is not likely to be mistaken for recurrent vascular headache.

Those aneurysms which do rupture evoke catastrophic headache, with associated neurological signs and symptoms, related to a sterile inflammatory reaction produced by the presence of blood in the subarachnoid space.

Is migraine a common feature of cerebral arteriovenous anastomoses? It is true that angiomas may leak briefly and repeatedly. Since the source of the bleeding is usually from anomalous blood vessels and is not arterial in type, the headache is often not so intense as in subarachnoid bleeding. If sufficient blood is liberated into the subarachnoid space, signs of meningeal irritation will also occur, indistinguishable from those which are associated with subarachnoid bleeding produced by the rupture of a typical berry aneurysm.

Hemispheric angiomas may produce almost any neurological sign or symptoms, related to bleeding, calcification, and the production of seizures. They are not considered to produce chronic headache.

Is headache therapy straightforward and easy, once the diagnosis is made? Successful treatment of a patient with headache may not be easily accomplished. The care and sympathy with which the physician relates to his patients is indispensable to effective management of each individual headache problem. Cures should not be promised. It is enough to advise the patient that attempts will be made to reduce the intensity and frequency of his headaches. The art of medical practice may be more important than scientific pharmacology. Patience and perseverance on the part of both physician and patient may be necessary. The physician may find that his therapeutic suggestions have not brought forth the desired result. It is important then not to become angry at the patient. Sometimes simple structuring of the environment will help the patient modify some of his life goals. At times the patient will demand a type of practical office psychotherapy, an informal program directed toward guidance and re-education of his emotional responses. With careful attention to the whole patient, some resolution of the problem can be achieved in the majority of headache complaints. If the physician suspects a serious thought disorder, psychiatric consultation is mandatory.

Allergy

Is migraine frequently caused by allergy? It has not been possible to demonstrate that migraine results from any significant or specific antigen-antibody reaction, whether the antigen be an inhaled pollen, an injected material, or food. There is no specific correlation between positive skin tests for various allergens and the appearance of migraine.

Dietary migraine may be related to the ingestion of vasoactive foods and materials. However, this is not an allergy, but simply a reaction to vasoactive substances in a person predisposed to overactivity of vasomotor responses. Thus, long trials of hyposensitization to presumed allergens are not indicated in the chronic treatment of migraine. Hives, allergic rhinitis, etopic eczema, bronchial asthma, and other manifestations of true allergic reactions cannot be equated with the migraine episode.

Brain Tumor

Is severe headache a common sign of brain tumor? Headache is certainly one of the cardinal signs of brain tumor, particularly of rapidly expanding tumors producing traction on the pain-sensitive structures of the head. This is especially the case if the ventricular system is compromised by obstruction of absorption or flow of cerebrospinal fluid, causing traction hydrocephalus. Headache is sometimes a prominent finding with increased intracranial pressure. But with more slowly growing tumors, headache may be transitory, or mild, or easily relieved by common analgesics, and the patient's description of his head pain in this situation may be desultory. The worst head pains are not usually related to tumor, but to vascular headaches or the major neuralgias. Some generalizations concerning headache and the localization of brain tumor seem justified.

1. Although the headache of brain tumor may be referred from a distant intracranial source, it approximately overlies the tumor in about one-third of all patients.

2. If the tumor is above the tentorium, the pain is frequently at the vertex, or in the frontal regions.

3. If the tumor is below the tentorium, the pain is occipital, and cervical muscle spasm may be present.

4. Headache is almost always present with posterior fossa tumor.

5. If the tumor is midline, it may be increased with cough or straining or sudden head movement. (This also occurs with migraine.)

6. If the tumor is hemispheric, the pain is usually appreciated on the same side of the head.

7. If the tumor is chiasmal, at the sella, the pain may be referred to the vertex.

How important are these clinical observations? Perhaps they are of modest value. The history of headache in patients with brain tumor is helpful most often when there is no previous history of headache; sudden appearance of headache in an adult should suggest an organic lesion of the brain. If the clinician feels that some pathological process is producing headache, then the work-up should be parsimonious and should search out suspected causes of headache in a logical fashion. The use of noninvasive techniques for the examination of the cranial contents is suggested. More aggressive and potentially damaging studies such as arteriograms and pneumoencephalograms, should not be done for the complaint of headache alone.

Is headache characteristic of chronic hydrocephalus? (normal pressure hydrocephalus). The clinical picture in occult hydrocephalus or the hydrocephalic syndromes includes disturbances of gait, mentation, and micturition. Almost all patients with this problem have a disturbance in gait, varying from slight disability to total inability to walk. Also, disturbance of gait is often the first sign of normal pressure hydrocephalus. When these patients are tested carefully by an experienced psychometrist, almost all of them will demonstrate significant mentational difficulties, particularly impairment of memory, distractibility, and inability to maintain attention and concentration span. Eventually, later on, the incontinence of sphincters occurs. It is not usually appreciated as urgency but almost always represents the incontinence of dementia, wherein concern for incontinence is lacking or reduced, or micturition may be performed in front of others, much in the manner of children. Problems with bowel incontinence are considerably less common, though flatus is often expelled without concern for social niceties. It should be emphasized that sphincter incontinence is almost always a late sign and is rarely seen early in the course of this disease.

Other symptoms of the hydrocephalic syndrome include dizziness, lightheadedness, faintness or weakness, falling spells, and brief episodes of unconsciousness. Complaints of headache, which is often the primary symptom of acute hydrocephalus, are absent.

Migraine Equivalents

Migraine may express itself in forms other than hemicranial pain, and these different modes of expression are known as migraine equivalents. The equivalents are paroxysmal, recurrent, symptom complexes characterized by the following:

1. No demonstrable organic lesion.
2. Previous history of typical migraine headache.
3. Replacement of headaches by the equivalent syndrome.
4. Absence of symptoms between attack.
5. Family history of migraine.
6. Relief from the equivalent syndrome using appropriate drugs.

Migraine equivalents may take many forms, including abdominal, ophthalmic, and psychic.

Abdominal migraine is characterized by recurrent episodes of vomiting and/or abdominal pain in association with symptoms of the migraine attack. It is the most common visceral manifestation of migraine. Although it has been reported in patients from infancy to old age, it is most common between the ages of two and eleven years and males are most often affected. Abdominal migraine is often characterized by a prodromal period of yawning, listlessness, drowsiness, or the typical aura of a migraine attack. The episode usually starts suddenly and is precipitated by a specific or stressful experience. The pain may be situated anywhere in the abdomen, but is usually epigastric or periumbilical. The individual bout of pain varies in severity, usually lasts l to 6 hr, and is frequently characterized by severe nausea and vomiting. There may also be associated a typical headache, constipation or diarrhea, lethargy, stuporous sleep, or irritability. Electroencephalography done during the attack may show a mild generalized dysrhythmia, with high-voltage slow waves, thought to be indicative of cerebral hypoxia.

Ophthalmic migraine is also a reasonably well recognized syndrome, characterized by temporary scotomas, amblyopias, or hemianopsias which mark the height of the migraine attack instead of acting as a prodrome to the unilateral headache. Many of these patients are men. Some may develop ophthalmic migraine without the subsequent headache.

Psychic migraine is probably more common than realized and is characterized by transient mood disorders or psychotic states which replace a typical unilateral headache. Often there is a short prodromal period of lethargy or vigor, followed by a mood disorder lasting from a few hours to days. Many patients experience similar symptoms prior to a typical migraine attack but in psychic migraine no headache occurs.

Various autonomic dysfunctions are common in patients with migraine. These include Raynaud's phenomenon, flushing, and even on occasion hemorrhage into the skin. Recurrent febrile episodes as a migraine equivalent have been reported. Recently three young women have been seen, with reasonably typical migraine, who have, in addition, a form of connective tissue disease, not clearly defined, perhaps a mixed connective tissue disease or Sjogren's syndrome.

Some of the migraine equivalents may be associated with intracranial vasoconstriction. For example, visual cortical ischemia almost certainly produces ophthalmic migraine, though the retinal artery may be involved as well. Cortical, subcortical, thalamic, or hypothalamic ischemia could evoke transient mood disorders. Ischemia in the thermal regulatory center could cause the febrile equivalent. Sensory and/or motor strip ischemia causes minor hemiplegic equivalents, with subsequent local cerebral edema causing the major hemiplegias. Ischemia in autonomic diencephalic centers would be capable of causing abdominal migraine.

INDEX

Abscess, intracranial, 297-98. *See also* Brain abscess
Acetanilid, 137, 216
Acetophenetidin, 137
Acetylcholine, 65, 100-101
Acetylsalicylic acid, 137. *See also* Aspirin
Acidosis, 124
Acoustic neurinoma, 451
Acoustic neuroma, 296
ACTH, 419
Acupuncture, 11, 428, 447
A-delta nerve fiber, 9-11, 18, 373
Adenoma, 353
Adenylate cyclase, 424
Adrenergic system, 424
Adrenocorticotropic hormone, 419
Affective disorders. *See also* Psychobiology
  biochemistry of, 418-26, 430-32
Aging
  effect on arteries, 172
  migraine and, 87, 151-52, 412
  pain tolerance and, 14, 18
  subarachnoid hemorrhage and, 178
  trigeminal neuralgia and, 233
Alcohol, 68, 164
  hangover, 213-14
Allergy, 66-67, 256-86
  angioedema, 277
  drug side effects in, 278-79
  and migraine, 67-68, 70, 149, 278-83, 459
  rhinitis, 259-60
  types of reactions, 256-59
  urticaria, 277
Alpha-methylparatyrosine, 421-22
Amicar, 180
Amitriptyline, 146, 425, 428, 431
Amphetamine, 423
Amyl nitrate, 62
Amyl nitrite, 71-73, 215-16, 373
Analgesic(s), 11-13, 455-56
  electrical stimulation, 261-53, 319
  in migraine therapy, 137-38
  use and abuse, 441-43
  withdrawal process, 443-44
Anaphylaxis, 256-58, 283

Anemia, 215
Anesthesia dolorosa, 318-19
Aneurysms, cerebral, 175-82, 450, 455, 458
  and ophthalmoplegic migraine, 111
  radiological investigations, 352, 354
Anger, suppressed, and migraine, 403
Angioedema, 277-78
Angiography, 345, 348-49, 351, 354-55, 357-59
Angioma, 458
Aniseikonia, 393-94
Anorexia, in migraine, 57
Anterior cerebral artery, 41-42, 53, 351
Anterior ethmoidal artery, 26
Anterior fossa, 28-29, 47, 355
Anterior-inferior cerebellar artery, 316
Anterior meningeal artery, 26, 28, 47
Antibodies, 256-58
Antidepressants, 146-47, 421, 423
Antifibrinolytics, 180
Antigens, 256-59
Antihistamines, 64-68
Antiserotonin, 64
Anturane, 67, 147-48
Anxiety, 16, 409-15, 431, 453
Apophyseal joints, 363, 368
Apoplexy, 180
Aqueduct of Sylvius, 44, 46
Arachnoid membrane, 364
Argyll Robertson pupil, 399, 401
Arteries. *See also* Cerebral arteries; Cranial arteries;
    Dural arteries; Vasoconstriction; Vasodilation;
    and *names of specific arteries*
  fluctuations in tone, 81-85
  innervation, 46-47
  pain sensitivity, 26-30, 39, 41-43, 47, 53, 221-23
Arteritis, 6-7, 220-32, 278
Aspirin, 64, 66-67, 147
Asthma, and migraine, 281-83
Astigmatism, 392
Atherosclerosis, 87
Atopy, 257, 281-82
Atypical facial neuralgia, 249-51
Australian antigenemia, 220
Autonomic reflex abnormalities, 189